CARDIOLOGY SECRETS

Third Edition

Glenn N. Levine, MD, FACC, FAHA
Professor of Medicine
Baylor College of Medicine
Houston, Texas
and
Director
Coronary Care Unit
Michael E. DeBakey VA Medical Center
Houston, Texas

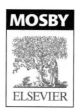

MOSBY

ELSEVIER

1600 John F. Kennedy Blvd.
Ste 1800
Philadelphia, PA 19103-2899

CARDIOLOGY SECRETS, THIRD EDITION

ISBN: 978-0-323-04525-4

NOTICE

Knowledge and best practice in this field are constantly changing. As new research and experience broaden our knowledge, changes in practice, treatment, and drug therapy may become necessary or appropriate. Readers are advised to check the most current information provided (i) on procedures featured or (ii) by the manufacturer of each product to be administered, to verify the recommended dose or formula, the method and duration of administration, and contraindications. It is the responsibility of the practitioner, relying on their own experience and knowledge of the patient, to make diagnoses, to determine dosages and the best treatment for each individual patient, and to take all appropriate safety precautions. To the fullest extent of the law, neither the Publisher nor the Editor assumes any liability for any injury and/or damage to persons or property arising out of or related to any use of the material contained in this book.

The Publisher

Library of Congress Cataloging-in-Publication Data

Cardiology secrets / [edited by] Glenn N. Levine. – 3rd ed.
   p. ; cm.
   Includes bibliographical references and index.
   ISBN 978-0-323-04525-4
   1. Cardiology–Miscellanea. I. Levine, Glenn N.
   [DNLM: 1. Heart Diseases–Examination Questions.
WG 18.2 C2697 2010]
   RC682.C397 2010
   616.1′2–dc22   2009014647

Acquisitions Editor: James Merritt
Developmental Editor: Barbara Cicalese
Project Manager: Mary Stermel
Marketing Manager: Allan McKeown

Working together to grow
libraries in developing countries

www.elsevier.com | www.bookaid.org | www.sabre.org

ELSEVIER   BOOK AID International   Sabre Foundation

Printed in the United States of America
Last digit is the print number: 9 8 7 6 5 4 3 2 1

CARDIOLOGY SECRETS

SECRETS

DEDICATION

To Lydia, who always has an optimistic and positive outlook on people and on life, and who inspires me to try to be a better person, and to our girls Sasha and Ginger, who were my constant companions through the many long nights of writing and editing this book (though they would often rather play fetch than just watch me write and edit!).

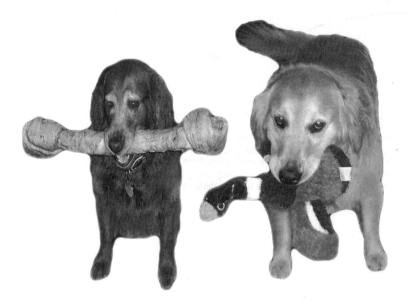

CONTENTS

III. CHEST PAINS, ANGINA, CAD, AND ACUTE CORONARY SYNDROMES

IV. CONGESTIVE HEART FAILURE, MYOCARDITIS, AND CARDIOMYOPATHIES

V. VALVULAR HEART DISEASE AND ENDOCARDITIS

VI. ARRHYTHMIAS

VII. PRIMARY AND SECONDARY PREVENTION

VIII. MISCELLANEOUS CARDIOVASCULAR SYMPTOMS AND DISEASES

IX. OTHER MEDICAL CONDITIONS WITH ASSOCIATED CARDIAC INVOLVEMENT

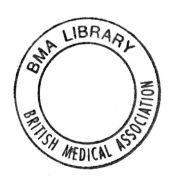

CONTRIBUTORS

Suhny Abbara, MD
Assistant Professor, Radiology, Harvard Medical School; Director of the Cardiovascular Imaging Section, Radiology, and Director of Education, Cardiac MR/PET/CT Program, Massachusetts General Hospital (Harvard Medical School), Boston, Massachusetts

Jameel Ahmed, MD
Clinical Fellow, Cardiovascular Medicine, Boston University School of Medicine; Cardiovascular Medicine, Boston Medical Center, Boston, Massachusetts

Ashish Aneja, MD
Clinical Instructor, General Internal Medicine, Case Western Reserve University; General Internal Medicine, University Hospitals, Case Medical Center, Case Western Reserve University, Cleveland, Ohio

Eric H. Awtry, MD
Assistant Professor, Cardiology, Boston University School of Medicine; Director of Clinical Cardiology, Boston Medical Center, Boston, Massachusetts

Jose L. Baez-Escudero, MD
Fellow, Cardiovascular Disease, Department of Medicine, Cardiology, Baylor College of Medicine, Houston, Texas

C. Noel Bairey Merz, MD, FACC, FAHA
Professor, Cardiology, David Geffen School of Medicine, University of California; Director of the Women's Heart Center and Preventive Cardiac Center, Women's Guild Endowed Chair in Women's Health, Department of Medicine, Cardiology, Cedars-Sinai Medical Center, Los Angeles, California

Faisal G. Bakaeen, MD
Assistant Professor, Department of Cardiothoracic Surgery, Baylor College of Medicine, Houston, Texas

Gary J. Balady, MD
Professor of Medicine, Boston University School of Medicine; Director of Preventive Cardiology, Boston Medical Center, Boston, Massachusetts

Luc M. Beauchesne, MD, FACC
Director of Adult Congenital Heart Disease Clinic, Division of Cardiology, University of Ottawa Heart Institute, Ottawa, Ontario, Canada

Sheilah A. Bernard, MD
Associate Professor of Medicine, Boston University School of Medicine; Director of Cardiac Ambulatory Services, Boston Medical Center, Boston, Massachusetts

Jean Bismuth, MD
Assistant Professor, Cardiovascular Surgery, Methodist Hospital, Houston, Texas

Fernando Boccalandro, MD, FACC, FSCAI
Internal Medicine, Texas Tech Health Science Center; Odessa Heart Institute, Odessa, Texas

Ann F. Bolger, MD, FACC, FAHA
William Watt Kerr Professor of Clinical Medicine, University of California, San Francisco School of Medicine; Director of Echocardiography, San Francisco General Hospital, San Francisco, California

Michael B. Bottorff, PharmD, FCCP, CLS
Professor, Clinical Pharmacy, University of Cincinnati, Cincinnati, Ohio

Biykem Bozkurt, MD, FACC
Professor, Cardiology, Baylor College of Medicine; Cardiology Section Chief, Cardiology, Michael E. DeBakey VA Medical Center, Houston, Texas

Blase A. Carabello, MD, FACC
Acting Chief of Staff of Medicine, Medical Care Line, Michael E. DeBakey VA Medical Center, Houston, Texas

Gustavo A. Cardenas, MD
Junior Staff, Department of Internal Medicine, Division of Cardiovascular Medicine, William Beaumont Hospital, Royal Oak, Michigan

Matthew A. Cavender, MD
Fellow, Division of Cardiovascular Medicine, Cleveland Clinic Foundation, Cleveland, Ohio

Danny Chu, MD, FACS
Assistant Professor of Surgery, Division of Cardiothoracic Surgery, Michael E. DeBakey VA Medical Center, Baylor College of Medicine, Houston, Texas

Anita Deswal, MD, MPH
Associate Professor, Cardiology, Winters Center for Heart Failure Research, Baylor College of Medicine and Michael E. DeBakey VA Medical Center, Houston, Texas

Amandeep Dhaliwal, MD
Baylor College of Medicine, Houston, Texas

José G. Díez, MD, FACC, FSCAI
Assistant Professor, Cardiology, Baylor College of Medicine; Staff Interventional Cardiologist, St. Luke's Episcopal Hospital/Texas Heart Institute, Houston, Texas

Hisham Dokainish, MD, FACC, FASE
Associate Professor, Cardiology, and Director of Echocardiography, Baylor College of Medicine; Director of Non-Invasive Cardiology, Ben Taub General Hospital, Houston, Texas

Michael E. Farkouh, MD, MSc, FACC
Associate Professor of Medicine and Director of Cardiovascular Clinical Trials Unit at Mount Sinai Heart, Mount Sinai School of Medicine, New York, New York

G. Michael Felker, MD, MHS, FACC
Director of Heart Failure Research, Cardiovascular Medicine, Duke University Medical Center, Durham, North Carolina

James J. Fenton, MD, FCCP
Associate Clinical Professor, Pulmonary Medicine, National Jewish Health, Denver, Colorado

Lee A. Fleisher, MD, FACC
Professor of Medicine and Robert Dunning Dripps Professor and Chair, Department of Anesthesiology and Critical Care, University of Pennsylvania School of Medicine; Professor of Medicine and Chair of Anesthesiology and Critical Care, Hospital of The University of Pennsylvania, Philadelphia, Pennsylvania

Joanne M. Foody, MD, FACC, FAHA
Associate Professor, Division of Cardiovascular Medicine, Brigham and Women's Hospital (Harvard Medical School), Boston, Massachusetts

Cindy L. Grines, MD, FACC
Corporate Vice Chief of Academic Affairs, Cardiovascular Medicine, William Beaumont Hospital, Royal Oak, Michigan

Gabriel B. Habib, Sr., MD, MS, FACC, FAHA, FCCP
Professor, Cardiology, Baylor College of Medicine; Associate Chief and Director of Educational Programs, Cardiology, Michael E. DeBakey VA Medical Center, Houston, Texas

Rudy M. Haddad, MD
Fellow, Cardiology, Department of Medicine, Baylor College of Medicine, Houston, Texas

J. Taylor Hays, MD
Associate Professor, General Internal Medicine, Mayo Clinic College of Medicine, Rochester, Minnesota

Bradley E. Hein, PharmD
Assistant Professor, Pharmacy, James L. Winkle College of Pharmacy, University of Cincinnati; Clinical Specialist, Internal Medicine, Pharmacy, The Christ Hospital, Cincinnati, Ohio

Stephan M. Hergert, MD
Division of Cardiology, University of California San Francisco General Hospital, San Francisco, California

Brian D. Hoit, MD
Professor of Medicine, Physiology, and Biophysics, Case Western Reserve University; Director of Echocardiography, University Hospitals Health System, Cleveland, Ohio

Joseph Huh, MD
Assistant Professor, Department of Cardiothoracic Surgery, Baylor College of Medicine, Houston, Texas

Hani Jneid, MD
Assistant Professor, Cardiology, Baylor College of Medicine; Interventional Cardiologist, Michael E. DeBakey VA Medical Center, Houston, Texas

Christof Karmonik, PhD
Assistant Professor, Radiology, Weill Medical College of Cornell University, New York, New York; Adjunct Assistant Professor, Computer Science, University of Houston, and Research Scientist, Radiology, Methodist Hospital Research Institute, Houston, Texas

Thomas A. Kent, MD
Professor, Department of Neurology, Baylor College of Medicine; Chief of Neurology, Neurology Care Line, Michael E. DeBakey VA Medical Center, Houston, Texas

Thomas J. Kiernan, MD, MRCPI
Interventional Fellow, Vascular Medicine and Interventional Cardiology, Massachusetts General Hospital (Harvard Medical School), Boston, Massachusetts

L. Veronica Lee, MD, FACC
Assistant Professor, Internal Medicine, Cardiology, Yale University; Yale New Haven Hospital, New Haven, Connecticut

Glenn N. Levine, MD, FACC, FAHA
Professor of Medicine, Baylor College of Medicine; Director of the Coronary Care Unit, Michael E. DeBakey VA Medical Center, Houston, Texas

Kaity Lin, MD
Fellow, Department of Medicine, Cardiology, Baylor College of Medicine, Houston, Texas

Alan B. Lumsden, MD, FACS
Professor and Chairman, Department of Cardiovascular Surgery, Methodist Hospital, Methodist DeBakey Heart and Vascular Center, Houston, Texas

Wilfred Mamuya, MD, PhD
Instructor, Medicine, Harvard Medical School; Division of Cardiology, Massachusetts General Hospital, Boston, Massachusetts

Salvatore Mangione, MD
Associate Professor of Medicine, Jefferson Medical College, Philadelphia, Pennsylvania

Sharyl R. Martini, MD, PhD
Resident, Neurology, University of Cincinnati; Resident, Neuroscience Institute, University Hospital, Cincinnati, Ohio

James McCord, MD
Heart and Vascular Institute, Henry Ford Hospital, Detroit, Michigan

Geno J. Merli, MD, FACP
Professor of Medicine, Jefferson Medical College; Chief Medical Officer, Thomas Jefferson University Hospital; Director, Jefferson Center for Vascular Diseases, Jefferson Medical College, Philadelphia, Pennsylvania

Arumina Misra, MD, FACC
Assistant Professor and Director of Nuclear Cardiology, Internal Medicine, Baylor College of Medicine; Assistant Professor and Director of Nuclear Cardiology and the Chest, Internal Medicine, Ben Taub General Hospital, Houston, Texas

John S. Nguyen, MD
Fellow, Cardiology, Department of Medicine, Baylor College of Medicine, Houston, Texas

E. Magnus Ohman, MD
Professor of Medicine and Director of the Program for Advanced Coronary Disease, Department of Medicine, Division of Cardiovascular Medicine, Duke University Medical Center, Durham, North Carolina

George J. Philippides, MD
Assistant Professor of Medicine, Internal Medicine, Boston University; Director of the Coronary Care Unit, Associate Chief for Clinical Affairs, and Chairman of the Critical Care Committee, Cardiology Section, Boston Medical Center, Boston, Massachusetts

Charles V. Pollack, Jr., MA, MD, FACEP, FAAEM, FAHA
Professor, Department of Emergency Medicine, University of Pennsylvania; Department of Emergency Medicine, Pennsylvania Hospital, Philadelphia, Pennsylvania

Allison M. Pritchett, MD
Assistant Professor, Department of Medicine, Cardiology, Baylor College of Medicine; Director of Outpatient Cardiology Services, Ben Taub General Hospital, Harris County Hospital District, Houston, Texas

Kumudha Ramasubbu, MD, FACC
Assistant Professor of Cardiology, Baylor College of Medicine; Cardiology, Michael E. DeBakey VA Medical Center, Houston, Texas

Christopher J. Rees, MD
Clinical Instructor, Emergency Medicine, University of Pennsylvania School of Medicine; Attending Physician, Emergency Department, Pennsylvania Hospital, Philadelphia, Pennsylvania

Kenneth A. Rosenfield, MD
Section Head, Vascular Medicine and Intervention, Cardiology Division, Massachusetts General Hospital (Harvard Medical School), Boston, Massachusetts

Zeenat Safdar, MD, FCCP
Assistant Professor of Medicine, Pulmonary-Critical Care Medicine, Baylor College of Medicine; Attending, Pulmonary-Critical Care Medicine, Methodist Hospital; Attending, Pulmonary-Critical Care Medicine, St. Luke's Episcopal Hospital, Houston, Texas

Ryan Seutter, MD
Fellow, Cardiovascular Medicine, Baylor College of Medicine; Fellow, Cardiovascular Medicine, Michael E. DeBakey VA Medical Center; Fellow, Cardiovascular Medicine, St. Luke's Episcopal Hospital, Houston, Texas

Nishant R. Shah, MD
Chief Medical Resident, Internal Medicine, Baylor College of Medicine, Houston, Texas

Gregg J. Stashenko, MD
Fellow, Pulmonary and Critical Care Medicine, Duke University Medical Center, Durham, North Carolina

Victor F. Tapson, MD
Professor of Medicine and Director of the Center for Pulmonary Vascular Disease, Pulmonary and Critical Care Medicine, Duke University Medical Center, Durham, North Carolina

Miguel Valderrábano, MD
Associate Professor, Weill College of Medicine at Cornell University, New York, New York; Director, Division of Cardiac Electrophysiology, Methodist Hospital, Houston, Texas

Jacobo Alejandro Vazquez, MD
Cardiology Fellow, Baylor College of Medicine, Houston, Texas

Matthew J. Wall, Jr., MD, FACS
Professor, Michael E. DeBakey Department of Surgery, Baylor College of Medicine; Deputy Chief of Surgery and Chief of Cardiothoracic Surgery, Ben Taub General Hospital, Houston, Texas

Brandi J. Witt, MD
Cardiovascular Consultants, North Memorial Medical Center, Robbinsdale, Minnesota

Bryan P. Yan, MBBS, FRACP
Interventional Fellow, Vascular Medicine and Interventional Cardiology, Massachusetts General Hospital (Harvard Medical School), Boston, Massachusetts

David Yao, MD
Fellow, Department of Medicine, Cardiology, Baylor College of Medicine, Houston, Texas

PREFACE

My hope is that this book will help educate health care providers in a didactic, interactive, interesting, and enjoyable manner on the optimal evaluation and management of patients with cardiovascular disease and, in doing so, will help to ensure that all patients with cardiovascular disease receive optimal preventive, pharmacologic, and device interventions and therapies. I welcome comments and suggestions from readers of this book: glevine@bcm.tmc.edu.

ACKNOWLEDGMENTS

I would like to acknowledge the many authors and editors who have pioneered the prior *Cardiology Secrets* and other *Secrets* books that have made this series so successful. I would like to extend my deep thanks to Barbara Cicalese for her outstanding editorial support, without which this book would never have come to fruition, and to James Merritt, who green-lighted this edition of the book.

I am indebted to the more than 60 chapter authors who have taken time from their many academic and clinical responsibilities to contribute to this book, and without whom this book would not have been possible.

I would also like to extend a deep personal thanks to the following:

- to Gary Balady, Joseph Vita, Alice Jacobs, Scott Flamm, and Doug Mann, who have been my academic and professional mentors and role models
- to my parents, who have always been supportive of my medical education, training, career, and aspirations
- to Lydia, whose always optimistic and positive outlook on people and on life serves as a model for me
- and to Sasha and Ginger, who have been my constant companions through the many long nights of writing and editing this book, constantly at my side (and often at my feet).

TOP 100 SECRETS

These secrets are 100 of the top board alerts. They summarize the concepts, principles, and most salient details of cardiology.

1. Coronary flow reserve (the increase in coronary blood flow in response to agents that lead to microvascular dilation) begins to decrease when a coronary artery stenosis is 50% or more luminal diameter. However, basal coronary flow does not begin to decrease until the lesion is 80% to 90% luminal diameter.

2. The most commonly used criteria to diagnose left ventricular hypertrophy (LVH) are R wave in V5-V6 + S wave in V1-V2 > 35 mm, or R wave in lead I plus S wave in lead III > 25 mm.

3. Causes of ST segment elevation include acute myocardial infarction (MI) as a result of thrombotic occlusion of a coronary artery, Prinzmetal's angina, cocaine-induced myocardial infarction, pericarditis, left ventricular aneurysm, left bundle branch block (LBBB), left ventricular hypertrophy with repolarization abnormalities, J point elevation, and severe hyperkalemia.

4. The initial electrocardiogram (ECG) manifestation of hyperkalemia is peaked T waves. As the hyperkalemia becomes more profound, there may be loss of visible P waves, QRS widening, and ST segment elevation. The preterminal finding is a sinusoidal pattern on the ECG.

5. The classic carotid arterial pulse in a patient with aortic stenosis is reduced *(parvus)* and delayed *(tardus)*.

6. The most common ECG finding in pulmonary embolus is sinus tachycardia. Other ECG findings that can occur include right atrial enlargement *(P pulmonale)*, right axis deviation, T-wave inversions in leads V1-V2, incomplete right bundle branch block (IRBBB), and a S1Q3T3 pattern (an S wave in lead I, a Q wave in lead III, and an inverted T wave in lead III).

7. The major *risk factors* for coronary artery disease (CAD) are family history of premature coronary artery disease (father, mother, brother, or sister who first developed clinical CAD at age younger than 45 to 55 for males and at age younger than 55 to 60 for females), hypercholesterolemia, hypertension, cigarette smoking, and diabetes mellitus.

8. Important causes of chest pain not related to atherosclerotic coronary artery disease include aortic dissection, pneumothorax, pulmonary embolism, pneumonia, hypertensive crisis, Printzmetal's angina, cardiac syndrome X, anomalous origin of the coronary artery, pericarditis, esophageal spasm or esophageal rupture (Boerhaave's syndrome), and shingles.

9. Kussmaul's sign is the paradoxical increase in jugular venous pressure (JVP) that occurs during inspiration. JVP normally decreases during inspiration because the inspiratory fall in intrathoracic pressure creates a *sucking effect* on venous return. Kussmaul's sign is observed when the right side of the heart is unable to accommodate an increased venous return, such as can occur with constrictive pericarditis, severe heart failure, cor pulmonale, restrictive cardiomyopathy, tricuspid stenosis, and right ventricular infarction.

10. Other causes of elevated cardiac troponin, besides acute coronary syndrome and myocardial infarction, that should be considered in patients with chest pains include pulmonary embolism, aortic dissection, myopericarditis, severe aortic stenosis, and severe chronic kidney disease.

11. Prinzmetal's angina, also called *variant angina*, is an unusual cause of angina caused by coronary vasospasm. Patients with Prinzmetal's angina are typically younger and often female. Treatment is based primarily on the use of calcium channel blockers and nitrates.

12. Cardiac syndrome X is an entity in which patients describe typical exertional anginal symptoms, yet are found on cardiac catheterization to have nondiseased, *normal* coronary arteries. Although there are likely multiple causes and explanations for cardiac syndrome X, it does appear that, at least in some patients, microvascular coronary artery constriction or dysfunction plays a role.

13. The three primary antianginal medications used for the treatment of chronic stable angina are beta-blockers, nitrates, and calcium channel blockers. Ranolazine, a newer antianginal agent, is generally used only as a third-line agent in patients with continued significant angina despite traditional antianginal therapy who have coronary artery disease not amenable to revascularization.

14. Findings that suggest a heart murmur is pathologic and requires further evaluation include the presence of symptoms, extra heart sounds, thrills, abnormal ECG or chest radiography, diminished or absent S2, holosystolic (or late systolic) murmur, any diastolic murmur, and all continuous murmurs.

15. The major categories of ischemic stroke are large vessel atherosclerosis (including embolization from carotid to cerebral arteries), small vessel vasculopathy or lacunar type, and cardioembolic.

16. Hemorrhagic strokes are classified by their location: subcortical (associated with uncontrolled hypertension in 60% of cases) versus cortical (more concerning for underlying mass, arteriovenous malformation, or amyloidosis).

17. Common radiographic signs of congestive heart failure include enlarged cardiac silhouette, left atrial enlargement, hilar fullness, vascular redistribution, linear interstitial opacities (Kerley's lines), bilateral alveolar infiltrates, and pleural effusions (right > left).

18. Classic ECG criteria for the diagnosis of ST-segment-elevation myocardial infarction (STEMI), warranting thrombolytic therapy, are ST segment elevation greater than 0.1 mV in at least two contiguous leads (e.g., leads III and aVF or leads V2 and V3) or new or presumably new left bundle branch block (LBBB).

19. *Primary percutaneous coronary intervention (PCI)* refers to the strategy of taking a patient who presents with STEMI directly to the cardiac catheterization laboratory to undergo mechanical revascularization using balloon angioplasty, coronary stents, and other measures.

20. The triad of findings suggestive of right ventricular infarction are hypotension, distended neck veins, and clear lungs.

21. Cessation of cerebral blood flow for as short a period as 6 to 8 seconds can precipitate syncope.

22. The most common causes of syncope in pediatric and young patients are neurocardiogenic syncope (vasovagal syncope, vasodepressor syncope), conversion reactions (psychiatric causes), and primary arrhythmic causes (e.g., long QT syndrome, Wolff-Parkinson-White

syndrome). In contrast, elderly patients have a higher frequency of syncope caused by obstructions to cardiac output (e.g., aortic stenosis, pulmonary embolism) and by arrhythmias resulting from underlying heart disease.

23. Preexisting renal disease and diabetes are the two major risk factors for the development of contrast nephropathy. Preprocedure and postprocedure hydration is the most established method of reducing the risk of contrast nephropathy.

24. During coronary angiography, flow down the coronary artery is graded using the *TIMI flow grade*, in which TIMI grade 3 flow is normal and TIMI grade 0 flow means there is no blood flow down the artery.

25. The National Cholesterol Education Program (NCEP) Adult Treatment Panel III (ATP III) recommends that all adults age 20 years or older should undergo the fasting lipoprotein profile every 5 years. Testing should include total cholesterol, low-density lipoprotein (LDL) cholesterol, high-density lipoprotein (HDL) cholesterol, and triglycerides.

26. Important *secondary* causes of hyperlipidemia include diabetes, hypothyroidism, obstructive liver disease, chronic renal failure/nephrotic syndrome, and certain drugs (progestins, anabolic steroids, corticosteroids).

27. The minimum LDL goal for secondary prevention in patients with established CAD, peripheral vascular disease, or diabetes is an LDL less than 100 mg/dl. A goal of LDL less than 70 mg/dl should be considered in patients with coronary heart disease at very high risk, including those with multiple major coronary risk factors (especially diabetes), severe and poorly controlled risk factors (especially continued cigarette smoking), and multiple risk factors of the metabolic syndrome and those with acute coronary syndrome.

28. Factors that make up *metabolic syndrome* include abdominal obesity (waist circumference in men larger than 40 inches/102 cm or in women larger than 35 inches/88 cm); triglycerides 150 mg/dl or higher; low HDL cholesterol (less than 40 mg/dl in men or less than 50 mg/dl in women); blood pressure 135/85 mm Hg or higher; and fasting glucose 110 mg/dl or higher.

29. Although optimal blood pressure is less than 120/80 mm Hg, the goal of blood pressure treatment is to achieve blood pressure levels less than 140/90 mm Hg in most patients with uncomplicated hypertension and less than 130/80 mm Hg in higher risk hypertensive patients with chronic kidney disease or diabetes mellitus.

30. Up to 5% of all hypertension cases are *secondary*, meaning that a specific cause can be identified. Causes of secondary hypertension include renal artery stenosis, renal parenchymal disease, primary hyperaldosteronism, pheochromocytoma, Cushing's disease, hyperparathyroidism, aortic coarctation, and sleep apnea.

31. Clinical syndromes associated with hypertensive emergency include hypertensive encephalopathy, intracerebral hemorrhage, unstable angina/acute myocardial infarction, pulmonary edema, dissecting aortic aneurysm, or eclampsia.

32. JNC-7 recommends that hypertensive emergencies be treated in an intensive care setting with intravenously administered agents, with an initial goal of reducing mean arterial blood pressure by 10% to 15%, but no more than 25%, in the first hour and then, if stable, to a goal of 160/100–110 mm Hg within the next 2 to 6 hours.

33. Common causes of depressed left ventricular systolic dysfunction and cardiomyopathy included coronary artery disease, hypertension, valvular heart disease, and alcohol abuse. Other causes include cocaine abuse, collagen vascular disease, viral infection, myocarditis, peripartum cardiomyopathy, human immunodeficiency virus/acquired immunodeficiency disease (HIV/AIDS), tachycardia-induced, hypothyroidism, anthracycline toxicity, and Chagas' disease.

34. The classic signs and symptoms of patients with heart failure are dyspnea on exertion (DOE), orthopnea, paroxysmal nocturnal dyspnea (PND), and lower extremity edema.

35. Heart failure symptoms are most commonly classified using the New York Heart Association (NYHA) classification system, in which class IV denotes symptoms even at rest and class I denotes the ability to perform ordinary physical activity without symptoms.

36. Patients with depressed ejection fractions (less than 40%) should be treated with agents that block the rennin-angiotensin-aldosterone system, in order to improve symptoms, decrease hospitalizations, and decrease mortality. Angiotensin-converting enzyme (ACE) inhibitors are first-line therapy; alternate or additional agents include angiotensin II receptor blockers (ARBs) and aldosterone receptor blockers.

37. The combination of high-dose hydralazine and high-dose isosorbide dinitrate should be used in patients who cannot be given or cannot tolerate ACE inhibitors or ARBs because of renal function impairment or hyperkalemia.

38. High-risk features in patients hospitalized with acute decompensated heart failure (ADHF) include low systolic blood pressure, elevated blood urea nitrogen (BUN), hyponatremia, history of prior heart failure hospitalization, elevated brain natriuretic peptide (BNP), and elevated troponin I or T.

39. Atrioventricular node reentry tachycardia (AVNRT) accounts for 65% to 70% of paroxysmal supraventriuclar tachycardias (SVTs).

40. Implantable cardioverter defibrillators (ICDs) should be considered for primary prevention of sudden cardiac death in patients whose left ventricular ejection fractions remains less than 30% to 35% despite optimal medical therapy or revascularization and who have good-quality life expectancy of at least 1 year.

41. The three primary factors that promote venous thrombosis *(Virchow's triad)* are (1) venous blood stasis; (2) injury to the intimal layer of the venous vasculature; and (3) abnormalities in coagulation or fibrinolysis.

42. *Diastolic heart failure* is a clinical syndrome characterized by the signs and symptoms of heart failure, a preserved left ventricular ejection fraction (greater than 45% to 50%), and evidence of diastolic dysfunction.

43. The four conditions identified as having the highest risk of adverse outcome from endocarditis for which prophylaxis with dental procedures is still recommended by the American Heart Association are prosthetic cardiac valve, previous infective endocarditis, certain cases of congenital heart disease, and cardiac transplantation recipients who develop cardiac valvulopathy.

44. Findings that should raise the suspicion for endocarditis include bacteremia/sepsis of unknown cause, fever, constitutional symptoms, hematuria/glomerulonephritis/suspected renal infarction, embolic event of unknown origin, new heart murmurs, unexplained new

atrioventricular (AV) nodal conduction abnormality, multifocal or rapid changing pulmonic infiltrates, peripheral abscesses, certain cutaneous lesions (Osler nodes, Janeway lesions), and specific ophthalmic manifestations (Roth spots).

45. Transthoracic echo (TTE) has a sensitivity of 60% to 75% in the detection of native valve endocarditis. In cases where the suspicion of endocarditis is higher, a negative TTE should be followed by a transesophageal echo (TEE), which has a sensitivity of 88% to 100% and a specificity of 91% to 100% for native valves.

46. The most common cause of culture-negative endocarditis is prior use of antibiotics. Other causes include fastidious organisms (HACEK group, *Legionella, Chlamydia, Brucella*, certain fungal infections) and noninfectious causes.

47. Indications for surgery in cases of endocarditis include acute aortic insufficiency or mitral regurgitation leading to congestive heart failure, cardiac abscess formation/perivalvular extension, persistence of infection despite adequate antibiotic treatment, recurrent peripheral emboli, cerebral emboli, infection caused by microorganisms with a poor response to antibiotic treatment (e.g., fungi), prosthetic valve endocarditis (particularly if hemodynamic compromise exists), "mitral kissing infection", and large (greater than 10 mm) mobile vegetations.

48. The main echocardiographic criteria for severe mitral stenosis are mean transvalvular gradient greater than 10 mm Hg, mitral valve area less than 1 cm^2, and pulmonary artery (PA) systolic pressure greater than 50 mm Hg.

49. The classic auscultatory findings in mitral valve prolapse (MVP) is a mid-systolic click and late systolic murmur, although the click may actually vary somewhat within systole, depending on changes in left ventricular dimension, and there may actually be multiple clicks. The clicks are believed to result from the sudden tensing of the mitral valve apparatus as the leaflets prolapse into the left atrium during systole.

50. In patients with pericardial effusions, echocardiography findings that indicate elevated intrapericardial pressure and tamponade physiology include diastolic indentation or collapse of the right ventricle (RV), compression of the right atrium (RA) for more than one third of the cardiac cycle, lack of inferior vena cava (IVC) collapsibility with deep inspiration, 25% or more variation in mitral or aortic Doppler flows, and 50% or greater variation of tricuspid or pulmonic valves flows with inspiration.

51. The causes of pulseless electrical activity (PEA) can be broken down to the *H's and T's* of PEA, which are hypovolemia, hypoxemia, hydrogen ion (acidosis), hyperkalemia/hypokalemia, hypoglycemia, hypothermia, toxins, tamponade (cardiac), tension pneumothorax, thrombosis (coronary and pulmonary), and trauma.

52. Hemodynamically significant atrial septal defects (ASDs) have a shunt ratio greater than 1.5, are usually 10 mm or larger in diameter, and are usually associated with right ventricular enlargement.

53. Findings suggestive of a hemodynamically significant coarctation include small diameter (less than 10 mm or less than 50% of reference normal descending aorta at the diaphragm), presence of collateral blood vessels, and a gradient across the coarctation of more than 20 to 30 mm Hg.

54. Tetralogy of Fallot (TOF) consists of four features: right ventricular outflow tract (RVOT) obstruction, a large ventricular septal defect (VSD), an overriding ascending aorta, and right ventricular hypertrophy.

55. The three *D*s of Ebstein's anomaly are an apically *displaced* tricuspid valve that is *dysplastic*, with a right ventricle that may be *dysfunctional*.

56. Systolic wall stress is described by the law of Laplace, which states that systolic wall stress is equal to:

    (arterial pressure (p) × radius (r)) / 2 × thickness (h), or $\sigma = (p \times r)/2h$

57. Echocardiographic findings suggestive of severe mitral regurgitation include enlarged left atrium or left ventricle, the color Doppler mitral regurgitation jet occupying a large proportion (more than 40%) of the left atrium, a regurgitant volume 60 ml or more, a regurgitant fraction 50% or greater, a regurgitant orifice 0.40 cm^2 or greater, and a Doppler vena contracta width 0.7 cm or greater.

58. The seven factors that make up the Thrombolysis in Myocardial Infarction (TIMI) Risk Score are age greater than 65 years; three or more cardiac risk factors; prior catheterization demonstrating CAD; ST-segment deviation; two or more anginal events within 24 hours; aspirin use within 7 days; and elevated cardiac markers.

59. The components of the GRACE Acute Cardiac Syndrome (ACS) Risk Model (at the time of admission) are age; heart rate; systolic blood pressure, creatinine; CHF Killip class, ST-segment deviation; elevated cardiac enzymes/markers; and present/absence of cardiac arrest at admission.

60. Myocarditis is most commonly caused by a viral infection. Other causes include nonviral infections (bacterial, fungal, protozoal, parasitic), cardiac toxins, hypersensitivity reactions, and systemic disease (usually autoimmune). Giant cell myocarditis is an uncommon but often fulminant form of myocarditis characterized by multinucleated giant cells and myocyte destruction.

61. Initial therapy for patients with non–ST-segment-elevation acute coronary syndrome (NSTE-ACS) should include antiplatelet therapy with aspirin and with clopidogrel or glycoprotein IIb/IIIa inhibitor, and antithrombin therapy with either unfractionated heparin, enoxaparin, fondaparinux, or bivalirudin (depending on the clinical scenario).

62. Important complications in heart transplant recipients include infection, rejection, vasculopathy (diffuse coronary artery narrowing), arrhythmias, hypertension, renal impairment, malignancy (especially skin cancer and lymphoproliferative disorders), and osteoporosis (caused by steroid use).

63. The classic symptoms of aortic stenosis are angina, syncope, and those of heart failure (dyspnea, orthopnea, paroxysmal nocturnal dyspnea, edema, etc.). Once any of these symptoms occur, the average survival without surgical intervention is 5, 3, or 2 years, respectively.

64. Class I indications for aortic valve replacement (AVR) include (1) development of symptoms in patients with severe aortic stenosis; (2) a left ventricular ejection fraction of less than 50% in the setting of severe aortic stenosis; and (3) the presence of severe aortic stenosis in patients undergoing coronary artery bypass grafting, other heart valve surgery, or thoracic aortic surgery.

65. The major risk factors for venous thromboembolism (VTE) include previous thromboembolism, immobility, cancer and other causes of hypercoagulable state (protein C or S deficiency, factor V Leiden, antithrombin deficiency), advanced age, major surgery, trauma, and acute medical illness.

66. The Wells Score in cases of suspected pulmonary embolism includes deep vein thrombosis (DVT) symptoms and signs (3 points); pulmonary embolism (PE) as likely as or more likely than alternative diagnosis (3 points); heart rate greater 100 beats/min (1.5 point); immobilization or surgery in previous 4 weeks (1.5 point); previous DVT or PE (1.5 point); hemoptysis (1.0 point); and cancer (1 point).

67. The main symptoms of aortic regurgitation (AR) are dyspnea and fatigue. Occasionally patients experience angina because reduced diastolic aortic pressure reduces coronary perfusion pressure, impairing coronary blood flow. Reduced diastolic systemic pressure may also cause syncope or presyncope.

68. The physical findings of aortic regurgitation (AR) include widened pulse pressure, a palpable dynamic left ventricular apical beat that is displaced downward and to the left, a diastolic blowing murmur heard best along the left sternal border with the patient sitting upward and leaning forward, and a low-pitched diastolic rumble heard to the left ventricular (LV) apex (*Austin Flint* murmur).

69. Class I indications for aortic valve replacement in patients with aortic regurgitation (AR) include (1) the presence of symptoms in patients with severe AR, irrespective of left ventricular systolic function; (2) chronic severe AR with left ventricular systolic dysfunction (ejection fraction 50% or less), even if asymptomatic; and (3) chronic, severe AR in patients undergoing coronary artery bypass grafting (CABG), other heart valve surgery, or thoracic aortic surgery.

70. Cardiogenic shock is a state of end-organ hypoperfusion caused by cardiac failure characterized by persistent hypotension with severe reduction in cardiac index (less than 1.8 L/min/m^2) in the presence of adequate or elevated filling pressure (left ventricular end-diastolic pressure 18 mm Hg or higher or right ventricular end-diastolic pressure 10 to 15 mm Hg or higher).

71. The rate of ischemic stroke in patients with nonvalvular atrial fibrillation (AF) is about 2 to 7 times that of persons without AF, and the risk increases dramatically as patients age. Both paroxysmal and chronic AF carry the same risk of thromboembolism.

72. In nuclear cardiology stress testing, a *perfusion defect* is an area of reduced radiotracer uptake in the myocardium. If the perfusion defect occurs during stress and improves or normalizes during rest, it is termed *reversible* and usually suggests the presence of inducible ischemia, whereas if the perfusion defect occurs during both stress and rest, it is termed *fixed* and usually suggests the presence of scar (infarct).

73. The main organ systems that need to be monitored with long-term amiodarone therapy are the lungs, the liver, and the thyroid gland. A chest radiograph should be obtained every 6 to 12 months, and liver function tests (LFTs) and thyroid function tests (thyroid-stimulating hormone [TSH] and free T4) should be checked every 6 months.

74. The target international normalized ratio (INR) for warfarin therapy in most cases of cardiovascular disease is 2.5, with a range of 2.0 to 3.0. In certain patients with mechanical heart valves (e.g., older valves, mitral position), the target is 3.0 with a range of 2.5 to 3.5.

75. Lidocaine may cause a variety of central nervous system symptoms including seizures, visual disturbances, tremors, coma, and confusion. Such symptoms are often referred to as *lidocaine toxicity*. The risks of lidocaine toxicity are increased in elderly patients, those with depressed left ventricular function, and those with liver disease.

76. The most important side effect of the antiarrhythmic drug sotalol is QT-segment prolongation leading to torsades de pointes.

77. The major complications of percutaneous coronary intervention (PCI) include periprocedural MI, acute stent thrombosis, coronary artery perforation, contrast nephropathy, access site complications (e.g., retroperitoneal bleed, pseudoaneurysm, arteriovenous fistula), stroke, and a very rare need for emergency CABG.

78. The widely accepted hemodynamic definition of pulmonary arterial hypertension (PAH) is a mean pulmonary arterial pressure of more than 25 mm Hg at rest or more than 30 mm Hg during exercise with a pulmonary capillary or left atrial pressure of less than 15 mm Hg.

79. Acute pericarditis is a syndrome of pericardial inflammation characterized by typical chest pain, a pathognomonic pericardial friction rub, and specific electrocardiographic changes (PR depression, diffuse ST-segment elevation).

80. Conditions associated with the highest cardiac risk in noncardiac surgery are unstable coronary syndromes (unstable or severe angina), decompensated heart failure, severe valvular disease (particularly severe aortic stenosis), and severe arrhythmias.

81. General criteria for surgical intervention in cases of thoracic aortic aneurysm are, for the ascending thoracic aorta, aneurysmal diameter of 5.5 cm (5.0 cm in patients with Marfan syndrome), and for the descending thoracic aorta, aneurismal diameter of 6.5 cm (6 cm in patients with Marfan syndrome).

82. Cardiac complications of advanced AIDS in untreated patients include myocarditis/cardiomyopathy (systolic and diastolic dysfunction), pericardial effusion/tamponade, marantic (thrombotic) or infectious endocarditis, cardiac tumors (Kaposi's sarcoma, lymphoma), and right ventricular dysfunction from pulmonary hypertension or opportunistic infections. Complications with modern antiretroviral therapy (ART) include dyslipidemias, insulin resistance, lipodystrophy, atherosclerosis, and arrhythmias.

83. The radiation dose of a standard cardiac computed tomography (CT) angiography depends on a multitude of factors and can range from 1 mSv to as high as 30 mSv. This compares to an average radiation dose from a nuclear perfusion stress test of 6 to 25 mSv (or as high as more than 40 mSv in thallium stress/rest tests) and an average dose from a simple diagnostic coronary angiogram of approximately 5 mSv.

84. The ankle-brachial index (ABI) is the ankle systolic pressure (as determined by Doppler examination) divided by the brachial systolic pressure. An abnormal index is less than 0.90. The sensitivity is approximately 90% for diagnosis of peripheral vascular disease (PVD). An ABI of 0.41 to 0.90 is interpreted as mild to moderate peripheral arterial disease; an ABI of 0.00 to 0.40 is interpreted as severe PAD.

85. Approximately 90% of cases of renal artery stenosis are due to atherosclerosis. Fibromuscular dysplasia (FMD) is the next most common cause.

86. In very general terms, in cases of carotid artery stenosis, indications for carotid endarterectomy (CEA) are: (1) symptomatic stenosis 50% to 99% diameter if the risk of perioperative stroke or death is less than 6%; and (2) asymptomatic stenosis greater than 60% to 80% diameter if the expected perioperative stroke rate is less than 3%.

87. The most common cardiac complications of systemic lupus erythematosus (SLE) are pericarditis, myocarditis, premature atherosclerosis, and Libman-Sacks endocarditis.

88. Cardiac magnetic resonance imaging (MRI) can be performed in most patients with implanted cardiovascular devices, including most coronary and peripheral stents, prosthetic heart valves, embolization coils, intravenous vena caval (IVC) filters, cardiac closure devices, and aortic stent grafts. Pacemakers and implantable cardioverter defibrillators are strong relative contraindications to MRI scanning, and scanning of such patients should be done under specific delineated conditions, only at centers with expertise in MRI safety and electrophysiology, and only when MRI imaging in particular is clearly indicated.

89. The clinical manifestations of symptomatic bradycardia include fatigue, lightheadedness, dizziness, presyncope, syncope, manifestations of cerebral ischemia, dyspnea on exertion, decreased exercise tolerance, and congestive heart failure.

90. Second-degree heart block is divided into two types: *Mobitz type I (Wenckebach)* exhibits progressive prolongation of the PR interval before an atrial impulse (P wave) is not conducted, whereas *Mobitz type II* exhibits no prolongation of the PR interval before an atrial impulse is not conducted.

91. Temporary or permanent pacing is indicated in the setting of acute MI, with or without symptoms, for (1) complete third-degree block or advanced second-degree block that is associated with block in the His-Purkinje system (wide complex ventricular rhythm) and (2) transient advanced (second-degree or third-degree) AV block with a new bundle branch block.

92. *Cardiac resynchronization therapy (CRT)* refers to simultaneous pacing of both ventricles (biventricular, or Bi-V, pacing). CRT is indicated in patients with advanced heart failure (usually NYHA class III or IV), severe systolic dysfunction (left ventricular ejection fraction 35% or less), and intraventricular conduction delay (QRS less than 120 msec) who are in sinus rhythm and have been on optimal medical therapy.

93. Whereas the left internal mammary artery (LIMA), when anastomosed to the left anterior descending artery (LAD), has a 90% patency at 10 years, for saphenous vein grafts (SVGs), early graft stenosis or occlusion of up to 15% can occur by 1 year, with 10-year patency traditionally cited at only 50% to 60%.

94. Myocardial contusion is a common, reversible injury that is the consequence of a nonpenetrating trauma to the myocardium. It is detected by elevations of specific cardiac enzymes with no evidence of coronary occlusion and by reversible wall motion abnormalities detected by echocardiography.

95. Causes of restrictive cardiomyopathy include infiltrative diseases (amyloidosis, sarcoidosis, Gaucher's disease, Hurler's disease), storage diseases (hemochromatosis, glycogen storage disease, Fabry's disease), and endomyocardial involvement from endomyocardial fibrosis, radiation, or anthracycline treatment.

96. Classical signs for cardiac tamponade include Beck's triad of (1) hypotension caused by decreased stroke volume, (2) jugulovenous distension caused by impaired venous return to the heart, and (3) muffled heart sounds caused by fluid inside the pericardial sac, as well as pulsus paradoxus and general signs of shock such as tachycardia, tachypnea, and decreasing level of consciousness.

97. The most common tumors that spread to the heart are lung (bronchogenic) cancer, breast cancer, melanoma, thyroid cancer, esophageal cancer, lymphoma, and leukemia.

98. Primary cardiac tumors are extremely rare, occurring in one autopsy series in less than 0.1% of subjects. Benign primary tumors are more common than malignant primary tumors, occurring approximately three times as often as malignant tumors.

99. Westermark's sign is the finding in pulmonary embolism of oligemia of the lung beyond the occluded vessel. If pulmonary infarction results, a wedge-shaped infiltrate may be visible.

100. Patients with cocaine-induced chest pain should be treated with intravenous benzodiazepines, which can have beneficial hemodynamic effects and relieve chest pain, and aspirin therapy, as well as nitrate therapy if the patient remains hypertensive. Beta-blockers (including labetolol) should not be administered in the acute setting of cocaine-induced chest pain.

I. GENERAL EXAMINATION

CARDIOVASCULAR PHYSICAL EXAMINATION

Salvatore Mangione, MD

Editor's Note to Readers: For an excellent and more detailed discussion of the cardiovascular physical examination, read *Physical Diagnosis Secrets*, ed 2, by Salvatore Mangione.

1. **What is the meaning of a slow rate of rise of the carotid arterial pulse?**
   A carotid arterial pulse that is reduced *(parvus)* and delayed *(tardus)* argues for *aortic valvular stenosis*. Occasionally this also may be accompanied by a palpable thrill. If ventricular function is good, a slower upstroke correlates with a higher transvalvular gradient. In left ventricular failure, however, *parvus* and *tardus* may occur even with mild aortic stenosis (AS).

2. **What is the significance of a brisk carotid arterial upstroke?**
   It depends on whether it is associated with *normal* or *widened* pulse pressure. If associated with *normal pulse pressure,* a brisk carotid upstroke usually indicates two conditions:
   - **Simultaneous emptying of the left ventricle into a high-pressure bed (the aorta) and a lower pressure bed:** The latter can be the right ventricle (in patients with ventricular septal defect [VSD]) or the left atrium (in patients with mitral regurgitation [MR]). Both will allow a rapid left ventricular emptying, which, in turn, generates a brisk arterial upstroke. The pulse pressure, however, remains normal.
   - **Hypertrophic cardiomyopathy (HCM):** Despite its association with left ventricular obstruction, this disease is characterized by a brisk and bifid pulse, due to the hypertrophic ventricle and its delayed obstruction.

   If associated with *widened pulse pressure,* a brisk upstroke usually indicates aortic regurgitation (AR). In contrast to MR, VSD, or HCM, the AR pulse has rapid upstroke *and* collapse.

3. **In addition to aortic regurgitaiton, which other processes cause rapid upstroke and widened pulse pressure?**
   The most common are the hyperkinetic heart syndromes (high output states). These include anemia, fever, exercise, thyrotoxicosis, pregnancy, cirrhosis, beriberi, Paget's disease, arteriovenous fistulas, patent ductus arteriosus, aortic regurgitation, and anxiety—all typically associated with rapid ventricular contraction and low peripheral vascular resistance.

4. **What is pulsus paradoxus?**
   Pulsus paradoxus is an exaggerated fall in systolic blood pressure during quiet inspiration. In contrast to evaluation of arterial contour and amplitude, it is best detected in a peripheral vessel, such as the radial artery. Although palpable at times, optimal detection of the pulsus paradoxus usually requires a sphygmomanometer. Pulsus paradoxus can occur in cardiac tamponade and other conditions.

5. **What is pulsus alternans?**
   Pulsus alternans is the alternation of strong and weak arterial pulses despite *regular rate and rhythm*. First described by Ludwig Traube in 1872, pulsus alternans is often associated with alternation of strong and feeble heart sounds (auscultatory alternans). Both indicate severe left ventricular dysfunction (from ischemia, hypertension, or valvular cardiomyopathy), with worse ejection fraction and higher pulmonary capillary pressure. Hence, they are often associated with an S_3 gallop.

6. **What is Duroziez's double murmur?**

   Duroziez's is a to-and-fro double murmur over a large central artery—usually the femoral, but also the brachial. It is elicited by applying gradual but *firm* compression with the stethoscope's diaphragm. This produces not only a systolic murmur (which is normal) but also a *diastolic* one (which is pathologic and typical of AR). Duroziez's has 58% to 100% sensitivity *and* specificity for AR.

7. **What is the carotid shudder?**

   Carotid shudder is a palpable thrill felt at the peak of the carotid pulse in patients with AS, AR, or both. It represents the transmission of the murmur to the artery and is a relatively specific but rather insensitive sign of aortic valvular disease.

8. **What is Corrigan's pulse?**

   Corrigan's is one of the various names for the bounding and quickly collapsing pulse of aortic regurgitation, which is both visible *and* palpable. Other common terms for this condition include *water hammer, cannonball, collapsing,* or *pistol-shot pulse.* It is best felt for by elevating the patient's arm while at the same time feeling the radial artery at the *wrist.* Raising the arm higher than the heart reduces the intraradial diastolic pressure, collapses the vessel, and thus facilitates the palpability of the subsequent systolic thrust.

9. **How do you auscultate for carotid bruits?**

   By placing your bell on the neck in a quiet room and with a relaxed patient. Auscultate from just behind the upper end of the thyroid cartilage to immediately below the angle of the jaw.

10. **What is the correlation between symptomatic carotid bruit and high-grade stenosis?**

    It's high. In fact, bruits presenting with transient ischemic attacks (TIAs) or minor strokes in the anterior circulation should be evaluated aggressively for the presence of high-grade (70%–99%) carotid stenosis, because endarterectomy markedly decreases mortality and stroke rates. Still, although presence of a bruit significantly increases the likelihood of high-grade carotid stenosis, its absence doesn't exclude disease. Moreover, a bruit heard over the bifurcation may reflect a narrowed *external* carotid artery and thus occur in angiographically normal or completely occluded *internal* carotids. Hence, surgical decisions should *not* be based on physical examination alone; imaging is mandatory.

11. **What is central venous pressure (CVP)?**

    The pressure within the right atrium/superior vena cava system (i.e., the right ventricular filling pressure). As pulmonary capillary wedge pressure reflects left ventricular end-diastolic pressure (in the absence of mitral stenosis), so central venous pressure reflects right ventricular end-diastolic pressure (in the absence of tricuspid stenosis).

12. **Which veins should be evaluated for assessing venous pulse and CVP?**

    Central veins, as much in direct communication with the right atrium as possible. The ideal one is therefore the internal jugular. Ideally the right internal jugular vein should be inspected, because it is in a more direct line with the right atrium and thus better suited to function as both a manometer for venous pressure and a conduit for atrial pulsations. Moreover, CVP may be spuriously higher on the left as compared with the right because of the left innominate vein's compression between the aortic arch and the sternum.

13. **Can the external jugulars be used for evaluating central venous pressure?**

    Theoretically not, practically yes. *Not* because:

- While going through the various fascial planes of the neck, they often become compressed.
- In patients with increased sympathetic vascular tone, they may become so constricted as to be barely visible.
- They are farther from the right atrium and thus in a less straight line with it. Yet both internal *and* external jugular veins can actually be used for estimating CVP because they yield comparable estimates.

Hence, if the only visible vein is the external jugular, do what Yogi Berra recommends you should do when coming to a fork in the road: take it.

14. What is a "cannon" A wave?

A "cannon" A wave is the hallmark of atrioventricular dissociation (i.e., the atrium contracts against a closed tricuspid valve). It is different from the other prominent outward wave (i.e., the presystolic giant A wave) insofar as it begins just after S_1, because it represents atrial contraction against a closed tricuspid valve.

15. How do you estimate the CVP?

- By positioning the patient so that you can get a good view of the internal jugular vein and its oscillations. Although it is wise to start at 45 degrees, it doesn't really matter which angle you will eventually use to raise the patient's head, as long as it can adequately reveal the vein. In the absence of a visible internal jugular, the external jugular may suffice.
- By identifying the highest point of jugular pulsation that is transmitted to the skin (i.e., the meniscus). This usually occurs during exhalation and coincides with the peak of "A" or "V" waves. It serves as a bedside pulsation manometer.
- By finding the sternal angle of Louis (the junction of the manubrium with the body of the sternum). This provides the standard zero for jugular venous pressure. (The standard zero for central venous pressure is instead the center of the right atrium.)
- By measuring in centimeters the vertical height from the sternal angle to the top of the jugular pulsation. To do so, place two rulers at a 90-degree angle: one horizontal (and parallel to the meniscus) and the other vertical to it and touching the sternal angle (Fig. 1-1). The extrapolated height between the sternal angle and meniscus represents the jugular venous pressure (JVP).
- By adding 5 to convert jugular venous pressure into central venous pressure. This method relies on the fact that the zero point of the entire right-sided manometer (i.e., the point where central venous pressure is, by convention, zero) is the center of the right atrium. This is vertically situated at 5 cm below the sternal angle, a relationship that is present in subjects of normal size and shape, regardless of their body position. Thus, using the sternal angle as the external reference point, the vertical distance (in centimeters) to the top of the column of blood in the jugular vein will provide the JVP. Adding 5 to the JVP will yield the CVP.

16. What is the significance of leg swelling without increased central venous pressure?

It reflects either bilateral venous insufficiency or noncardiac edema (usually hepatic or renal). This is because any cardiac (or pulmonary) disease resulting in right ventricular failure would manifest itself through an increase in central venous pressure. Leg edema *plus ascites* in the absence of increased CVP argues in favor of a hepatic or renal cause (patients with cirrhosis do *not* have high CVP). Conversely, a high CVP in patients with ascites and edema argues in favor of an underlying cardiac etiology.

17. What is Kussmaul's sign?

Kussmaul's sign is the paradoxical increase in JVP that occurs during inspiration. Jugular venous pressure normally *decreases* during inspiration because the inspiratory fall in

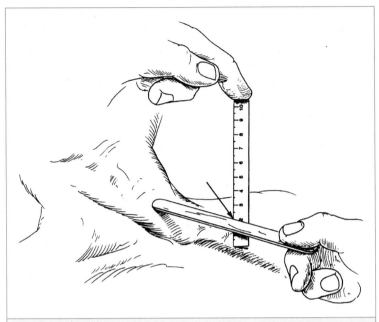

Figure 1-1. Measurement of jugular venous pressure. (From Adair OV: *Cardiology secrets*, ed 2, Philadelphia, 2001, Hanley & Belfus.)

intrathoracic pressure creates a "sucking effect" on venous return. Thus, Kussmaul's sign is a true physiologic paradox. This can be explained by the inability of the right side of the heart to handle an increased venous return.

Disease processes associated with a positive Kussmaul's are those that interfere with venous return and right ventricular filling. The original description was in a patient with constrictive pericarditis. (Kussmaul's is still seen in one third of patients with severe and advanced cases, in whom it is often associated with a positive abdominojugular reflux.) Nowadays, however, the most common cause is severe heart failure, independent of etiology. Other causes include cor pulmonale (acute or chronic), constrictive pericarditis, restrictive cardiomyopathy (such as sarcoidosis, hemochromatosis, and amyloidosis), tricuspid stenosis, and right ventricular infarction.

18. **What is the "venous hum"?**
Venous hum is a *functional* murmur produced by turbulent flow in the internal jugular vein. It is *continuous* (albeit louder in diastole) and at times strong enough to be associated with a palpable thrill. It is best heard on the right side of the neck, just above the clavicle, but sometimes it can become audible over the sternal/parasternal areas, both right and left. This may lead to misdiagnoses of carotid disease, patent ductus arteriosus, or AR/AS. The mechanism of the venous hum is a mild compression of the internal jugular vein by the transverse process of the atlas, in subjects with strong cardiac output and increased venous flow. Hence, it is common in young adults or patients with a high output state. A venous hum can be heard in 31% to 66% of normal children and 25% of young adults. It also is encountered in 2.3% to 27% of adult outpatients. It is especially common in situations of arteriovenous fistula, being present in 56% to 88% of patients undergoing dialysis and 34% of those *between* sessions.

19. **Which characteristics of the apical impulse should be analyzed?**
   - **Location:** Normally over the fifth left interspace midclavicular line, which usually (but not always) corresponds to the area just below the nipple. *Volume loads* to the left ventricle (such as aortic or mitral regurgitation) tend to displace the apical impulse downward and laterally. Conversely, *pressure loads* (such as aortic stenosis or hypertension) tend to displace the impulse more upward and medially—at least initially. Still, a failing and decompensated ventricle, independent of its etiology, will typically present with a downward and lateral shift in point of maximal impulse (PMI). Although not too sensitive, this finding is very specific for cardiomegaly, low ejection fraction, and high pulmonary capillary wedge pressure. Correlation of the PMI with anatomic landmarks (such as the left anterior axillary line) can be used to better characterize the displaced impulse.
   - **Size:** As measured in left lateral decubitus, the normal apical impulse is the size of a dime. Anything larger (nickel, quarter, or an old Eisenhower silver dollar) should be considered pathologic. A diameter greater than 4 cm is quite specific for cardiomegaly.
   - **Duration and timing:** This is probably one of the most important characteristics. A normal apical duration is brief and never passes midsystole. Thus, a *sustained impulse* (i.e., one that continues into S_2 and beyond—often referred to as a "heave") should be considered pathologic until proven otherwise and is usually indicative of pressure load, volume load, or cardiomyopathy.
   - **Amplitude:** This is not the length of the impulse, but its *force*. A *hyperdynamic* impulse (often referred to as a "thrust") that is forceful enough to lift the examiner's finger can be encountered in situations of volume overload and increased output (such as aortic regurgitation and ventricular septal defect) but may also be felt in normal subjects with very thin chests. Similarly, a *hypodynamic* impulse can be due to simple obesity but also to congestive cardiomyopathy. In addition to being hypodynamic, the precordial impulse of these patients is large, somewhat sustained, and displaced downward/laterally.
   - **Contour:** A normal apical impulse is single. Double or triple impulses are clearly pathologic.
   - Hence, a normal apical impulse consists of a single, dime-sized, brief (barely beyond S_1), early systolic, and nonsustained impulse, localized over the fifth interspace midclavicular line.

20. **What is a thrill?**
   A palpable vibration associated with an audible murmur. A thrill automatically qualifies the murmur as being more than 4/6 in intensity and thus pathologic.

BIBLIOGRAPHY, SUGGESTED READINGS, AND WEBSITES

1. On Doctoring: Physical Examination Movies: http://dms.dartmouth.edu/ed_programs/course_resources/ondoctoring_yr2/
2. The Cardiac Examination: http://www.meded.virginia.edu/courses/pom1/pexams/CardioExam/
3. Basta LL, Bettinger JJ: The cardiac impulse. *Am Heart J* 197:96-111, 1979.
4. Constant J: Using internal jugular pulsations as a manometer for right atrial pressure measurements, *Cardiology* 93:26-30, 2000.
5. Cook DJ, Simel N: Does this patient have abnormal central venous pressure? *JAMA* 275:630-634, 1996.
6. Davison R, Cannon R: Estimation of central venous pressure by examination of the jugular veins, *Am Heart J* 87:279-282, 1974.
7. Drazner MH, Rame JE, Stevenson LW, et al: Prognostic importance of elevated jugular venous pressure and a third heart sound in patients with heart failure, *N Engl J Med* 345:574-581, 2001.
8. Ellen SD, Crawford MH, O'Rourke RA: Accuracy of precordial palpation for detecting increased left ventricular volume, *Ann Intern Med* 99:628-630, 1983.
9. Mangione S: *Physical diagnosis secrets*, ed 2, Philadelphia, 2008, Mosby.

10. McGee SR: Physical examination of venous pressure: a critical review, *Am Heart J* 136:10-18, 1998.
11. O'Neill TW, Barry M, Smith M, et al: Diagnostic value of the apex beat, *Lancet* 1:410-411, 1989.
12. Sauve JS, Laupacis A, Ostbye T, et al: The rational clinical examination. Does this patient have a clinically important carotid bruit? *JAMA* 270:2843-2845, 1993.

CHAPTER 2

HEART MURMURS

Salvatore Mangione, MD

Editor's Note to Readers: For an excellent and more detailed discussion of heart murmurs, read *Physical Diagnosis Secrets*, ed 2, by Salvatore Mangione.

1. **What are the auscultatory areas of murmurs?**
   Auscultation typically starts in the aortic area, continuing in clockwise fashion: first over the pulmonic, then the mitral (or apical), and finally the tricuspid areas (Fig. 2-1). Because murmurs may radiate widely, they often become audible in areas outside those historically assigned to them. Hence, "inching" the stethoscope (i.e., slowly dragging it from site to site) can be the best way to avoid missing important findings.

2. **What is the Levine system for grading the intensity of murmurs?**
   The intensity or loudness of a murmur is traditionally graded by the Levine system (no relation to this book's editor) from 1/6 to 6/6. Everything else being equal, increased intensity usually reflects increased flow turbulence. Thus, a louder murmur is more likely to be pathologic and severe.
   - **1/6:** a murmur so soft as to be heard only intermittently and always with concentration and effort. Never immediately
   - **2/6:** a murmur that is soft but nonetheless audible immediately and on every beat
   - **3/6:** a murmur that is easily audible and relatively loud
   - **4/6:** a murmur that is relatively loud and associated with a palpable thrill (always pathologic)
   - **5/6:** a murmur loud enough that it can be heard even by placing the edge of the stethoscope's diaphragm over the patient's chest
   - **6/6:** a murmur so loud that it can be heard even when the stethoscope is not in contact with the chest, but held slightly above its surface

3. **What are the causes of a systolic murmur?**
   - **Ejection** (i.e., increased "forward" flow over the aortic or pulmonic valve): This can be:
     - **Physiologic:** normal valve, but flow high enough to cause turbulence (anemia, exercise, fever, and other hyperkinetic heart syndromes)
     - **Pathologic:** abnormal valve, with or without outflow obstruction (i.e., aortic stenosis versus aortic sclerosis)
   - **Regurgitation:** "backward" flow from a high- into a low-pressure bed. Although this is usually due to incompetent atrioventricular (AV) valves (mitral/tricuspid), it also can be due to ventricular septal defect.

4. **What are functional murmurs?**
   They are benign findings caused by turbulent ejection into the great vessels. Functional murmurs have no clinical relevance, other than getting into the differential diagnosis of a systolic murmur.

5. **What is the most common systolic ejection murmur of the elderly?**
   The murmur of aortic sclerosis. This early peaking systolic murmur is extremely age related, affecting 21% to 26% of persons older than 65 and 55% to 75% of octogenarians. (Conversely, the prevalence of aortic stenosis in these age groups is 2% and 2.6%, respectively.) The murmur

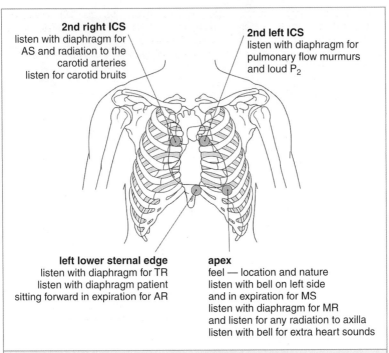

2nd right ICS
listen with diaphragm for
AS and radiation to the
carotid arteries
listen for carotid bruits

2nd left ICS
listen with diaphragm for
pulmonary flow murmurs
and loud P₂

left lower sternal edge
listen with diaphragm for TR
listen with diaphragm patient
sitting forward in expiration for AR

apex
feel — location and nature
listen with bell on left side
and in expiration for MS
listen with diaphragm for MR
and listen for any radiation to axilla
listen with bell for extra heart sounds

Figure 2-1. Sequence of auscultation of the heart. *AR,* Aortic regurgitation; *AS,* aortic stenosis; *ICS,* intercostal space; *MR,* mitral regurgitation; *MS,* mitral stenosis; *TR,* tricuspid regurgitation. (From Baliga R: *Crash course cardiology,* St. Louis, 2005, Mosby.)

of aortic sclerosis may be due to either a degenerative change of the aortic valve or abnormalities of the aortic root. Senile degeneration of the aortic valve includes thickening, fibrosis, and occasionally calcification. This can stiffen the valve and yet not cause a transvalvular pressure gradient. In fact, commissural fusion is typically absent in aortic sclerosis. Abnormalities of the aortic root may be diffuse (such as a tortuous and dilated aorta) or localized (like a calcific spur or an atherosclerotic plaque that protrudes into the lumen, creating a turbulent bloodstream).

6. **How can physical examination help differentiate functional from pathologic murmurs?**
   There are two golden and three silver rules:
   - The first golden rule is to always judge (systolic) murmurs like people: by the company they keep. Hence, murmurs that keep bad company (like symptoms; extra sounds; thrill; and abnormal arterial or venous pulse, electrocardiogram [ECG], or chest radiograph) should be considered pathologic until proven otherwise. These murmurs should receive lots of evaluation, including technology based.
   - The second golden rule is that a diminished or absent S₂ usually indicates a poorly moving and abnormal semilunar (aortic or pulmonic) valve. This is the hallmark of pathology. As a flip side, functional systolic murmurs are always accompanied by a well-preserved S₂, with normal split.

   The three silver rules are:
   - All holosystolic (or late systolic) murmurs are pathologic.
   - All diastolic murmurs are pathologic.
   - All continuous murmurs are pathologic.

Thus, functional murmurs should be systolic, short, soft (typically less than 3/6), early peaking (never passing mid-systole), predominantly circumscribed to the base, and associated with a well-preserved and normally split-second sound. They should have an otherwise normal cardiovascular examination and often disappear with sitting, standing, or straining (as, for example, following a Valsalva maneuver).

7. **How much reduction in valvular area is necessary for the aortic stenosis (AS) murmur to become audible?**
At least 50% (the minimum for creating a pressure gradient at rest). Mild disease may produce loud murmurs, too, but usually significant hemodynamic compromise (and symptoms) does not occur until a 60% to 70% reduction in valvular area exists. This means that early to mild AS may be subtle at rest. Exercise, however, may intensify the murmur by increasing the output and gradient.

8. **What factors may suggest severe aortic stenosis?**
   - Murmur intensity and timing (the louder and later peaking the murmur, the worse the disease)
   - A single S_2
   - Delayed upstroke/reduced amplitude of the carotid pulse (pulsus parvus and tardus)

9. **What is a thrill?**
It is a palpable vibratory sensation, often compared to the purring of a cat, and typical of murmurs caused by very high pressure gradients. These, in turn, lead to great turbulence and loudness. Hence, thrills are only present in pathologic murmurs whose intensity is greater than 4/6.

10. **What is isometric hand grip, and what does it do to AS and mitral regurgitation (MR) murmurs?**
Isometric hand grip is carried out by asking the patient to lock the cupped fingers of both hands into a grip and then trying to pull them apart. The resulting increase in peripheral vascular resistance intensifies MR (and ventricular septal defect) while softening instead AS (and aortic sclerosis). Hence, a positive hand grip argues strongly in favor of MR.

11. **What is the Gallavardin phenomenon?**
One noticed in some patients with AS, who may exhibit a dissociation of their systolic murmur into two components:
   - A typical AS-like murmur (medium to low pitched, harsh, right parasternal, typically radiated to the neck, and caused by high-velocity jets into the ascending aorta)
   - A murmur that instead mimics MR (high pitched, musical, and best heard at the apex)
This phenomenon reflects the different transmission of AS: its medium frequencies to the base and its higher frequencies to the apex. The latter may become so prominent as to be misinterpreted as a separate apical "cooing" of MR.

12. **Where is the murmur of hypertrophic cardiomyopathy (HCM) best heard?**
It depends. When septal hypertrophy obstructs not only left but also right ventricular outflow, the murmur may be louder at the left lower sternal border. More commonly, however, the HCM murmur is louder at the apex. This may often cause a differential diagnosis dilemma with the murmur of MR.

13. **What are the characteristics of a ventricular septal defect (VSD) murmur?**
VSD murmurs may be holosystolic, crescendo-decrescendo, crescendo, or decrescendo. A crescendo-decrescendo murmur usually indicates a defect in the muscular part of the septum. Ventricular contraction closes the hole toward the end of systole, thus causing the decrescendo phase of the murmur. Conversely, a defect in the membranous septum will enjoy no systolic

reduction in flow and thus produce a murmur that remains constant and holosystolic. VSD murmurs are best heard along the left lower sternal border, often radiating left to right across the chest. VSD murmurs always start immediately after S_1.

14. **What is a systolic regurgitant murmur?**
One characterized by a pressure gradient that causes a retrograde blood flow across an abnormal opening. This can be (1) a ventricular septal defect, (2) an incompetent mitral valve, (3) an incompetent tricuspid valve, or (4) fistulous communication between a high-pressure and a low-pressure vascular bed (such as a patent ductus arteriosus).

15. **What are the auscultatory characteristics of systolic regurgitant murmurs?**
They tend to start immediately after S_1, often extending into S_2. They also may have a musical quality, variously described as "honk" or "whoop." This is usually caused by vibrating vegetations (endocarditis) or chordae tendineae (mitral valve prolapse, dilated cardiomyopathy) and may help separate the more musical murmurs of AV valve regurgitation from the harsher sounds of semilunar stenosis. Note that in contrast to systolic ejection murmurs like AS or VSD, systolic regurgitant murmurs do not increase in intensity after a long diastole.

16. **What are the characteristics of the MR murmur?**
It is loudest at the apex, radiated to the left axilla or interscapular area, high pitched, plateau, and extending all the way into S_2 (holosystolic). S_2 is normal in intensity but often widely split. If the gradient is high (and the flow is low), the MR murmur is high pitched. Conversely, if the gradient is low (and the flow is high) the murmur is low pitched. In general, the louder (and longer) the MR murmur, the worse the regurgitation.

17. **What are the characteristics of the acute MR murmur?**
The acute MR murmur tends to be very short, and even absent, because the left atrium and ventricle often behave like a common chamber, with no pressure gradient between them. Hence, in contrast to that of chronic MR (which is either holosystolic or late systolic), the acute MR murmur is often early systolic (exclusively so in 40% of cases) and is associated with an S_4 in 80% of the patients.

18. **What are the characteristics of the mitral valve prolapse murmur?**
It is a mitral regurgitant murmur—hence, loudest at the apex, mid to late systolic in onset (immediately following the click), and usually extending all the way into the second sound (A_2). In fact, it often has a crescendo shape that peaks at S_2. It is usually not too loud (never greater than 3/6), with some musical features that have been variously described as whoops or honks (as in the honking of a goose). Indeed, musical murmurs of this kind are almost always due to mitral valve prolapse (MVP).

19. **How are diastolic murmurs classified?**
By their timing. Hence, the most important division is between murmurs that start just after S_2 (i.e., early diastolic—reflecting aortic or pulmonic regurgitation) versus those that start a little later (i.e., mid to late diastolic, often with a presystolic accentuation—reflecting mitral or tricuspid valve stenosis) (Fig. 2-2).

20. **What is then the best strategy to detect the mitral stenosis (MS) murmur?**
The best strategy consists of listening over the apex, with the patient in the left lateral decubitus position, at the end of exhalation, and after a short exercise. Finally, applying the bell with very light pressure also may help. (Strong pressure will instead completely eliminate the low frequencies of MS.)

Phonocardiogram (inspiration unless noted)	Description

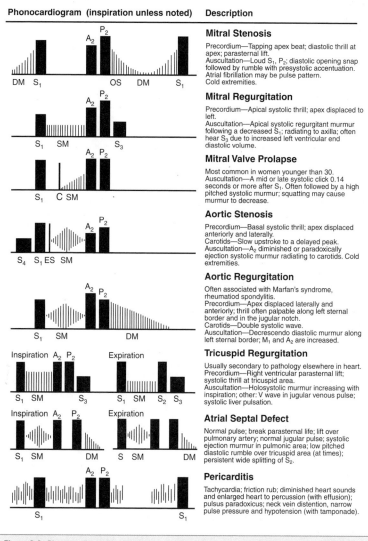

Mitral Stenosis

Precordium—Tapping apex beat; diastolic thrill at apex; parasternal lift.
Auscultation—Loud S_1, P_2; diastolic opening snap followed by rumble with presystolic accentuation. Atrial fibrillation may be pulse pattern. Cold extremities.

Mitral Regurgitation

Precordium—Apical systolic thrill; apex displaced to left.
Auscultation—Apical systolic regurgitant murmur following a decreased S_1; radiating to axilla; often hear S_3 due to increased left ventricular end diastolic volume.

Mitral Valve Prolapse

Most common in women younger than 30.
Auscultation—A mid or late systolic click 0.14 seconds or more after S_1. Often followed by a high pitched systolic murmur; squatting may cause murmur to decrease.

Aortic Stenosis

Precordium—Basal systolic thrill; apex displaced anteriorly and laterally.
Carotids—Slow upstroke to a delayed peak.
Auscultation—A_2 diminished or paradoxically ejection systolic murmur radiating to carotids. Cold extremities.

Aortic Regurgitation

Often associated with Marfan's syndrome, rheumatiod spondylitis.
Precordium—Apex displaced laterally and anteriorly; thrill often palpable along left sternal border and in the jugular notch.
Carotids—Double systolic wave.
Auscultation—Decrescendo diastolic murmur along left sternal border; M_1 and A_2 are increased.

Tricuspid Regurgitation

Usually secondary to pathology elsewhere in heart.
Precordium—Right ventricular parasternal lift; systolic thrill at tricuspid area.
Auscultation—Holosystolic murmur increasing with inspiration; other: V wave in jugular venous pulse; systolic liver pulsation.

Atrial Septal Defect

Normal pulse; break parasternal life; lift over pulmonary artery; normal jugular pulse; systolic ejection murmur in pulmonic area; low pitched diastolic rumble over tricuspid area (at times); persistent wide splitting of S_2.

Pericarditis

Tachycardia; friction rub; diminished heart sounds and enlarged heart to percussion (with effusion); pulsus paradoxicus; neck vein distention, narrow pulse pressure and hypotension (with tamponade).

Figure 2-2. Phonocardiographic description of pathologic cardiac murmurs. (From James EC, Corry RJ, Perry JF: *Principles of basic surgical practice*, Philadelphia, 1987, Hanley & Belfus.)

21. **What are the typical auscultatory findings of aortic regurgitation (AR)?**
Depending on severity, there may be up to three murmurs (one in systole and two in diastole) plus an ejection click. Of course, the typical auscultatory finding is the diastolic tapering murmur, which, together with the brisk pulse and the enlarged/displaced point of maximal impulse (PMI), constitutes the bedside diagnostic triad of AR. The diastolic tapering murmur is usually best heard over Erb's point (third or fourth interspace, left parasternal line) but at times also over the aortic area, especially when a tortuous and dilated root pushes the ascending aorta anteriorly and to the right. The decrescendo diastolic murmur of AR is best heard by

having the patient sit up and lean forward while holding breath in exhalation. Using the diaphragm and pressing hard on the stethoscope also may help because this murmur is rich in high frequencies. Finally, increasing peripheral vascular resistances (by having the patient squat) will also intensify the murmur. A typical, characteristic early diastolic murmur argues very strongly in favor of the diagnosis of AR.

An accompanying systolic murmur may be due to concomitant AS but most commonly indicates severe regurgitation, followed by an increased systolic flow across the valve. Hence, this accompanying systolic murmur is often referred to as *comitans* (Latin for "companion"). It provides an important clue to the severity of regurgitation. A second diastolic murmur can be due to the rumbling diastolic murmur of Austin Flint (i.e., functional mitral stenosis). The Austin Flint murmur is a mitral stenosis–like diastolic rumble, best heard at the apex, and is due to the regurgitant aortic stream preventing full opening of the anterior mitral leaflet.

22. What is a mammary soufflé?
Not a fancy French dish but a systolic-diastolic murmur heard over one or both breasts in late pregnancy and typically disappearing at end of lactation. It is caused by increased flow along the mammary arteries, which explains why its systolic component starts just a little after S_1. It can be obliterated by pressing (with finger or stethoscope) over the area of maximal intensity.

BIBLIOGRAPHY, SUGGESTED READINGS, AND WEBSITES

1. Heart Sounds and Cardiac Arrhythmias: An excellent audiovisual tutorial on heart sounds. http://www.blaufuss.org/
2. Heart Sounds and Murmurs: http://depts.washington.edu/physdx/heart/index.html
3. Constant J, Lippschutz EJ: Diagramming and grading heart sounds and murmurs, *Am Heart J* 70:326-332, 1965.
4. Danielsen R, Nordrehaug JE, Vik-Mo H: Clinical and haemodynamic features in relation to severity of aortic stenosis in adults, *Eur Heart J* 12:791-795, 1991.
5. Etchells E, Bell C, Robb K: Does this patient have an abnormal systolic murmur? *JAMA* 277:564-571, 1997.
6. Mangione S: *Physical diagnosis secrets*, ed 2, Philadelphia, 2008, Mosby.

CHAPTER 3

ELECTROCARDIOGRAM

Glenn N. Levine, MD, FACC, FAHA

1. **What are the most commonly used criteria to diagnose left ventricular hypertrophy (LVH)?**
   - R wave in V5-V6 + S wave in V1-V2 > 35 mm
   - R wave in lead I + S wave in lead III > 25 mm

2. **What are the most commonly used criteria to diagnose right ventricular hypertrophy (RVH)?**
   - R wave in V1 ≥ 7 mm
   - R/S wave ratio in V1 > 1

3. **What criteria are used to diagnose left atrial enlargement (LAE)?**
   - P wave total width of > 0.12 sec (3 small boxes) in the inferior leads, usually with a double-peaked P wave
   - Terminal portion of the P wave in lead V1 ≥ 0.04 sec (1 small box) wide and ≥ 1 mm (1 small box) deep

4. **What electrocardiogram (ECG) finding suggests right atrial enlargement?**
   - P-wave height in the inferior leads (II, III, and aVF) ≥ 2.5 to 3 mm (2.5–3 small boxes) (Fig. 3-1)

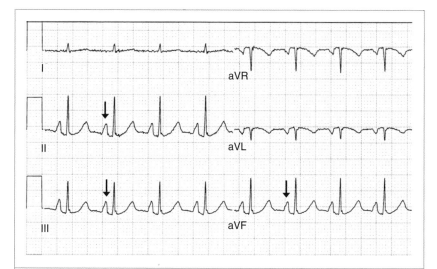

Figure 3-1. Right atrial enlargement. The tall P waves in the inferior leads (II, III, and avF) are more than 2.5 to 3 mm high.

5. **What is the normal rate of a junctional rhythm?**
The normal rate is 40 to 60 beats/min. Rates of 61 to 99 beats/min are referred to as *accelerated junctional rhythm,* and rates of 100 beats/min or higher are referred to as *junctional tachycardia.*

6. **How can one distinguish a junctional escape rhythm from a ventricular escape rhythm in a patient with complete heart block?**
Junctional escape rhythms usually occur at a rate of 40 to 60 beats/min and will usually be narrow complex (unless the patient has a baseline bundle branch block), whereas ventricular escape rhythms will usually occur at a rate of 30 to 40 beats/min and will be wide complex.

7. **Describe the three types of heart block.**
   - **First-degree heart block:** The PR interval is a fixed duration of more than 0.20 seconds.
   - **Second-degree heart block:** In Mobitz type I (Wenkebach), the PR interval increases until a P wave is nonconducted (Fig. 3-2). The cycle then resets and starts again. Mobitz type I second-degree heart block is sometimes due to increased vagal tone and is usually a relatively benign finding. In Mobitz type II, the PR interval is fixed and occasional P waves are nonconducted. Mobitz type II second-degree heart block usually indicates structural disease in the atrioventricular (AV) node or His-Purkinje system and is an indication for pacemaker implantation.
   - **Third-degree heart block:** All P waves are nonconducted, and there is either a junctional or ventricular escape rhythm. To call a rhythm third-degree or complete heart block, the atrial rate (as evidenced by the P waves) should be faster than the ventricular escape rate (the QRS complexes). Third-degree heart block is almost always an indication for a permanent pacemaker.

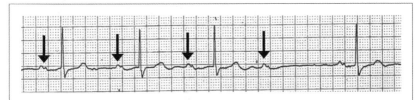

Figure 3-2. Wenkebach (Mobitz type I second-degree AV block). The PR interval progressively increases until there is a nonconducted P wave.

8. **What are the causes of ST segment elevation?**
   - Acute myocardial infarction (MI) due to thrombotic occlusion of a coronary artery
   - Prinzmetal's angina (variant angina), in which there is vasospasm of a coronary artery
   - Cocaine-induced MI, in which there is vasospasm of a coronary artery, with or without additional thrombotic occlusion
   - Pericarditis, in which there is usually diffuse ST segment elevation
   - Left ventricular aneurysm
   - Left bundle branch block (LBBB)
   - Left ventricular hypertrophy with repolarization abnormalities
   - J point elevation, a condition classically seen in young African-American patients but that can be seen in any patient, which is felt due to "early repolarization"
   - Severe hyperkalemia

9. **What are the electrocardiographic findings of hyperkalemia?**
Initially, a "peaking" of the T waves is seen (Fig. 3-3). As the hyperkalemia becomes more profound, "loss" of the P waves, QRS widening, and ST segment elevation may occur. The preterminal finding is a sinusoidal pattern on the ECG (Fig. 3-4).

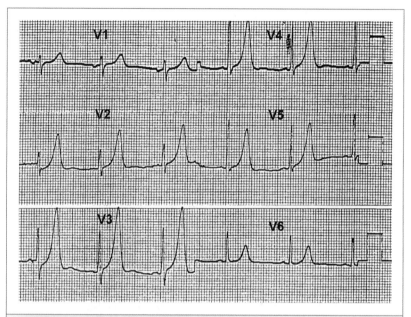

Figure 3-3. Hyperkalemia. Peaked T waves are seen in many of the precordial leads. (Adapted with permission from Levine GN, Podrid PJ: *The ECG workbook: a review and discussion of ECG findings and abnormalities,* New York, Futura Publishing Company, 1995. p. 405)

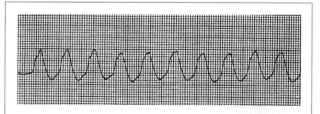

Figure 3-4. Severe hyperkalemia. The rhythm strip demonstrates the preterminal rhythm sinusoidal wave seen in cases of severe hyperkalemia. (Adapted with permission from Levine GN, Podrid PJ: *The ECG workbook: a review and discussion of ECG findings and abnormalities,* New York, Futura Publishing Company, 1995. p. 503)

10. **What are the ECG findings in pericarditis?**
The first findings are believed by some to be PR segment depression caused by repolarization abnormalities of the atria. This may be fairly transient and is often not present by the time the patient is seen for evaluation. Either concurrent with PR segment depression or shortly following PR segment depression, diffuse ST segment elevation occurs (see ECG example in Chapter 53 on Pericarditis). At a later time, diffuse T-wave inversions may develop.

11. **What is electrical alternans?**
In the presence of large pericardial effusions, the heart may "swing" within the large pericardial effusion, resulting in an alteration of the amplitude of the QRS complex (Fig. 3-5).

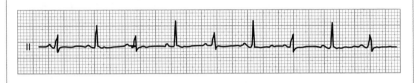

Figure 3-5. Electrical alternans in a patient with a large pericardial effusion. Note the alternating amplitude of the QRS complexes. (From Manning WJ: Pericardial disease. In Goldman L: *Cecil medicine,* ed 23, Philadelphia, Saunders, 2008.)

12. **What is the main ECG finding in hypercalcemia and hypocalcemia?**
With hypercalcemia the QT interval shortens. With hypocalcemia, prolongation of the QT interval occurs as a result of delayed repolarization (Fig. 3-6).

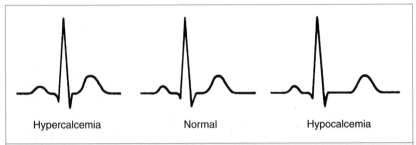

Hypercalcemia   Normal   Hypocalcemia

Figure 3-6. Electrocardiographic findings of hypercalcemia and hypocalcemia. With hypercalcemia, the QT interval shortens. With hypocalcemia there is prolongation of the QT interval due to delayed repolarization. (From Park MK, Guntheroth WG: *How to read pediatric ECGs,* ed 4, Philadelphia, Mosby, 2006.)

13. **What ECG findings may be present in pulmonary embolus?**
- Sinus tachycardia (the most common ECG finding)
- Right atrial enlargement (P pulmonale)—tall P waves in the inferior leads
- Right axis deviation
- T wave inversions in leads V1-V2
- Incomplete right bundle branch block (IRBBB)
- S1Q3T3 pattern—an S wave in lead I, a Q wave in lead III, and an inverted T wave in lead III. Although this is only occasionally seen with pulmonary embolus, it is said to be quite suggestive that a pulmonary embolus has occurred.

14. **What is torsades de pointes?**

Torsades de pointes is a ventricular arrhythmia that occurs in the setting of QT prolongation, usually when drugs that prolong the QT interval have been administered. It may also occur in the setting of prolonged QT syndrome and other conditions. The term was reported coined by Dessertenne to describe the arrhythmia, in which the QRS axis appears to twist around the isoelectric line (Fig. 3-7). It is usually a hemodynamically unstable rhythm that can further degenerate and lead to hemodynamic collapse.

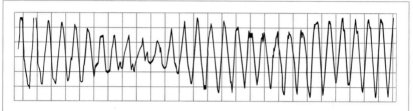

Figure 3-7. Torsades de pointes, in which the QRS axis seems to rotate about the isoelectric point. (From Olgin JE, Zipes DP: Specific arrhythmias: diagnosis and treatment. In Libby P, Bonow R, Mann D, et al: *Braunwald's heart disease: a textbook of cardiovascular medicine,* ed 8, Philadelphia, Saunders, 2008.)

15. **What are cerebral T waves?**

Cerebral T waves are strikingly deep and inverted T waves, most prominently seen in the precordial leads, that occur with central nervous system diseases, most notably subarachnoid and intracerebral hemorrhages. They are believed to be due to prolonged and abnormal repolarization of the left ventricle, presumably as a result of autonomic imbalance. They should not be mistaken for evidence of active cardiac ischemia (Fig. 3-8).

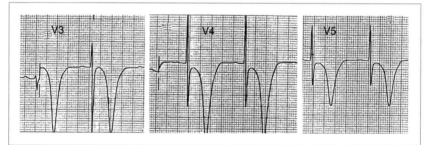

Figure 3-8. Cerebral T waves. The markedly deep and inverted T waves are seen with central nervous system disease, particularly subarachnoid and intracerebral hemorrhages. (Reproduced with permission from Levine GN, Podrid PJ: *The ECG workbook: a review and discussion of ECG findings and abnormalities,* New York, Futura Publishing Company, 1995. p. 437)

BIBLIOGRAPHY, SUGGESTED READINGS, AND WEBSITES

1. ECG Library: http://www.ecglibrary.com/ecghome.html
2. ECG Tutorial: http://www.uptodate.com
3. Electrocardiogram Rhythm Tutor: http://www.coldbacon.com/mdtruth/more/ekg.html
4. Electrocardiography: An On-Line Tutorial: http://www.drsegal.com/medstud/ecg/
5. Dublin D: *Rapid interpretation of EKGs*, Tampa, Fla, 2000, Cover Publishing.
6. Levine GN: *Diagnosing (and treating) arrhythmias made easy*, St. Louis, 1998, Quality Medical Publishers.
7. Levine GN, Podrid PJ: *The ECG workbook*, Armonk, NY, 1995, Futura Publishing.
8. Mason JW, Hancock EW, Gettes LS: Recommendations for the standardization and interpretation of the electrocardiogram: part II: electrocardiography diagnostic statement list, a scientific statement from the American Heart Association Electrocardiography and Arrhythmias Committee, Council on Clinical Cardiology; the American College of Cardiology Foundation; and the Heart Rhythm Society Endorsed by the International Society for Computerized Electrocardiology, *J Am Coll Cardiol* 49(10):1128-1135, 2007.
9. Wagner GS: *Marriot's practical electrocardiography*, Philadelphia, 2008, Lippincott Williams & Wilkins.

CHAPTER 4

CHEST RADIOGRAPHS

James J. Fenton, MD, FCCP and Glenn N. Levine, MD, FACC, FAHA

1. **Describe a systematic approach to interpreting a chest radiograph (chest x-ray [CXR]) (Fig. 4-1).**
    Common recommendations are to:
    1. Begin with general characteristics such as the age, gender, size, and position of the patient.
    2. Next examine the periphery of the film, including the bones, soft tissue, and pleura. Look for rib fractures, rib notching, bony metastases, shoulder dislocation, soft tissue masses, and pleural thickening.
    3. Then evaluate the lung, looking for infiltrates, pulmonary nodules, and pleural effusions.
    4. Finally, concentrate on the heart size and contour, mediastinal structures, hilum, and great vessels. Also note the presence of pacemakers and sternal wires.

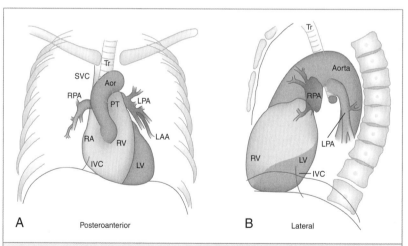

Figure 4-1. Diagrammatic representations of the anatomy of the chest radiograph. *Aor*, Aorta; *IVC*, inferior vena cava; *LAA*, left atrial appendage; *LPA*, left pulmonary artery; *LV*, left ventricle; *PT*, pulmonary trunk; *RA*, right atrium; *RPA*, right pulmonary artery; *RV*, right ventricle; *SVC*, superior vena cava; *Tr*, trachea; *IVC*, inferior vena cava; *LPA*, left pulmonary artery; *LV*, left ventricle; *RPA*, right pulmonary artery; *RV*, right ventricle; *Tr*, trachea. (From Inaba AS: Cardiac disorders. In Marx J, Hockberger R, Walls R: *Rosen's emergency medicine: concepts and clinical practice*, ed 6, Philadelphia, 2006, Mosby.)

2. **Identify the major cardiovascular structures that form the silhouette of the mediastinum (Fig. 4-2).**
   - **Right side:** Ascending aorta, right pulmonary artery, right atrium, right ventricle
   - **Left side:** Aortic knob, left pulmonary artery, left atrial appendage, left ventricle

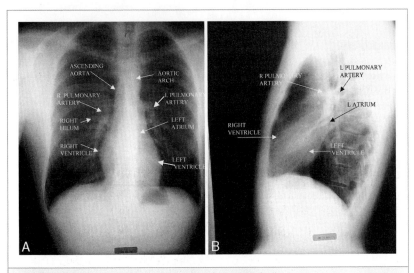

Figure 4-2. Major cardiovascular structures evident on chest radiograph.

3. **How is heart size measured on a chest radiograph?**
   Identification of cardiomegaly on a CXR is subjective, but if the heart size is equal to or greater than twice the size of the hemithorax, then it is enlarged. Remember that a film taken during expiration, in a supine position, or by a portable AP technique will make the heart appear larger.

4. **What factors can affect heart size on the chest radiograph?**
   - **Size of the patient:** Obesity decreases lung volumes and enlarges the appearance of the heart.
   - **Degree of inspiration:** Poor inspiration can make the heart appear larger.
   - **Emphysema:** Hyperinflation changes the configuration of the heart, making it appear smaller.
   - **Contractility:** Systole or diastole can make up to a 1.5-cm difference in heart size. In addition, low heart rate and increased cardiac output lead to increased ventricular filling.
   - **Chest configuration:** Pectus excavatum can compress the heart and make it appear larger.
   - **Patient positioning:** The heart appears larger if the film is taken in a supine position.
   - **Type of examination:** On an anteroposterior (AP) projection, the heart is farther away from the film and closer to the camera. This creates greater beam divergence and the appearance of an increased heart size.

5. **What additional items should be reviewed when examining a chest radiograph from the intensive care unit (ICU)?**
On portable cardiac care unit (CCU) and ICU radiographs, particular attention should be paid to:
  - Placement of the endotracheal tube
  - Central lines
  - Pulmonary arterial catheter
  - Pacing wires
  - Defibrillator pads
  - Intraaortic balloon pump
  - Feeding tubes
  - Chest tubes

A careful inspection should be made for pneumothorax (Fig. 4-3), subcutaneous emphysema, and other factors that may be related to instrumentation and mechanical ventilation.

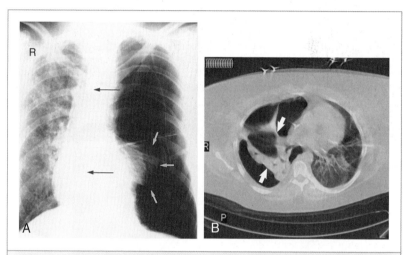

Figure 4-3. Tension pneumothorax. On a posteroanterior chest radiograph **(A)** the left hemithorax is very dark or lucent because the left lung has collapsed completely *(white arrows)*. The tension pneumothorax can be identified because the mediastinal contents, including the heart, are shifted toward the right and the left hemidiaphragm is flattened and depressed. **B,** A computed tomography scan done on a different patient with a tension pneumothorax shows a completely collapsed right lung *(arrows)* and shift of the mediastinal contents to the left. (From Mettler: *Essentials of radiology,* ed 2, Philadelphia, 2005, Saunders.)

6. **How can one determine which cardiac chambers are enlarged?**
  - **Ventricular enlargement:** usually displaces the lower heart border to the left and posteriorly. Distinguishing right ventricular (RV) from left ventricular (LV) enlargement requires evaluation of the outflow tracts. In RV enlargement the pulmonary arteries are often prominent and the aorta is diminutive. In LV enlargement the aorta is prominent and the pulmonary arteries are normal.
  - **Left atrial (LA) enlargement:** creates a convexity between the left pulmonary artery and the left ventricle on the frontal view. Also, a *double density* may be seen inferior to the carina. On the lateral view, LA enlargement displaces the descending left lower lobe bronchus posteriorly.
  - **Right atrial enlargement:** causes the lower right heart border to bulge outward to the right.

7. **What are some of the common causes of chest pain that can be identified on a chest radiograph?**
   - Aortic dissection
   - Pneumonia
   - Pneumothorax
   - Pulmonary embolism
   - Subcutaneous emphysema
   - Pericarditis (if a large pericardial effusion is suggested by the radiograph)
   - Esophageal rupture
   - Hiatal hernia

   All patients with chest pain should undergo a CXR even if the cause of the chest pain is suspected myocardial ischemia.

8. **What are the causes of a widened mediastinium?**
   There are multiple potential causes of a widened mediastinum (Fig. 4-4). Some of the most concerning causes of mediastinal widening include aortic dissection/rupture and mediastinal bleeding from chest trauma or misplaced central venous catheters. One of the most common causes of mediastinal widening is thoracic lipomatosis in an obese patient. Tumors should also be considered as a cause of a widened mediastinum—especially germ cell tumors, lymphoma, and thymomas. The mediastinum may also appear wider on a portable AP film compared with a standard posteroanterior/lateral chest radiograph.

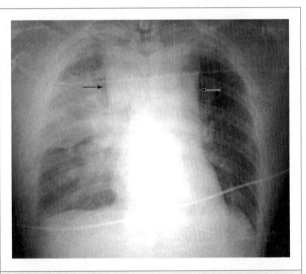

Figure 4-4. Widened mediastinum *(arrows)*. (From Marx J, Hockberger R, Walls R: *Rosen's emergency medicine: concepts and clinical practice*, ed 6, Philadelphia, 2006, Mosby.)

9. **What are the common radiographic signs of congestive heart failure?**
   - Enlarged cardiac silhouette
   - Left atrial enlargement
   - Hilar fullness
   - Vascular redistribution
   - Linear interstitial opacities (Kerley's lines)
   - Bilateral alveolar infiltrates
   - Pleural effusions (right greater than left)

10. **What is vascular redistribution? When does it occur in congestive heart failure?**
Vascular redistribution occurs when the upper-lobe pulmonary arteries and veins become larger than the vessels in the lower lobes. The sign is most accurate if the upper lobe vessels are increased in diameter greater than 3 mm in the first intercostal interspace. It usually occurs at a pulmonary capillary occlusion pressure of 12–19 mm Hg. As the pulmonary capillary occlusion pressure rises above 19 mm Hg, interstitial edema develops with bronchial cuffing, Kerley's B lines, and thickening of the lung fissures. Vascular redistribution to the upper lobes is probably most consistently seen in patients with chronic pulmonary venous hypertension (mitral valve disease, left ventricular dysfunction) because of the body's attempt to maintain more normal blood flow and oxygenation in this area. Some authors believe that vascular redistribution is a cardinal feature of congestive heart failure, but it may be a particularly unhelpful sign in the ICU patient with acute congestive failure. In these patients, all the pulmonary arteries look enlarged, making it difficult to assess upper and lower vessel size. In addition, the film is often taken supine, which can enlarge the upper lobe pulmonary vessels because of stasis of blood flow and not true redistribution.

11. **How does LV dysfunction and RV dysfunction lead to pleural effusions?**
    - LV dysfunction causes increased hydrostatic pressures, which lead to interstitial edema and pleural effusions. Right pleural effusions are more common than left pleural effusions, but the majority are bilateral.
    - RV dysfunction leads to system venous hypertension, which inhibits normal reabsorption of pleural fluid into the parietal pleural lymphatics.

12. **How helpful is the chest radiograph at identifying and characterizing a pericardial effusion?**
The CXR is not sensitive for the detection of a pericardial effusion, and it may not be helpful in determining the extent of an effusion. Smaller pericardial effusions are difficult to detect on a CXR but can still cause tamponade physiology if fluid accumulation is rapid. A large *hourglass* cardiac silhouette (Fig. 4-5), however, may suggest a large pericardial effusion. Distinguishing pericardial fluid from chamber enlargement is often difficult.

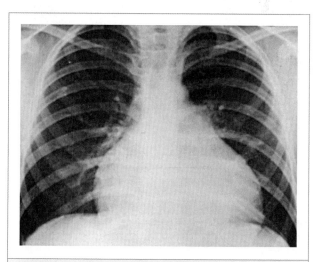

Figure 4-5. The *water bottle* configuration that can be seen with a large pericardial effusion. (From Kliegman RM, Behrman RE, Jenson HB, et al: *Nelson textbook of pediatrics*, ed 18, Philadelphia, 2007, Saunders.)

13. **What are the characteristic radiographic findings of significant pulmonary hypertension?**
    Enlargement of the central pulmonary arteries with rapid tapering of the vessels is a characteristic finding in patients with pulmonary hypertension (Fig. 4-6). If the right descending pulmonary artery is greater than 17 mm in transverse diameter, it is considered enlarged. Other findings of pulmonary hypertension include cardiac enlargement (particularly the right ventricle) and calcification of the pulmonary arteries. Pulmonary arterial calcification follows atheroma formation in the artery and represents a rare but specific radiographic finding of severe pulmonary hypertension.

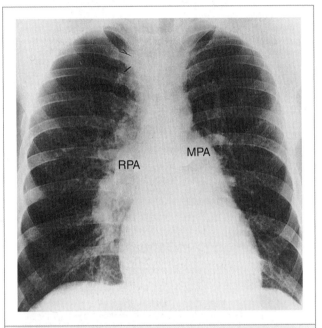

Figure 4-6. Pulmonary arterial hypertension. Marked dilation of the main pulmonary artery (MPA) and right pulmonary artery (RPA) is noted. Rapid tapering of the arteries as they proceed peripherally is suggestive of pulmonary hypertension and is sometimes referred to as *pruning*. (From Mettler FA: *Essentials of radiology,* ed 2, Philadelphia, 2005, Saunders.)

14. **What is Westermark's sign?**
    Westermark's sign is seen in patients with pulmonary embolism and represents an area of oligemia beyond the occluded pulmonary vessel. If pulmonary infarction results, a wedge-shaped infiltrate may be visible (Fig. 4-7).

15. **What is rib notching?**
    Rib notching is erosion of the inferior aspects of the ribs (Fig. 4-8). It can be seen in some patients with coarctation of the aorta and results from a compensatory enlargement of the intercostal arteries as a means of increasing distal circulation. It is most commonly seen between the fourth and eighth ribs. It is important to recognize this life-saving finding because aortic coarctation is treatable with percutaneous or open surgical intervention.

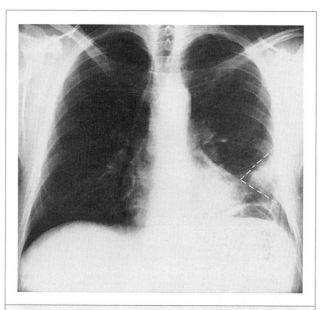

Figure 4-7. A peripheral wedge-shaped infiltrate *(white dashed lines)* seen after a pulmonary embolism has lead to infarction. (From Mettler FA: *Essentials of radiology,* ed 2, Philadelphia, Saunders, 2005.)

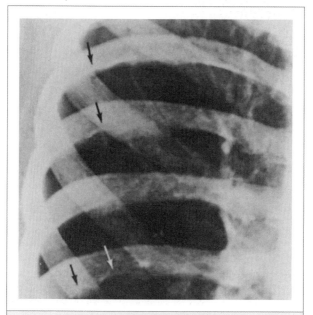

Figure 4-8. Rib notching in a patient with coarctation of the aorta. (From Park MK: *Pediatric cardiology for practitioners,* ed 5, Philadelphia, 2008, Mosby.)

16. **What does the finding in Figure 4-9 suggest?**
    The important finding in this figure is pericardial calcification. This can occur in
    diseases that affect the pericardium, such as tuberculosis. In a patient with signs and symptoms
    of heart failure, this finding would be highly suggestive of the diagnosis of constrictive
    pericarditis.

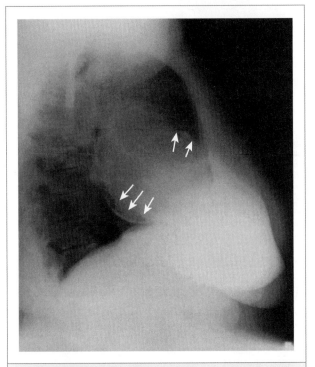

Figure 4-9. Pericardial calcification *(arrows)*. In a patient with signs and
symptoms of heart failure, this findings would strongly suggest the diagnosis
of constrictive cardiomyopathy. (From Libby P, Bonow RO, Mann DL, et al:
Braunwald's heart disease, ed 8, Philadelphia, 2008, Saunders.)

BIBLIOGRAPHY, SUGGESTED READINGS, AND WEBSITES

1. Hollander JE, Chase M: Evaluation of Chest Pain in the Emergency Department:
   http://www.utdol.com
2. Chandraskhar AJ: Chest X-ray Atlas:
   http://www.meddean.luc.edu/lumen/MedEd/medicine/pulmonar/cxr/atlas/cxratlas_f.htm
3. Baron MG: Plain film diagnosis of common cardiac anomalies in the adult, *Radiol Clin North Am* 37:401-420,
   1999.
4. MacDonald SLS, Padley S: The mediastinum, including the pericardium. In Adam A, Dixon AK, editors: *Grainger
   & Allsion's diagnostic radiology,* ed 5, Philadelphia, 2008, Churchill Livingstone.

5. Meholic A: *Fundamentals of chest radiology*, Philadelphia, 1996, Saunders.
6. Mettler FA: Cardiovascular system. In Mettler FA, editors: *Essentials of radiology*, ed 2, Philadelphia, 2005, Saunders.
7. Newell J: Diseases of the thoracic aorta: a symposium, *J Thorac Imag* 5:1-48, 1990.

II. DIAGNOSTIC PROCEDURES

HOLTER MONITORS, EVENT MONITORS, AND IMPLANTABLE LOOP RECORDERS

Ryan Seutter, MD and Glenn N. Levine, MD, FACC, FAHA

1. **What are the major indications for ambulatory electrocardiography monitoring?**

   Ambulatory electrocardiography monitoring (AECG) allows the noninvasive evaluation of a suspected arrhythmia during normal daily activities. It aids in the diagnosis, documentation of frequency, severity, and correlation of an arrhythmia with symptoms such as palpitations, lightheadedness, or overt syncope. AECG monitoring can be extremely helpful in excluding an arrhythmia as a cause for a patient's symptoms if there is no associated event during monitoring. AECG can also be used to assess antiarrhythmic drug response in patients with defined arrhythmias. Occasionally AECG is also used in other situations. The current major indications for AECG monitoring, from the American College of Cardiology/American Heart Association (ACC/AHA), are given in Box 5-1.

BOX 5-1. SUMMARY OF THE AMERICAN COLLEGE OF CARDIOLOGY/AMERICAN HEART ASSOCIATION GUIDELINES FOR AMBULATORY ELECTROCARDIOGRAPHY INDICATIONS FOR AECG MONITORING

Class I (Recommended)
- Patients with unexplained syncope, near syncope, or episodic dizziness in whom the cause is not obvious
- Patients with unexplained recurrent palpitations
- To assess antiarrhythmic drug response in individuals with well-characterized arrhythmias
- To aid in the evaluation of pacemaker and implantable cardioverter defibrillator (ICD) function and guide pharmacologic therapy in patients receiving frequent ICD therapy

Class IIa (Weight of Evidence/Opinion Is in Favor of Usefulness/Efficacy)
- To detect proarrhythmic responses to patients receiving antiarrhythmic therapy
- Patients with suspected variant angina

Class IIb (Usefulness/Efficacy Is Less Well Established by Evidence/Opinion)
- Patients with episodic shortness of breath, chest pain, or fatigue that is not otherwise explained
- Patients with symptoms such as syncope, near syncope, episodic dizziness, or palpitation in whom a probable cause other than an arrhythmia has been identified but in whom symptoms persist despite treatment
- To assess rate control during atrial fibrillation
- Evaluation of patients with chest pain who cannot exercise
- Preoperative evaluation for vascular surgery of patients who cannot exercise
- Patients with known coronary artery disease and atypical chest pain syndrome
- To assess risk in asymptomatic patients who have heart failure or idiopathic hypertrophic cardiomyopathy or in post–myocardial infarction patients with ejection fraction less than 40%
- Patients with neurologic events when transient atrial fibrillation or flutter is suspected

---

CHAPTER 5

2. **What are the different types of ambulatory ECG monitoring available?**

The major types of ambulatory electrocardiography (ECG) monitoring include Holter monitors, event monitors, and implantable loop recorders (ILRs). The type and duration of monitoring is dependent on the frequency and severity of symptoms. Most modern devices have the capability for transtelephonic transmission of ECG data during or after a detected arrhythmia. Each system has advantages and disadvantages; selection must be tailored to the individual. With any system, however, patients must record in some fashion (e.g., diary) symptoms and activities during the monitored period.

- A Holter monitor constantly monitors and records two to three channels of ECG data for 24 to 48 hours. It is ideal for patients with episodes that occur daily.
- An event monitor constantly monitors two to three channels of ECG data for 30 to 60 days. However, it will only record events when the patient experiences a symptom and presses a button that triggers the event monitor to store ECG data 1 to 4 minutes before and 1 to 2 minutes after the event. Some event monitors will also store arrhythmias that are detected by the monitor itself, based on preprogrammed parameters. An event monitor is appropriate for patients with episodes that occur weekly or monthly.
- An ILR is an invasive monitoring device allowing long-term monitoring and recording of a single ECG channel for over a year. It records events similar to an event monitor based on patient's symptoms or automatically based on heart rate. It is best reserved for patients with more infrequent episodes occurring greater than 1 month apart from each other.

3. **What is an implantable loop recorder?**

An ILR is a surgically placed, long-term monitoring device used to record and identify potentially life-threatening arrhythmias. It is commonly placed subcutaneously below the left shoulder and continuously monitors bipolar electrocardiographic signals for up to 14 months. The patient may use a magnetic activator held over the device to trigger an event at the time of symptoms. In addition, the device automatically records episodes of bradycardia and tachycardia (Fig. 5-1). The device is then interrogated with an external programmer and recorded events reviewed in a similar manner to a permanent pacemaker. After a diagnosis is obtained, the device is surgically extracted. In patients with unexplained syncope, an ILR yields a diagnosis in more than 90% of patients after 1 year.

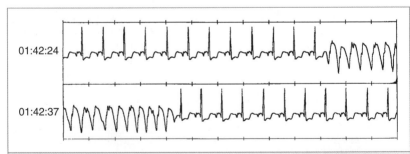

Figure 5-1. Representative printout from an interrogated implantable loop recorder (ILR) demonstrated a run of nonsustained ventricular tachycardia.

4. **When is Holter or event monitoring considered abnormal?**

It is not uncommon to identify several arrhythmias that are not necessarily abnormal during ambulatory electrocardiographic monitoring. These include sinus bradycardia during rest or sleep, sinus arrhythmia with pauses less than 3 seconds, sinoatrial exit block, Wenckebach atrioventricular (AV) block (type I second-degree AV block), wandering atrial pacemaker, junctional escape complexes, and premature atrial or ventricular complexes.

Of concern are frequent and complex atrial and ventricular rhythm disturbances that are less commonly observed in normal subjects, including second-degree AV block type II, third-degree AV block, sinus pauses longer than 3 seconds, marked bradycardia during waking hours, and tachyarrhythmias. One of the most important factors for any documented arrhythmia is the correlation with symptoms. In some situations, even some "benign" rhythms may warrant treatment if there are associated symptoms.

5. **How often are arrhythmias detected during ambulatory ECG monitoring?**
Approximately 25% to 50% of patients experience a complaint or symptom during a 24-hour recording. Of such symptoms, only 2% to 15% correlate with or are believed to be caused by arrhythmia. Approximately 35% of patients will log a symptom without a corresponding ECG abnormality. Extending the period of monitoring can increase the yield of identifying symptomatic events. In patients with presyncope or syncope, the incidence of symptomatic events can be increased to 50% at 3 days and to 75% at 5 to 21 days of ambulatory ECG monitoring.

6. **How often are ventricular arrhythmias identified in apparently healthy subjects during ambulatory ECG monitoring?**
Ventricular arrhythmias are found in 40% to 75% of normal persons as assessed by 24- to 48-hour Holter monitors. The incidence and frequency of ventricular ectopy increases with age, but this has no impact on long-term prognosis in apparently healthy subjects.

7. **What is the role of ambulatory ECG monitoring in patients with known ischemic heart disease?**
Although ejection fraction after myocardial infarction is one of the strongest predictors of survival, ambulatory ECG monitoring can be helpful in further risk stratification. Ventricular arrhythmias occur in 2% to 5% of patients after transmural infarction in long-term follow-up. In the post–myocardial infarction patient, the occurrence of frequent premature ventricular contractions (PVCs) (more than 10 per hour) and nonsustained ventricular tachycardia (VT) by 24-hour monitoring is associated with a 1.5- to 2.0-fold increase in death during the 2- to 5-year follow-up, independent of left ventricular (LV) function.

8. **Can Holter monitors assist in the diagnosis of suspected ischemic heart disease?**
Yes. Transient ST-segment depressions 0.1 mV or greater for more than 30 seconds are rare in normal subjects and correlate strongly with myocardial perfusion scans that show regional ischemia.

9. **What have Holter monitors demonstrated about angina and its pattern of occurrence?**
Holter monitoring has shown that the majority of ischemic episodes that occur during normal daily activities are silent (asymptomatic) and that symptomatic and silent episodes of ST-segment depression exhibit a circadian rhythm, with ischemic ST changes more common in the morning. Studies also have shown that nocturnal ST-segment changes are a strong indicator of significant coronary artery disease.

10. **What is a signal-averaged ECG?**
A signal-averaged ECG (SAECG) is a unique type of ECG initially developed to identify patients at risk for sudden cardiac death and complex ventricular arrhythmias. In patients susceptible to VT and ventricular fibrillation (VF), there can be slowing of electrical potentials through diseased myocardium, resulting in small, delayed electrical signals (late potentials) not easily visible on a normal ECG. Through the use of amplification and computerized signal averaging, these microvolt late potentials can be visualized on a SAECG and potentially assist in risk-stratifying patients susceptible to certain arrhythmias.

11. **When should a signal-averaged ECG be considered?**
    The use of SAECG to identify late potentials and those post–myocardial infarction patients at greatest risk for sudden death has been extensively evaluated. Although an association exists between late potentials and increased risk of ventricular arrhythmias after myocardial infarction, the positive predictive value of SAECG is low. In the Coronary Artery Bypass Graft (CABG) Patch Trial, patients with an abnormal SAECG and depressed ejection fraction who were to undergo cardiac surgery were randomized to implantable cardioverter defibrillator (ICD) implantation or no implantation and then followed for an average of 32 months. The study could detect no benefit for ICD implantation in this patient population with abnormal SAECGs. A study of SAECG use in patients treated with reperfusion, mainly primary percutaneous coronary intervention (PCI), did not find SAECG to be a useful risk stratification tool in this patient population. In current practice, the test is rarely used for risk stratification.

12. **What is microvolt T-wave alternans and does it predict outcomes in certain patients?**
    Microvolt T-wave alternans (MTWA) is a technique used to measure very small beat-to-beat variability in T-wave voltage not generally detectable on a standard ECG. Significant MTWA changes are associated with increased risk of sudden cardiac death and complex ventricular arrhythmias. The benefit of MTWA for risk stratification is greatest in patients with a history of coronary artery disease and reduced ejection fraction. A positive MTWA test predicts nearly a fourfold risk of ventricular arrhythmias compared with MTWA-negative patients. The ACC/AHA/ESC guidelines on ventricular arrhythmias and prevention of sudden cardiac death state that it is reasonable to use T-wave alternans for improving the diagnosis and risk stratification of patients with ventricular arrhythmias or who are at risk for developing life-threatening ventricular arrhythmias (class IIa; level of evidence A).

13. **Is heart-rate variability useful in certain patients?**
    Diminished heart-rate variability is an independent predictor of increased mortality after myocardial infarction and results from decreased beat-to-beat vagal modulation of heart rate. The predictive value of heart-rate variability is low after myocardial infarction. It is recommend by the ACC as a class IIb recommendation to assess risk for future events in asymptomatic patients who:
    - Are post–myocardial infarction with LV dysfunction
    - Have heart failure
    - Have idiopathic hypertrophic cardiomyopathy

BIBLIOGRAPHY, SUGGESTED READINGS, AND WEBSITES

1. Narayan SM: T-Wave (Repolarization) Alternans: Clinical Aspects: http://www.utdol.com
2. Narayan SM, Cain ME: Clinical Applications of the Signal-Averaged Electrocardiogram: Overview: http://www.utdol.com
3. Assar MD, Krahn AD, Klein GJ, et al: Optimal duration of monitoring in patients with unexplained syncope. *Am J Cardiol* 92:1231-1233, 2003.
4. Bass EB, Curtiss EI, Arena VC, et al: The duration of Holter monitoring in patients with syncope: is 24 hours enough? *Arch Intern Med* 50:1073, 1990.
5. Bigger JT Jr: Prophylactic use of implanted cardiac defibrillators in patients at high risk for ventricular arrhythmias after coronary-artery bypass graft surgery. Coronary Artery Bypass Graft (CABG) Patch Trial investigators, *N Engl J Med* 337:1569-1575, 1997.
6. Chow T, Kereiakes DJ, Bartone C, et al: Microvolt T-wave alternans identifies patients with ischemic cardiomyopathy who benefit from implantable cardioverter-defibrillator therapy, *J Am Coll Cardiol* 49:50-58, 2007.
7. Crawford MH, Bernstein SJ, Deedwania PC, et al: ACC/AHA guidelines for ambulatory electrocardiography: executive summary and recommendations: a report of the American College of Cardiology/American Heart

Association Task Force on Practice Guidelines (Committee to Revise the Guidelines for Ambulatory Electrocardiography), *J Am Coll Cardiol* 34:912-948, 1999.

8. Epstein AE, Hallstrom AP, Rogers WJ, et al: Mortality following ventricular arrhythmia suppression by encainide, flecainide, and moricizine after myocardial infarction. The original design concept of the Cardiac Arrhythmia Suppression Trial (CAST), *JAMA* 270(20):2451-2455, 1993.

9. Kennedy HL, Whitlock JA, Sprague MK, et al: Long-term follow-up of asymptomatic healthy subjects with frequent and complex ventricular ectopy, *N Engl J Med* 312:193, 1985.

10. Maggioni AP, Zuanetti G, Franzosi MG, et al: Prevalence and prognostic significance of ventricular arrhythmias after acute myocardial infarction in the fibrinolytic era. GISSI-2 results, *Circulation* 87:312-322, 1993.

11. Signal-averaged electrocardiography: ACC Expert Consensus Document. *J Am Coll Cardiol* 27:238, 1996.

12. Zeldis SM, Levine BJ, Michaelson EL, et al: Cardiovascular complaint. Correlation with cardiac arrhythmias on 24 hour electrocardiographic monitoring, *Chest* 78:456, 1980.

13. Zipes DP, Camm AJ, Borggrefe M, et al: ACC/AHA/ESC 2006 guidelines for management of patients with ventricular arrhythmias and the prevention of sudden cardiac death, *J Am Coll Cardiol* 48:1064-1108, 2006.

CHAPTER 6

ECHOCARDIOGRAPHY

Hisham Dokainish, MD, FACC, FASE

1. **How does echocardiography work?**

   Echocardiography uses transthoracic and transesohageal probes that emit ultrasound directed at cardiac structures. Returning ultrasound signals are received by the probe, and the computer in the ultrasound machine uses algorithms to reconstruct images of the heart. The time it takes for the ultrasound to return to the probe determines the depth of the structures relative to the probe because the speed of sound in soft tissue is relatively constant (1540 msec). The amplitude (intensity) of the returning signal determines the density and size of the structures with which the ultrasound comes in contact.

   The probes also perform Doppler, which measures the frequency shift of the returning ultrsound signal to determine the speed and direction of moving blood through heart structures (e.g., through the aortic valve) or in the myocardium itself (tissue Doppler imaging).

   Appropriateness criteria for obtaining an echocardiogram are given in Box 6-1.

2. **What is the difference between echocardiography and Doppler?**

   Echocardiography usually refers to two-dimensional (2D) ultrasound interrogation of the heart in which the brightness mode is utilized to image cardiac structures based on their density and location relative to the chest wall (Fig. 6-1). Two-dimensional echocardiography is particularly useful for identifying cardiac anatomy and morphology, such as identifying a pericardial effusion, left ventricular aneurysm, or cardiac mass.

   Doppler refers to interrogation of the movement of blood in and around the heart, based on the shift in frequency *(Doppler shift)* that ultrasound undergoes when it comes in contact with a moving object (usually red blood cells). Doppler has three modes:

   - Pulsed Doppler (Fig. 6-2, *A*), which can localize the site of flow acceleration but is prone to aliasing
   - Continuous-wave Doppler (Fig. 6-2, *B*), which cannot localize the level of flow acceleration but can identify very high velocities without aliasing
   - Color Doppler (Fig. 6-3), which utilizes different colors (usually red and blue) to identify flow toward and away from the transducer, respectively, and identify flow acceleration qualitatively by showing a mix of color to represent high velocity or aliased flow

   Doppler is particularly useful for assessing the hemodynamic significance of cardiac stuctural disease, such as the severity of aortic stenosis (see Fig. 6-2), degree of mitral regurgitation (see Fig. 6-3), flow velocity across a ventricular septal defect, or severity of pulmonary hypertension.

   The great majority of echocardiograms are ordered as *echocardiography with Doppler* to answer cardiac morphologic and hemodynamic questions in one study (e.g., a mitral stenosis murmur; 2D echo to identify the restricted, thickened, and calcified mitral valve (see Fig. 6-1); and Doppler to analyze its severity based on transvalvular flow velocities and gradients.

3. **How is systolic function assessed using echocardiography?**

   The most commonly used measurement of left ventricular (LV) systolic function is left ventricular ejection fraction (LVEF), which is defined by:

   $$LVEF = \frac{(\text{End-diastolic volume} - \text{End-systolic volume})}{\text{End-diastolic volume}}$$

BOX 6-1. APPROPRIATENESS CRITERIA FOR ECHOCARDIOGRAPHY

Appropriate indications include, but are not limited to:
- Symptoms possibly related to cardiac etiology, such as dyspnea, shortness of breath, lightheadedness, syncope, cerebrovascular events.
- Initial evaluation of left-sided ventricular function after acute myocardial infarction.
- Evaluation of cardiac murmur in suspected valve disease.
- Sustained ventricular tachycardia or supraventricular tachycardia.
- Evaluation of suspected pulmonary artery hypertension.
- Evaluation of acute chest pain with nondiagnostic laboratory markers and electrocardiogram.
- Evaluation of known native or prosthetic valve disease in a patient with change of clinical status.

Uncertain indications for echocardiography:
- Cardiovascular source of embolic event in a patient who has normal transthoracic echocardiogram (TTE) and electrocardiogram findings and no history of atrial fibrillation or flutter.

Inappropriate indications for echocardiography:
- Routine monitoring of known conditions, such as heart failure, mild valvular disease, hypertensive cardiomyopathy, repair of congenital heart disease, or monitoring of an artificial valve, when the patient is clinically stable.
- Echocardiography is also not the test of choice in the initial evaluation for pulmonary embolus and should not be routinely used to screen asymptomatic hypertensive patients for heart disease.

Appropriate indications for transesophageal echocardiography (TEE) as the initial test instead of TTE:
- Evaluation of suspected aortic pathology including dissection.
- Guidance during percutaneous cardiac procedures including ablation and mitral valvuloplasty.
- To determine the mechanism of regurgitation and suitability of valve repair.
- Diagnose or manage endocarditis in patients with moderate-high probability of endocarditis.
- Persistent fever in a patient with an intracardiac device.
- TEE is *not* appropriate in evaluation for a left atrial thrombus in the setting of atrial fibrillation when it has already been decided to treat the patient with anticoagulant drugs.

Modified from Douglas PS, Khandheria B, Stainback RF, et al: ACCF/ASE/ACEP/ASNC/SCAI/SCCT/SCMR 2007 appropriateness criteria for transthoracic and transesophageal echocardiography. *J Am Coll Cardiol* 50:187-204, 2007.

- Simpson's method (method of discs), in which the LV endocardial border of multiple *slices* of the left ventricle is traced in systole and diastole and the end-diastolic and end-systolic volumes are computed from these tracings, is one of the most common methods of calcuating LVEF.
- The Teicholz method, in which the shortening fraction:

$$\frac{(\text{LV end-diastolic dimension} - \text{LV end-systolic dimension})}{\text{LV end-diastolic dimension}}$$

is multiplied by 1.7, can also be used to estimate LVEF, although this method is inaccurate in patients with regional wall motion abnormalities.
- Visual estimation of LVEF by expert echocardiography readers is also commonly used.

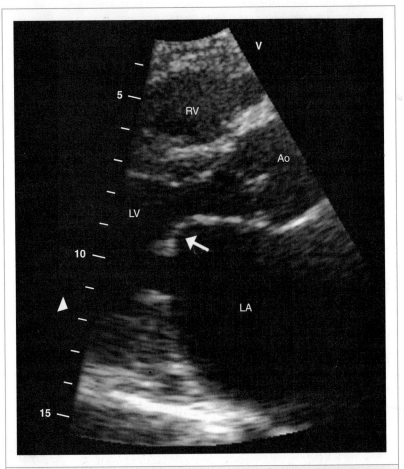

Figure 6-1. Parasternal long axis view showing typical *hockey stick* appearance of the mitral valve *(arrow)* in rheumatic mitral stenosis. *Ao,* Aortic valve; *LA,* left atrium; *LV,* left ventricle; *RV,* right ventricle.

- Increasingly, state-of-the-art full volume acqusition using three-dimensional echocardiography can be used to provide accurate LVEF.
- Systolic dysfunction in the presence of preserved LVEF (more than 50%)—such as in patients with hypertrophic hearts, ischemic heart disease, or infiltrative cardiomyopathies—can be identified by depressed systolic tissue Doppler velocities.

4. **What is an echocardiographic diastolic assessment? What information can it provide?**
   A diastolic assessment does two things: identifies LV relaxation and estimates LV filling pressures. LV relaxation is described as the time it takes for the LV to relax in diastole to accept blood from the left atrium (LA) through an open mitral valve. A normal heart is very elastic *(lussitropic)* and readily accepts blood during LV filling. When relaxation is impaired, the LV cannot easily accept increased volume, and this increased LV preload results in increases in LA presssure, which in turn results in pulmonary edema.

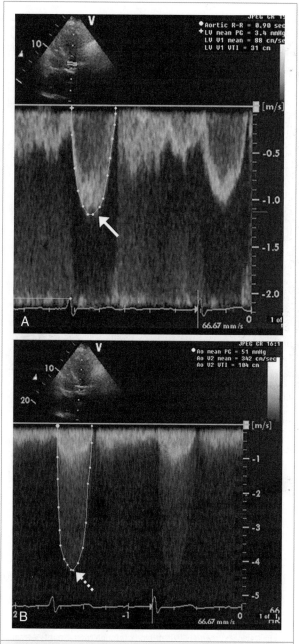

Figure 6-2. A, shows pulsed Doppler in the left ventricular outflow tract in a patient with aortic stenosis. The peak velocity of the spectral tracing *(arrow)* is 1.2 msec, indicating normal flow velocity proximal to the aortic valve. **B,** shows continuous Doppler across the aortic valve revealing a peak velocity of 4.5 msec *(dashed arrow)*. Therefore, the blood-flow velocity nearly quadrupled across the stenotic aortic valve, consistent with severe aortic stenosis.

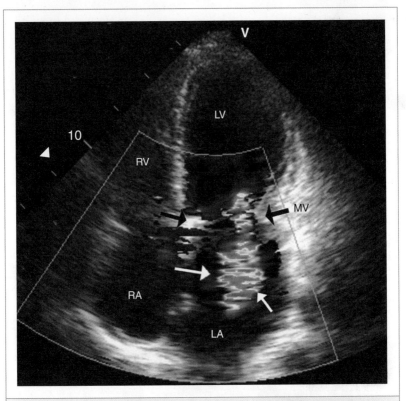

Figure 6-3. Apical four-chamber view with color Doppler *(white arrows)* revealing severe mitral regurgitation. Note that in *real life,* this Doppler image displays mitral regurgitation and other abnormalities in shades of blue and red. *Black arrows* point to the mitral valve. *MV,* Mitral valve; *LA,* left atrium; *LV,* left ventricle; *RA,* right atrium; *RV,* right ventricle. (Courtesy Hisham Dokainish.)

- LV relaxation is usually best determined using tissue Doppler imaging, which assesses early diastolic filling velocity (Ea) of the LV myocardium. Normal hearts have Ea 10 cm/sec or greater; impaired relaxation is present when Ea is less than 10 cm/sec.
- An indicator of LV preload is peak transmitral early diastolic filling velocity (E), which measures the velocity of blood flow across the mitral valve. An estimate of the LV filling pressure can be made using the ratio of blood flow velocity across the mitral valve (E) to the velocity of myocardial tissue during early diastole. A high ratio (e.g., E/Ea ≥ 15) indicates elevated LV filling pressure (LA pressure ≥ 15 mm Hg); a lower ratio (e.g., E/Ea ≤ 10) indicates normal LV filling pressure (LA pressure < 15 mm Hg).

5. **How can echocardiography with Doppler be used to answer cardiac hemodynamic questions?**
   - Stroke volume and cardiac output can be obtained with measurements of the LV outflow tract and time-velocity integral (TVI) of blood through the LV outflow tract.
   - Doppler evaluation of right ventricular outflow tract diameter and TVI similarly allow measurement of right ventricular output.
   - Tricuspid regurgitation peak gradient can be added to estimate of right atrial pressure to in turn estimate pulmonary artery systolic pressure.

- Mitral inflow velocities, deceleration time, pulmonary venous parameters, and tissue Doppler imaging of the mitral annulus can give accurate assessment of LV diastolic function, including LV filling pressures.
- Measurement of TVI and valve annular diameters can be used to assess intracardiac shunts (QP/QS) and regurgitant flow volumes.
- Pressure gradients across native and prosthetic valves and across cardiac shunts can be used to assess hemodynamic severity of valve stenosis, regurgitation, or shunt severity, respectively.
- Respiratory variation in valvular flow can aid in the diagnosis of cardiac tamponade or constrictive pericarditis.

6. **How is echocardiography used to evaluate valvular disease?**
    - Two-dimensional echocardiography can provide accurate visualization of valve structure to assess morphologic abnormalities (calcification, prolapse, flail, rheumatic disease, endocarditis). See Fig. 6-1, demonstrating the restricted movement of the mitral valve in a patient with mitral stenosis.
    - Color Doppler can provide semiquantitative assessment of the degree of valve regurgitation (mild, moderate, severe) in any position (aortic, mitral, pulmonic, tricuspid).
    - Pulsed Doppler can help pinpoint the location of a valular abnormalitity (e.g., subaortic versus aortic versus supraortic stenosis). Pulsed Doppler can also be used to quantitate regurgitant volumes and fractions using the continuity equation.
    - Continuous-wave Doppler is useful for determining the hemodynamic severity of stenotic lesions, such as aortic or mitral stenosis.

7. **How can echocardiography help diagnose and manage patients with suspected pericardial disease?**
    - Echocardiography can diagnose pericardial effusions (Fig. 6-4) as fluid in the pericardial space readily transmits ultrasound (appears black on echo).

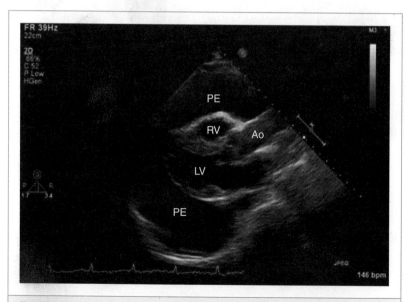

Figure 6-4. Parasternal long-axis view showing a large pericardial effusion (PE) surrounding the heart. *LV,* Left ventricle; *RV,* right ventricle. (From Kabbani SS, LeWinter M: Cardiac constriction and restriction. In Crawford MH, DiMarco JP: *Cardiology,* St. Louis, Mosby, 2001.)

- Two-dimensional echocardiography and Doppler are pivotal in determining the hemodynamic impact of pericardial fluid; that is, whether the patient has elevated intraperidial pressure or frank cardiac tamponade.
- The following are indicators of elevated intrapericardial pressure in the setting of pericardial effusion:
  - Diastolic indentation or collapse of the right ventricle (RV)
  - Compression of the right atrium (RA) for more than one third of the cardiac cycle
  - Lack of inferior vena cava (IVC) collapsability with deep inspiration
  - 25% or greater variation in mitral or aortic Doppler flows
  - 50% or greater variation of triscuspid or pulmonic valves flows with inspiration
- Echocardiographic signs of constrictive pericarditis include: thickened or calcified pericardium, diastolic *bounce* of the interventricular septum, restrictive mitral filling pattern with 25% or greater respiratory variation in peak velocities, and lack of inspiratory collapsibility of the inferior vena cava.
- Echocardiography is additionally useful for guiding precutaneous needle pericardiocentesis by identifying the transthoracic or subcostal window with the largest fluid *cushion,* monitoring decrease of fluid during pericardiocentsis, and in follow-up studies, assessing for reaccumulation of fluid.

8. **What is the role of echocardiography in patients with ischemic stroke?**
   The following are echocardiographic findings that may be associated with a cardiac embolic cause in patients with stroke:
   - Depressed LV ejection fraction, generally less than 40%
   - Left ventricular or left atrial clot (Fig. 6-5)
   - Intracardiac mass such as tumor or endocarditis

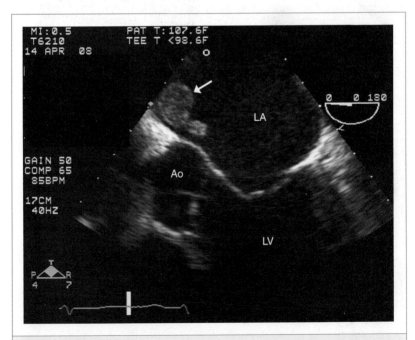

Figure 6-5. Tranesophageal echocardiography showing a left atrial thrombus *(arrow)*. *Ao,* Aortic valve; *LA,* left atrium; *LV,* left ventricle.

- Mitral stenosis (especially with a history of atrial fibrillation)
- Prosthetic valve in the mitral or aortic position
- Significant atherosclerotic disease in the aortic root, ascending aorta, or aortic arch
- Saline contrast study indicating a signficant right to left intracardiac shunt, such as atrial septal defect

Note: A normal transthoracic echocardiogram in a patient without atrial fibrillation generally excludes a cardiac embolic source of clot and generally obviates the need for transesophageal echocardiography (TEE).

9. **What are the echocardiographic findings in hypertrophic cardiomyopathy (HCM)?**
   - Septal, concentric, or apical hypertrophy (walls greater than 1.5 cm in diameter)
   - The presence of systolic anterior motion (SAM) of the mitral valve in some cases of obstructive hypertrophic cardiomyopathy
   - Dynamic left ventricular outflow tract (LVOT) gradients caused by SAM, midcavitary obliteration, or apical obliteration

10. **What are the common indications for transesophageal echocardiography?**
    - Significant clinical suspicion of endocarditis in patients with suboptimal transthoracic windows
    - Significant clinical suspicion of endocarditis in patients with prosthetic heart valve
    - Suspected aortic dissection (Fig. 6-6)
    - Suspected atrial septal defect (ASD) or patent foramen ovale in patients with cryptogenic embolic stroke

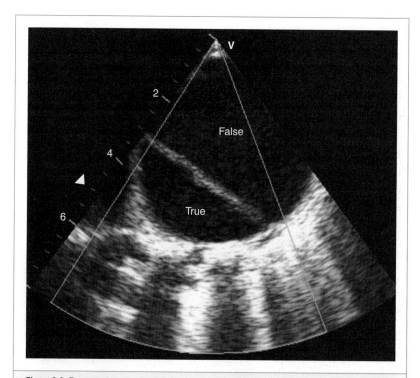

Figure 6-6. Transesophageal echocardiography revealing dissection of the descending thoracic aorta. The true aortic lumen (*true*) is seen separated from the false lumen (*false*) by the dissection.

- Embolic stroke with nondiagnostic transthoracic echo
- Endocarditis with suspected valvular complications (abscess, fistula, pseudoaneurysm)
- Evaluation of the mitral valve in cases of possible surgical mitral valve
- Intracardiac shunt in which the location is not well seen on transthoracic echocardiography
- Assessment of the left atria and left atrial appendage for the presence of thrombus (clot) (see Fig. 6-5) prior to planned cardioversion

11. **What is contrast echocardiography?**

    Contrast echocardiography involves injection of either saline contrast or synthetic microbubbles (perflutren bubbles) into a systemic vein, then imaging the heart using ultrasound. Saline contrast, because of its relatively large size, does not cross the pulmonary capillary bed, and it therefore is confined to the right heart. Therefore, rapid appearance of saline contrast in the left heart indicates an intracardiac shunt.

    Because synthetic microbubbles are smaller than saline bubbles, they cross the pulmonary capillaries and are used to image left heart structures. Most commonly, synthetic microbubbles are used to achieve better endocardial border definition in patients with suboptimal echocardiographic windows. Contrast is also used to better visualize structures such as possible LV clots or other masses.

    Both synthetic and saline contrast can be used to augment Doppler signals, for example, in patients with pulmonary hypertension in whom a tricuspid regurgitation jet is needed to estimate pulmonary artery pressure.

12. **What is stress echocardiography?**

    Stress echocardiography involves imaging the heart first at rest and subsequently during either exercise (treadmill or bike) or pharmacologic (usually dobutamine) stress to identify left ventricular (LV) wall motion abnormalities resulting from the presence of flow-limiting coronary artery disease. Other uses of stress echocardiography include:

    - Assessment of mitral or aortic valve disease in patients who have moderate disease at rest but significant symptoms with exercise
    - Assessment of patients with suspected exerise-induced diastolic dysfunction
    - Assessment of viability in patients with depressed ejection fractions. Improvement in left ventricular functon with infusion of low-dose dobutamine (<10 μg/kg/min) suggests viable myocadium.
    - Distinguishing between true aortic stenosis and *pseudo* aortic stenosis in patients with mild-moderate aortic stenosis at rest and depressed ejeciticon fraction with low cardiac output

BIBLIOGRAPHY, SUGGESTED READINGS, AND WEBSITES

1. Abraham TP, Dimaano VL, Liang HY: Role of tissue Doppler and strain echocardiography in current clinical practice, *Circulation* 116:2597-2609, 2007.
2. Armstrong WF, Zoghbi WA: Stress echocardiography: current methodology and clinical applications, *J Am Coll Cardiol* 45:1739-1747, 2005.
3. Douglas PS, Khandheria B, Stainback RF, et al: ACCF/ASE/ACEP/ASNC/SCAI/SCCT/SCMR 2007 appropriateness criteria for transthoracic and transesophageal echocardiography, *J Am Coll Cardiol* 50:187-204, 2007.
4. Evangelista A, Gonzalez-Alujas MT: Echocardiography in infective endocarditis, *Heart* 90:614-617, 2004.
5. Grayburn PA: How to measure severity of mitral regurgitation: valvular heart disease, *Heart* 94:376-383, 2008.
6. Kirkpatrick JN, Vannan MA, Narula J, et al: Echocardiography in heart failure: applications, utility, and new horizons, *J Am Coll Cardiol* 50:381-396, 2007.
7. Lang RM, Mor-Avi V, Sugeng L, et al: Three-dimensional echocardiography: the benefits of the additional dimension, *J Am Coll Cardiol* 48:2053-2069, 2006.

8. Lester SJ, Tajik AJ, Nishimura RA, et al: Unlocking the mysteries of diastolic function: deciphering the Rosetta Stone 10 years later, *J Am Coll Cardiol* 51:679-689, 2008.

9. Otto CM: Valvular aortic stenosis: disease severity and timing of intervention, *J Am Coll Cardiol* 47:2141-2151, 2006.

10. Peterson GE, Brickner ME, Reimold SC: Transesophageal echocardiography: clinical indications and applications, *Circulation* 107:2398-2402, 2003.

11. Stewart MJ: Contrast echocardiography, *Heart* 89:342-348, 2003.

CHAPTER 7

EXERCISE STRESS TESTING

Fernando Boccalandro, MD, FACC, FSCAI

1. **How can a patient exercise during stress testing?**

   Exercise stress testing (EST) is routinely performed to diagnose myocardial ischemia and to assess cardiopulmonary reserve. They are accomplished with a treadmill, bicycle ergometer, or, rarely, with an arm ergometer and may involve ventilatory gas analysis (the latter is called a cardiopulmonary stress test). Different protocols of progressive cardiovascular workload have been developed specifically for EST (e.g., Bruce, Cornell, Balke-Ware, ACIP, mAICP, Naughton, Weber). Bicycle ergometers are less expensive and smaller than treadmills and produce less motion of the upper body, but early fatigue of the lower extremities is a common problem that limits reaching maximal exercise capacity. As a result, treadmills are more commonly used in the United States for EST. Much of the reported data are based on the Bruce Protocol, which is performed on a treadmill and has become the most commonly protocol used in clinical practice. Exercise stress tests may involve only electrocardiographic (ECG) monitoring or may employ in addition echocardiography or nuclear myocardial perfusion imaging, improving the sensitivity and specificity of the test.

2. **What is the difference between a maximal and submaximal exercise stress test?**
   - *Maximal EST or symptoms-limited EST* is the preferred way to perform an exercise stress test and attempts to achieve the maximal tolerated exercise capacity of the patient. It is terminated based on patient symptoms (e.g., fatigue, angina, shortness of breath); an abnormal ECG (e.g., significant ST depression or elevation, arrhythmias); or an abnormal hemodynamic response (e.g., abnormal blood pressure response). A goal of maximal EST is to achieve a heart rate response of at least 85% the maximal predicted heart rate (see Question 9).
   - *Submaximal EST* is performed when the goal is lower than the individual maximal exercise capacity. Reasonable targets are: 70% of the maximal predicted heart rate, 120 beats per minute, or 5 to 6 metabolic equivalents (METs) of exercise capacity (see Question 12). Submaximal EST is used early after myocardial infarction (see Question 8).

3. **How helpful is an exercise stress test in the diagnosis of coronary artery disease?**

   Multiple studies have been reported comparing the accuracy of exercise stress testing with coronary angiography. However, different criteria have been used to define a significant coronary stenosis, and this lack of standardization has complicated the issue. A meta-analysis of 24,074 patients reported a mean sensitivity of 68% and a mean specificity of 77%. The sensitivity increases to 81% and the specificity decreases to 66% for multivessel disease, and to 86% and 53%, respectively, for left main disease or three-vessel coronary artery disease. The diagnostic accuracy of EST can be improved by adding imaging techniques, including echocardiography or myocardial perfusion imaging.

4. **What are the risks associated with exercise stress testing?**

   When supervised by an adequately trained physician the risks are very low. In the general population, the mortality is less than 0.01%, and the morbidity is less than 0.05%. A survey of 151,944 patients 4 weeks after a myocardial infarction showed slight increased mortality and morbidity of 0.03% and 0.09%, respectively. According to the national survey of exercise stress testing facilities, myocardial infarction and death can be expected in 1 per 2,500 tests.

5. **What are the indications for exercise stress testing?**
The most common indications for EST, according to the current American College of Cardiology (ACC) and American Heart Association (AHA) guidelines, are summarized in Box 7-1.

BOX 7-1. INDICATIONS FOR EXERCISE STRESS TESTING

- When diagnosing suspected obstructive coronary artery disease (CAD) based on age, gender, and clinical presentation, including those with right bundle branch block and less than 1 mm of resting ST depression
- For risk stratification, functional class assessment, and prognosis in patients with suspected or known CAD based on age, gender, and clinical presentation
- When evaluating patients with known CAD who witnessed a significant change in their clinical status
- To evaluate patients with vasoespastic angina
- To evaluate patients with low- or intermediate-risk unstable angina after they had been stabilized and who had been free of active ischemic symptoms or heart failure
- After myocardial infarction for prognosis assessment, physical activity prescription, or evaluation of current medical treatment before discharge with a submaximal stress test 4 to 6 days after myocardial infarction or after discharge with a symptoms-limited EST at least 14 to 21 days after myocardial infarction
- To detect myocardial ischemia in patients considered for revascularization
- After discharge for physical activity prescription and counseling after revascularization as part of a cardiac rehabilitation program
- n patients with chronic aortic regurgitation to assess the functional capacity and symptomatic responses in those with a history of equivocal symptoms
- When evaluating the proper settings in patients who received rate-responsive pacemakers
- When investigating patients with known or suspected exercise-induced arrhythmias

---

6. **Should asymptomatic patients undergo exercise stress tests?**
In general, asymptomatic patients should not undergo EST because the pretest probability of coronary artery disease in this population is low, leading to a significant amount of false-positive results, requiring unnecessary follow-up tests and expenses without well-documented benefit. Individually, some asymptomatic patients may be selectively considered for EST (e.g., diabetic patients planning to enroll in a vigorous exercise program, certain high-risk occupations).

7. **What are contraindications for exercise stress testing?**
The contraindications for EST according to the current ACC/AHA guidelines are summarized in Box 7-2.

8. **What parameters are monitored during an exercise stress test?**
During EST three principal parameters are monitored and reported: the clinical response of the patient to exercise (e.g., shortness of breath, dizziness, chest pain, angina pectoris, Borg Scale score), the hemodynamic response (e.g., heart rate, blood pressure response, etc.), and the ECG changes that occur during exercise and the recovery phase of EST.

9. **What is an adequate heart rate to ellicit an ischemic response?**
When a significant coronary artery stenosis exists, it is accepted that a heart rate of 85% of the maximal predicted heart rate for the age of the patient is sufficient to elicit an ischemic response and is considered an adequate heart rate for a diagnostic exercise EST.

BOX 7-2. CONTRAINDICATIONS FOR EXERCISE STRESS TESTING

Absolute Contraindications
Acute myocardial infarction within 2 days
Unstable angina
Uncontrolled cardiac arrhythmias causing symptoms or hemodynamic compromise
Symptomatic, severe aortic stenosis
Acute aortic dissection
Uncontrolled, symptomatic heart failure
Acute pulmonary embolism or infarction
Acute myocarditis or pericarditis

Relative Contraindications
Left main coronary stenosis
Moderate aortic stenosis
Electrolyte abnormalities
Uncontrolled hypertension
Arrhythmias
Hypertrophic cardiomyopathy and other forms of left ventricular outflow obstruction
Mental or physical impairment leading to inability to exercise adequately
High-degree atrioventricular block

---

10. **How do I calculate the predicted maximal heart rate?**
    The maximal predicted heart rate can be estimated with the following formula:

    $$\text{Maximal predicted heart rate} = 220 - \text{Age}$$

11. **What is the Borg scale?**
    The Borg Scale is a numeric scale of perceived patient exertion commonly used during EST. Values of 7 to 9 reflect light work and 13 to 17 hard work; a value above 18 is close to the maximal exercise capacity. Readings of 14 to 16 reach the anaerobic threshold. The Borg Scale is particularly useful when evaluating the patient functional capacity during EST.

12. **What is a metabolic equivalent?**
    Metabolic equivalents are defined as the caloric consumption of an active individual compared with the resting basal metabolic rate at rest. They are used during EST as an estimate of functional capacity. One MET is defined as 1 kilocalorie per kilogram per hour and is the caloric consumption of a person while at complete rest (i.e., 2 METs will correspond to an activity that is twice the resting metabolic rate). Activities of 2 to 4 METs (light walking, doing household chores, etc.) are considered light, whereas running or climbing can yield 10 or more METs. A functional capacity below 5 METs during treadmill EST is associated with a worse prognosis, whereas higher METs during exercise are associated with better outcomes.

13. **What is considered a hypertensive response to exercise?**
    The current ACC/AHA guidelines for exercise stress testing suggest a hypertensive response to exercise is one in which systolic blood pressure rises to more than 250 mm Hg or diastolic blood pressure rises to more than 115 mm Hg.

14. **Can I order an exercise stress test in a patient taking beta-blockers?**
    Exercise stress test in patients taking beta-blockers may have reduced diagnostic and prognostic value because of inadequate heart rate response. Nonetheless, according to the current ACC/AHA guidelines for exercise testing, stopping beta-blockers before EST is discouraged to avoid "rebound" hypertension or anginal symptoms.

15. **What baseline ECG findings interfere with the interpretation of an exercise stress test?**

Patients with left bundle branch block (LBBB), ventricular pacing, more than 1 mm baseline ST depression, and those with preexcitation syndromes (Wolf-Parkinson-White syndrome) should be considered for imaging stress testing because their baseline ECG abnormalities prevent an adequate ECG interpretation during exercise. Right bundle branch block does not reduce significantly the accuracy of the EST for the diagnosis of ischemia. Digoxin may also cause false-positive ST depressions during exercise and is also an indication of image stress testing.

16. **When can an exercise stress test be performed after an acute myocardial infarction?**

Submaximal EST is occasionally recommended after myocardial infarction as early as 4 days after the acute event. This can be followed by later (3–6 weeks) symptom-limited EST. Exercise stress testing in this circumstance assists in formulating a prognosis, determining activity levels, assessing medical therapy, and planning cardiac rehabilitation. It is unclear if asymptomatic patients who had an acute myocardial infarction (MI) with a consequent revascularization procedure benefit from follow-up exercise stress testing after myocardial infarction, although one small study demonstrated that physicians were more apt to allow patients to return earlier to various activities after a negative stress test.

17. **Are the patient's sex and age considerations for exercise stress testing?**

Women appear to have more false-positive ST-segment depression during EST than men, which may limit the sensitivity of EST for the detection of coronary artery disease in this population. This problem reflects differences in exercise physiology, body habitus, coronary physiology, prevalence of coronary artery disease, and ECG response to exercise. Based on this, the use of imaging EST (i.e., nuclear or echocardiography EST) traditionally have been favored for women. Age is not an important consideration for EST if the patient is fit to complete an exercise protocol adequately.

18. **When is an exercise stress test interpreted as *positive*?**

It is important for the physician supervising the test to consider the pretest probability of the patient undergoing EST to have underlying coronary artery disease while interpreting the results and to consider not only the ECG response but all the information provided by the test, including functional capacity and hemodynamic and clinical response to exercise. Electrocardiographic changes consisting of greater than or equal to 1 mm of horizontal or down-sloping ST-segment depression or elevation at least 60 to 80 msec after the end of the QRS complex during EST are considered positive for myocardial ischemia (Fig. 7-1). Also the occurrence of angina is important, particularly if it forces early termination of the test. Abnormalities in exercise capacity, blood pressure, and heart rate response to exercise are also important to report.

19. **What are the indications to terminate an exercise stress test?**

The *absolute indications* to stop EST according to the current ACC/AHA guidelines include a drop of more than 10 mm Hg in the systolic blood pressure despite an increased workload in addition to other signs of ischemia, ST elevation of more than 1 mm in leads without diagnostic Q waves (other than V1 and aVR), moderate to severe angina, increased autonomic nervous system symptoms (e.g., ataxia, dizziness, near syncope), signs of poor perfusion (cyanosis or pallor), difficulties monitoring the ECG or blood pressure, patient request to stop the test, and sustained ventricular tachycardia.

Relative indications include a drop of more than 10 mm Hg in the systolic blood pressure despite an increased workload in the absence of other evidence of ischemia; excessive ST depression (more than 2 mm of horizontal or downsloping ST depression) or marked QRS axis shift; arrhythmias other than sustained ventricular tachycardia; fatigue, shortness of breath, wheezing, leg cramps, or claudication; development of bundle branch block or intraventricular conduction delay that cannot be distinguished from ventricular tachycardia; hypertensive response to exercise; and increasing nonanginal chest pain.

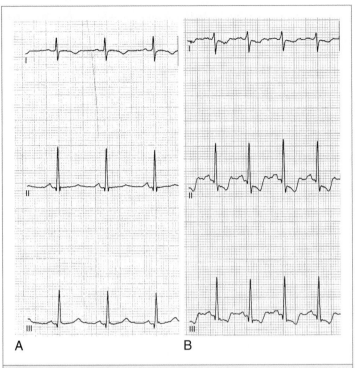

Figure 7-1. Abnormal electrocardiographic response to exercise in a patient found to have a severe stenosis of the right coronary artery. **A,** Normal baseline ECG. **B,** Abnormal ECG response at peak exercise with marked downsloping ST depression and T-wave inversion.

20. **What is a cardiopulmonary exercise stress test?**
    During a cardiopulmonary EST the patient's ventilatory gas exchange is monitored in a closed circuit and measurements of gas exchange are obtained during exercise (i.e., oxygen uptake, carbon dioxide output, anaerobic threshold), in addition to the information provided during routine EST.

21. **What are the indications for a cardiopulmonary exercise stress test?**
    Cardiopulmonary EST is indicated to differentiate cardiac versus pulmonary causes of exercise-induced dyspnea or impaired exercise capacity. It is also used in the follow-up of patients with heart failure or who are being considered for heart transplantation.

22. **Can one obtain a stress test if a patient cannot exercise?**
    If the patient is unable to exercise, pharmacologic methods can detect ischemia with the use of echocardiography and myocardial nuclear perfusion imaging. Both stress imaging methods increase the accuracy for detection of coronary artery disease compared with EST alone but cannot predict functional capacity.

BIBLIOGRAPHY, SUGGESTED READINGS, AND WEBSITES

1. ACC/AHA 2002 Guideline Update for Exercise Testing: Summary Article http://circ.ahajournals.org/cgi/content/full/106/14/1883
2. AHA Scientific Statement: Exercise Testing in Asymptomatic Adults http://circ.ahajournals.org/cgi/content/full/112/5/771

3. Lee TH, Boucher CH: Noninvasive tests in patients with stable coronary artery disease, *N Engl J Med* 344:1840-1845, 2001.

4. Libby P, Bonow R, Zipes D, et al: Exercise stress testing. In *Braunwald's heart disease edition*, ed 8, Philadelphia, Saunders, 2008.

5. Mayo Clinic Cardiovascular Working Group on Stress Testing: Cardiovascular stress testing: a description of the various types of stress tests and indications for their use, *Mayo Clinic Proc* 71:43-52, 1996.

6. Gibbons RJ, Balady GJ, Beasley JW, et al: ACC/AHA 2002 guideline update for exercise testing. Summary article. A report of the American College of Cardiology/American Heart Association Task Force on Practice Guidelines, *Circulation* 106(14):1883-1892, 2002.

7. Lauer M, Sivarajan EF, Williams M, et al: Exercise testing in asymptomatic adults, *Circulation* 112:771-776, 2005.

CHAPTER 8

NUCLEAR CARDIOLOGY

Arumina Misra, MD, FACC

1. **What is nuclear cardiology?**
   Nuclear cardiology is a field of cardiology that encompasses cardiac radionuclide imaging, which uses radioisotopes to assess myocardial perfusion or myocardial function in different clinical settings, as well as radionuclide angiography, metabolic and receptor imaging, and positron emission tomography.

2. **What is myocardial perfusion imaging?**
   Myocardial perfusion imaging (MPI) is a noninvasive method that utilizes radioisotopes to assess regional myocardial blood flow, function, and viability. The basis for MPI rests on the ability of this technique to demonstrate inhomogenity of blood flow during stress compared with rest, thereby identifying ischemic regions.

   During the *stress* portion of the test, exercise or a pharmacologic agent is used to produce vasodilation in the coronary vascular bed. Whereas a normal vessel can vasodilate and increase coronary blood flow up to four times basal blood flow, a diseased or stenotic vessel cannot. Because radiotracer uptake into the myocardium is dependent on blood flow, the areas that are supplied by normal vessels in which there is maximally increased blood flow will take up more radiotracer than areas supplied by the stenotic vessel with relatively less blood flow. Therefore, there will be heterogeneous radiotracer uptake, which will be seen as a perfusion defect.

3. **Define a perfusion defect and differentiate between a reversible and fixed defect.**
   A perfusion defect is an area of reduced radiotracer uptake in the myocardium.

   If the perfusion defect occurs during stress and improves or normalizes during rest, it is termed *reversible* (Fig. 8-1). Generally, a reversible perfusion defect suggests the presence of ischemia.

   If the perfusion defect occurs during both stress and rest, it is termed *fixed*. Generally, a fixed defect suggests the presence of scar. However, in certain settings a fixed defect may not be scar. Instead, a fixed defect may represent viable tissue that is hibernating due to chronic stenosis. Hibernating myocardium alters its metabolism in order to conserve energy. Therefore, it appears underperfused and has hypokinetic or akinetic function.

4. **What are the different uses of myocardial perfusion imaging?**
   - MPI is used to diagnose coronary artery disease (CAD) in patients with intermediate risk for CAD who present with chest pain or its equivalent.
   - MPI can be used to localize and quantify perfusion abnormalities or physiologic ischemia in patients with known CAD.
   - MPI can be used to assess the presence of viability in areas of fixed defects using rest and redistribution studies with thallium.
   - MPI can also be used for risk assessment and determination of prognosis with regard to cardiovascular events. It can be used as a prognostic tool in post MI patients, including patients with and without ST elevation, to identify further areas of myocardium at risk.
   - MPI can also be used in preoperative assessment to identify perioperative or postoperative cardiovascular risk. The extent and severity of perfusion defects are proportional to the risk of perioperative cardiac events.

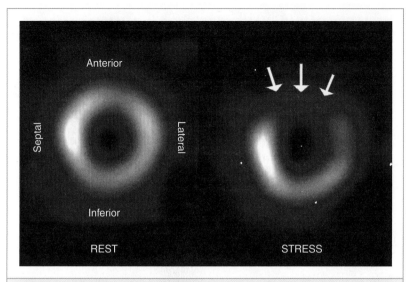

Figure 8-1. Nuclear stress testing short-axis view demonstrating a reversible perfusion defect. Normal myocardial perfusion occurred during resting images *(left panel)*, but a large anterior wall perfusion defect *(arrows)* was seen during previous stress imaging *(right panel)*. (Modified from http://www. texasheartinstitute.org/HIC/Topics/Diag/dinuc.cfm.)

5. **Is MPI the most sensitive and specific test for diagnosing CAD?**
   The ischemic cascade suggests that MPI would be a more sensitive test to detect ischemia because in the setting of ischemia, a perfusion abnormality occurs before a wall motion abnormality. The sensitivity of an MPI is slightly better than stress echocardiography (85% versus 75%, respectively) and the specificity slightly worse (79% versus 88%). This results in similar accuracy for both types of stress tests. Both modalities are more sensitive and specific than treadmill or exercise electrocardiography testing, although according to the American Heart Association/American College of Cardiology (AHA/ACC) guidelines, the latter should be the first-line test for the diagnosis of CAD in someone who can exercise and has a relatively normal electrocardiogram (ECG).

6. **List the different perfusion agents used in myocardial perfusion imaging.**
   For an agent to be an effective radiopharmaceutical, its distribution has to be proportional to regional blood flow and it has to have a high level of extraction by the organ of interest and rapid clearance from the blood. The two most important physiologic factors that affect myocardial uptake of a radiotracer are variations in regional blood flow and the myocardial extraction of the radiotracer. In other words, there will be more uptake of a radiotracer in areas of increased blood flow and less in areas supplied by diseased or stenosed vessels. Importantly, because myocardial extraction is an active process with regard to thallium-201 and a mitochondrial-dependent process with regard to the technetium-99m agents, it can only occur if the cells in that region are viable. The relative advantages and disadvantages of thallium-201 and technitium-99 are summarized in Table 8-1.
   - **Thallium-201** (Tl-201) is a potassium analog used for MPI. It is the oldest and best studied of the present-day agents. Thallium distribution is dependent on blood flow and tracer extraction by the myocardium. It enters the myocardium by active transport of membrane-bound $Na^+K^+ATPase$. One of the most important characteristics of Tl-201 is its myocardial

TABLE 8-1. RELATIVE ADVANTAGES OF TC-99M AND TL-201 IN NUCLEAR CARDIOLOGY STRESS TESTING

Advantages of Tc-99m Compared with Tl-201	Advantages of Tl-201 Compared with Tc-99m
■ Shorter half-life allows for higher dose, resulting in better count statistics	■ Redistribution allows for single-injection studies and viability assessment
■ Less radiation exposure	■ Less expensive
■ Less attenuation effects	■ Less abdominal and hepatic uptake during exercise
■ Higher energy level allows for improved resolution with gamma camera, especially in gated SPECT studies	■ Diagnostic and prognostic value of lung uptake of Tl-201
■ Faster imaging protocols due to reinjection	

SPECT, Single-photon emission computed tomography.

redistribution. A dynamic quality to the uptake of Tl-201 gives it the ability to redistribute over time. There is continued influx of Tl-201 over time from the blood-pool activity and a clearance or washout from the myocardium. This phenomenon results in normalization or reversibility in areas that are ischemic, and over additional time improvement or normalization can occur in areas that are viable but appeared as scar during the first rest imaging.

- **Technetium-99m** (Tc-99m) comprises many radiotracers. Some agents include Tc-99m sestamibi, Tc-99m teboroxime (not used clinically at present), Tc-99m tetrofosmin, and Tc-99m N-NOET.

- **Tc-99m sestamibi** (or MIBI or Cardiolite) is the third of the isonitriles to be developed but the first of the Tc-99m agents to be approved for commercial use. It contains a hydrophilic cation and the isonitrile hydrophobic portion that allows for the necessary interactions with the cell membrane for uptake into the myocardioum. The uptake of MIBI is dependent on mitochondrial-derived membrane electrochemical gradient, cellular pH, and intact energy production. Unlike Tl-201, MIBI does not possess a strong redistribution quality. The reason for this is that the clearance of MIBI is slow even though continued uptake occurs during the rest phase of a study. Therefore, there may be some improvement in 2 to 3 hours between stress and rest, but the degree of redistribution is slower and less complete than Tl-201. Importantly, however, only viable tissue can extract and uptake MIBI.

- **Tc-99m tetrofosmin** (Myoview) is the newest of the Tc-99m agents to be approved for clinical use. Its properties are similar to MIBI, although the mechanism by which myocardial uptake occurs is not well elucidated; however, uptake is dependent on intact mitochondrial potentials (i.e., viable cells). Studies show similar characteristics to MIBI, with a more rapid clearance from the liver allowing for faster imaging times.

- **Tc-99m furifosmin** is similar to Tc-99m tetrofosmin but is not currently approved for clinical use.

- **Tc-99m N-NOET** is a newer investigational agent that has similar physical and imaging properties to that of other Tc-99m agents but also favorable redistribution qualities similar to Tl-201.

7. **How is stress produced for MPI in the evaluation of CAD?**
   Stress can be produced in different ways. The goal of myocardial perfusion imaging is to
   produce vasodilation in order to assess the presence of diseased or stenotic vessels, which will
   vasodilate to a lesser extent than healthy, nonstenotic vessels. Forms of stress are either
   exercise or pharmacologic (Table 8-2).

TABLE 8-2. STRESS AGENTS USED FOR MYOCARDIAL PERFUSION IMAGING AND
THEIR INDICATIONS, CONTRAINDICATIONS, ADVANTAGES, AND DISADVANTAGES

Stress Agents for MPI			
	Indications	Contraindications	Pros	Cons
---	---	---	---	---
Exercise	Diagnose CAD, assess risk for those who can exercise but whose ECG is abnormal	Can't exercise, have LBBB on ECG, or comorbid condition such as severe AS, CHF (see guidelines)	Assess FS, diagnosis and prognosis for CAD	None
Adenosine	Diagnose CAD, assess risk for those who can't exercise	Bronchospastic COPD or asthma, heart block, hypotension	Produces excellent vasodilation greater than that of exercise	Cannot assess FS
Dipyridamole	Diagnose CAD, assess risk for those who can't exercise	Bronchospastic COPD or asthma, heart block, hypotension	Produces excellent vasodilation greater than that of exercise	Cannot assess FS
Dobutamine	Diagnose CAD, assess risk for those who can't exercise	Tachyarrhythmias, uncontrolled hypertension, AS (similar to those for exercise)	Reserved for those who need pharmacologic MPI but who have bronchospastic disease	Does not produce good vasodilation and cannot assess FS

AS, aortic stenosis; *CHF*, congestive heart failure; *COPD*, chronic obstructive pulmonary disease; *FS*,
functional status; *LBBB*, left bundle branch block.

- Exercise can include treadmill, supine or erect bicycle, dynamic arm, or isometric handgrip.
  Generally, because of its diagnostic and prognostic value, the treadmill is used most
  often. Functional capacity can be determined. In addition, prognosis for cardiac events can
  be determined using the Duke treadmill score when using the Bruce protocol. Exercise
  increases myocardial blood flow and metabolic demand.
- Pharmacologic agents include dobutamine, dipyridamole, and adenosine.
  - Dobutamine is a β-1 agonist that increases heart rate and contractility and thereby
    produces an indirect increase in myocardial blood flow as a result of increased
    metabolic demand. This agent is used for nuclear stress MPI when vasodilators are
    contraindicated, such as in bronchospastic lung disease or bradycardia and heart block.
  - Dipyridamole and adenosine are both vasodilators. They purely produce vasodilation by
    acting on the adenosine receptors. Dipyridamole does this by increasing the
    endogenous levels of adenosine by preventing its breakdown, whereas adenosine is
    given exogenously to increase levels. They do not affect myocardial metabolic demand.

8. **How much radiation exposure does a patient get from a typical myocardial perfusion imaging study? How does it compare to other cardiac studies?**
It depends on the radiotracer used and the protocol. Exposure can vary from about 10 mSv to upwards of 30 mSv. Table 8-3 summarizes radiation exposure from various tests.

TABLE 8-3. RADIATION EXPOSURE FROM VARIOUS STUDIES	
PA chest film	0.02 mSv
Background radiation	3 mSv
Coronary catheterization	5 mSv
CT angiography	10–14 mSv
CT coronary angiography 64 slice	17 mSv
CT of the body	20–40 mSv
Tc-99m MIBI (10/27.5 mCi)	14.6 mSv
Tl-201 (3.5 mCi)	29 mSv
Calcium scoring	2.6 mSv

CT, Computed tomography; *mCi*, milliCurriè; *mSv*, milliSievert; *PA*, posteroanterior.

9. **Is it possible to assess both myocardial perfusion and left ventricular function with one study?**
Yes. Both Tc-99m agents and Tl-201 have been validated in assessing left ventricular (LV) volumes and left ventricular ejection fraction (LVEF) using gated single-photon emission computed tomography (SPECT) imaging. Thus, one can gate stress and rest portions of the MPI when using gated SPECT technology. Gating is a method of stopping cardiac motion that allows for the assessment of the different phases of the cardiac cycle. This triggering of the imaging camera at the onset of the R wave over multiple cardiac cycles provides an 8- or 16-frame average of multiple cardiac beats, which are needed to accurately assess wall motion and thickening. Gated studies improve specificity by helping to differentiate fixed defects caused by attenuation versus scar.

10. **Functional assessment of cardiac performance is determined using which nuclear cardiology techniques?**
The term *radionuclide angiography* encompasses both the first-pass bolus technique and gated equilibrium blood pool imaging, both of which can be used to assess LV function.
   ▪ First-pass radionuclide angiography (FPRNA) uses a bolus technique and rapid acquisition to track the tracer bolus through the right atrium, right ventricle, pulmonary arteries, lungs, left atrium, left ventricle, and finally aorta. The first-pass technique can be used to assess both left and right ventricular ejection fraction, regional wall motion, and cardiopulmonary shunts. FPRNA can be done both at rest and during exercise.
   ▪ Gated equilibrium blood pool imaging or multiple gated acquisition (MUGA) can also be used to assess left ventricular function and ejection fraction. The right ventricle is not easily assessed with this technique because of overlap of cardiac structures but can be done if care is taken in imaging. The technique is performed after a sample of the patient's red

blood cells is labeled with Tc-99m sodium pertechnetate and then reinjected for planar imaging in three different views. The gating is done similar to SPECT gating; however, instead of a standard number of frames per cardiac cycle, there can be a variable number depending on the R to R cycle length or heart rate. The cardiac images are then compiled into summed images. They are then processed and displayed as a continuous cinematic loop. From the cinematic loop, one can assess wall motion in the different views, including left anterior oblique (LAO), lateral, and anterior. The data from the LAO view is also displayed as still images so that the counts in the region of interest (the left ventricle) at end-systole and end-diastole can be used to calculate the end-diastolic volume (EDV) and end-systolic volume (ESV) and subsequently the ejection fraction.

$$LVEF = \frac{(EDV - \text{background counts}) - (ESV - \text{background counts})}{(EDV - \text{background counts})} \times 100$$

Importantly, this technique can be done both at rest and during stress to give accurate volumetric information for comparison.

11. Why should one use radionuclide angiography to assess LVEF?

- It is a precise and accurate measure of LVEF that is more reproducible than echocardiography, especially when doing serial studies to look for changes in LVEF caused by cardiotoxic agents, valvular heart disease, and new therapeutic agents in clinical trials.
- It is less expensive and more feasible than magnetic resonance imaging for evaluation of LVEF.
- On a more practical level, radionuclide angiography can be used to assess LVEF when other methods are not possible because of poor images as a result of body habitus, lung disease, or chest wall deformities.
- LVEF is an independent predictor of cardiac events and thus serves as a valid prognostic index in many clinical settings.

12. What is the role of positron emission tomography (PET) in the assessment of the heart, in particular CAD?

PET has many capabilities, including assessing myocardial blood flow, glucose utilization, fatty acid metabolism, oxidative metabolism, oxygen consumption, and adrenergic neuronal activity and β-receptor densities.

Tracers used to assess myocardial blood flow include O-15 water, Rb-82, and N-13 ammonia. Tracers used to assess metabolism include F-18-fluoro-2-deoxyglucose (F-18 FDG), carbon-11-labeled palmitate and acetate, and molecular oxygen-15.

The most useful tool that PET provides in the assessment of CAD is identifying viable tissue. The issue of viability is raised when a myocardial segment appears as scar such that it has reduced perfusion and contractility in both stress and rest imaging. Combined PET imaging with N-13 ammonia or rubidium perfusion and F-18 FDG for glucose metabolism is considered the gold standard to assess myocardial viability. Viable myocardium is identified on the basis of myocardial blood flow and preserved or enhanced substrate utilization. First a segment with impaired contractility is identified. Then the relative blood flow to that region is assessed, followed by determination of the regional metabolic activity. The importance of assessing viability is illustrated by outcomes after revascularization of viable and nonviable regions. Table 8-4 summarizes the interpretation of PET testing for myocardial viability.

TABLE 8-4. INTERPRETATION OF MYOCARDIAL VIABILITY WITH PET IMAGING

Interpretation of Viability in PET Imaging

Regional Wall Motion	Blood Flow	FDG Uptake	Diagnosis
Normal	Normal	Normal	Normal myocardium
Reduced	Normal	Normal	Stunned myocardium (blood flow intact; function should recover with time)
Reduced	Abnormal	Normal	Hibernating myocardium (blood flow impaired, function may improve with revascularization)
Reduced	Abnormal	Reduced	Scar tissue/infarction with no viability

BIBLIOGRAPHY, SUGGESTED READINGS, AND WEBSITES

1. Baghdasarian SB, Heller GV: The role of myocardial perfusion imaging in the diagnosis of patients with coronary artery disease: developments over the past year, *Curr Opin Cardiol* 20:369-374, 2005.

2. Berman DS, Shaw LJ, Hachamovitch, R, et al: Comparative use of radionuclide stress testing, coronary artery calcium scanning, and noninvasive coronary angiography for diagnostic and prognostic cardiac assessment, *Semin Nucl Med* 37:2-16, 2007.

3. Bourque JM, Velasquez EJ, Tuttle RJ, et al: Mortality risk associated with ejection fraction differs across resting nuclear perfusion findings, *J Nucl Cardiol* 14:165-173, 2007.

4. Brindis RG, Douglas PS, Hendel RC, et al: ACCF/ASNC appropriateness criteria for single-photon emission computed tomography myocardial perfusion imaging (SPECT MPI), *J Am Cardiol* 51:1127-1147, 2005.

5. Hachamovitch R, Berman DS: The use of nuclear cardiology in clinical decision making, *Semin Nucl Med* 35: 62-72, 2005.

6. Hachamovitch R, Hayes SW, Friedman JD, et al: Comparison of the short-term survival benefit associated with revascularization compared with medical therapy in patients with no prior coronary artery disease undergoing stress myocardial perfusion single photon emission computed tomography, *Circulation* 107:2900-2906, 2003.

7. Iskanderian AE, Verani MS. *Nuclear cardiac imaging principles and applications*, ed 3, New York, 2003, Oxford University Press.

8. Klocke FJ, Baird MG, Bateman TM, et al: ACC/AHA/ASNC guidelines for the clinical use of cardiac radionuclide imaging, *J Am Cardiol* 42:1318-1333, 2003.

9. Metz LD, Beattie M, Hom R, et al: The prognostic value of normal exercise myocardial perfusion imaging and exercise echocardiography, *J Am Coll Cardiol* 49:227-237, 2007.

10. Miller TD, Redberg RF, Wackers FJT: Screening asymptomatic diabetic patients for coronary artery disease, why not? *J Am Coll Cardiol* 48:761-764, 2006.

11. Shaw LJ, Berman DS, Maron DJ, et al: Optimal medical therapy with or without percutaneous coronary intervention to reduce ischemic burden: results from the Clinical Outcomes Utilizing Revascularization and Aggressive Drug Evaluation (COURAGE) trial nuclear substudy, *Circulation* 117:1283-1291, 2008.

12. Travin MI, Bergman SR: Assessment of myocardial viability, *Semin Nucl Med* 35:2-16, 2005.

CARDIAC MAGNETIC RESONANCE IMAGING

Glenn N. Levine, MD, FACC, FAHA

1. **Does cardiac magnetic resonance imaging (MRI) expose the patient to any radiation?**

   No. MRI uses an extremely strong static magnet 1.5–3.0 tesla (equivalent to 30,000–60,000 times the strength of the earth's magnetic field), pulsed radiofrequency energy, and gradient magnetic fields to image the body. Most imaging uses positively charged hydrogen protons, most of which are in water molecules, as the means to image body structures. The pulse sequences actually used for the static and dynamic imaging of the heart are quite complex and far beyond the scope of this chapter. In very simple terms, many pulse sequences are based on either gradient echo *(bright blood)* or spin echo *(black blood)* sequences, as well as steady-state free precession imaging, which is used during cine cardiac MR imaging.

2. **What are the primary indications for cardiac MRI?**

   Although echocardiography is usually the first-line imaging modality for questions of left ventricular function and assessment of valvular disease, cardiac MRI still has many important potential uses and advantages:

   Assessment of left ventricular function, volume, and mass: Cardiac MRI allows for a reproducible and accurate assessment of left ventricular (LV) ejection fraction. Given its ability to image three-dimensional structures in any plane, it can produce accurate assessments of left ventricular end-systolic and end-diastolic volumes from which ejection fraction, as well as stroke volume and cardiac output, can be calculated. Unlike echocardiography, a patient's body habitus does not affect image quality; therefore, issues like obesity or expanded lungs in patients with chronic obstructive pulmonary disease (COPD) are usually not an issue.

   Cardiac MRI is considered by almost all as the gold standard for the measurement of ejection fraction (EF), LV volumes, and LV mass. It is generally felt to be more accurate and reproducible than echocardiography (at least two-dimensional echocardiography) and provides vastly more information than radionuclide imaging. Clinical studies, particularly those involving only limited numbers of patients, increasingly use cardiac MRI for the serial assessment of LVEF, volume, and mass.

   Assessment of myocardial infarction and myocardial viability: Using a technique called *late gadolinium enhancement,* in which gadolinium is injected and then approximately 10 minutes later the heart is imaged using special sequences, infarcted myocardium can be imaged. This technique can very accurately detect and delineate infarcted myocardium (Fig. 9-1). Using this technique, infarcted myocardium appears bright; noninfarcted, viable myocardium appears dark.

   This technique is very useful in assessing potentially hibernating myocardium in patients with depressed ejection fraction and multivessel disease who are being considered for bypass surgery. Kim and Judd have demonstrated that in a given area of the left ventricle in patients with multivessel disease, areas in which transmural infarction is demonstrated are unlikely to improve contractility after revascularization, whereas areas that show little or no demonstrated infarction are much more likely to improve contractility after revascularization. This modality is at least as good as if not better than nuclear or echocardiographic imaging in predicting functional recovery of contractile function after revascularization.

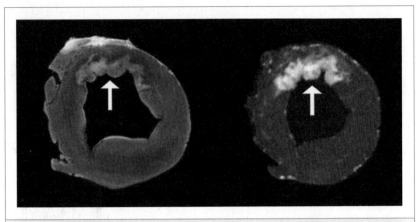

Fig. 9-1. Correlation between myocardial infarction as demonstrated by gross pathology and tissue staining and gadolinium-enhanced delayed MRI imaging. Left figure shows experimentally induced subendocardial infarction *(arrow)*. Right figure demonstrates gadolinium-enhanced delayed hyperenhancement *(arrow)*, corresponding almost exactly to the actual pathology. (Modified from Libby P, Bonow RO, Mann DL, et al: *Braunwald's heart disease: a textbook of cardiovascular medicine,* ed 8, Philadelphia, 2008, Saunders. Courtesy Dr. R. J. Kim and Dr. R. M. Judd.)

Stress myocardial perfusion imaging: Just as adenosine is used to dilate the coronary arteries and increase blood flow in nonstenosed vessels during nuclear stress testing, adenosine can be used during MR stress imaging. Typically, the patient is treated with intravenous adenosine for 3 minutes. An intravenous bolus of gadolinium is then administered. The heart is imaged in real time. Gadolinium will cause normally perfused myocardium to appear *bright,* whereas nonperfused areas remain dark. Areas of relative or absolute perfusion defects can be easily detected (Fig. 9-2). Dobutamine stress testing can also be performed using cardiac MRI to assess for improvement in wall motion or decrease in wall motion (e.g., normally contracting wall during rest becomes hypokinetic during stress).

Valvular heart disease: Although echocardiography remains the first-line test in the evaluation of valvular disease, cardiac MRI can also be used for valvular assessment, especially

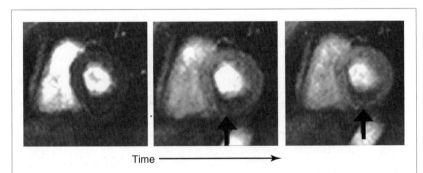

Time ⟶

Fig. 9-2. Stress perfusion imaging. The patient is first treated with adenosine for 3 minutes. A bolus of gadolinium is then administered. The gadolinium leads to perfused myocardium appearing bright, whereas nonperfused myocardium remains dark *(arrow).* (Courtesy Dr. Scott Flamm and Dr. Benjamin Chung.)

in patients with poor echocardiographic windows and those who are not candidates for or refuse to undergo transesophageal echocardiography (TEE).

Assessment of infiltrative diseases and inflammatory processes: Using gadolinium enhancement, infiltrative diseases (e.g., sarcoidosis; Fig. 9-3) and active inflammatory processes, such as myocarditis, can be visualized. Cardiac MRI is the procedure of choice in patients with suspected infiltrative diseases or myocarditis.

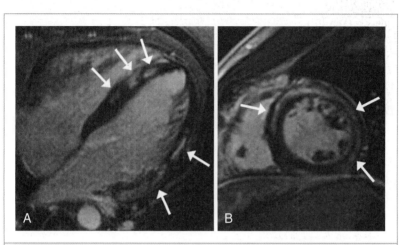

Fig. 9-3. Gadolinium-enhanced delayed MRI of a 23–year-old patient with known sarcoidosis demonstrating cardiac sarcoidosis. The left ventricular myocardium should appear uniformly black, but patchy bright areas *(arrows)* are visible in both the horizontal long-axis view **(A)** and the short-axis view **(B)** as a result of the presence of sarcoid infiltration. (Modified from Hunold P, Schlosser T, Vogt FM, et al: Myocardial late enhancement in contrast-enhanced cardiac MRI: distinction between infarction scar and non–infarction-related disease, *Am J Roentegenol* 184:1420-1426, 2005.)

Coronary artery imaging: Cardiac MRI can be used to visualize the coronary arteries. Due to issues such as cardiac motion and the size of the coronary arteries, coronary magnetic resonance angiography (MRA) is not currently as reliable and accurate as coronary computed tomography (CT) angiography, and images as good as Figure 9-4 are not always obtained. Coronary MRA is, however, an excellent technique to assess for aberrant origin of the coronary arteries and the course of such arteries (e.g., between the aorta and pulmonary artery). It is particularly useful in young patients, avoiding the radiation exposure of cardiac CT.

Assessment of tumors: Cardiac MRI is an excellent modality for the assessment of tumors (Fig. 9-5). Although initial hopes that it could definitely noninvasively characterize tumor tissue (e.g., a *noninvasive biopsy*) have not quite come to fruition, cardiac MRI is still helpful in determining whether a tumor is more likely to be benign or malignant and may be able to more specifically suggest the specific tumor type. It is also excellent in defining the borders of the tumor and can be used to further assess any mass visualized on echocardiography, many of which will turn out to be benign findings or pseudotumors.

Congenital heart disease: MRI is the test of choice in patients with suspected or known congenital heart disease. MRI allows both anatomic and physiologic assessment of lesions, defects, and shunts.

Arrhythmogenic right ventricular dysplasia/cardiomyopathy: Arrhythmogenic right ventricular dysplasia/cardiomyopathy (ARVD/C) is a rare condition in which fibrosis and fatty infiltration of the right ventricle are present, predisposing the patient to potentially lethal ventricular arrhythmias. MRI is the study of choice in assessing for this condition.

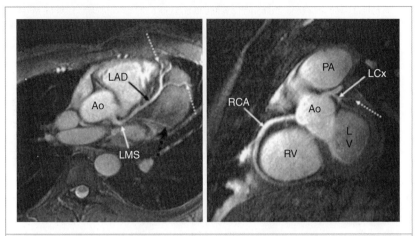

Fig. 9-4. Coronary magnetic resonance angiography. Coronary cardiovascular magnetic resonance (CMR) at 3 Tesla. *Left panel*, Left coronary artery and branches *(dotted arrows)*. *Right panel*, Right coronary artery (RCA). *Ao*, Aorta; *LAD*, left anterior descending artery; *LCx*, left circumflex artery; *LMS*, left main stem; *LV*, left ventricle; *PA*, pulmonary artery; *RV*, right ventricle. (From Stuber M, Botnar RM, Fischer SE, et al: Preliminary report on in vivo coronary MRA at 3 Tesla in humans, *Magn Reson Med* 48(3):425-429, 2002. Reprinted with permission of Wiley-Liss, Inc. a subsidiary of John Wiley & Sons, Inc.)

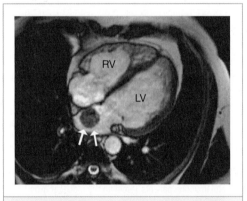

Fig. 9-5. Cardiac MRI demonstrating a left atrial myxoma.

3. **Can MRI be performed in patients with implanted cardiovascular devices?**
   Most implanted cardiovascular devices are nonferromagnetic or only weakly ferromagnetic. This includes most commonly used coronary stents, peripheral vascular stents, inferior vena cava (IVC) filters, prosthetic heart valves, cardiac closure devices, aortic stent grafts, and embolization coils. Pacemakers and implantable cardioverter defibrillators are strong relative contraindications to MRI scanning, and scanning of such patients should be done under specific delineated conditions, only at centers with expertise in MRI safety and electrophysiology, and only when MRI imaging in particular is clearly indicated.

   A statement on the safety of scanning patients with cardiovascular devices was published by the American Heart Association, giving guidelines of the timing and safety of device scanning. (See the Websites box and Bibliography at the end of this chapter.) Before MRI scanning is performed, the safety of scanning that particular device should always be verified based on manufacturer device information and dedicated websites. (See the Websites box and Bibliography at the end of this chapter.) Particular care has to be taken in the case of patients with intracranial implants, in which an inappropriate MRI could have fatal consequences.

4. What is nephrogenic systemic fibrosis?

For many years, administration of gadolinium was considered to be completely safe in patients with chronic kidney disease. Over the last decade, it has become apparent that a rare condition called nephrogenic systemic fibrosis (NSF) can occur in patients with severe or end-stage renal insufficiency who are administered gadolinium (most commonly those on dialysis). The syndrome, which was previously called nephrogenic fibrosing dermopathy, involves fibrosis of the skin (hence the prior name), joints, skeletal muscles, and internal organs. Clinical involvement is usually noted in the first several months after exposure. Both the Food and Drug Administration (FDA) and radiology experts have issued recommendations on the issue of gadolinium administration in patients with chronic kidney disease. The risks and benefits of gadolinium-enhanced MRI scans should be carefully weighted in patients with more severe renal disease or end-stage renal disease, and clinicians should consult with radiology services regarding the best imaging modality for a particular clinical circumstance. (Refer to the articles by Kanal et al and the FDA statement on the subject listed in the Websites box and Bibliography at the end of this chapter.)

BIBLIOGRAPHY, SUGGESTED READINGS, AND WEBSITES

1. U.S. Food and Drug Administration: Information for Healthcare Professionals: Gadolinium-Based Contrast Agents for Magnetic Resonance Imaging (Marketed as Magnevist, MultiHance, Omniscan, OptiMARK, ProHance): http://www.fda.gov/cder/drug/InfoSheets/HCP/gcca_200705HCP.pdf
2. Kanal E, Barkovich AJ, Bell C, et al: ACR guidance document for safe MR practices: 2007, *Am J Roentgenol* 188(6):1447-1474, 2007.
3. Kanal E, Broome DR, Martin DR, et al: Response to the FDA's May 23, 2007, nephrogenic systemic fibrosis update, *Radiology* 246:11-14, 2008.
4. Kim RJ, Wu E, Rafael A, et al: The use of contrast-enhanced magnetic resonance imaging to identify reversible myocardial dysfunction, *N Engl J Med* 343(20):1445-1453, 2000.
5. Levine GN, Gomes AS, Arai AE, et al: Safety of magnetic resonance imaging in patients with cardiovascular devices: an American Heart Association scientific statement from the Committee on Diagnostic and Interventional Cardiac Catheterization, Council on Clinical Cardiology, and the Council on Cardiovascular Radiology and Intervention: endorsed by the American College of Cardiology Foundation, the North American Society for Cardiac Imaging, and the Society for Cardiovascular Magnetic Resonance, *Circulation* 116(24): 2878-2891, 2007.
6. Lin D, Kramer C: Late gadolinium-enhanced cardiac magnetic resonance, *Curr Cardiol Rep* 10(1):72-78, 2008.
7. Sen-Chowdhry S, McKenna WJ: The utility of magnetic resonance imaging in the evaluation of arrhythmogenic right ventricular cardiomyopathy, *Curr Opin Cardiol* 23(1):38-45, 2008.

CHAPTER 10

CARDIAC CT ANGIOGRAPHY

Suhny Abbara, MD and Wilfred Mamuya, MD, PhD

1. **What are the contraindications for cardiac CT?**
    An inability to breath-hold or follow instructions are contraindications to cardiac computed tomographic angiography (CTA). A history of anaphylactic reaction to intravenous iodinated contrast is also considered a contraindication. Often, severe anaphylactic reactions can be confused with other, less severe contrast reactions. In the latter case, computed tomography (CT) is possible if the patient has been adequately premedicated (local premedication policies vary). According to the most recent *appropriateness criteria,* ongoing acute coronary syndrome is a contraindication to performing cardiac CTA.

2. **Is it necessary to administer beta-blockers during acquisition?**
    With the advent of dual-source scanners and 320-detector scanners, we have witnessed a significant increase in temporal resolution and z-axis coverage, respectively. Thus, beta-blockers are no longer necessary before an acquisition on certain scanners (dual-source CT) but remain necessary on conventional single-source 64-slice scanners. In any case, a slower heart rate is still desirable because of increased image quality and lower radiation exposure when a *prospective-triggered* mode of acquisition is used. Target heart rates are typically 60 or below.

3. **What are the three most challenging cardiac CT (CCT) artifacts?**
    - Coronary artery motion artifact, especially at high heart rates, leads to blurring and potentially leads to the segment to be nondiagnostic for assessment of obstruction. The mid-right coronary artery is commonly affected. Low heart rates and scanners with fast temporal resolution help minimize the prevalence of motion artefact.
    - Calcium deposition within coronary arteries is most influenced by increasing age. Calcium usually results in a blooming artifact and may render segments of coronary arteries nonevaluable for underlying stenosis.
    - Other potential sources of image artifacts include slab artifacts from reconstruction kernels, respiratory motion artifacts, and cardiac motion secondary to heart rate variability or premature ventricular contractions (PVCs), as well as beam hardening artifact from pacer wires, implantable cardioverter defibrillators (ICDs), artificial valves, surgical clips, and other devices.

4. **What is the radiation dose of a standard cardiac CT examination?**
    The radiation dose of a standard cardiac CTA depends on a multitude of factors and can range from 1 mSv to as high as 30 mSv. To put things in perspective, the average dose from a nuclear perfusion stress test is 6 to 25 mSv (or as high as 40 mSv or more in thallium stress/ rest tests), and the average dose from a simple diagnostic coronary angiogram is approximately 5 mSv. Factors affecting the radiation dose of a cardiac CT include the type of scanner (single-source versus dual-source), the number of detectors (z-axis coverage), the body habitus of the patient and the selection of kVp and mAs, and the scan mode (triggered versus gated with or without tube modulation). General measures to reduce the radiation dose to

the patient should be used whenever possible according to the as low as reasonably achievable (ALARA) principle. Tube modulation routinely should be applied if retrospective gating is selected, unless a specific reason prohibits its use. If only coronary anatomy is needed, prospective triggering is preferred if clinically feasible (low and regular heart rate).

5. **What are volume-rendered three-dimensional (3D) images (VRT)? And are volume-rendered images diagnostically useful in the assessment of coronary artery disease?**
Volume-rendered images are images that have been generated using a reconstruction algorithm to render a 3D volumetric image of the entire dataset. They are not suitable for an assessment of the severity of coronary artery disease. However, they are particularly useful in a rapid evaluation of course and number of coronary artery bypass grafts and the evaluation of coronary fistulas, collaterals, and coronary aneurysms. However, use of 3D VRT images does still require review of the two-dimensional (2D) dataset in axial and multiplanar modes.

6. **Is there a calcium score above which a cardiac CT acquisition would be contraindicated?**
There is no data demonstrating a clear calcium score cutoff above which a cardiac CT would be contraindicated. However, it is clear that the higher the calcium score, the higher the probability that one or more coronary artery segments might be rendered nonevaluable for stenosis exclusion secondary to blooming artifacts. A number often bandied around in the literature is an Agatston calcium score of 1000, but again many sites do not use any cutoff value that would preclude from acquiring a coronary CTA. Because of the limited prognostic value, performance of calcium scores on patients who have been previously revascularized (stents or bypass grafts) is not indicated.

7. **Is a calcium score useful in a 67-year-old man who is a smoker with diabetes?**
A calcium score is useful in a patient with an intermediate pretest probability of disease because it has been shown to be able to change the classification of such a patient and potentially affect therapy. This patient has a high pretest probability of disease (ATP III/Framingham) and should be treated accordingly to current guidelines. The information from a calcium score CT would not have incremental value in this setting and should therefore be considered "not indicated."

8. **What is the role of cardiac CT in patients presenting for noncoronary cardiac surgery?**
A cardiac CT in this setting is quite useful for the assessment of coronary arteries for obstructive disease in young and middle-aged patients presenting for noncoronary cardiac surgery such as valve repair, resection of cardiac masses, and aortic surgery. Older patients, however, tend to have a higher calcium score, and up to 10% to 25% of studies in octogenarians may not allow definitive exclusion of obstructive coronary artery disease because of one or more nonevaluable segments (Fig. 10-1).

9. **What is the diagnostic accuracy and clinical utility of plaque characterization by cardiac CT?**
Cardiac CT is excellent for detection and quantification of calcified portions of coronary plaque (Agatston score) and for differentiation of calcified, mixed, and noncalcified plaques. However, when compared with the gold standard of intravascular ultrasound (IVUS), CT is only modestly accurate in the detection and quantification of the volume of noncalcified plaques (stable fibrous or potentially vulnerable lipid rich), and differentiation of the two subtypes is not reliably possible. Plaque characterization remains a work in progress, and currently there is no demonstrable utility of plaque characterization in prognosis or in directing medical therapy.

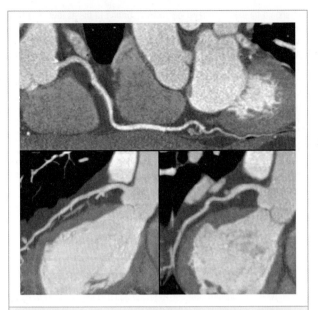

Figure 10-1. Cardiac gated CTA with curved multiplanar reconstructions of the right *(top)*, left anterior descending *(bottom left)*, and left circumflex *(bottom right)* coronary arteries show absence of coronary plaque or stenosis. A negative CT with good image quality has a very high negative predictive value and may spare a patient a diagnostic invasive angiogram.

10. **Is cardiac CT safe and useful in patients presenting with newly diagnosed heart failure?**
    Coronary angiography is usually performed in patients with dilated cardiomyopathy and heart failure, in order to exclude multivessel coronary artery disease as a cause. Cardiac CTA has been shown to be safe and sensitive in excluding multivessel coronary artery disease in this group of patients, with a negative predictive value approaching 97% to 99%. In intermediate-risk to high-risk patients with chest pain or heart failure and a cardiac ultrasound demonstrating classic Tako-Tsubo features, a cardiac CT may be useful in excluding superimposed coronary artery disease.

11. **Is cardiac CT useful in the assessment and management of asymptomatic postbypass patients?**
    Cardiac CT should not be performed in asymptomatic patients. However, it is excellent in assessing graft patency in symptomatic post-bypass patients, and it is useful for the assessment of native coronary artery disease progression and in the assessment of postoperative complications such as graft aneurysms, sternal integrity, and aortotomy dissections.

12. **A 74-year-old diabetic, who underwent stenting of his second obtuse marginal artery with a 2.5-mm drug-eluting stent a year ago, has new-onset exertional chest pain. Is cardiac CT an appropriate modality for his initial evaluation?**
    Current scanner technology limits adequate evaluation of in-stent restenosis in stents that are smaller than 3 mm in diameter. Technical factors include metallic artifacts, calcium and motion artifacts, stent material, and strut design. However, cardiac CTA is useful in the assessment of stent patency, in the detection of other complications such as stent fractures, and in assessment of patients with large proximal stents (e.g., 3.5-mm left main stent).

13. **What is the role of cardiac CT in patients with ST-segment elevation myocardial infarction (STEMI)?**

Cardiac CTA is not indicated in patients with STEMI. However, because of its superior negative predictive value, it has been shown to be an excellent tool in the triage of patients in the emergency room whose presenting symptoms include chest pain, negative biomarkers, and a nondiagnostic ECG. Patients with a negative CT (in absence of substantial artifacts) can be safely discharged from the emergency room with no significant negative short-term outcomes after 30-day and 6-month follow-up.

14. **Can cardiac CT be used to differentiate between a subacute and an old myocardial infarction?**

An acute myocardial infarction appears as a hypoperfused, akinetic area of myocardium, with normal thickness. An old myocardial infarction is usually distinguished by wall thinning, aneurysm formation, fatty metaplasia, calcium deposition, and hyperenhancement on delayed imaging (Fig. 10-2). Functional evaluation may reveal normal contraction (if small nontransmural infarct is present), hypokinesis, or dyskinesis.

15. **Should noncoronary structures be reviewed and reported on during cardiac CT examination?**

The current consensus and standard of care is to include in the final report all significant findings noted in the acquired data set, using a wide *field of view*. Everything that is part of the originally acquired data set should be reviewed and reported on if potentially significant (Fig. 10-3).

16. **Summarize the current consensus of indications for cardiac CT in the management of coronary artery disease.**

Cardiac CT is indicated in intermediate-risk patients with symptoms suggestive of coronary artery disease who are unable to exercise, have an uninterpretable ECG, or have an equivocal stress test. It is also indicated in low-risk to intermediate-risk patients with acute chest pain being treated in an emergency room in the setting of negative biomarkers and a nondiagnostic ECG. Cardiac CT is the modality of choice in the evaluation of the origin and course of coronary anomalies and can accurately exclude coronary artery disease in patients with a left bundle branch block or a dilated cardiomyopathy with heart failure. It is also useful in the assessment of symptomatic postintervention patients (coronary artery bypass grafts [CABG] and stents), in preoperative assessment before repeat CABG, and in the assessment of pulmonary and coronary veins before or after electrophysiologic procedures.

17. **In the evaluation of the pericardium, what are the advantages of cardiac CT when compared with cardiac magnetic resonance imaging (MRI) and cardiac ultrasound?**

Cardiac CT is superior to the other modalities in the identification and delineation of the extent of calcium deposition within the pericardium and thus is useful in the detection of a patchy constrictive pericardial process. Moreover, it is useful in the delineation of accompanying findings such as a dilated inferior vena cava (IVC), dilated hepatic veins, ascites, and mottled enhancement of the hepatic parenchyma. MRI is superior for detection of pericardial enhancement/fibrosis and pericardial adhesions (tagged cine views).

18. **What are the indications for performing cardiac CT after coronary angiography?**

Cardiac CT is ideal in the delineation of the origin and course of coronary anomalies. It is also useful in the serial assessment of coronary artery aneurysms and aneurysms of the sinus of Valsalva. It is useful in the assessment of coronary, pulmonary, and systemic fistulas and collaterals (Fig. 10-4).

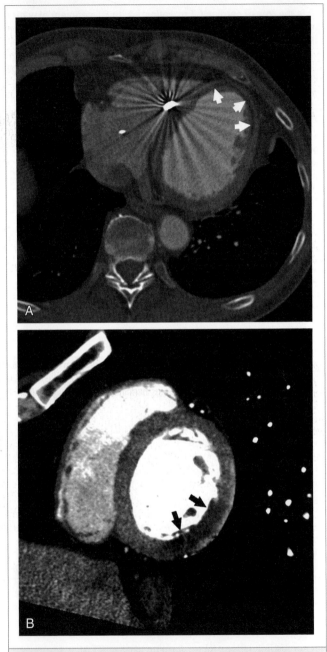

Figure 10-2. A, Cardiac gated axial CT shows apical myocardial thinning and deposition of subendocardial low attenuation material *(arrows)* measuring -15 Hounsfield units, indicating fatty metaplasia in a patient with remote left anterior descending myocardial infarction. **B,** Cardiac gated CT in left ventricular short axis shows inferolateral subendocardial hypoenhancement that measures 35HU *(arrows)* and normal myocardial wall thickness, representing a perfusion defect in a patient with acute left circumflex myocardial infarction.

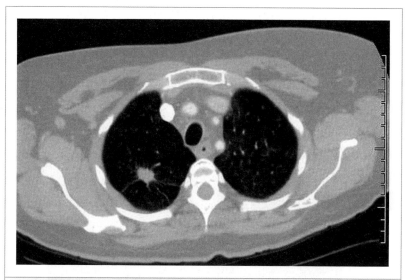

Figure 10-3. Cardiac CT reveals spiculated 1.5-cm mass in the right upper lobe, suspicious for malignancy.

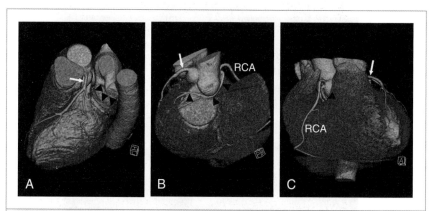

Figure 10-4. Volume-rendered 3D views: **A,** superior view; **B,** posterior view with atria removed; **C,** anterior view) of coronary CTA demonstrate LAD *(white arrow)* arising directly from left sinus of Valsalva. A benign left circumflex anomaly is present where the LCX arises from the right sinus of Valsalva and courses posterior to the aortic root toward the left *(black arrowheads).*

19. **Would cardiac CT be an appropriate first modality in the assessment of a 29-year-old woman with suspected Turner's syndrome with presenting symptoms of dyspnea, a murmur, and hypertension?**
    Patients with suspected Turner's syndrome may have multiple congenital anomalies, including a bicuspid aortic valve, coarctation of the thoracic aorta, an atrial septal defect (ASD) or ventricular septal defect (VSD), or partial anomalous pulmonary venous return.
    A comprehensive cardiac CT examination is capable of identifying all these potential cardiac congenital anomalies in a single study (Figs 10-5 to 10-7).

CHAPTER 11

BEDSIDE HEMODYNAMIC MONITORING

Jameel Ahmed, MD and George J. Philippides, MD

1. **What is a Swan-Ganz catheter?**
   A Swan-Ganz catheter is a relatively soft, flexible catheter with an inflatable balloon at its tip that is used in right-sided heart catheterization. The balloon tip allows the catheter to *float* with the flow of blood from the great veins through the right-sided heart chambers and into the pulmonary artery, before *wedging* in a distal branch of the pulmonary artery.

2. **How is a Swan-Ganz catheter constructed?**
   The basic Swan-Ganz catheter in current clinical use has four lumens. One is connected to the distal port of the catheter, allowing for measurement of pulmonary artery pressure when the balloon is deflated and pulmonary artery wedge pressure (PAWP) when the balloon is inflated. The second lumen is attached to a temperature-sensing thermocouple 5 cm proximal to the catheter tip and is used for measurement of cardiac output (CO) by thermodilution. The third lumen is connected to a port 15 cm proximal to the catheter tip, allowing for measurement of pressure in the right atrium and for infusion of drugs or fluids into the central circulation. The fourth lumen is used to inflate the balloon with air when initially floating the catheter into position and later to reinflate the balloon for intermittent measurement of PAWP. Many catheters contain an additional proximal port for infusion of fluids and drugs. Some catheters have an additional lumen through which a temporary pacing electrode can be passed into the apex of the right ventricle for internal cardiac pacing.

3. **What information can be gained from a Swan-Ganz catheter?**
   Direct measurements obtained from the catheter include vascular pressures and oxygen saturations within the cardiac chambers, cardiac output, and systemic venous oxygen saturation (SvO_2). These hemodynamic measurements can be used to calculate other hemodynamic parameters, such as systemic vascular resistance and pulmonary vascular resistance.

4. **How is a Swan-Ganz catheter inserted?**
   At the bedside, venous access is usually obtained by introducing an 8.5 French sheath into the internal jugular or subclavian vein using the Seldinger technique. The right internal jugular or left subclavian veins are preferred sites because the natural curve of the catheter will allow easier flotation into the pulmonary artery. Less commonly, the antecubital or femoral veins are used.

   Next, a 7.5 French Swan-Ganz catheter is passed through the introducer sheath and advanced approximately 15 cm to exit the sheath into the central vein. The balloon is then inflated with 1.5 cc air, and the catheter is advanced slowly, allowing the balloon to float through the right atrium, right ventricle, and pulmonary artery, and finally achieving a wedge position in a distal branch of the pulmonary artery that is smaller in diameter than the balloon itself. The wedge position is usually achieved when the catheter has advanced a total of 35 to 55 cm, depending on which central vein is cannulated.

5. **Describe the normal pressure waveforms along the path of an advancing Swan-Ganz catheter.**
   The *a wave* is produced by atrial contraction and follows the electrical P wave on electrocardiogram (ECG). The *x descent* reflects atrial relaxation. The *c wave* is produced at the beginning of ventricular systole as the closed tricuspid valve bulges into the right atrium. The *x′ descent* is

thought to be the result of the descent of the atrioventricular ring during ventricular contraction and continued atrial relaxation. The *v wave* is caused by venous filling of the atrium during ventricular systole, when the tricuspid valve is closed. This should correspond with the electrical T wave. However, at the bedside, because of a lag in pressure transmission, the *a wave* will align with the QRS complex and the v wave will follow the T wave. Finally, the *y descent* is produced by rapid atrial emptying, when the tricuspid valve opens at the onset of diastole.

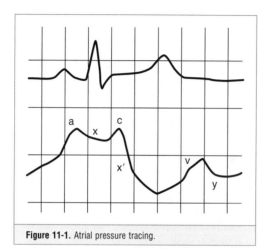

Figure 11-1. Atrial pressure tracing.

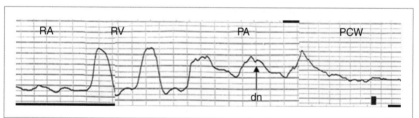

Figure 11-2. Pressure tracings as the catheter is advanced through the right-sided chambers. As the catheter moves from the right atrium to the right ventricle, a ventricular wave form is seen representing isovolumic contraction, ejection, and diastole. When the catheter passes into the pulmonary artery, the diastolic pressure rises. The dicrotic notch *(dn)* is produced by the closure of the pulmonic valve. If the catheter is advanced farther, it attains the wedge position.

6. How is the location of the catheter determined?
At the bedside, continuous monitoring of pressure tracings from the distal port and simultaneous ECG tracings allow the operator to determine the catheter's position and to detect any arrhythmias caused by the catheter as it passes through the right ventricle. Fluoroscopy can be used in the cardiac catheterization laboratory to guide placement. The use of fluoroscopy should especially be considered if a Swan-Ganz catheter is placed via the femoral or brachial veins or in patients with dilated right ventricles.

7. How do we know that the catheter is in the true wedge position?
There are three ways to confirm that the catheter is in the wedge position. At the bedside, an atrial tracing (reflecting left atrial pressure) will be seen when the catheter is in the wedge

position. Secondly, if the catheter is withdrawn from the wedge position, the mean arterial pressure should be observed to rise from the wedge pressure (reflecting a physiologic gradient between the mean pulmonary artery and mean wedge pressure). Gentle aspiration of blood from the distal port should reveal highly oxygenated blood if the catheter is truly wedged. Additionally, in the catheterization laboratory, fluoroscopy can be used to determine that the catheter is in a distal pulmonary arteriole, immobile in the wedge position.

8. **What does the PAWP signify?**

When the catheter is in the wedge position (Fig. 11-3, *B*), proximal blood flow is occluded and a static column of blood is created between the catheter tip and the distal cardiac chambers. With the balloon shielding the catheter tip from the pressure in the pulmonary artery proximally, the pressure transducer measures pressure distally in the pulmonary arterioles. This pressure closely approximates left atrial pressure. When the mitral valve is open at end diastole, left ventricular end-diastolic pressure is measured (Fig. 11-3, *C*), assuming that there is no obstruction between the catheter tip and the left ventricle (i.e., mitral stenosis). The PAWP can be used to approximate left ventricular preload.

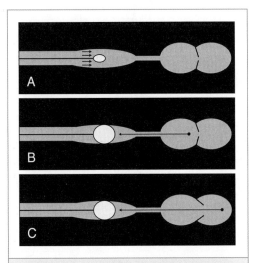

Figure 11-3. A, With the balloon tip deflated, the pressure transducer at the catheter tip sees blood flow from the proximal pulmonary artery. **B,** With the balloon tip inflated, proximal blood flow is occluded and a static column of blood is created between the catheter tip and the distal cardiac chamber. With the mitral valve closed, left atrial pressure is approximated. **C,** With the mitral valve open at end diastole, left ventricular end-diastolic pressure can be measured, assuming there is no significant mitral stenosis.

9. **How is cardiac output determined?**

Cardiac output can be determined either by the measured thermodilution method or the calculated Fick method.

With **thermodilution,** 5 to 10 ml of normal saline is injected rapidly via the proximal port into the right atrium. The injectate mixes completely with blood and causes a drop in temperature that is measured continuously by a thermocouple near the catheter tip. The area under the curve is calculated and is inversely related to cardiac output (Figure 11-4). This method of measurement is not reliable in patients with low cardiac output or significant tricuspid regurgitation. In a

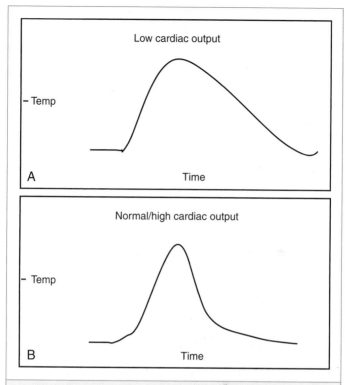

Figure 11-4. Area under the curve is inversely proportional to cardiac output. **A,** Illustration depicts larger area under the curve (AUC) in patient with low cardiac output. **B,** Temperature equilibrates faster in a patient with a higher cardiac output, resulting in a smaller AUC.

low-cardiac-output state, blood is rewarmed by the walls of the cardiac chambers and surrounding tissue, resulting in an overestimation of cardiac output.

Alternatively, the **Fick method** can be used to calculate cardiac output.

$$CO = \frac{\text{oxygen consumption (ml/min)}}{\text{Arterial-venous O}_2 \text{ difference} \times \text{Blood O}_2 \text{ capacity}}$$

$$= \frac{\text{Measured O}_2 \text{ consumption (ml/min)}}{\text{A-V difference} \times \text{Hb(gm \%)} \times 1.36 \text{ (ml O}_2/\text{gm of Hb)} \times 10}$$

This method is based on the principle that the consumption of a substance (oxygen) by any organ is determined by the arterial-venous (A-V) difference of the substance and the blood flow (CO) to that organ. The consumption of oxygen by a patient can be measured using a covered hood in the cardiac catheterization laboratory, and the A-V difference can be measured by obtaining blood samples from the right atrium and pulmonary artery. This method is more accurate in patients with atrial fibrillation, tricuspid regurgitation, and low cardiac output than the thermodilution method. Common sources of error include improper collection of blood samples.

At the bedside, use of a covered hood can be cumbersome and impractical. For this reason, some laboratories assume that resting oxygen consumption is 125 ml/meter^2 and calculate cardiac output based on an assumed Fick equation. However, studies have shown that there is wide variability in resting oxygen consumption among patients, particularly in those patients who are critically ill. As expected, use of an assumed Fick calculation can introduce significant error into the estimation of cardiac output.

10. **What are normal values for intravascular pressures and hemodynamic parameters?**

TABLE 11-1.   NORMAL HEMODYNAMIC MEASUREMENTS

	Normal Values (mm Hg)	Units
Measured Intravascular Pressures		
Right atrium	0–4	
Right ventricle	15–30/0–4	
Pulmonary artery	15–30/6–12	
Pulmonary artery mean	10–18	
Pulmonary artery wedge	6–12	
Derived Hemodynamic Parameters		
Cardiac index	2–4	$1/min/m^2$
Stroke volume index	36–48	$m1/beat/m^2$
Right ventricular (RV) stroke work index	7 10	$gm-m/m^2$
Left ventricular (LV) stroke work index	44–56	$gm-m/m^2$
Pulmonary vascular resistance index	80–240	$Dyne-sec/cm^5/m^2$
Systemic vascular resistance index	1200–2500	$Dyne-sec/cm^5/m^2$
Oxygen delivery	500–600	$ml/min/m^2$
Oxygen uptake	110–160	$ml/min/m^2$
Oxygen extraction ratio	22–32	—

11. **Why are cardiac output and left ventricular (LV) preload important?**
In certain clinical situations, the knowledge of cardiac output and PAWP (surrogate of LV preload; see Question 8) can help to make diagnoses and/or guide management (see Question 12). PAWP can be applied to the Starling curve and help to predict whether cardiac output may improve if filling pressures are altered.

12. **When is placing a Swan-Ganz catheter clinically indicated, and do all patients derive clinical benefit?**
Other situations in which a Swan-Ganz catheter can considered include the following:

Heart Failure/Shock

- Differentiation between cardiogenic and noncardiogenic pulmonary edema when a trial of diuretic and/or vasodilator therapy has failed
  - It is *not* indicated for the routine management of pulmonary edema.
- Differentiation of causes of shock and guide management when a trial of intravascular volume expansion has failed (see Question 15)
- Determination of whether pericardial tamponade is present when clinical assessment is inconclusive and echocardiography is unavailable
- Assessment of valvular heart disease

- Determination of reversibility of pulmonary vasoconstriction in patients being considered for heart transplantation
- Management of congestive heart failure refractory to standard medical therapy, especially in the setting of acute myocardial infarction
  - Of note, a major, randomized trial, Evaluation Study of Congestive Heart Failure and Pulmonary Artery Catheterization Effectiveness (ESCAPE), showed no significant difference in endpoints of mortality and days out of hospital at 6 months in this category of patients.

Acute Myocardial Infarction

American College of Cardiology/American Heart Association (ACC/AHA) guidelines state that Swan-Ganz catheters should be used in those patients who have progressive hypotension unresponsive to fluids and in patients with suspected mechanical complications of ST-elevation myocardial infarction (MI) if an echocardiogram has not been performed (class I). However, mortality benefit has not been demonstrated in a randomized trial.

The use of Swan-Ganz catheters can also be considered in the following situations:

- Diagnosis of mechanical complications of myocardial infarction (i.e., mitral regurgitation, ventricular septal defect)
- Diagnosis of intracardiac shunts and to establish their severity before surgical correction (see Question 16)
- Guidance of management of cardiogenic shock with pharmacologic or mechanical support
- Guidance of management of right ventricular infarction with hypotension or signs of low cardiac output not responding to intravascular volume expansion or low doses of inotropic drugs
- Short-term guidance of pharmacologic or mechanical management of acute mitral regurgitation before surgical correction

Perioperative Use

A 2003 randomized trial in high-risk surgical patients showed no significant difference in mortality with the use of Swan-Ganz catheters. Although the routine use of Swan-Ganz catheters perioperatively remains of unclear benefit, it should be considered in the following situations:

- In patients undergoing cardiac surgery, to differentiate between causes of low cardiac output or to differentiate between right and left ventricular dysfunction, when clinical assessment and echocardiography is inadequate
- Guidance of perioperative management in selected patients with decompensated heart failure undergoing intermediate or high-risk noncardiac surgery

Pulmonary Hypertension

- Exclusion of postcapillary causes of pulmonary hypertension (i.e., elevated PAWP)
- To establish diagnosis and assess severity of primary pulmonary hypertension (normal PAWP)
- Selection and establishment of safety and efficacy of long-term vasodilator therapy based on acute hemodynamic response

Use in Intensive Care Units

- Many studies have shown that clinical data predict PAWP and CO poorly and that insertion of the catheter often changes patient management. However, despite widespread use of these devices in intensive care units, only a few observational studies have shown their use to decrease mortality. A 2005 meta-analysis of several randomized trials showed that the use of Swan-Ganz catheters was associated with neither benefit nor or increased mortality. Current thinking is reflected in a 1997 pulmonary artery consensus statement recommending that the decision to insert a Swan-Ganz catheter be made on an individual basis, such that the potential risks and benefits are considered in each case.

13. **What are absolute and relative contraindications to placement of a Swan-Ganz catheter?**

Absolute Contraindications

- Right-sided endocarditis
- Mechanical tricuspid or pulmonic valve prosthesis
- Presence of thrombus or tumor in a right-sided heart chamber

Relative Contraindications

- Coagulopathy
- Recent implantation of a permanent pacemaker or cardioverter defibrillator
- Left bundle branch block
- Bioprosthetic tricuspid or pulmonic valve

14. **What diagnoses can the catheter help make?**
   The characteristic waveform of the Swan-Ganz catheter is altered in several disease states.
   - In pericardial tamponade, equalization of diastolic pressures across all chambers is seen (Fig. 11-5).
   - In atrial fibrillation, the *a wave* disappears from the right atrial pressure tracing, whereas in atrial flutter, mechanical flutter waves occur at a rate of 300/min.
   - *Cannon a waves* occur when the atria contract against closed valves due to atrioventricular dissociation. Irregular *cannon a waves* during a wide-complex tachycardia strongly suggest ventricular tachycardia.
   - Complications of myocardial infarction can be detected on the PAWP tracing, such as giant v waves seen with acute mitral insufficiency, and the *dip and plateau* pattern of the right ventricular (RV) pressure tracing seen with RV infarction.

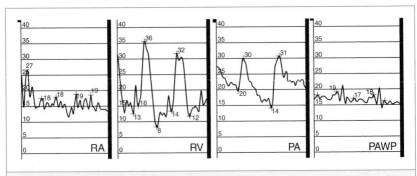

Figure 11-5. Pressure tracings in cardiac tamponade.

15. How can causes of shock be differentiated by Swan-Ganz catheterization?

TABLE 11-2. HEMODYNAMIC PARAMETERS IN DIFFERENT CAUSES OF SHOCK						
Cause	RA	RV	PA	PCWP	CO	SVR
Hypovolemic	↓	↓	↓	↓	↓	↑
Cardiogenic	↑↑	↑↑	↑↑	↑↑	↓	↑
Septic	↔	↔	↔	↔	↑	↓

RA, right atrium; *RV*, right ventricle; *PA*, pulmonary artery; *PCWP*, pulmonary capillary wedge pressure; *CO*, cardiac output; *SVR*, systemic vascular resistance.

16. How can left-to-right intracardiac shunts be diagnosed by Swan-Ganz catheterization?

An intracardiac shunt results in flow of blood from left-sided to right-sided cardiac chambers or vice versa. Left-to-right shunts results in flow from the left-sided chambers to right-sided chambers. With ventricular septal defects, flow is often left-to-right as a result of higher left-sided pressures. Atrial septal defects can result in a shunt in either direction. Because of the flow of oxygenated blood into right-sided chambers, a sudden increase in oxygen saturation in right-sided chambers is observed. A step-up in mean oxygen saturation of 7% between the caval chambers and the right atrium is diagnostic of an atrial septal defect. A step-up of 5% between the right atrium and right ventricle is diagnostic for a ventricular septal defect.

17. What complications are associated with use of a Swan-Ganz catheter?
   - All complications of central venous cannulation, including bleeding and infection
     - Local infection rates range from 18% to 63% in patients with catheter in place for an average of 3 days.
     - Bloodstream infection has been reported in up to 5% of patients.
   - Transient right bundle branch block
   - Complete heart block (especially in patients with preexisting left bundle branch block)
   - Ventricular tachyarrhythmias
     - Clinically insignificant ventricular arrhythmias can occur in up to 30% to 60% of patients.
     - Sustained arrhythmias usually occur in patients with myocardial ischemia or infarction.
   - Pulmonary infarction (incidence 0% to 1.3%)
   - Pulmonary artery rupture
     - Risk factors include pulmonary hypertension and recent cardiopulmonary bypass.
   - Thrombophlebitis
   - Venous or intracardiac thrombus formation
   - Endocarditis
   - Catheter knotting

18. How can complications be minimized?
   - The use of fluoroscopy should be considered for placement of the catheter, particularly if access is obtained from a nontraditional site or if the patient has a dilated right ventricle.
   - Consideration should be given to removing the catheter after the first set of data is obtained.
   - The duration the catheter is kept in place should be minimized because infectious and thrombotic complications increase significantly after 3 to 4 days.
   - Use of the introducer side arm for infusion of medications should be minimized.
   - Manipulation of the catheter should only be performed by trained personnel.

19. **The wedge tracing is abnormal. What do I do?**
    - Check a chest radiograph for proper catheter position. The tip should lie in lung zone 3, below the level of the left atrium.
    - Aspirate and flush the catheter to remove clots and bubbles.
    - Check all connecting lines and stopcocks.
    - Confirm that the pressure transducers are zeroed to the level of the right atrium.
    - Check that the balloon is not overinflated; try letting out the air and refilling it slowly.
    - Consider the possibility that the tracing really is a wedge tracing with a giant v wave, as is seen in acute mitral insufficiency and several other conditions.

20. **The cardiac output doesn't make sense. What is wrong?**
    - Check that at least three values were averaged and that the range of these values is no greater than 20% of the mean.
    - Check the chest radiograph: Is the distal tip of the catheter in the pulmonary artery and the proximal port in the right atrium?
    - Check to see if the computer is calibrated to the proper temperatures.
    - If the computer can display the time versus temperature curve, check that the curve is shaped properly.

BIBLIOGRAPHY, SUGGESTED READINGS, AND WEBSITES

1. Baim DS: *Grossman's cardiac catheterization, angiography, and intervention*, Philadelphia, 2006, Lippincott Williams & Wilkins.
2. Binanay C, Califf RM, Hasselblad V, et al: Evaluation study of congestive heart failure and pulmonary artery catheterization effectiveness: the ESCAPE trial, *JAMA* 294:1625, 2005.
3. Leatherman JW, Marini JJ: Clinical use of the pulmonary artery catheter. In *Principles of critical care*, ed 2, New York, 1998, McGraw-Hill.
4. Mueller HS, Chatterjee K, Davis KB, et al: American College of Cardiology consensus statement. Present use of bedside right heart catheterization in patients with cardiac disease, *J Am Coll Cardiol* 32:840, 1998.
5. Pulmonary Artery Catheter Consensus Conference Participants: Pulmonary artery catheter consensus conference: consensus statement, *Crit Care Med* 25(6):910-925, 1997.
6. Robin ED: The cult of the Swan-Ganz catheter, *Ann Intern Med* 103:445-449, 1985.
7. Sandham JD, Hull RD, Brant RF, et al: A randomized, controlled trial of the use of pulmonary-artery catheters in high-risk surgical patients, *N Engl J Med* 348:5, 2003.
8. Shah MR, Hasselblad V, Stevenson LW, et al: Impact of the pulmonary artery catheter in critically ill patients: meta-analysis of randomized clinical trials, *JAMA* 294:1664, 2005.
9. Sharkey SW: Beyond the wedge: clinical physiology and the Swan Ganz catheter, *Am J Med* 83:111-122, 1987.
10. Sise MJ, Hollingsworth P, Brimm JE, et al: Complications of the flow-directed pulmonary-artery catheter: a prospective analysis of 219 patients, *Crit Care Med* 9:315-318, 1981.
11. Walston A, Kendall ME: Comparison of pulmonary wedge and left atrial pressure in man, *Am Heart J* 86:159-164, 1973.
12. Zipes DP, Libby P, Bonow RO, Braunwald E: *Braunwald's heart disease*, Philadelphia, 2005, Saunders.

CHAPTER 12

CARDIAC CATHETERIZATION AND ANGIOGRAPHY

Glenn N. Levine, MD, FACC, FAHA

1. **What are generally accepted indications for cardiac catheterization?**
   Although recommendations are consistently evolving, those listed here are generally accepted as reasonable indications for cardiac catheterization. Cardiac catheterization is a relatively safe procedure; however, life-threatening complications can rarely occur (see later), so there needs to be a clearly thought out and documented indication for catheterization and a plan for how to use the information obtained during catheterization for patient management.
   - Class III-IV angina despite medical treatment or intolerance of medical therapy
   - High-risk results on noninvasive stress testing
   - Sustained (more than 30 seconds) monomorphic ventricular tachycardia or nonsustained (less than 30 seconds) polymorphic ventricular tachycardia
   - Sudden cardiac death survivors
   - Most patients with non–ST-segment elevation acute coronary syndrome (NSTE-ACS) who have high-risk features and no contraindications to early cardiac catheterization and revascularization
   - Systolic dysfunction and stress testing results suggesting multivessel disease and potential benefit from revascularization
   - Recurrent typical angina within 9 months of percutaneous coronary revascularization
   - For assessment of valvular dysfunction or other hemodynamic assessment when the results of echocardiography are indeterminate
   - As part of primary percutaneous coronary intervention (PCI) for ST-segment elevation myocardial infarction (STEMI)
   - Patients s/p STEMI (with or without thrombolytic therapy) with high-risk features, depressed ejection fraction, or high-risk results on subsequent stress testing
   - Within 36 hours of STEMI in appropriate patients who develop cardiogenic shock
   - In select patients who are to undergo valve replacement/repair

2. **What are the risks of cardiac catheterization?**
   The risks of cardiac catheterization will depend to some extent on the individual patient. For "all comers," the risk of death is approximately 1 in 1000, with the risk of myocardial infarction or stroke rarer than 1 in 1000. The risk of any major complication in "all comers" is approximately 2%. These risks are summarized in Table 12-1.

3. **How are coronary lesions assessed?**
   Coronary lesions are most commonly assessed in day-to-day practice based on subjective visual impression (Fig. 12-1). Lesions are subjectively given a percent stenosis, ideally based on ocular assessment of at least two orthogonal images of the lesion. Studies have shown interobserver and intraobserver variability in judging coronary stenosis from as little as 7% to as much as 50%. Quantitative coronary angiography (QCA) more objectively assesses the lesion severity than "ocular judgment" but is not commonly used in day-to-day practice. QCA generally grades lesions as less severe than subjective ocular judgment of a lesion's severity. Intravascular ultrasound (IVUS) can more accurately assess the total plaque burden and severity of a lesion than ocular judgment or QCA. IVUS is often used when the results of angiography alone still leave doubt as to the "significance" of the lesion (Fig. 12-2).

TABLE 12-1. RISKS OF CARDIAC CATHETERIZATION AND CORONARY ANGIOGRAPHY

Complication	Risk (%)
Mortality	0.11
Myocardial infarction	0.05
Cerebrovascular accident	0.07
Arrhythmia	0.38
Vascular complications	0.43
Contrast reaction	0.37
Hemodynamic complications	0.26
Perforation of heart chamber	0.03
Other complications	0.28
Total of major complications	1.70

(From Scanlon PJ, Faxon DP, Audet AM, et al: ACC/AHA guidelines for coronary angiography: a report of the American College of Cardiology/American Heart Association Task Force on Practice Guidelines [Committee on Coronary Angiography], *J Am Coll Cardiol* 33:1760, 1999.)

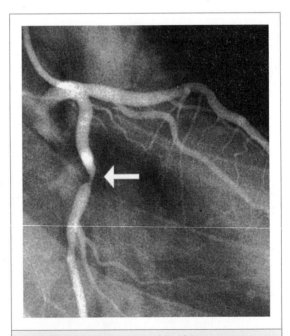

Figure 12-1. Coronary angiography of the left coronary artery demonstrates an approximate 90% lesion *(arrow)* in the left coronary artery.

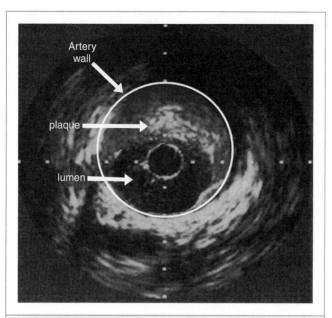

Figure 12-2. Intravascular ultrasound (IVUS) demonstrating plaque occluding greater than 60% of the arterial lumen. Coronary angiography had demonstrated only mild narrowing in this segment of coronary artery.

4. **What is considered a "significant" stenosis?**
   The classification of *significant stenosis* depends on the clinical context and what one considers "significant." Coronary flow reserve (the increase in coronary blood flow in response to agents that lead to microvascular dilation) begins to decrease when a coronary artery stenosis is 50% or more of the luminal diameter. However, basal coronary flow does not begin to decrease until the lesion is 80% to 90% of the luminal diameter.

5. **During cardiac catheterization, how is aortic or mitral regurgitation graded?**
   For aortic regurgitation, an aortogram is performed in the ascending thoracic aorta above the aortic valve and the amount of contrast that regurgitates in to the left ventricle is noted. For mitral regurgitation, a left ventriculogram is performed and the amount of contrast that regurgitates in to the left atrium is noted. The systems used to grade the degree of regurgitation are similar for the two valvular abnormalities, and based on a 1+ to 4+ system, where 1+ is little if any regurgitation and 4+ is profound or severe regurgitation. Regurgitation of 3+ or 4+ is often considered "surgical" regurgitation, although the criteria for surgery are more complex than this (see Chapters 32 and 33 on aortic valve disease and on mitral valve disease). Table 12-2 summarizes the grading of regurgitant lesions as assessed by cardiac catheterization and "ballpark" regurgitant fractions for each degree of regurgitation.

6. **What is TIMI flow grade?**
   Thrombolysis in myocardial infarction (TIMI) flow grade is a system for qualitatively describing blood flow down a coronary artery. It was originally derived to describe blood flow down the

TABLE 12-2. VISUAL ASSESSMENT OF VALVULAR REGURGITATION AND APPROXIMATE CORRESPONDING REGURGITANT FRACTION*

Visual Appearance of Regurgitation	Designated Grading/Severity of Valvular Regurgitation	Approximate Corresponding Regurgitant Fraction
Minimal regurgitant jet seen; clears rapidly from proximal chamber with each beat	1+	<20%
Moderate opacification of proximal chamber, clearing with subsequent beats	2+	21%–40%
Intense opacification of proximal chamber, becoming equal to that of the distal chamber	3+	41%–60%
Intense opacification of proximal chamber, becoming more dense than that of the distal chamber; opacification often persists over entire series of images obtained	4+	>60%

*These regurgitant fraction values are dependent on numerous factors and should be taken only as rough estimates.

Adapted from Davidson CJ, Bonow RO: Cardiac catheterization. In Libby P, Bonow R, Mann D, et al: *Braunwald's heart disease: a textbook of cardiovascular medicine*, ed 8, Philadelphia, 2008, Saunders.

infarct-related artery in patients with STEMI. Reportedly it was originally written down on a napkin or the back of an envelope during an airplane flight. The grades are based on observing contrast flow down the coronary artery after injection of the contrast, and are as follows:

- TIMI grade 3: normal flow down the entire artery
- TIMI grade 2: contrast (blood) flows through the entire artery but at a delayed rate compared with flow in a normal (TIMI grade 3 flow) artery
- TIMI grade 1: contrast (blood) flows beyond the area of vessel occlusion but without perfusion of the distal coronary artery and coronary bed
- TIMI grade 0: complete occlusion of the infarct-related artery

7. **What are the different methods of describing the aortic transvalvular gradient in a patient undergoing cardiac catheterization for the evaluation of aortic stenosis?**

Three terms are variably used. Figure 12-3 illustrates these terms and what they imply.

- *Peak instantaneous gradient:* The maximal pressure difference between the left ventricular pressure and aortic pressure assessed at the exact same time
- *Peak-to-peak gradient:* The difference between the maximal left ventricular pressure and the maximal aortic pressure
- *Mean gradient:* The integral of the pressure difference between the left ventricle and the aorta during systole

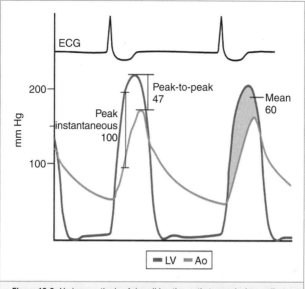

Figure 12-3. Various methods of describing the aortic transvalvular gradient. (From Bashore TM: *Invasive cardiology: principles and techniques,* Philadelphia, 1990, BC Decker, p. 258.)

8. **Which patients should be premedicated to prevent allergic reactions to iodine-based contrast?**

   In patients with a history of prior true allergic reaction (e.g., hives, urticaria, bronchoconstriction) to iodine-based contrast, the risk of repeat anaphylactoid reaction to contrast agents is reported to be 17% to 35%. Such patients should be premedicated before angiography. The usual regimen is 60 mg orally (PO) of prednisone the night before and morning of the procedure and 50 mg oral diphenhydramine the morning of the procedure. There is actually a surprising dearth of data supporting the belief that previous adverse reactions to shellfish or seafood are associated with increased risk of future anaphylactoid reactions to iodine-based contrast.

9. **What are the major risk factors for contrast nephropathy?**

   Preexisting renal disease and diabetes are the two major risk factors for the development of contrast nephropathy. Preprocedure and postprocedure hydration is the most established method of reducing the risk of contrast nephropathy. Regimens vary, but one suggested regimen is ½ normal saline at 1 ml/kg of body weight beginning 12 hours preprocedure and continuing until 12 hours postprocedure. Acetylcysteine (Mucomyst) probably has at best modest protective effects (if any at all). However, given its low risk of side effects, many practitioners will use it in high-risk patients. The most common dosing regimen is 600 mg PO twice a day (BID) the day before and day of the procedure. Small studies have suggested that sodium bicarbonate infusion or ultrafiltration may be of benefit in select high-risk patients.

10. **What are the major vascular complications with cardiac catheterization?**

    In general, major vascular complications are uncommon with diagnostic cardiac catheterization and more common with percutaneous coronary intervention, which often requires larger sheath placement, venous sheath placement, and more intense or prolonged anticoagulation. Nevertheless, practitioners and patients should be aware of the following potential vascular complications:

- **Retroperitoneal hematoma:** This should be suspected in cases of flank, abdominal, or back pain, with unexplained hypotension, or with a marked decrease in hematocrit. Diagnosis is by computed tomography (CT) scan.
- **Pseudoaneurysm:** A pseudoaneurysm results from the failure of the puncture site to seal properly. Pseudoaneurysm is a communication between the femoral artery and the overlying fibromuscular tissue, resulting in a blood-filled cavity. Pseudoaneurysm is suggested by the finding of groin tenderness, palpable pulsatile mass, or new bruit in the groin area. Pseudoaneurysm is diagnosed by Doppler flow imaging.
- **Arterovenous (AV) fistula:** An AV fistula can result from sheath-mediated communication between the femoral artery and the femoral vein. AV fistula is suggested by the presence of a systolic and diastolic bruit in the groin area. Diagnosis is confirmed by Doppler ultrasound.
- **Stroke:** Stroke may be due to many factors. A proportion of strokes may be due to embolization of atherosclerotic material in the aorta.
- **Cholesterol Emboli Syndrome:** This is a rare and potentially catastrophic complication that results from plaque disruption in the aorta, with distal embolization in to the kidneys, lower extremities, and other organs.

11. **What is intracardiac echo?**
    Intracardiac echo (ICE) is the direct imaging of cardiac structures via transvenous insertion of a miniaturized echo probe. Most commonly, the device is inserted via the femoral vein and threaded up to the right atrium. ICE is used to visualize the interatrial septum and fossa ovalis, aiding with transseptal puncture, percutaneous treatment of atrial septal defect (ASD) or patent foramen ovale (PFO), and during electrophysiolgocial procedures, imaging the fossa ovalis and pulmonary veins.

BIBLIOGRAPHY, SUGGESTED READINGS, AND WEBSITES

1. Carrozza JP: Complications of Diagnostic Cardiac Catheterization: http://www.uptodate.com
2. Kern MJ: Quantitative Coronary Arteriography: Clinical applications: http://www.uptodate.com
3. Olade R, Safi A, Kesari S: Cardiac Catheterization (Left Heart): http://www.emedicine.com
4. Baim DS: *Grossman's cardiac catheterization, angiography, and intervention*, ed 7, Philadelphia, 2005, Lippincott Williams & Wilkins.
5. Davidson CJ, Bonow RO: Cardiac catheterization. In Libby P, Bonow R, Mann D, et al, editors: *Braunwald's heart disease: a textbook of cardiovascular medicine*, ed 8, Philadelphia, Saunders, 2008.
6. Kern MJ: *The cardiac catheterization handbook*, ed 4, St. Louis, 2007, Mosby.
7. Levine GN, Kern MJ, Berger PB, et al: Management of patients undergoing percutaneous coronary revascularization, *Ann Intern Med* 139: 123-136, 2003.
8. Scanlon PJ, Faxon DP, Audet AM, et al: ACC/AHA guidelines for coronary angiography, *J Am Coll Cardiol* 33(6): 1756-824, 1999.

III. CHEST PAINS, ANGINA, CAD, AND ACUTE CORONARY SYNDROMES

CHAPTER 13

CHEST PAINS AND ANGINA

Glenn N. Levine, MD, FACC, FAHA

1. Are most ER visits for chest pain caused by acute coronary syndromes?
No. Acute coronary syndromes (e.g., unstable angina, myocardial infarction) account for only a small percentage of emergency room (ER) visits for chest pain. Depending on the study, only a small percentage of patients (1%–11%) will be diagnosed as having chest pains caused by coronary artery disease (CAD) or acute coronary syndrome (ACS). *ACS* is the term now used to describe the continuum of syndromes that include *unstable angina* and *myocardial infarction* (MI).

2. What are the other important causes of chest pains besides chronic stable angina and acute coronary syndrome?
The differential for chest pains include the following:
- Aortic dissection
- Severe aortic stenosis
- Hypertrophic cardiomyopathy
- Printzmetal's angina
- Cardiac syndrome X
- Hypertensive crisis
- Musculoskeletal pain and cervical radiculopathies
- Pleurisy
- Pericarditis
- Pneumonia
- Pneumothorax
- Pulmonary embolism
- Gastrointestinal (GI) causes (reflux, esophagitis, esophageal spasm, peptic ulcer disease, gallbladder disease, and esophageal rupture [Boerhaave's syndrome])
- Dermatologic (such as shingles)

It is important not to assume that all chest pains are due to angina or ACS, even if someone else has made such a preliminary diagnosis. This is particularly important as time-to-diagnosis is critical for aortic dissection, where the mortality rate increases by approximately 1% every hour from presentation to diagnosis and treatment. Additionally, the treatment of aortic dissection is dramatically different from the treatment of ACS, and anticoagulation is contraindicated with aortic dissection.

3. Does an elevated troponin level make the diagnosis ACS?
Not necessarily. Although troponin elevations are fairly sensitive and specific for myocardial necrosis, it is well known that other conditions can also be associated with elevations in cardiac troponins. Importantly, troponin elevation can occur with pulmonary embolus and is in fact associated with a worse prognosis in cases of pulmonary embolus in which the troponin levels are elevated. Myopericarditis (inflammation of the myocardium and pericardium) may also cause elevated troponin levels. In addition, aortic dissection that involves the right coronary artery may lead to secondary myocardial infarction. Further, troponins may be modestly chronically elevated in patients with severe chronic kidney disease.

4. **What is angina?**
   Angina is the term used to denote the discomfort associated with myocardial ischemia or myocardial infarction. Angina occurs when myocardial oxygen demand exceeds myocardial oxygen supply, usually as a result of a severely stenotic or occluded coronary artery. Patients with angina most commonly describe a *chest pain, chest pressure,* or *chest tightness* sensation. They may also use words such as *heaviness, discomfort, squeezing,* or *suffocating.* The discomfort is more commonly over a fist or larger sized region than just a pinpoint (though this distinction is not enough to confidently distinguish anginal from nonanginal pain in itself). The discomfort classically occurs over the left precordium but may manifest as right-sided chest discomfort, retrosternal discomfort, or discomfort in other areas of the chest. Some persons may experience the discomfort only in the upper back, in the arm or arms, or in the neck or jaw.

5. **What are the associated symptoms that persons with angina may experience in addition to chest discomfort?**
   Patients with angina may experience one or more of the following symptoms. Some patients do not experience classic chest discomfort, but instead manifest only one or more of these associated symptoms.
   - Shortness of breath
   - Diaphoresis
   - Nausea
   - Radiating pains. Patients may describe pains or discomfort that *radiate* to the back (typically midscapula), the neck, the jaw, or down one or both arms. They may also describe a *numbness*-type sensation in the arm.

6. **What are the major risk factors for coronary artery disease?**
   - Family history of premature coronary artery disease. This is traditionally defined as a father, mother, brother, or sister who first developed clinical CAD at age younger than 45 to 55 years for men and at age younger than 55 to 60 for women.
   - Hypercholesterolemia
   - Hypertension
   - Cigarette smoking
   - Diabetes mellitus

   Other factors that have been associated with an increased risk of CAD include inactivity (lack of regular exercise), elevated C-reactive protein, and obesity (specifically, large abdominal girth).

7. **What symptoms and findings make it more (or less) likely that the patient's chest pains are due to angina (or that the patient has acute coronary syndrome)?**
   The answer to this question is given below. Tables 13-1 and 13-2 are taken from an excellent review article on this subject in the *Journal of the American Medical Association (JAMA)* and summarize many of the relevant questions and value of the chest pain characteristics in distinguishing angina and ACS/MI pain from other causes.
   - **Quality and characteristics of the chest discomfort:** Patients who describe a chest *tightness* or *pressure* are more likely to have angina. Pain that is stabbing, pleuritic, positional or reproducible is less likely to be angina and is often categorized as *atypical chest pain,* although the presence of such symptoms does not 100% rule out that the pain may be due to coronary artery disease. Although it is generally accepted that a more diffuse area of discomfort is suggestive of angina, whereas a coin-sized, very focal area of discomfort is more likely to be noncardiac, this distinction in itself is not enough to confidently dismiss very focal pain as noncardiac. The severity of the pain or discomfort is not helpful in distinguishing angina from other causes of chest pain. Chest pain that is sudden in onset and maximal intensity at onset is suggestive of aortic dissection. Patients

Continued on p. 98.

TABLE 13-1.   SPECIFIC DETAILS OF THE CHEST PAIN HISTORY HELPFUL IN DISTINGUISHING ANGINAL CHEST PAIN IN PATIENTS WITH MYOCARDIAL INFARCTION FROM NONCARDIAC CAUSES

Element	Question	Comments
Chest Pain Characteristics		
Quality	In your own words, how would you describe the pain? What adjectives would you use?	Pay attention to language and cultural considerations; use interpreter if necessary.
Location	Point with your finger to where you are feeling the pain.	Can elicit size of chest pain area with the same question.
Radiation	If the pain moves out of your chest, trace where it travels with your finger.	Patient may need to point to examiner's scapula or back.
Size of area or distribution	With your finger, trace the area on your chest where the pain occurs.	Focus on distinguishing between a small coin-sized area and a larger distribution.
Severity	If 10 is the most severe pain you have ever had, on this 10-point scale, how severe was this pain?	Patient may need to be coached in this: pain of fetal delivery, kidney stone, bony fracture are good references for 10.
Time of onset and is it continuing	Is the pain still present? Has it gotten better or worse since it began? When did it begin?	Ongoing pain a concern: it is worthwhile to obtain an initail ECG while pain is present.
Duration	Does the pain typically last seconds, minutes, or hours? Roughly, how long is a typical episode?	Focus on the most recent (especially if ongoing) and the most severe episode; be precise: if the patient says "seconds," tap out 4 seconds.
First occurrence	When is the first time you ever had this pain?	Interest should focus on this recent episode, that is, the last few days or weeks.
Frequency	How many times per hour or per day has it been occuring?	Relevant only for recurring pain: a single index episode is not uncommon.
Similar to previous cardiac ischemic episodes	If you have had a heart attack or angina in the past, is this pain similar to the pain you had then? Is it more or less severe?	Follow-up questions elicit how the diagnosis of CAD was confirmed and whether any intervention occurred.
Precipitating or Aggravating Factors		
Pleuritic	Is the pain worse if you take a deep breath or cough?	Distinguish between whether these maneuvers only partially or completely reproduce the pain and if it reproduces the pain only some or all of the time.
Positional	Is the pain made better or worse by your changing body position? If so, what position makes the pain better or worse?	Distinguish between whether these maneuvers only partially or completely reproduce the pain: on physical examination, turn the chest wall, shoulder, and back.

(Continued)

TABLE 13-1. SPECIFIC DETAILS OF THE CHEST PAIN HISTORY HELPFUL IN DISTINGUISHING ANGINAL CHEST PAIN IN PATIENTS WITH MYOCARDIAL INFARCTION FROM NONCARDIAC CAUSES (CONTINUED)

Element	Question	Comments
Palpable	If I press on your chest wall, does that reproduce the pain?	Distinguish between whether these maneuvers only partially or completely reproduce the pain: ask the patient to lead you to the area of pain; then palpate.
Exercise	Does the pain come back or get worse if you walk quickly, climb stairs, or extert yourself?	Helpful to quantify a change in pattern, e.g., the number of stairs or distance walked before the pain began.
Emotional stress	Does becoming upset affect the pain?	Are there other stress-related symptoms, e.g., acroparesthesias?
Relieving factors	Are there any things that you can do to relieve the pain, once it has begun?	In particular, ask about response to nitrates, antacids, ceasing strenuous activity.
Associated symptoms	Do you typically get other symptoms when you get this chest pain?	After asking question in open-ended way, ask specifically about nausea or vomiting and about sweating.

CAD, coronary artery disease; *ECG*, electrocardiogram.

Adapted from Swap CJ, et al: Specific details of the chest pain history, *JAMA* 294:2623-2629, 2005.

with aortic dissection may describe the pain as *tearing* or *ripping* and may describe pain radiating to the back.

- **Duration of the discomfort:** Angina usually lasts on the order of minutes, not seconds or hours (unless the patient is suffering a myocardial infarction) or days. Typically, patients will describe the anginal pain as lasting approximately 5 to 30 minutes. Pain that truly lasts just several seconds is usually not angina, though one has to be careful because some patients will initially describe the pain as lasting seconds when on further questioning it becomes clear it has really lasted minutes. Pain that lasts continuously (not off and on) for a day or days is usually not angina.
- **The Levine sign:** The Levine sign (pronounced *La Vine*, and no relationship to this book's editor) is when the patient spontaneously clenches his or her fist and puts it over the chest while describing the chest discomfort.
- **Precipitating factors:** Because angina results from a mismatch between myocardial oxygen demand and supply, activities that increase myocardial oxygen demand or decrease supply may cause angina. Discomfort that is brought on by exercise or exertion is highly suggestive of angina. Mental stress or anger may not only increase heart rate and blood pressure but may also lead to coronary artery vasoconstriction, precipitating angina. One has to be careful in not ruling out angina as the cause of the chest discomfort in patients who experience chest discomfort at rest, without precipitation, however, as this may be due to acute coronary syndrome, where the problem is primarily thrombus formation in the coronary artery, leading to decreased myocardial oxygen supply.

TABLE 13-2. VALUE OF SPECIFIC COMPONENTS OF THE CHEST PAIN HISTORY FOR THE DIAGNOSIS OF ACUTE MYOCARDIAL INFARCTION (AMI)

Pain Descriptor	Positive Likelihood Ratio (95% CI)
Increased Likelihood of AMI	
Radiation to right arm or shoulder	4.7 (1.9–12)
Radiation to both arms or shoulders	4.1 (2.5–6.5)
Associated with exertion	2.4 (1.5–3.8)
Radiation to left arm	2.3 (1.7–3.1)
Associated with diaphoresis	2.0 (1.9–2.2)
Associated with nausea or vomiting	1.9 (1.7–2.3)
Worse than previous angina or similar to previous MI	1.8 (1.6–2.0)
Described as pressure	1.3 (1.2–1.5)
Decreased Likelihood of AMI	
Described as pleuritic	0.2 (0.1–0.3)
Described as positional	0.3 (0.2–0.5)
Described as sharp	0.3 (0.2–0.5)
Reproducible with palpation	0.3 (0.2–0.4)
Inframammary location	0.8 (0.7–0.9)
Not associated with exertion	0.8 (0.6–0.9)

AMI, acute myocardial infarction; *CI*, confidence interval.

Adapted from Swap CJ, et al: Value of specific components of the chest pain history for the diagnosis of acute myocardial infarction (AMI), *JAMA* 294:2623-2629, 2005.

- **Relief with sublingual nitroglycerin (SL NTG) or rest:** Nitroglycerin is a coronary artery vasodilator. Patients who report partial or complete relief of their chest discomfort within 2 to 5 minutes of taking SL NTG are more likely to be experiencing angina as the cause of their chest discomfort. One has to question patients carefully because some will report that the SL NTG decreased their discomfort, but on further questioning one learns that the discomfort only decreased 30 to 60 minutes after taking the SL NTG. Because SL NTG exerts its effect within minutes, this does not necessarily imply that the chest discomfort was *relieved* by the SL NTG. However, in patients experiencing myocardial infarction caused by an occluded coronary artery, the fact that the chest discomfort is not relieved with SL NTG does not necessarily make it less likely that the pain is due to coronary artery disease. Patients who describe that when they experience the chest discomfort, they then sit or rest for minutes and the chest discomfort gradually resolves, are more likely to have angina.
- **Probability of having CAD:** In patients with multiple risk factors for CAD or with known CAD, the occurrence of chest pains is more likely to be due to angina.
- **Associated symptoms:** The presence of one or more associated symptoms, such as shortness of breathe, diaphoresis, nausea, or radiating pain, increase the likelihood that the discomfort is due to angina.

- **Electrocardiogram (ECG) abnormalities:** ST-segment depressions or elevations, or T-wave inversions, increase the likelihood that the discomfort is due to angina. However, the lack of these findings should not rule out angina as a cause of the chest discomfort. The initial ECG has only a 20% to 60% sensitivity for myocardial infarction, let alone merely the presence of coronary artery disease.
- **Troponin elevation:** The finding of an elevated troponin level significantly increases the likelihood that the discomfort is due to angina and CAD. However, the lack of an elevated troponin does not rule out angina and CAD as a cause of the discomfort. Further, as discussed earlier, other conditions besides angina can cause an elevated troponin.

8. **If one is still in doubt as to the diagnosis of CAD, should a stress test be obtained?**
Yes. Stress testing for diagnostic purposes is best in patients who, after initial evaluation, have an intermediate probability of having CAD. For example, in a patient with a pretest probability of having CAD of 50%, a *positive* exercise stress test makes the post-test probability of CAD 83%, whereas a *negative* exercise stress test makes the post-test probability of CAD just 36%. Stress testing may also be used for prognostic purposes. Stress testing is discussed in greater detail in the chapters on exercise stress testing (Chapter 7), nuclear cardiology (Chapter 8), echocardiography (Chapter 6), and magnetic resonance imaging (Chapter 9). Coronary computed tomography (CT) angiography is an emerging alternate form of diagnosis and is discussed in Chapter 10.

9. **Can one be sure that patients with chest pains, without typical anginal symptoms, do not have coronary artery disease?**
No! It is well known that women often do not present with *typical* anginal symptoms. In fact, women are often misdiagnosed because of a lower suspicion by doctors that they have coronary artery disease and the fact that they often experience discomfort that is not *classic* for angina. Older patients may have difficulty in remembering or describing their chest discomfort and so also may not describe *classic* anginal symptoms. Some diabetic patients appear to have an impaired sensation of chest discomfort when the heart experiences myocardial ischemia. Thus, some diabetic patients may not report chest discomfort but rather only one or more associated symptoms, such as shortness of breath or diaphoresis.

10. **Who first described angina, and when?**
This question is in here primarily so you can *pimp* your attending for a change! The association between chest pain (angina pectoris) and heart disease was first described by Heberden in 1772. He described this sensation of a *strangling sensation in the chest*.

11. **What is Prinzmetal's angina?**
Prinzmetal's angina, also called *variant angina*, is an unusual type of angina caused by coronary vasospasm. The coronary artery is believed to spasm, severely reducing myocardial oxygen supply to the affected myocardium. Although the spasm can occur in either a *normal* or a diseased coronary artery, it most commonly occurs within 1 cm of an atherosclerotic plaque. Prinzmetal's angina usually does not occur with physical exertion or stress but occurs during rest, most typically between midnight and 8 AM. The pain can be severe, and if an ECG is obtained during an episode, it may demonstrate ST-segment elevations. Patients with Prinzmetal's angina are typically younger, often female. Treatment is based primarily on the use of calcium channel blockers, as well as nitrates.

12. **What is cardiac syndrome X?**
Cardiac syndrome X is an entity in which patients describe epicardial exertional anginal symptoms, yet are found on cardiac catheterization to have nondiseased *normal* coronary arteries. They may also have ST-segment depressions on exercise stress testing and even

perfusion defects with nuclear stress testing. Unlike Prinzmetal's angina, they do not have spontaneous coronary spasm and do not have provocable coronary spasm. Although there are likely multiple causes and explanations for cardiac syndrome X, it does appear that, at least in some patients, microvascular coronary artery constriction or dysfunction plays a role. Treatment is usually individually tailored to the patient; no one standardized recipe has been established.

BIBLIOGRAPHY, SUGGESTED READINGS, AND WEBSITES

1. Alaeddini J: Angina Pectoris: http://www.emedicine.com
2. Chest Pain: Approach to the Cardiac Patient: http://www.merck.com/mmpe
3. Delehanty JM: Cardiac Syndrome X: Angina Pectoris with Normal Coronary Arteries: http://www.utdol.com
4. Delehanty JM: Variant Angina: http://www.utdol.com
5. Meisel JL: Diagnostic Approach to Chest Pains in Adults: http://www.utdol.com
6. Warnica JW: Angina Pectoris: http://www.merck.com/mmpe
7. Cohn JK, Cohn PF: Chest pain, *Circulation* 106:530, 2002.
8. Haro LH, Decker WW, Boie ET, et al: Initial approach to the patient who has chest pain, *Cardiol Clin* 24(1):1-17, 2006.
9. Lanza GA: Cardiac syndrome X: a critical overview and future perspectives, *Heart* 93:159-166, 2007.
10. Mayer S, Hillis LD: Prinzmetal's variant angina, *Clin Cardiol* 21:243-246, 1998.
11. Ringstrom E, Freedman J: Approach to undifferentiated chest pain in the emergency department: a review of recent medical literature and published practice guidelines, *Mt Sinai J Med* 73(2):499-505, 2006.
12. Swap CJ, Nagurney JT: Value and limitations of chest pain history in the evaluation of patients with suspected acute coronary syndromes, *JAMA* 23:294(20):2623-2629, 2005.

CHAPTER 14

CHRONIC STABLE ANGINA

Glenn N. Levine, MD, FACC, FAHA

1. **What is the most common cause of angina?**
   Angina is the sensation of discomfort experienced during periods of myocardial ischemia or myocardial infarction. It may occur when myocardial oxygen demand exceeds myocardial oxygen supply. Myocardial ischemia and angina are most commonly the result of significant stenosis of one or more coronary arteries. Typically, coronary artery stenosis that is 70% or more of the coronary artery diameter is flow restricting and may cause angina. In patients with chronic stable angina, myocardial ischemia results when myocardial oxygen demand increases, such as during physical exertion. Coronary vasoconstriction, particularly at the site of a preexisting stenosis, can also contribute to myocardial ischemia and produce angina.

2. **What other conditions can cause anginal pain?**
   - Aortic stenosis
   - Hypertrophic cardiomyopathy
   - Hypertensive crisis
   - Tachyarrhythmias and tachycardia (such as caused by hyperthyroidism)
   - Coronary artery anomaly
   - Severe anemia (as a result of decreased oxygen-carrying capacity of the blood)
   - Severe hypoxemia
   - Coronary vasospasm (Prinzmetal's angina or cocaine induced)
   - Cardiac syndrome X

3. **How is chronic stable angina classified or graded?**
   The most commonly used system is the Canadian Cardiovascular Society system, in which angina is graded on a scale of I to IV. These grades and this system are described in Box 14-1.

4. **What are the three primary antianginal medications used for the treatment of chronic stable angina?**
   - Beta-blockers
   - Nitrates
   - Calcium channel blockers

5. **What are the principal issues regarding the use of beta-blockers?**
   The most commonly used beta-blockers are metoprolol and atenolol, although many others are used. Both generic and brand names are available for many of these agents. Beta-blockers' principal effects are negative chronotropic (slow heart rate) and, to a variable extent, negative inotropic (decrease cardiac contractility). Both these actions serve to decrease cardiac oxygen demand. Beta-blockers are usually started at a low dose, then titrated upward as tolerated. Primary side effects include excessive bradycardia, prolongation of the PR interval and heart block, exacerbation of congestive heart failure, and exacerbation of severe reactive airway disease. Thus, generally they are not initiated in patients with baseline bradycardia, significantly prolonged PR interval (more than 220–240 msec), acute decompensated heart failure as a result of systolic dysfunction, and severe reactive airway disease. In general, the dose is titrated to control of symptoms or resting heart rate in the 60s (beats/min).

> ## BOX 14-1. GRADING OF ANGINA PECTORIS BY THE CANADIAN CARDIOVASCULAR SOCIETY CLASSIFICATION SYSTEM
>
> ### Class I
>
> Ordinary physical activity, such as walking and climbing stairs, does not cause angina. Angina occurs with strenuous, rapid, or prolonged exertion at work or recreation.
>
> ### Class II
>
> Slight limitation of ordinary activity. Angina occurs on walking or climbing stairs rapidly, walking uphill, walking or stair climbing after meals, in cold, in wind, under emotional stress, or only during the few hours after awakening. Angina occurs on walking more than two blocks on level ground and climbing more than one flight of ordinary stairs at a normal pace and in normal condition.
>
> ### Class III
>
> Marked limitations of ordinary physical activity. Angina occurs on walking one to two blocks on level ground and climbing one flight of stairs in normal conditions and at a normal pace.
>
> ### Class IV
>
> Inability to carry on any physical activity without discomfort—anginal symptoms may be present at rest.
>
> Modified from Ferri FF: *Ferri's clinical advisor, 2008*, Philadelphia, 2008, Mosby.

6. **When should one primarily use a peripherally acting calcium channel blocker (amlodipine or felodipine), and when should one use a calcium channel blocker that has effects on both the heart and the periphery (verapamil, diltiazem)?**
Amlodipine and felodipine are used primarily as second- or third-line antianginal agents in patients already on beta-blockers (and often, also long-acting nitrates). They act mainly as vasodilators, lowering blood pressure and likely having some coronary vasodilating effects. Verapamil and diltiazem, in addition to having vasodilating effects, also have negative chronotropic and negative inotropic effects and can block atrioventricular (AV) conduction. Thus, they may be used instead of beta-blockers in patients with severe reactive airway disease. Generally they are not used in patients already on beta-blockers and are contraindicated in patients with depressed ejection fractions (less than 40%) because of their negative inotropic effects and because studies in the 1980s suggested a worse outcome with their use in such patients.

7. **When does one prescribe a long-acting nitrate?**
Long-acting nitrates are often prescribed along with beta-blockers as the initial treatments in patients with chronic stable angina (Table 14-1). A *nitrate-free interval,* usually overnight, is necessary to prevent the development of tolerance to these agents. Once-a-day, long-acting nitrate preparations are ideal in terms of avoidance of nitrate tolerance and patient compliance.

8. **When should one consider using ranolazine?**
Ranolazine is a newer antianginal agent unlike previous agents. It does not work by affecting heart rate or blood pressure or by coronary artery vasodilation. Its mechanism of action is still not completely understood. In clinical trials (MARISA, CARISA, ERICA), it leads to a modest

TABLE 14-1. ANTIANGINAL CLASSES, EFFECTS, SIDE EFFECTS, AND CONTRAINDICATIONS

Class	Effects	Side Effects	Contraindications
Beta-blockers	• Negative chronotropy • Negative inotropy	• Extreme bradycardia • AV node block and PR prolongation • Exacerbation of acute heart failure • Bronchospasm • Blood pressure reduction	• Resting bradycardia • Prolonged PR interval (>220–240 msec) • Acute decompensated heart failure • Severe reactive airway disease • Baseline hypotension
Long-acting nitrates	• Coronary vasodilation • Venodilation	• Headache • Venous pooling	• Use of erectile dysfunction medications
Calcium-channel blockers: verapamil and diltiazem	• Peripheral vasodilation • Coronary vasodilation • Negative chronotropy • Negative inotropy	• Extreme bradycardia • AV node block and PR prolongation • Blood pressure reduction • Exacerbation of chronic and acute heart failure	• Resting bradycardia • Prolonged PR interval (>220–240 msec) • Baseline low blood pressure • Acute decompensated heart failure • Ejection fraction < 40% • Usually, patients already on beta-blockers
Calcium-channel blockers: amlodipine and felodipine	• Peripheral vasodilation • Coronary vasodilation • Coronary vasodilation • No net negative chronotropic or inotropic effects	• Blood pressure reduction • Peripheral edema	• Baseline low blood pressure

increase in exercise tolerance (approximately 30 seconds) and decreases in angina and sublingual nitroglycerin (SL NTG) use. It is generally a third-line agent in patients with continued significant angina despite traditional antianginal therapy. Its major side effect is QT prolongation. Thus, it should not be used in patients with baseline QT prolongation or those on other medications that can prolong the QT interval. Patients initiated on this drug should have their QT duration monitored periodically with 12-lead electrocardiograms (ECGs). The usual starting dose is 500 mg orally twice a day (PO BID), which can be increased to 1000 mg PO BID. Generally this drug should be prescribed only by cardiologists.

9. **Should everyone with chronic stable angina be prescribed sublingual nitroglycerin (or nitroglycerin spray)?**
Yes. This is the standard of care. Patients should be instructed on how to use SL NTG— generally one pill every 5 minutes up to a maximum of three tablets. Patients with chronic stable angina should be instructed to call 911 and seek immediate medical attention if their angina is not relieved after three pills or 15 minutes (or after one pill or 5 minutes in the case of patients with a history of acute coronary syndrome [ACS]).

10. **Which patients with chronic stable angina should be referred for stress testing or cardiac catheterization?**
The two purposes of stress testing are diagnosis of coronary artery disease (CAD) and prognosis in patients with presumed or known CAD. If the pretest likelihood of CAD is extremely high (e.g., a 64-year-old man with multiple cardiac risk factors and classic exertional anginal symptoms has a pretest probability of CAD of at least 94%), there is little diagnostic value in stress testing, because even a *negative* stress test would not significantly change the true probability that the patient has CAD. For example, in patients with a pretest probability of having CAD of 90%, a *negative* exercise stress test lowers the post-test probability of CAD to only 83%.

Many experts and the American College of Cardiology/American Heart Association (ACC/AHA) guidelines on chronic stable angina advocate in many cases obtaining a stress test for prognostic reasons—if the stress test reveals *low-risk* findings, then the patient can be managed medically, whereas if the stress test reveals *high-risk* findings, the patient is referred for cardiac catheterization. Although this latter strategy is often used, it is important to note that percutaneous coronary intervention has never been shown to reduce the risk of myocardial infarction (MI) or death in patients with chronic stable angina. Referral for cardiac catheterization is appropriate if the patient's symptoms cannot be adequately controlled with antianginal medications, the patient develops unstable symptoms, or the patient has a depressed ejection fraction (less than 40%).

Stress testing performed for diagnostic purposes is usually performed with the patient off antianginal therapy, whereas stress testing performed for prognostic purposes may sometimes be performed with the patient on antianginal agents.

11. **What other medications, besides antianginal medications, should patients with chronic stable angina be prescribed?**
   - Sublingual nitroglycerin, as described earlier
   - Aspirin (75–325 mg qD)
   - Statin therapy to lower low-density lipoprotein (LDL) cholesterol levels to less than 70 to 100 mg/dl
   - Angiotensin-converting enzyme (ACE) inhibitor if diabetic, hypertension, chronic kidney disease, and left ventricular ejection fraction is less than 40%, unless contraindicated
   - Clopidogrel after an episode of acute coronary syndrome and after bare-metal stent implantation, usually for 1 year, and after drug-eluting stent implantation for at least 1 year. Other newer antiplatelet agents that block the P2Y12 platelet receptor may be used instead

of clopidogrel at the physician's discretion. The CHARISMA study, which assessed long-term clopidogrel use (in addition to aspirin) in patients with atherosclerosis or with high-risk features, demonstrated no overall benefit of this strategy, although it did show a trend toward benefit in those with preexisting atherosclerosis. However, this latter finding in this subgroup analysis was not statistically significant, and the general approach to indefinitely treating all patients with atherosclerosis with long-term dual antiplatelet treatment has not been embraced by most of the medical community.

- Annual influenza vaccination

12. Is chelation therapy of any benefit in patients with coronary artery disease?
No.

BIBLIOGRAPHY, SUGGESTED READINGS, AND WEBSITES

1. Alaeddini J: Angina Pectoris: http://www.emedicine.com
2. Warnica JW: Angina Pectoris: http://www.merck.com/mmpe
3. 2007 Chronic Angina Focused Update of the ACC/AHA 2002 Guidelines for the Management of Patients with Chronic Stable Angina: http://www.my.americanheart.org
4. ACC/AHA 2002 Guideline Update for the Management of Patients With Chronic Stable Angina: http://www.my.americanheart.org
5. Kannam JP, Aroesty JM, Gersh JB: Overview of the Management of Stable Angina Pectoris: http://www.utdol.com
6. Abrams J: Chronic stable angina, *N Engl J Med* 352;2524-2533, 2005.
7. Bhatt DL, Fox KA, Hacke W, et al: Clopidogrel and aspirin versus aspirin alone for the prevention of atherothrombotic events, *N Engl J Med* 354:1706-1717, 2006.
8. Chaitman BR, Pepine CJ, Parker JO, et al: Effects of ranolazine with atenolol, amlodipine, or diltiazem on exercise tolerance and angina frequency in patients with severe chronic angina: a randomized controlled trial, *JAMA* 21:291:309-316, 2004.
9. Fox K, Garcia MAA, Ardissino D, et al: Guidelines on the management of stable angina pectoris, *Eur Heart J* 27:1341-1381, 2006.

NON–ST-SEGMENT ELEVATION ACUTE CORONARY SYNDROME

Glenn N. Levine, MD, FACC, FAHA

1. **What is non–ST-segment elevation acute coronary syndrome?**

   It is now recognized that unstable angina, non–Q-wave myocardial infarction (MI), non–ST-segment elevation MI, and ST-segment elevation myocardial infarction (STEMI) are all part of a continuum of the pathophysiologic process in which a coronary plaque ruptures, thrombus formation occurs, and partial or complete, transient or more sustained vessel occlusion may occur (Fig. 15-1). This process is deemed acute coronary syndrome when it is clinically recognized and causes symptoms. Acute coronary syndromes can be subdivided for treatment purposes into non–ST-segment elevation acute coronary syndrome (NSTE-ACS) and ST-segment elevation acute coronary syndrome (STE-ACS).

   The American College of Cardiology/American Heart Association (ACC/AHA) guidelines use the terms *unstable angina/non–ST-elevation MI* when referring to patients with NSTE-ACS, whereas the European Society of Cardiology (ESC) guidelines prefers the term *NSTE-ACS*. In this chapter, we will use this latter term, but the reader should recognize that we are also discussing patients who have been referred to as having unstable angina or non–ST-segment-elevation MI.

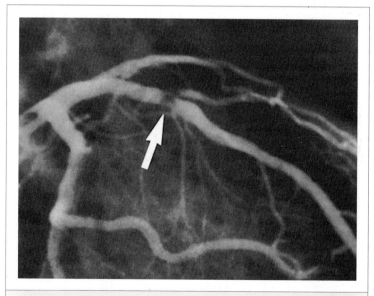

Figure 15-1. Plaque rupture in the proximal left anterior descending (LAD) has led to thrombus formation *(arrow)* and partial occlusion of the vessel. (Reproduced with permission from Cannon CP, Braunwald E: Unstable angina and non-ST elevation myocardial infarction. In Libby P, Bonow R, Mann D, et al: *Braunwald's heart disease: a textbook of cardiovascular medicine*, ed 8, Philadelphia, 2008, Saunders.)

2. **What is the current definition of a myocardial infarction?**
   According to the 2007 joint European Society of Cardiology/American College of Cardiology Foundation/American Heart Association/World Heart Federation statement, the term *myocardial infarction* should be used "when there is evidence of myocardial necrosis in a clinical setting consistent with myocardial ischemia." For patients with acute coronary syndromes, this includes detection of the rise or fall of cardiac biomarkers (preferably troponin) with at least one value above the ninety-ninth percentile of the upper reference limit, together with evidence of myocardial ischemia with at least one of the following:
   - Symptoms of ischemia
   - Electrocardiogram (ECG) changes indicative of new ischemia (new ST-T changes or new left bundle branch block)
   - Development of pathologic Q waves in the ECG
   - Imaging evidence of new loss of viable myocardium or new regional wall motion abnormalities

   Note that using this definition, patients admitted with anginal chest pains and troponin elevations of as little as 0.04 to 0.08 ng/ml may now be diagnosed as having myocardial infarction, depending on locally established ninety-ninth percentile ranges of troponin values.

3. **What other conditions besides epicardial coronary artery disease and acute coronary syndrome can cause elevations in troponin?**
   Although troponins have extremely high myocardial tissue specificity, numerous conditions besides epicardial coronary artery disease and acute coronary syndromes may cause elevations of troponins, including the following:
   - Pulmonary embolism and pulmonary hypertension
   - Acute decompensated heart failure
   - Cardiac contusion
   - Coronary vasospasm
   - Hypertensive crisis
   - "Demand ischemia" (e.g., tachyarrhythmias, hypotension, severe systemic illness, hypertensive crisis)
   - Myocarditis
   - Cardioversion/defibrillation or ablation procedures
   - Renal failure
   - Acute neurologic disease (cerebrovascular accident [CVA], subarachnoid hemorrhage)
   - Infiltrative heart disease
   - Critical illness (sepsis, respiratory failure, burns)
   - Apical ballooning syndrome
   - Aortic dissection

4. **What are the factors that make up the *TIMI Risk Score*?**
   The seven factors that make up the TIMI Risk Score are shown in the list here. Each factor counts as 1 point. A sum score of 0 to 2 is a low TIMI Risk Score and is associated with a 4.7% to 8.3% 2-week risk of adverse cardiac events; a sum score of 3 to 5 is an intermediate TIMI Risk Score and is associated with a 13.2 to 26.2% 2-week risk of adverse cardiac events; and a score of 6 to 7 is a high TIMI Risk Score and is associated with a 40.9% risk of adverse cardiac events.
   - Age greater than 65 years
   - Three or more risk factors for coronary artery disease (CAD)
   - Prior catheterization demonstrating CAD
   - ST-segment deviation
   - Two or more anginal events within 24 hours
   - Acetylsalicylic acid (ASA) use within 7 days
   - Elevated cardiac markers

5. **What are the components of the GRACE ACS Risk Model (at the time of admission)?**

   The components of the Global Registry of Acute Coronary Events (GRACE) ACS Risk Model at the time of admission are given here. Scores are calculated based on established criteria. Calculation algorithms are easily downloadable to computers and handheld devices (http://www. outcomes-umassmed.org/grace/acs_risk.cfm). A low-risk score is considered 108 or less and is associated with a less than 1% risk of in-hospital death. An intermediate score is 109 to 140 and is associated with a 1% to 3% risk of in-hospital death. A high risk score is greater than 140 and associated with a more than 3% risk of in-hospital death.
   - Age
   - Heart rate (HR)
   - Systolic blood pressure (SBP)
   - Creatinine
   - Congestive heart failure Killip class
   - Cardiac arrest at admission (yes/no)
   - ST-segment deviation (yes/no)
   - Elevated cardiac enzymes/markers

6. **What other biomarkers and measured blood levels have been shown to correlate with increased risk of adverse cardiovascular outcome?**

   Multiple biomarkers and measured blood levels, besides creatine kinase–MB (CK-MB) and troponin levels, recently have been shown to be independent predictors of adverse cardiovascular outcome. How these findings should be used in clinical practice is subject to continued investigation and debate. Among such biomarkers and measured blood levels are C-reactive protein (CRP), B-type naturetic peptide (BNP), white blood cell count, myeloperoxidase (MPO), creatinine, and glucose. Additional other markers will no doubt emerge over the next several years.

7. **What do the classification of recommendations actually mean in the guidelines from the American College of Cardiology/American Heart Association (ACC/AHA) and European Society of Cardiology (ESC)?**

   Although the terminology is slightly different between the ACC/AHA and ESC guidelines, the following summarizes the terminology used by these organizations.
   - **Class I:** Procedure/treatment should be performed/administered; evidence and/or general agreement that a given treatment or procedure is beneficial, useful, and effective.
   - **Class IIa:** It is reasonable to perform procedure/administer treatment; the procedure/ treatment is probably recommended or indicated; the weight of evidence/opinion is in favor of usefulness/efficacy.
   - **Class IIb:** Procedure/treatment may be considered; usefulness or efficacy is unknown/ unclear/uncertain or not well established by evidence/opinion.
   - **Class III:** Evidence or general agreement that procedure/treatment should not be performed/administered because it is not helpful and may be harmful.

8. **What does *Level of Evidence,* as used in the guidelines, mean?**

   In addition to giving a class of the recommendation, both the ACC/AHA and ESC classify the level of evidence that supports their class I, IIa, IIb, or III recommendations. Again, the schemes are slightly different, but can be summarized as follows:
   - **Level of Evidence A:** Multiple studies (e.g., randomized trials, meta-analyses, large registries) support the recommendation.
   - **Level of Evidence B:** Limited number of studies or a single randomized trial support the recommendation.
   - **Level of Evidence C:** Single study, retrospective studies, or only registries support the recommendation; recommendation may predominantly be based on *consensus expert opinion*.

9. **What antiplatelet agents are recommended by the ACC/AHA and ESC guidelines?**

Both organizations agree that aspirin should be administered and that in patients with true aspirin allergies or aspirin contraindications, clopidogrel should be administered as a substitute for aspirin. The ACC/AHA recommends that either clopidogrel or a glycoprotein (GP) IIb/IIIa inhibitor (in addition to aspirin) should be administered (and one can consider administering both), whereas the ESC guidelines forcefully recommend that all patients receive clopidogrel (in addition to aspirin) and also recommend the additional use of GP IIb/IIIa inhibitors in intermediate-risk to high-risk patients. The antiplatelet recommendations of the organizations are summarized in Table 15-1. Antiplatelet therapies are discussed further in Chapter 17, Oral and Intravenous Antiplatelet Therapies.

10. **What antithrombin agents are recommended by the ACC/AHA and ESC guidelines?**

The ACC/AHA guidelines give a class I recommendation to unfractionated heparin (UFH), enoxaparin, fondaparinux, and bivalirudin. The ESC guidelines place a strong emphasis on prevention of bleeding complications and preferentially recommend fondaparinux in patients who are not to undergo an *urgent invasive* strategy; for those who undergo an *urgent invasive strategy*, the guidelines give class I recommendations to UFH and bivalirudin and a class IIa recommendation to enoxaparin. The antithrombin recommendations of the organizations are summarized in Table 15-2. Antithrombin therapies are discussed further in Chapter 18, Anticoagulant Therapy.

11. **What is the recommended dosing of unfractionated heparin?**

The dosing recommendations vary slightly between ACC/AHA and ESC, as well as with the American College of Chest Physicians (ACCP).

- ACC/AHA: 60 U/kg bolus (max. 4000 U), then initial infusion of 12 U/kg (max. initial infusion 1000 U/hr). Target anti-Xa 0.3 to 0.7; target activated partial thromboplastin time (aPTT) 1.5 to 2.5 times control (60–80 seconds per ACCP guidelines).
- ESC: 60 to 70 U/kg bolus (max. 5000 U), then initial infusion of 12 to 15 U/kg (initial max. 1000 U/hr). Target aPTT 50 to 75 sec (1.5–2.5 times control).

12. **Which patients with NSTE-ACS should be treated with a strategy of early catheterization and revascularization?**

Early studies (TIMI IIIb, VANQWISH, MATE) performed in the 1980s comparing a strategy of early catheterization and revascularization with a strategy of initial medical therapy failed to show a benefit of the early catheterization and revascularization strategy. More recent studies (e.g., TACTICS, FRISC II, RITA-3, ISAR-COOL) have demonstrated a benefit of a strategy of early catheterization and revascularization in appropriately selected patients. In current practice, *early* is taken to denote within 48 to 72 hours of admission and in real-world practice most commonly occurs *the next day*. Patients who should be treated with this strategy are those without clear contraindications to catheterization and revascularization and with intermediate-risk to high-risk features that place them at elevated risk for clinical events.

The ACC/AHA criteria for elevated risk for clinical events include recurrent angina/ischemia, elevated troponin, ST depression, CHF, high-risk findings on noninvasive testing, hemodynamic instability, sustained ventricular tachycardia (VT), percutaneous coronary intervention (PCI) within 6 months, prior coronary artery bypass graft (CABG), and high risk score (TIMI, GRACE).

The ESC criteria of intermediate to high risk features includes: elevated troponin, dynamic ST or T-wave changes, diastolic murmur (DM), reduced renal function (glomerular filtration rate [GFR] less than 60), ejection fraction (EF) less than 40%, post-MI angina, PCI within the past 6 months, prior CABG, and intermediate to high GRACE risk score.

TABLE 15-1. ACC/AHA AND ESC GUIDELINES FOR ANTIPLATELET THERAPIES IN PATIENTS WITH NSTE-ACS*

I	IIa	IIb	III	
ACC/AHA Guidelines				
A				Aspirin
A				Clopidogrel if ASA allergic/intolerant
A				Clopidogrel in addition to ASA if initial conservative strategy
A				Clopidogrel or GP IIb/IIIa (in addition to ASA) upstream if early invasive strategy
	B			Clopidogrel *and* GP IIb/IIIa (in addition to ASA) upstream if early invasive strategy
	B			Reasonable to omit GP IIb/IIIa if early invasive strategy and patient treated with bivalirudin and with clopidogrel (>6 hr)
	C			For initial conservative strategy, if already on ASA and clopidogrel and has recurrent ischemia, add GP IIb/IIIa
ESC Guidelines				
A				Aspirin
B				Clopidogrel for patients with ASA contraindications
A				Clopidogrel (in addition to ASA) *for all patients* (300 mg, then 75 mg daily)
	B			In patients considered for invasive procedure/PCI, 600 mg loading dose may be used
	A			GP IIb/IIIa (in addition to oral antiplatelet agents) in intermediate-to high-risk patients
A				In high-risk patients not pretreated with GP IIb/IIIa, proceeding to PCI, abciximab recommended
	B			Eptifibatide and tirofiban in this setting are less well established
	B			Bivalirudin may be used as an alternative to GP IIb/IIIa inhibitors plus UFH/LMWH
			C	NSAIDs (nonselective and COX-2) should not be administered in combination with either ASA or clopidogrel
		C		Routine assessment of platelet aggregation inhibition therapy with ASA and/or clopidogrel is not recommended

*The first four columns represent the level of recommendation; the letters *A*, *B*, and *C* within those columns represent the level of evidence supporting the recommendation.

PCI, Percutaneous coronary intervention.

Modified from Anderson JL, Adams CD, Antman EM, et al: ACC/AHA 2007 guidelines for the management of patients with unstable angina/non–ST-elevation myocardial infarction, *J Am Coll Cardiol* 50(7): e1-e157, 2007; and Task Force for Diagnosis and Treatment of Non-ST-Segment Elevation Acute Coronary Syndromes of European Society of Cardiology: guidelines for the diagnosis and treatment of non–ST-segment elevation acute coronary syndromes, *Eur Heart J* 28(13):1598-1660, 2007.

TABLE 15-2. ACC/AHA AND ESC GUIDELINES FOR ANTITHROMBIN THERAPIES IN PATIENTS WITH NSTE-ACS*

I	IIa	IIb	III	
ACC/AHA Guidelines				
A				UFH (early invasive or initial conservative strategies)
A				Enoxaparin (early invasive or initial conservative strategies)
B				Fondaparinux (early invasive or initial conservative strategies)
B				Bivalirudin (early invasive strategy only)
B				Fondaparinux preferred for conservative strategy in patients with increased risk of bleeding
	B			For initial conservative treatment, enoxaparin or fondaparinux preferred over UFH
ESC Guidelines				
B				Anticoagulant should be selected according to risk of both ischaemic and bleeding events
B				Choice of anticoagulant depends on initial strategy
				For "urgent invasive" strategy:
C				▪ UFH
	B			▪ Enoxaparin
B				▪ Bivalirudin
				For "nonurgent situation":
A				▪ Fondaparinux recommended on basis of most favorable efficacy safety profile
	B			▪ Enoxaparin with less favorable efficacy/safety profile than fondaparinux should be used only if bleeding risk low
	B			▪ Other LMWH and UFH cannot be recommended over fondaparinux because of lack of head-to-head data
				At time of PCI, initial anticoagulant should be maintained during procedure for:
C				▪ UFH
	B			▪ Enoxaparin
B				▪ Bivalirudin
B				In conservative treatment, fondaparinux and LMWH may be maintained up to hospital discharge

*The first four columns represent the level of recommendation; the letters *A*, *B*, and *C* within those columns represent the level of evidence supporting the recommendation.

LMWH, Low-molecular-weight heparin.

Modified from Anderson JL, Adams CD, Antman EM, et al: ACC/AHA 2007 guidelines for the management of patients with unstable angina/non–ST-elevation myocardial infarction, *J Am Coll Cardiol* 50(7): e1-e157, 2007; and Task Force for Diagnosis and Treatment of Non-ST-Segment Elevation Acute Coronary Syndromes of European Society of Cardiology: guidelines for the diagnosis and treatment of non–ST-segment elevation acute coronary syndromes, *Eur Heart J* 28(13):1598-660, 2007.

13. **Should patients with diabetes who present with NSTE-ACS be treated with** *up-front* **(e.g., at the time of admission) glycoprotein IIB/IIIA inhibitors?**
Yes. In the ACC/AHA guidelines this is a class I recommendation (level of evidence B), and in the ESC guidelines this is a class IIa recommendation (level of evidence B). These recommendations are based predominantly on subgroup analyses of the GP IIb/IIIa studies performed in the past decade, as well as bench-level research demonstrating that diabetics are more apt to have activated "angry" platelets.

14. **Should nonsteroidal antiinflammatory drugs (NSAIDS) or COX-2 inhibitors (other than aspirin) be continued in patients admitted for NSTE-ACS?**
No. Recent data suggest potential adverse effects of these agents, and it is now recommended to stop such therapy in patients admitted for NSTE-ACS.

15. **Can nitrate therapy be administered to patients currently taking erectile dysfunction agents?**
No. Concurrent use of nitrates and currently available erectile dysfunction (ED) agents may lead to profound hypotension because of increased levels of the vasodilator nitric oxide. Patients who have taken an ED agent should not be treated with nitrates for the following periods:
- **Sildenafil (Viagra):** 24 hours
- **Tadalafil (Cialis):** 48 hours
- **Vardenafil (Levitra):** not established at the time of this writing, but common sense would dictate at least 24 hours and perhaps a little longer

16. **Can statin therapy be safely started in patients admitted with acute coronary syndromes?**
Yes. The Myocardial Ischemia Reduction with Acute Cholesterol Lowering (MIRACL) and Pravastatin or Atorvastatin Evaluation and Infection Therapy—Thrombolysis in Myocardial Infarction (22PROVE IT–TIMI 22) trials demonstrated a very low incidence of liver function test (LFT) elevation and rhabdomyolysis in appropriately selected patients who presented with acute coronary syndrome and were started on high-dose/high-intensity lipid therapy (e.g., atorvastatin 80 mg). Based on these and other studies, it is now recommended that statin therapy, when appropriate, be initiated in hospital.

17. **What are the recommendations regarding drug discontinuation in patients who are to undergo CABG?**
The following recommendations have been made regarding these medications commonly used in patients with NSTE-ACS who are to undergo CABG:
- Discontinue clopidogrel **5 to 7 days** before CABG when possible.
- Discontinue GP IIb/IIIa **4 hours** before CABG.
- Discontinue enoxaparin **12 to 24 hours** before CABG and dose with UFH.
- Discontinue fondaparinux **24 hours** before CABG and dose with UFH.
- Discontinue bivalirudin **3 hours** before CABG and dose with UFH.

BIBLIOGRAPHY, SUGGESTED READINGS, AND WEBSITES

1. Breall JA, Aroesty JM, Simons M: Overview of the Management of Unstable Angina and Acute Non-ST Elevation (Non-Q Wave) Myocardial Infarction: http://www.utdol.com
2. GRACE Risk Calculator: http://www.outcomes-umassmed.org/grace/acs_risk.cfm
3. Tan WA, Moliterno DJ: Unstable Angina: http://www.emedicine.com
4. Anderson JL, Adams CD, Antman EM, et al: ACC/AHA 2007 guidelines for the management of patients with unstable angina/non–ST-elevation myocardial infarction, *J Am Coll Cardiol* 50(7):e1-e157, 2007.

5. Cannon CP, Braunwald E: Unstable angina and non–ST-elevation myocardial infarction. In Libby P, Bonow R, Mann D, et al, editors: *Braunwald's heart disease: a textbook of cardiovascular medicine*, ed 8, Philadelphia, 2008, Saunders.

6. Task Force for Diagnosis and Treatment of Non-ST-Segment Elevation Acute Coronary Syndromes of European Society of Cardiology. Guidelines for the diagnosis and treatment of non–ST-segment elevation acute coronary syndromes, *Eur Heart J* 28(13):1598-660, 2007.

7. Thygesen K, Alpert JS, White HD: Universal definition of myocardial infarction, *Circulation* 116(22):2634-2653, 2007.

CHAPTER 16

ST-SEGMENT ELEVATION MYOCARDIAL INFARCTION

Glenn N. Levine, MD, FACC, FAHA

1. **What are the electrocardiograph (ECG) criteria for the diagnosis of ST-segment elevation myocardial infarction (STEMI)?**

   Unofficial *criteria* for the diagnosis of STEMI can be based on established criteria for the administration of thrombolytic therapy, which evolved in the late 1980s and 1990s. These criteria include symptoms suggestive of myocardial infarction (MI) within the prior 12 hours and the following:

   - ST-segment elevation greater than 0.1 mV (one small box) in at least two contiguous leads (e.g., leads III and aVF, or leads V2 and V3). Note that the European Society of Cardiology (ESC) STEMI guidelines require 0.2 mV or greater ST elevation when analyzing leads V1-V3 (but similarly 0.1 mV elevation for other leads/territories).
   - New or presumably new left bundle branch block (LBBB)

2. **Is intracoronary thrombus common in STEMI?**

   Yes. The majority of STEMI is due to plaque rupture, fissure, or disruption, leading to superimposed thrombus formation and vessel occlusion. Angioscopy demonstrates coronary thrombus in more than 90% of patients with STEMI (as opposed to 35% to 75% of patients with non–ST-segment-elevation acute coronary syndrome [NSTE-ACS] and 1% of patients with stable angina).

3. **What is *primary PCI*?**

   Primary percutaneous coronary intervention (PCI) refers to the strategy of taking a patient who presents with STEMI directly to the cardiac catheterization laboratory to undergo mechanical revascularization using balloon angioplasty, coronary stents, and other measures. Patients are not treated with thrombolytic therapy in the emergency room (or ambulance) but preferentially taken directly to the cardiac catheterization laboratory for primary PCI. Studies have demonstrated that primary PCI is superior to thrombolytic therapy when it can be performed in a timely manner by a skilled interventional cardiologist with a skilled and experienced catheterization laboratory team.

4. **What are considered to be contraindications to thrombolytic therapy?**

   Several absolute contraindications to thrombolytic therapy and several relative contraindications (or cautions) must be considered in deciding whether to treat a patient with lytic agents. As would be expected, these are based on the risks and consequences of bleeding resulting from thrombolytic therapy. These contraindications and cautions are given in Table 16-1.

5. **What is door-to-balloon time?**

   Door-to-balloon time is a phrase that denotes the time it takes from when a patient with STEMI sets foot in the emergency room until the time that a balloon is inflated in the occluded, culprit coronary artery. More recently, the concept of *medical contact-to-balloon time* has been emphasized, given that STEMI may first be diagnosed in the transporting ambulance in some cases. The generally accepted door-to-balloon time goal is 90 minutes or less.

TABLE 16-1. CONTRAINDICATIONS AND CAUTIONS/RELATIVE CONTRAINDICATIONS FOR FIBRINOLYTIC THERAPY, AS GIVEN BY THE AMERICAN COLLEGE OF CARDIOLOGY/AMERICAN HEART ASSOCIATION (ACC/AHA)) AND BY THE EUROPEAN SOCIETY OF CARDIOLOGY (ESC)

ACC/AHA	ESC
Absolute Contraindications: ■ Any prior intracranial hemorrhage (ICH) ■ Known structural cerebral vascular lesion (e.g., arterovenous malformation) ■ Known malignant intracranial neoplasm (primary or metastatic) ■ Ischemic stroke within 3 months (except acute ischemic stroke within 3 hours) ■ Suspected aortic dissection ■ Active bleeding (excluding menses) or bleeding diathesis ■ Significant closed-head or facial trauma within 3 months	**Absolute Contraindications:** ■ Hemorrhagic stroke or stroke of unknown origin at any time ■ Ischemic stroke in preceding 6 months ■ Central nervous system (CNS) damage or neoplasms ■ Recent major trauma/surgery/head injury (within preceding 3 weeks) ■ Gastrointestinal bleeding within the last month ■ Known bleeding disorder ■ Aortic dissection
Cautions/Relative Contraindications: ■ History of chronic, severe, poorly controlled hypertension ■ Severe uncontrolled hypertension of presentation (systolic blood pressure [SBP] >180 mm Hg or diastolic blood pressure [DBP] >110 mm Hg) ■ Traumatic or prolonged (>10 minutes) cardiopulmonary resuscitation (CPR) or major surgery within 3 weeks ■ Recent (within 2–4 weeks) internal bleeding ■ Noncompressible vascular punctures ■ Pregnancy ■ Active peptic ulcer ■ Current use of anticoagulants with high international normalized ratio (INR); the higher the INR, the higher the risk of bleeding ■ For streptokinase or anistreplase: prior exposure (more than 5 days ago) or prior allergic reaction to these agents	**Relative Contraindications:** ■ Transient ischemic attach in preceding 6 months ■ Oral anticoagulant therapy ■ Pregnancy or within 1 week post-partum ■ Non-compressible punctures ■ Traumatic resuscitation ■ Refractory hypertension (SBP > 180 mm Hg) ■ Advanced liver disease ■ Infective endocarditis ■ Active peptic ulcer

Modified from Antman EM, Anbe DT, Armstrong PW, et al: ACC/AHA guidelines for the management of patients with ST-elevation myocardial infarction. *J Am Coll Cardiol* 44(3):E1-E211, 2004, and from Van de Werf F, Ardissino D, Betriu A, et al: Management of acute myocardial infarction in patients presenting with ST-segment elevation. The Task Force on the Management of Acute Myocardial Infarction of the European Society of Cardiology. *Eur Heart J* 24(1):28-66, 2003.

6. **What is door-to-needle time?**
Door-to-needle time is a phrase that denotes the time it takes from when a patient with STEMI sets foot in the emergency room until the beginning of thrombolytic therapy administration (Table 16-2). The generally accepted goal for door-to-needle time is 30 minutes or less.

7. **In patients treated with thrombolytic therapy, how long should antithrombin therapy be continued?**
Patients who are treated with unfractionated heparin (UFH) should be treated for 48 hours. Studies of low-molecular-weight heparins (EXTRACT, CREATE) and of direct thrombin inhibitors

TABLE 16-2.	ACC/AHA GUIDELINES FOR STEMI			
I	IIa	IIb	III	
A				Aspirin (162-325 mg, chewed)
B				Clopidogrel 75 mg orally (PO) qD (in addition to aspirin) for at least 14 days in those treated with fibrinolytic therapy or without reperfusion therapy
	C			Loading dose of clopidogrel 300 mg in those < 75 years of age who receive fibrinolytic therapy or who do not receive reperfusion therapy
C				Sublingual (SL) nitroglycerin (0.4 mg) for ongoing ischemic discomfort q5 min x 3 doses
C				IV nitroglycerin for relief of ongoing ischemic discomfort, control of hypertension, or pulmonary edema
C				Morphine sulfate (2-4 mg IV initially, then 2-8 mg IV q5-15 minutes) for pain associated with STEMI
B				Oral beta blockers for those without contraindications (see text)
	B			IV beta blockers to patients who are hypertensive and are without contraindications (see text)
		C		In patients undergoing fibrinolytic therapy, unfractionated heparin therapy for 48 hours
A/B				In patients undergoing fibrinolytic therapy, enoxaparin or fondaparinux for the duration of hospitalization (up to 8 days)
A				Primary PCI within 90 minutes of first medical contact (as a systems goal)
B				Fibrinolytic therapy if primary PCI not readily available; lytic therapy within 30 minutes of hospital presentation
			C	Nonselective nonsteroidal anti-inflammatory drugs (NSAIDS) (except aspirin) and COX-2 inhibitors should not be administered during hospitalization
A				In-hospital initiation of lipid therapy with goal of low-density lipoprotein (LDL) < 100 mg/dL
	A			In-hospital initiation of lipid therapy with goal of LDL < 70 mg/dL

Modified from Antman EM, Hand M, Armstrong PW, et al: 2007 focused update of the ACC/AHA 2004 guidelines for the management of patients with ST-elevation myocardial infarction. *J Am Coll Cardiol* 51(2):210-47, 2008, and from Antman EM, Anbe DT, Armstrong PW, et al: ACC/AHA guidelines for the management of patients with ST-elevation myocardial infarction. *J Am Coll Cardiol* 44(3):E1-E211, 2004.

(OASIS-6) have suggested that patients treated with these agents should be treated throughout their hospitalizations, up to 8 days maximum.

8. **What is facilitated PCI?**
   Facilitated PCI refers to a strategy of planned PCI immediately or shortly after administration of an initial pharmacologic regimen intended to improve coronary artery patency before the PCI procedure. Such regimens have included full-dose or reduced-dose thrombolytic therapy, glycoprotein IIb/IIIa inhibitors, antithrombin agents, and combinations of agents. The concept is to restore at least some coronary blood flow as the cardiac catheterization laboratory is getting activated and the patient is being transported to the hospital's catheterization laboratory. Although this strategy is intuitively appealing, studies of such a strategy generally have not demonstrated any advantage of facilitated PCI over primary PCI.

9. **What is rescue PCI?**
   Rescue PCI is the performance of PCI after a patient has *failed* thrombolytic therapy. Studies of rescue PCI versus medical management generally have shown a modest benefit with rescue PCI in appropriately selected patients. The problem with rescue PCI is that clinical and electrocardiographic criteria for predicting which patients have actually failed thrombolytic therapy (have not had successful lysis of coronary thrombosis and restoration of coronary perfusion) are imprecise. Thus, some patients with continued occluded arteries may not be referred for rescue PCI and some patients with successful reperfusion will be referred for unnecessary cardiac catheterization. At present, rescue PCI is recommended (class I) or is reasonable (class IIa) in the following situations:
   - Development of cardiogenic shock (class I if younger than 75 years; class IIa if 75 years or older and a suitable candidate for revascularization)
   - Severe congestive heart failure/pulmonary edema (class I)
   - Hemodynamically compromising ventricular arrhythmias (class I)
   - Hemodynamic or electrical instability (class IIa)
   - Persistent ischemic symptoms (class IIa)
   - Less than 50% resolution of maximal ST-segment elevation at 90 minutes and a moderate to large area of myocardium at risk (anterior MI, or inferior MI with right ventricular enlargement or precordial ST-segment depression)

10. **Which patients should not be treated with beta-blocker therapy?**
    Beta-blockers have been a mainstay of STEMI therapy for decades. However, in the Clopidogrel and Metoprolol in Myocardial Infarction Trial/Second Chinese Cardiac (COMMIT/CCS-2) study, the potential benefits of beta-blocker therapy were offset by an increased incidence of cardiogenic shock and shock-related death with beta-blocker therapy. Therefore, in patients with signs of heart failure, evidence of a low-output state, or increased risk for cardiogenic shock, beta-blocker therapy should not be initiated. Risk factors for cardiogenic shock include age older than 70 years, systolic blood pressure less than 120 mm Hg, sinus tachycardia greater than 110 beats/min, and heart rate less than 60 beats/min. Other contraindications to initiating beta-blocker therapy include PR interval more than 0.24 seconds, second- or third-degree heart block, active asthma, or severe reactive airway disease.

11. **Which patients should be treated with nitrate therapy?**
    Sublingual (S/L) nitroglycerin (0.4 mg) every 5 minutes, up to three doses, should be administered for ongoing ischemic discomfort. Intravenous nitroglycerin is indicated for relief of ongoing ischemic discomfort that responds to nitrate therapy, for control of hypertension, and for management of pulmonary edema. Nitrates should not be administered to patients who have received a phosphodiesterase inhibitor for erectile dysfunction within 24 to 48 hours (depending on the specific agent). Nitrates should also not be administered to those with suspected right ventricular (RV) infarction, systolic blood pressure less than 90 mm Hg (or 30 mm Hg or more below baseline), severe bradycardia (less than 50 beats/min), or tachycardia (more than 100 beats/min).

12. **Should clopidogrel be given to patients with STEMI?**
The answer is a qualified yes. The COMMIT-CCS 2 trial was a large clinical trial of patients with acute MI that demonstrated that administration of clopidogrel, 75 mg daily, decreased ischemic endpoints (including death). Clopidogrel as Adjunctive Reperfusion Therapy—Thrombolysis in Myocardial Infarction 28 (CLARITY-TIMI 28) was primarily an angiographic study that demonstrated more favorable angiographic findings in those who received a 300-mg loading dose of clopidogrel. Based on these studies, the American College of Cardiology/American Heart Association (ACC/AHA) guidelines now recommend clopidogrel administration to those patients with STEMI. Administration of 75 mg daily is a class I recommendation; administration of a 300-mg loading dose to those less than 75 years of age is a class IIa recommendation. There are no specific trials at the time of this writing assessing the potential benefit of clopidogrel administration in those with STEMI who are to undergo primary PCI. For the time being, this will likely be a decision made by individual operators and institutions.

13. **Should patients with STEMI be continued on nonselective NSAIDS (other than aspirin) or COX-2 inhibitors?**
No. Use of these agents has been associated with increased risk of reinfarction, hypertension, heart failure, myocardial rupture, and death. Therefore, such agents should be discontinued at the time of admission.

14. **What are the main mechanical complications of myocardial infarction?**
    - **Free wall rupture:** Acute free wall rupture is almost always fatal within minutes. In some cases of *subacute free wall rupture,* only a small quantity of blood initially reaches the pericardial cavity and begins to cause signs of pericardial tamponade. Emergent echocardiography and immediate surgery are indicated.
    - **Ventricular septal rupture:** A ventricular septal defect (VSD) caused by myocardial infarction and septal rupture occurred in 1% to 2% of all patients with infarction in older series, though the incidence in the fibrinolytic age is 0.2% to 0.3%. Patients may complain of a chest pain somewhat different than their MI pain and will usually develop cardiogenic shock. A new systolic murmur may be audible, often along the left sternal border. Mortality without surgery is 54% in the first week and up to 92% within the first year.
    - **Papillary muscle rupture:** Papillary muscle rupture leads to acute and severe mitral regurgitation. It occurs in approximately 1% of STEMIs. Because of the abrupt elevation in left atrial pressure, there may not be an audible murmur of mitral regurgitation. Pulmonary edema and cardiogenic shock usually develop. Treatment is urgent/emergent mitral valve replacement (or in rare cases, mitral valve repair).

15. **What are the triad of findings suggestive of right ventricular infarction?**
The triad of findings suggestive of RV infarction are hypotension, distended neck veins, and clear lungs. Clinical RV infarction occurs in approximately 30% of inferior MIs. Because the infarcted right ventricle is dependent on preload, administration of nitroglycerin (or morphine), which leads to venous pooling and decreased blood return to the right ventricle, may lead to profound hypotension. When such hypotension occurs, patients should be placed in reverse Trendelenburg position (legs above chest and head) and treated with extremely aggressive administration of several liters of fluid through large-bore intravenous needles. Those who do not respond to such therapy may require treatment with such agents as dopamine.
In patients with inferior MI, a *right-sided* ECG should be obtained. The precordial leads are placed over the right side of the chest in a mirror-image pattern to normal. The finding of 1 mm or greater ST elevation in leads RV4-RV6 is highly suggestive of RV infarction (Fig. 16-1), although the absence of this often-transient finding should not be used to dismiss a diagnosis of RV infarction made on clinical grounds.

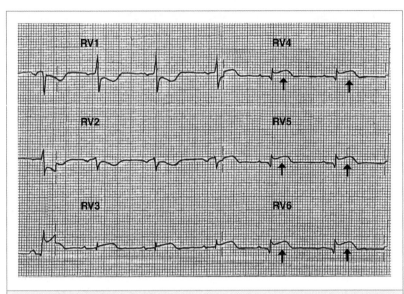

Figure 16-1. Right-sided leads demonstrating ST-segment elevation *(arrows)* in leads RV4-RV6, highly suggestive of right ventricular infarction.

BIBLIOGRAPHY, SUGGESTED READINGS, AND WEBSITES

1. Garas S, Zafari AM: Myocardial Infarction: http://www.emedicine.com

2. Gibson CM, Carrozza JP, Laham RJ: Primary PCI versus Fibrinolysis (Thrombolysis) in Acute ST Elevation (Q Wave) Myocardial Infarction: Clinical Trials: http://www.utdol.com

3. Reeder GS, Kennedy HL, Rosenson RS: Overview of the Management of Acute ST Elevation (Q Wave) Myocardial Infarction: http://www.utdol.com

4. Antman EM: ST-elevation myocardial infarction: management. In Libby P, Bonow R, Mann D et al, editors: *Braunwald's heart disease: a textbook of cardiovascular medicine*, ed 8, Philadelphia, 2008, Saunders.

5. Antman EM, Anbe DT, Armstrong PW, et al: ACC/AHA guidelines for the management of patients with ST-elevation myocardial infarction: a report of the American College of Cardiology/American Heart Association Task Force on Practice Guidelines (Committee to Revise the 1999 Guidelines for the Management of Patients with Acute Myocardial Infarction), *J Am Coll Cardiol* 44(3):E1-E211, 2004.

6. Antman EM, Hand M, Armstrong PW, et al: 2007 focused update of the ACC/AHA 2004 guidelines for the management of patients with ST-elevation myocardial infarction: a report of the American College of Cardiology/American Heart Association Task Force on Practice Guidelines, *J Am Coll Cardiol* 51(2):210-47, 2008.

7. Van de Werf F, Ardissino D, Betriu A, et al: Management of acute myocardial infarction in patients presenting with ST-segment elevation. The Task Force on the Management of Acute Myocardial Infarction of the European Society of Cardiology, *Eur Heart J* 24(1):28-66, 2003.

ORAL AND INTRAVENOUS ANTIPLATELET THERAPIES

Glenn N. Levine, MD, FACC, FAHA

1. **Why is antiplatelet therapy important in the treatment of cardiac disease?**
   In simple terms, whereas venous thrombosis is regarded as primarily a manifestation of the coagulation cascade and involves *red thrombus,* arterial thrombosis is driven to a significant extent by platelet activation and aggregation, producing *white thrombus*. In reality there is an extremely complex interaction between platelets, the coagulation cascade, and the vessel wall, but the role of platelet activation and aggregation figures more prominently in arterial thrombosis than in venous thrombosis. Platelets can be activated by many different stimuli, including arachodonic acid, adenosine diphosphate (ADP), collagen, and thrombin. When activated, in addition to aggregating, platelets can release many mediators of coagulation and inflammation. Approximately 10^{11} platelets are produced each day, though this level of production can increase up to tenfold when necessary. Platelets have a maximal circulating life span of approximately 10 days. Thus, antiplatelet agents that irreversibly inhibit platelet activation will have effects on the circulation for days after they are discontinued.

2. **What is the usual minimum daily dose of aspirin in the prevention and treatment of arterial thrombosis?**
   Doses of 75 to 100 mg daily are generally regarded as the low end of daily aspirin therapy, though there continues to be debate about what is the ideal dose of aspirin. This lower end range of therapy has been shown in at least some retrospective analyses to lead to less bleeding complications than higher dose aspirin (e.g., 325 mg daily), including when aspirin and clopidogrel are used together for intermediate to long-term therapy. The 2007 iterations of the American College of Cardiology/American Heart Association (ACC/AHA) guidelines on chronic stable angina recommend a daily dose of 75 to 162 mg. Note, however, that some studies of aspirin plus clopidogrel therapy for the prevention of stent thrombosis were performed using higher doses of aspirin, so many interventionalists will discharge patients after stent implantation on higher doses of aspirin, at least for the initial weeks or months of therapy. Doses of 162 to 325 mg are generally used in acute settings, where rapid and complete inhibition of thromboxane A_2-dependent platelet aggregation is critical, and this initial dose range is recommended in the 2007 iterations of the ACC/AHA guidelines on unstable angina/non–ST-segment-elevation myocardial infarction (MI) (e.g., non–ST-segment elevation acute coronary syndrome).

3. **Should aspirin therapy be used in patients who have undergone coronary artery bypass grafting (CABG)?**
   Yes. Aspirin has been shown to significantly reduce saphenous vein graft closures during the first postoperative year. It is continued indefinitely in post-CABG patients given its proven benefits in secondary prevention in patients with coronary artery disease. The use of warfarin or the addition of dipyridimole does not add any protection from vein graft closure. The use of clopidogrel plus aspirin, as opposed to aspirin alone, has not been prospectively specifically studied for the prevention of vein graft closure.

4. **How does clopidogrel work?**
Clopidogrel irreversibly inhibits ADP-mediated platelet activation by blocking the $P2Y_{12}$ receptor on the platelet surface (this is one of the reasons one now hears the term *$P2Y_{12}$ receptor blocker* more commonly than *ADP receptor blocker*). Because it irreversibly inhibits platelet, it is recommended that, when possible, clopidogrel be discontinued for approximately 5 to 7 days before cardiac surgery, because of the increased risks of bleeding complications during such surgery. Clopidogrel requires hepatic transformation to an active metabolite in order to exert its antiplatelet effects.

5. **Should clopidogrel be given to patients with ST-segment-elevation myocardial infarction (STEMI)?**
The answer is a qualified yes. The Clopidogrel and Metoprolol in Myocardial Infarction/Second Chinese Cardiac Study (COMMIT-CCS 2) trial was a large clinical trial of patients with acute MI that demonstrated that administration of clopidogrel, 75 mg daily, decreased ischemic endpoints (including death). Clopidogrel as Adjunctive Reperfusion Therapy—Thrombolysis in Myocardial Infarction 28 (CLARITY-TIMI 28) was primarily an angiographic study that demonstrated more favorable angiographic findings in those who received a 300-mg loading dose of clopidogrel. Based on these studies, the ACC/AHA guidelines now recommend clopidogrel administration to patients with STEMI. Administration of 75 mg daily is a class I recommendation; administration of a 300-mg loading dose to those less than 75 years old is a class IIa recommendation. There are no specific trials at the time of this writing assessing the potential benefit of clopidogrel administration in those with STEMI who are to undergo primary percutaneous coronary intervention (PCI). For the time being, this will likely be a decision made by individual operators and institutions.

6. **How do the glycoprotein IIB/IIIA inhibitors work?**
Once platelets become activated, the glycoprotein IIb/IIIa receptors located on the platelet membrane surface undergo a conformational change that allows them to bind to fibrin and other substances. When other activated platelets also bind to the fibrin molecules, the platelets begin to aggregate, ultimately leading to thrombus formation. Eptifibatide (Integrilin) and tirofiban (Aggrastat) reversibly bind to these glycoprotein IIb/IIIa receptors, preventing the platelet from binding with fibrin and thus inhibiting platelet aggregation. Abciximab (ReoPro) is an antibody fragment that more tightly and less reversibly binds to the glycoprotein IIb/IIIa receptor, inhibiting platelet aggregation in a similar manner. When used at appropriate doses, the IIb/IIIa inhibitors inhibit approximately 80% to 99% of platelet aggregation.

7. **Do the doses of the glycoprotein IIB/IIIA inhibitors eptifibatide (integrilin) and tirofiban (aggrastat) need to be adjusted in patients with chronic kidney disease?**
Yes. Both eptifibatide and tirofiban have significant renal excretion. The dosing regimens are as follows:
   - **Eptifibatide:** For creatinine clearance less than 50 ml/min, decrease maintenance infusion rate to 1 µg/kg/min. The bolus dose (or doses during PCI) remains the same.
   - **Tirofiban:** For creatinine clearance less than 30 ml/min, the infusion rates should be halved (0.2 µg/kg/min for the first 30 minutes then 0.05 µg/kg/min subsequently).

8. **Is routine testing for degree of platelet inhibition recommended in patients treated with antiplatelet agents?**
Testing of platelet inhibition has demonstrated that a variable number of patients are *hyporesponders* or *nonresponders* to treatment with aspirin and/or clopidogrel. Several studies have suggested that those with lesser degrees of platelet inhibition are at increased risk of stent thrombosis. One PCI study demonstrated that those with lesser degrees of platelet inhibition after GP IIb/IIIa therapy were at increased risks of ischemic complications in the

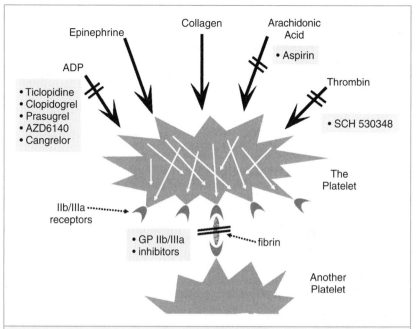

Figure 17-1. The upper half of the illustration shows the many agents (e.g., ADP, thrombin) that can lead to platelet activation and the drugs that block such agent-mediated activation. The lower half of the illustration shows how activated platelet glycoprotein IIb/IIIa receptors bind to fibrin (as well as other substances), leading to platelet aggregation. This binding of fibrin to the IIb/IIIa receptor and platelet aggregation can be inhibited at this level by the glycoprotein IIb/IIIa inhibitors. *ADP,* Adenosine diphosphate.

peri-PCI period. Despite these findings, there is at present little data demonstrating that more aggressively treating those with lesser degrees of platelet inhibition results in a better clinical outcome (one large study to assess this, GRAVITIS, is in progress at the time of this writing). Complicating matters is the fact that there are numerous different devices that test platelet inhibition, which use different methods to measure different parameters of platelet inhibition. Further, there are at present many different definitions of *hyporesponsiveness* or *nonresponsiveness* used in studies. Thus, most experts and ad hoc expert documents have recommended against routine testing of platelet inhibition until a gold standard for testing and degree of inhibition has been identified and until clinical studies demonstrate the clinical benefit of routine platelet testing.

9. **What are some of the newer antiplatelet agents, and how do they work?**
   - Prasugrel is an oral third-generation thienopyridine antiplatelet agent that, like clopidogrel, blocks the P2Y$_{12}$ platelet receptor from binding with ADP, preventing platelet activation. Compared with clopidogrel, it has a faster onset of action and a greater and more uniform degree of platelet inhibition. In the Trial to Assess Improvement in Therapeutic Outcomes by Optimizing Platelet Inhibition with Prasugrel–Thrombolysis in Myocardial Infarction (TRITON) study of patients undergoing coronary stenting, compared with clopidogrel therapy, prasugrel therapy led to fewer ischemic complications and stent thromboses but to more bleeding complications, particularly in those with a history of prior stroke or transient ischemic attack (TIA), older than 75 years, and less than 60 kg in body weight. The dose of prasugrel used in the study was a 60-mg loading dose, followed by 10 mg daily.

Prasugrel has recently been approved by the FDA. It is contraindicated in patients with a prior stroke or transient ischemic attack.

- AZD6140 (it has no other designated name at the time of this writing) is an oral non-thienopyridine reversible P2Y12 receptor blocker that also inhibits ADP-mediated platelet activation. It has rapid onset of action. Once discontinued, most of the abilities of the platelets to become activated and aggregate should occur within 1 to 2 days. It has been shown to have greater and more consistent inhibition of ADP-induced platelet aggregation compared with clopidogrel. At the time of this writing, it is being compared with clopidogrel treatment in the large Percutaneous Left Atrial Appendage Transcatheter Occlusion (PLAATO) study and several smaller studies. The dosing regimen being studied in PLAATO is a 180-mg loading dose, followed by a maintenance regimen of 90 mg twice a day.

- Cangrelor is an intravenously administered P2Y12 platelet inhibitor with a very short onset and offset (half-life of 3–5 minutes). At the time of this writing, it is being tested in patients undergoing PCI in the study, CardioMEMS Heart Sensor Allows Monitoring of Pressure to Improve Outcomes in NYHA Class III Patients (CHAMPION), and may emerge as an alternative to clopidogrel or the glycoprotein IIb/IIIa inhibitors.

- SCH 530348 (it has no other designated name at the time of this writing) is an oral PAR-1 antagonist compound, blocking thrombin-mediated platelet activation. It is being tested in patients with coronary artery disease and acute coronary syndrome.

BIBLIOGRAPHY, SUGGESTED READINGS, AND WEBSITES

1. Lincoff AM: Antiplatelet Agents in Acute ST-Elevation (Q Wave) Myocardial Infarction: http://www.utdol.com

2. Simons M. Antiplatelet Agents in Unstable Angina and Acute Non–ST-Elevation (Non-Q Wave) Myocardial Infarction: http://www.utdol.com

3. http://my.americanheart.org/portal/professional/guidelines

4. http://www.cardiosource.com/guidelines/index.asp

5. http://www.escardio.org/knowledge/guidelines/

6. Anderson JL, Adams CD, Antman EM, et al: American College of Cardiology, American Heart Association Task Force on Practice Guidelines (Writing Committee to Revise the 2002 Guidelines for the Management of Patients With Unstable Angina/Non-ST-Elevation Myocardial Infarction), *J Am Coll Cardiol* 50(7):e1-e157, 2007.

7. Antman EM, Hand M, Armstrong PW, et al: 2007 Focused Update of the ACC/AHA 2004 Guidelines for the Management of Patients With ST-Elevation Myocardial Infarction: a report of the American College of Cardiology/American Heart Association Task Force on Practice Guidelines, *Circulation* 117(2):296-329, 2008.

8. Fourth Joint Task Force of the European Society of Cardiology and Other Societies on Cardiovascular Disease Prevention in Clinical Practice: European guidelines on cardiovascular disease prevention in clinical practice: executive summary, *Eur Heart J* (19):2375-414, 2007.

9. Fraker TD Jr, Fihn SD: 2007 chronic angina focused update of the ACC/AHA 2002 guidelines for the management of patients with chronic stable angina: a report of the American College of Cardiology/American Heart Association Task Force on Practice Guidelines Writing Group to develop the focused update of the 2002 guidelines for the management of patients with chronic stable angina, *J Am Coll Cardiol* 50(23):2264-2274, 2007.

10. Gurbel PA, Becker RC, Mann KG, et al: Platelet function monitoring in patients with coronary artery disease, *J Am Coll Cardiol* 50(19):1822-1834, 2007.

11. King SB 3rd, Smith SC Jr, Hirshfeld JW Jr, et al: 2007 Focused Update of the ACC/AHA/SCAI 2005 Guideline Update for Percutaneous Coronary Intervention: a report of the American College of Cardiology/American Heart Association Task Force on Practice Guidelines: 2007 Writing Group to Review New Evidence and Update the ACC/AHA/SCAI 2005 Guideline Update for Percutaneous Coronary Intervention, writing on behalf of the 2005 Writing Committee, *Circulation* 117(2):261-295, 2008.

12. Steinhubl SR, Schneider DJ, Berger PB, et al: Determining the efficacy of antiplatelet therapies for the individual: lessons from clinical trials, *J Thromb Thrombolysis* 2007.

13. Task Force for Diagnosis and Treatment of Non-ST-Segment Elevation Acute Coronary Syndromes of European Society of Cardiology. Guidelines for the diagnosis and treatment of non-ST-segment elevation acute coronary syndromes, *Eur Heart J* (13):1598-1660, 2007.

14. Task Force for Percutaneous Coronary Interventions of the European Society of Cardiology. Guidelines for percutaneous coronary interventions. The Task Force for Percutaneous Coronary Interventions of the European Society of Cardiology, *Eur Heart J* (8):804-847, 2005.

CHAPTER 18

ANTICOAGULANT THERAPY

José G. Díez, MD, FACC, FSCAI

1. **How does thrombus form?**

   Classically, the coagulation system mechanisms have been compartmentalized into the *intrinsic* pathway (with all the required factors present in the blood), the *extrinsic* pathway (with at least some requisite extravascular factors), and the *common* pathway (into which both former pathways feed). In recent years, however, a new perspective of coagulation has evolved that details three steps: initiation, amplification, and propagation (Fig. 18-1).

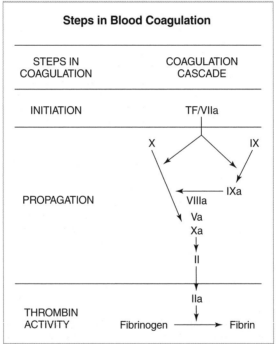

Steps in Blood Coagulation

Figure 18-1. Coagulation is triggered by the tissue factor/factor VIIa complex (TF/VIIa), which activates factor IX (IX) and factor X (X). Activated factor IX (IXa) propagates coagulation by activating factor X in a reaction that use activated factor VIII (VIIIa) as a cofactor. Activated factor X (Xa), with activated factor V (Va) as a cofactor, converts prothrombin (II) to thrombin (IIa). Thrombin then converts fibrinogen to fibrin. (Modified from Ferguson JJ, Wilson JM, Díez J: Antithrombotic therapy and the transition to the catheterization laboratory in UA/NSTEMI, *Minerva Cardioangiol* 55(5):529-556, 2007.)

2. **At what levels of the coagulation cascade do unfractionated heparin (UFH) and low-molecular-weight heparin (LMWH) work?**

Pharmacologic agents can affect the coagulation cascade at different levels. The heparinoids UFH and LMWH are not only antithrombotic agents (thrombin = factor II) but also inhibitors of factor Xa (FXa), an important component of the coagulation cascade. Coagulation is triggered by tissue factor (TF), a cellular receptor for activated factor VII (FVIIa), which has little enzymatic activity until it binds to TF. Once it is bonded, FVIIa triggers activated factors IX (FIXa) and X (FXa), respectively. The latter converts small amounts of prothrombin to thrombin, sufficient enough to activate platelets and factors V and VIII, the key cofactors of coagulation (see Fig. 18-1).

3. **How does unfractionated heparin (UFH) work?**

UFH is a heterogeneous mixture of polysaccharides of varying chain lengths, ranging in molecular weight from 5000 to 30,000 daltons. UFH exerts its anticoagulant effect by binding via a specific pentasaccharide sequence to antithrombin (an endogenous regulator of coagulation), which results in conformational changes in antithrombin, enhancing its affinity for its regulatory targets, thrombin and factor Xa.

4. **What is the recommended dosing of unfractionated heparin for acute coronary syndromes?**

The dosing recommendations vary slightly between the American College of Cardiology/ American Heart Association (ACC/AHA) and the European Society of Cardiology (ESC), as well as with the American College of Chest Physicians (ACCP).

- ACC/AHA: 60 U/kg bolus (max. 4000 U), then initial infusion of 12 U/kg (max. initial infusion 1000 U/hr). Target anti-Xa 0.3 to 0.7; target activated partial thromboplastin time (aPTT) 1.5 to 2.5 times control (60–80 seconds per ACCP guidelines)
- ESC: 60 to 70 U/kg bolus (max. 5000 U), then initial infusion of 12 to 15 U/kg (initial max. 1000 U/hr). Target aPTT 50 to 75 seconds (1.5–2.5 times control)

5. **How do the low-molecular-weight heparins work?**

The LMWHs are derived from chemical cleavage of longer unfractionated heparin chains, producing shorter saccharide chains (molecular weight ranging from 4000 to 6000 daltons). These shorter chains result in a greater degree of factor Xa inhibition (and hence inhibition of thrombin generation) relative to thrombin inhibition. These shorter chains are also less prone to binding by non–coagulation-related proteins, and therefore there is more potent, predictable, and sustained anticoagulation. LMWHs carry the additional advantage of maintaining some downstream antithrombin activity (because of retention of some longer chains) and therefore still may significantly block thrombin activity if large amounts of thrombin are not present. The most commonly used LMWH in cardiology is enoxaparin (Lovenox). Numerous studies have compared enoxaparin with UFH (TIMI 11B, ESSENCE, A-to-Z, INTERACT, SYNERGY). In general, in most studies and overviews enoxaparin leads to slightly fewer ischemic complications and slightly more bleeding complications compared with UFH. In patients with ST-segment-elevation myocardial infarction (STEMI) undergoing fibrinolytic therapy, a treatment strategy using enoxaparin has been shown to be superior to using UFH (EXTRACT).

6. **Does the dose of enoxaparin need to be adjusted in patients with chronic kidney disease?**

Yes. Enoxaparin is cleared to a greater degree by the kidneys than unfractionated heparin. In patients with creatinine clearance less than 30 ml/min, the dosing regimen should be 1 mg/kg every 24 hours (as opposed to every 12 hours). In patients with severely impaired renal function and acute coronary syndrome (ACS), particularly those who are to undergo cardiac catheterization and possible revascularizaiton, it makes more sense to use UFH.

7. **What is a pentasacharide anti-XA inhibitor?**

A pentasaccharide is derived from the 5 saccharide moiety of heparin that binds to antithrombin. Because is has no remaining *tail* of saccharides, it cannot facilitate the binding of thrombin to antithrombin; thus, it is generally regarded as a *pure* Xa inhibitor, although it may have other minor upstream effects on coagulation. Nevertheless, it still acts indirectly against factor Xa (like UFH and LMWH) in that it requires the intermediary of AT. It is not known to induce the formation of heparin-PF4 complexes and consequently is not associated with a risk of heparin-induced thrombocytopenia (HIT). The most-studied and most commonly used anti-Xa inhibitor is fondaparinux (Arixtra), which was demonstrated to be effective in non–ST-segment ACS (OASIS-5) and in STEMI (OASIS-6). Fondaparinux should not be used in patients with severely impaired renal function.

8. **How do direct thrombin inhibitors work?**

In contrast to heparin and heparin derivatives, which act indirectly via antithrombin, the direct thrombin inhibitors directly and specifically inhibit the autocatalytic actions of thrombin and the conversion of fibrinogen to fibrin. Additionally, thrombin inhibitors block the amplification feedback actions of thrombin and interfere with thrombin-mediated platelet activation. Importantly, unlike heparin, the direct-acting thrombin antagonists do no require antithrombin cofactor for their activity against thrombin, thus allowing for concentration-dependent activity. Direct thrombin inhibitors also do not cause heparin-Induced thrombocytopenia. Four direct thrombin antagonists are currently commercially available: desirudin, lepirudin, bivalirudin, and argatroban. Bivalirudin (Angiomax) is currently commonly used during percutaneous coronary angiography (REPLACE-2), including primary percutaneous coronary intervention (PCI) (HORIZONS), and has also been demonstrated to be an effective agent in the treatment of non–ST-segment-elevation ACS (NSTE-ACS) (ACUITY); it is also being studied in patients undergoing coronary artery bypass grafting (CABG). Argatroban is often used in patients with HIT being treated medically or undergoing CABG.

9. **Which agents can be used in the treatment of NSTE-ACS?**

The most recent ACC/AHA unstable angina/non–ST-segment-elevation myocardial infarction (UA/NSTEMI, or NSTE-ACS) guidelines have emphasized that multiple options are available, and no one agent can be recommended over the others in all cases. In reference to antithrombin therapy, the ACC/AHA guidelines give a class I recommendation to the use of all four current alternatives (UFH, enoxaparin, fondaparinux, and bivalirudin). The guidelines note that there are more data in support of enoxaparin and UFH (level of evidence [LOE] A) than for fondaparinux and bivalirudin (LOE B). Bivalirudin is only recommended for early-invasive-strategy patients. The ACC/AHA guidelines mention that for an initial invasive strategy using bivalirudin, it is reasonable to omit upstream GP IIb/IIIa inhibitor therapy if bivalirudin is used *only* if at least 300 mg of clopidogrel was administered at least 6 hours earlier than planned catheterization or PCI (class IIa, LOE B). For initial conservative-strategy patients, enoxaparin and fondaparinux are preferred over UFH (class IIa, LOE B), and fondaparinux is preferred for conservative-strategy patients with increased risk of bleeding (class I, LOE B).

The ESC guidelines emphasize that the choice of anticoagulant depends on the initial strategy and that the anticoagulant should be selected according to the risk of both ischemic and bleeding events. The ESC guidelines preferentially recommend fondaparinux in patients who are not to undergo an *urgent invasive* strategy. For *urgent invasive situations,* UFH (class I, LOE C), enoxaparin (class IIa, LOC B), and bivalirudin (class I, LOE B) are recommended.

BIBLIOGRAPHY, SUGGESTED READINGS, AND WEBSITES

1. CRUSADE Q4 2006 Results: http://www.crusadeqi.com/main/Slidesets.shtml
2. ACC/AHA 2007 Guidelines for the management of patients with unstable angina/non–ST-elevation myocardial infarction: a report of the American College of Cardiology/American Heart Association Task Force on Practice Guidelines, *Circulation* 116:e148-e304, 2007.

3. Antman EM, Morrow DA, McCabe CH, et al: Enoxaparin versus unfractionated heparin with fibrinolysis for ST-elevation myocardial infarction, *N Engl J Med*, 2006; 354(14):1477-1488.

4. Bassand JP, Hamm CW, Ardissino D, et al: Guidelines for the diagnosis and treatment of non–ST-segment elevation acute coronary syndromes: the Task Force for the Diagnosis and Treatment of Non–ST-Segment Elevation Acute Coronary Syndromes of the European Society of Cardiology, *Eur Heart J* 28:1598-1660, 2007.

5. Bhatt DL, Lee BI, Casterella PJ, et al: Safety of concomitant therapy with eptifibatide and enoxaparin in patients undergoing percutaneous coronary intervention: results of the Coronary Revascularization Using Integrilin and Single Bolus Enoxaparin Study, *J Am Coll Cardiol* 41:20-25, 2003.

6. Blazing MA, de Lemos JA, White HD, et al: Safety and efficacy of enoxaparin vs. unfractionated heparin in patients with non–ST-segment elevation acute coronary syndromes who receive tirofiban and aspirin: a randomized controlled trial, *JAMA* 292:55-64, 2004.

7. Brieger DB, Mak K-H, Kottke-Marchant K, et al: Heparin-induced thrombocytopenia, *J Am Coll Cardiol* 31:1449-1459, 1998.

8. Direct Thrombin Inhibitor Trialists' Collaborative Group: Direct thrombin inhibitors in acute coronary syndromes: principal results of a meta-analysis based on individual patients' data, *Lancet* 359:294-302, 2002.

9. Eikelboom JW, Anand SS, Malmberg K, et al: Unfractionated heparin and low-molecular-weight heparin in acute coronary syndrome without ST elevation: a meta-analysis [see comments], *Lancet* 355:1936-1942, 2000.

10. Eikelboom JW, Quinlan DJ, Mehta SR, et al: Unfractionated and low-molecular-weight heparin as adjuncts to thrombolysis in aspirin-treated patients with ST-elevation acute myocardial infarction: a meta-analysis of the randomized trials, *Circulation* 112:3855-3867, 2005.

11. Ferguson JJ, Califf RM, Antman EM, et al: Enoxaparin vs unfractionated heparin in high-risk patients with non–ST-segment elevation acute coronary syndromes managed with an intended early invasive strategy: primary results of the SYNERGY randomized trial, *JAMA* 292:45-54, 2004.

12. Gibson CM, Murphy SA, Montalescot G, et al: Percutaneous coronary intervention in patients receiving enoxaparin or unfractionated heparin after fibrinolytic therapy for ST-segment elevation myocardial infarction in the ExTRACT-TIMI 25 trial, *J Am Coll Cardiol* 49:2238-2246, 2007.

13. Hirsh J, Anand SS, Halperin JL, et al: Guide to anticoagulant therapy: heparin, *Circulation* 103:2994-3018, 2001.

14. Lefkovits J, Topol E: Direct thrombin inhibitors in cardiovascular medicine, *Circulation* 90:1522-1536, 1994.

15. OASIS 5 Investigators. Comparison of fondaparinux and enoxaparin in acute coronary syndromes, *N Engl J Med* 354:1464-1476, 2006.

16. OASIS 6 Trial Group: Effects of fondaparinux on mortality and reinfarction in patients with acute ST-segment elevation myocardial infarction: The OASIS-6 Randomized Trial, *JAMA* 295:1519-1530, 2006.

17. Simoons ML, Bobbink IW, Boland J, et al: A dose-finding study of fondaparinux in patients with non–ST-segment elevation acute coronary syndromes: the pentasaccharide in unstable angina (PENTUA) study, *J Am Coll Cardiol* 43:2183-2190, 2004.

18. Stone GW, McLaurin BT, Cox DA, et al: Bivalirudin for patients with acute coronary syndromes, *N Engl J Med* 355:2203-2216, 2006.

19. Stone GW, White HD, Magnus Ohman E, et al: Bivalirudin in patients with acute coronary syndromes undergoing percutaneous coronary intervention: a subgroup analysis from the Acute Catheterization and Urgent Intervention Triage strategy (ACUITY) trial, *Lancet* 369: 907-919, 2007.

20. Stone GW, Witzenbichler B, Guagliumi G, et al: HORIZONS-AMI Trial Investigators. Bivalirudin during primary PCI in acute myocardial infarction, *N Engl J Med* 358(21):2218-2230, 2008.

21. Turpie AG: Pentasaccharides, *Semin Hematol* 39:158-171, 2002.

CHAPTER 19

CARDIOGENIC SHOCK

Hani Jneid, MD

1. **Define cardiogenic shock.**
   Cardioegnic shock is a state of end-organ hypoperfusion due to cardiac failure and the inability of the cardiovascular system to provide adequate blood flow to the extremities and vital organs. In general, patients with cardiogenic shock manifest persistent hypotension (systolic blood pressure less than 80 to 90 mm Hg or a mean arterial pressure 30 mm Hg below baseline) with severe reduction in cardiac index (less than 1.8 L/min/m^2) in the presence of adequate or elevated filling pressure (left ventricular end-diastolic pressure more than 18 mm Hg or right ventricular end diastolic pressure more than 10 to 15 mm Hg).

2. **What are the various types of shock?**
   Blood flow is determined by three entities: blood volume, vascular resistance, and pump function. There are three main types of shock: (1) hypovolemic, (2) vasogenic or distributive, and (3) cardiogenic. Examples of causes of *hypovolemic shock* include gastrointestinal bleeding, severe hemorrhage, and severe diabetic ketoacidosis (as a result of volume depletion). Examples of *vasogenic shock* include septic shock, anaphylactic shock, neurogenic shock, and shock from pharmacologic causes. There are many causes of *cardiogenic shock,* although acute myocardial infarction (MI) is the most common. Cardiogenic shock can be separated into *true cardiac causes*, such as MI, and *extracardiac causes* caused by obstruction to inflow (tension pneumothorax, cardiac tamponade) or outflow (pulmonary embolus).

3. **Describe the clinical signs observed in cardiogenic shock and other types of shock.**
   The medical history and clinical examination help in making the diagnosis of cardiogenic shock. Feeling the extremities and examining the jugular veins provide vital clues: warm skin is suggestive of a vasogenic cause; cool, clammy skin reflects enhanced reflex sympathoadrenal discharge leading to cutaneous vasoconstriction, suggesting hypovolemia or cardiogenic shock. On the other hand, distended jugular veins, rales, and an S3 gallop suggest a cardiogenic cause rather than hypovolemia.

   It is important to note that the clinical examination and chest radiograph may not be reliable predictors of the pulmonary capillary wedge pressure (PCWP). Neither detect elevated PCWP in up to 30% of cardiogenic shock patients. In addition, both cardiac tamponade and massive pulmonary embolism can present as cardiogenic shock without associated pulmonary congestion. Right-sided heart catheterization with intracardiac pressure and cardiac pressure measurements is important to confirm the diagnosis of cardiogenic shock. In 2004 the American College of Cardiology/American Heart Association (ACC/AHA) concluded that pulmonary artery catheterization is considered useful (a class IIa recommendation) in patients with cardiogenic shock.

4. **Do all patients with cardiogenic shock have an increased heart rate?**
   No. Patients with cardiogenic shock related to third-degree heart block or drug overdose (such as beta-blockers and calcium channel antagonists overdose) can present with bradycardia and require temporary transvenous pacemaker implantation.

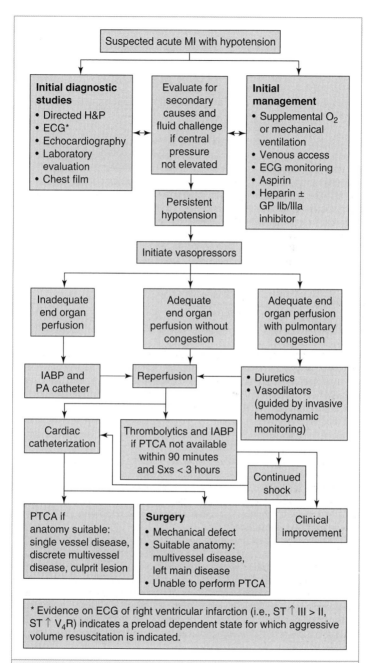

Figure 19-1. Evaluation and treatment algorithm for cardiogenic shock. (Modified from Hollenberg SM, Kavinsky CJ, Parillo JE: Cardiogenic shock. *Ann Intern Med* 131:47, 1999.)

5. **What are the determinants of central venous pressure?**
The normal central venous pressure (CVP) is 5 to 12 cm H_2O. Intravascular volume, intrathoracic pressure, right ventricular function, and venous tone all affect the CVP. To reduce variability caused by intrathoracic pressure, CVP should be measured at the end of expiration.

6. **What is the significance of a loud holosystolic murmur in a patient with shock after acute myocardial infarction?**
Loud holosystolic murmurs with MI indicates either papillary muscle rupture or an acute ventricular septal defect (VSD). These may be indistinguishable, but acute VSD usually occurs with an anteroseptal MI and has an associated palpable thrill. Papillary rupture often does not have a thrill and is usually seen in inferior MI. These often cause shock on the basis of reduced forward blood flow and can be differentiated by echocardiography or pulmonary artery catheterization. Both require emergent cardiothoracic surgery for early repair. Note that in some patients, particularly those who develop acute mitral regurgitation, the murmur may be soft or inaudible (as a result of a small pressure gradient between the left ventricule and left atrium [or right ventricle]).

7. **How can one differentiate cardiogenic from septic shock?**
In classic septic shock, the systemic vascular resistance (SVR) and the PCWP are reduced and the cardiac output is increased. These are usually opposite to the findings in cardiogenic shock. However, a significant decrease in cardiac output may occur in advanced and late stages of sepsis (*cold* septic shock, which carries a very high mortality rate). Many patients with cardiogenic shock may have normal SVR (i.e., relatively low), even while on vasopressor therapy. Patients with cardiogenic shock may also become *dry* (normal or low PCWP) with overzealous diuresis. Conversely, septic shock patients may become *wet* (normal or high PCWP) with overzealous volume replacement. It is therefore ill advised to depend solely on the aforementioned hemodynamic criteria to differentiate cardiogenic shock from septic shock.

8. **What is the most common cause of cardiogenic shock?**
Acute MI remains the leading cause of cardiogenic shock in the United States. In fact, despite the decline in its incidence with progressive use of timely primary PCI, cardiogenic shock still occurs in 5% to 8% of hospitalized patients with ST-segment-elevation myocardial infarction (STEMI). Unlike what is commonly believed, cardiogenic shock may also occur in up to 2% to 3% of patients with non–ST-segment-elevation myocardial infarction (NSTEMI). Overall, 40,000 to 50,000 cases of cardiogenic shock occur annually in the United States.

9. **Describe the pathophysiology of cardiogenic shock among patients with acute myocardial infarction?**
Left ventricular (LV) pump failure is the primary insult in most forms of cardiogenic shock. The degree of myocardial dysfunction that initiates cardiogenic shock is often, but not always, severe. Hypoperfusion causes release of catecholamines, which increase contractility and peripheral blood flow, but this comes at the expense of increased myocardial oxygen demand and its proarrhythmic and cardiotoxic effects. The decrease in cardiac output triggers also the release of vasopressin and angiotensin II levels, which lead to improvement in coronary and peripheral perfusion at the cost of increased afterload. Neurohormonal activation also promotes salt and water retention, which may improve perfusion but exacerbates pulmonary edema.

On the other hand, the reflex mechanism of increased SVR is not fully effective, and many patients have normal SVR even while on vasopressor therapy. Systemic inflammation, including expression of inducible nitric oxide synthase and generation of excess nitric oxide, is believed to contribute to the pathogenesis and inappropriate vasodilatation of persistent cardiogenic shock.

10. **Describe other mechanisms that cause or contribute to cardiogenic shock after myocardial infarction.**

It is critical to exclude mechanical complications after MI, which may cause or excacerbate cardiogenic shock in these patients. These include ventricular septal rupture, ventricular free wall rupture, and papillary muscle rupture. Two-dimensional (2D) echocardiography is the preferred diagnostic modality and should be promptly performed when mechanical complications are suspected. Among STEMI patients with suspected mechanical complications in whom a 2D echocardiogram is not available, diagnostic pulmonary artery catheterization should be performed (class I recommendation by the 2004 ACC/AHA guidelines). The detection of mechanical complications before coronary angiography may help in dictating the revascularization strategy (surgical revascularization/repair rather than primary PCI).

Additional contributing factors to shock after MI include hemorrhage, infection, and bowel ischemia (the latter may be related to embolization after large anterior MI or presistent hypotension or may be a complication of prolonged intraaortic balloon pump placement).

11. **Can right ventricular dysfunction result in cardiogenic shock?**

Right ventricular (RV) dysfunction may cause or contribute to cardiogenic shock. Predominant RV shock represents 5% of all cardiogenic shock cases complicating MI. RV failure may limit LV filling via a decrease in the cardiac output, ventricular interdependence, or both. Treatment of patients with RV dysfunction and shock has traditionally focused on ensuring adequate right-sided filling pressures to maintain cardiac output and adequate left ventricular preload. However, caution should be undertaken not to overfill the RV and compromise LV filling (via ventricular interdependence).

Shock caused by isolated RV dysfunction carries nearly as high a mortality as LV shock and benefits equally from revascularization.

12. **List the other major causes of cardiogenic shock.**
   - Valvular stenosis (rheumatic mitral, aortic stenosis)
   - Valvular regurgitation (endocarditis, chordal rupture, arotic dissection with acute aortic regurgitation)
   - Cardiac tamponade
   - Massive pulmonary embolism
   - Chronic congestive cardiomyopathy
   - Hypertrophic cardiomyopathy
   - Tako-Tsubo cardiomyopathy
   - Acute myopericarditis
   - Arrhythmias
   - Left atrial myxoma
   - Toxins, drugs
   - Traumatic cardiogenic shock (cardiac penetration with subsequent tamponade, myocardial contusion, tension pneumothorax)

13. **What is the mainstay therapy for patients with cardiogenic shock complicating myocardial infarction?**

Acute reperfusion and prompt revascularization for cardiogenic shock improves survival substantially and is considered the mainstay therapy for cardiogenic shock after acute MI. The Should We Emergently Revascularize Occluded Coronaries for Cardiogenic Shock (SHOCK) study was an a landmark trial (1993–1998) enrolling patients with acute MI complicated by cardiogenic shock and randomizing them to emergency revascularization (152 patients) or initial medical stabilization (150 patients). Six-month mortality was lower in the early revascularization group than in the medical-therapy group (50% versus 63%, P = 0.03). At 1 year, survival was 47% for patients in the early revascularization group compared with 34% in the initial medical stabilization group (P < 0.03). The benefits of early revascularization persisted at long-term follow-up, and the strategy of early revascularization was associated with 67% relative improvement in 6-year survival compared with initial medical stabilization. Currently, the ACC/AHA guidelines recommend early revascularization in cardiogenic shock for those 75 years or younger (class I recommendation) and for suitable candidates older than 75 years (class IIa recommendation). Prasugrel has recently been approved by the FDA. It is contraindicated in patients with a prior stroke or transient ischemic attack.

14. **Which is the best revascularization strategy in patients with cardiogenic shock, complicating myocardial infarction?**
Among patients assigned to revascularization in the SHOCK trial, PCI accounted for 64% of initial revascularization attempts and coronary artery bypass grafting (CABG) for 36%. Although those treated with CABG had more diabetes and worse coronary disease, survival rates were similar with both revascularization strategies. Therefore, emergency CABG is an important treatment strategy in patients with cardiogenic shock and should be considered a complementary revascularization option to PCI in patients with extensive coronary disease.
    The ACC/AHA guidelines recommend CABG in cardiogenic shock patients with multivessel coronary artery disease. However, staged multivessel PCI may be performed if surgery is not an option. A single-stage procedure may be considered if the patient remains in shock after PCI of the infarct-related artery and if the other vessel has a critical flow-limiting lesion and supplies a large myocardium at risk. When cardiogenic shock patients are undergoing PCI, stenting and glycoprotein IIb/IIIa inhibitors improve acute outcomes and are strongly recommended.

15. **Does the timing of revascularization matter in the treatment of cardiogenic shock?**
It is essential that revascularization and reperfusion are conducted promptly. Among patients with STEMI and cardiogenic shock, primary PCI is should be done within a timely door-to-balloon time (less than 90 minutes). Although fibrinolytic therapy is less effective, it is indicated when timely PCI is unlikely to occur and when MI and cardiogenic shock onset are within 3 hours. Unlike what is commonly believed, prompt CABG is feasible. In the SHOCK trial, patients underwent CABG at a median time of 2.7 hours after randomization. It is also important to emphasize that approximately three fourths of patients with cardiogenic shock after MI develop shock after hospital admission. Therefore, prompt revascularization and early reperfusion after acute MI may serve as a strategy to prevent the occurrence of cardiogenic shock.

16. **Describe the common medical therapies for cardiogenic shock.**
Antiplatelet and antithrombotic therapies with aspirin and heparin should be administered to all patients with MI. Although somewhat controversial, some advocate to defer clopidogrel until after emergency coronary angiography is done. This is important in cases where CABG must be performed immediately. Intravenous glycoprotein IIb/IIIa inihibitors (predominantly abciximab) should be used as an adjunct in most PCI procedures. Negative inotropes and vasodilators (including nitroglycerin) should be avoided. Optimal oxygenation and a low threshold to institute mechanical ventilation are neeed. Intensive insulin therapy is recommended for use in complicated MI (while avoiding hypoglycemia). Antiarrhythmic therapies (intravenous amiodarone) should be instituted when needed.
    Pharmacologic support with inotropic and vasopressor agents may be needed for short-term hemodynamic improvement. Although inotropic agents have a central role in cardiogenic shock treatment because the initiating event involves contractile failure, these agents increase myocardial adenosine triphosphate (ATP) consumption and hence their short-term hemodynamic benefits occur at the cost of increased oxygen demand. Higher vasopressor doses have also been associated with poorer survival. Therefore, these agents should be used in the lowest possible doses and for the shortest time possible. The ACC/AHA guidelines

recommend norepinephrine for more severe hypotension because of its high potency. Often, dobutamine is needed as an addition inotropic agent.

17. **What is the mainstay mechanical therapy for cardiogenic shock?**
Intraaortic balloon counterpulsation (IABP) has long been the mainstay of mechanical therapy for cardiogenic shock. IABP support should be instituted promptly, even before transfer for revascularization. IABP improves coronary and peripheral perfusion via diastolic balloon inflation (perfusion augmentation) and augments LV performance via systolic balloon deflation (afterload reduction). Thus, accurate timing of IABP inflation and deflation is important for the optimal hemodynamic support of the failing heart. IABP was performed in 86% of patients in the SHOCK trial. The overall and major complication rates were 7% and 3%, respectively, and were more evident among women and in patients with small body size and peripheral arterial disease.

18. **What is the role of total circulatory support in cardiogenic shock?**
Temporary mechanical circulatory support with LV assist devices (LVADs) interrupts the vicious cycles of ischemia, hypotension, and myocardial dysfunction and allows the recovery of stunned and hibernating myocardium and reversal of neurohormonal derangements. LVAD support involves circulation of oxygenated blood through a device that drains blood from the left side of the heart and returns blood to the systemic arteries with pulsatile or continuous flow. These devices are advocated as a bridge to surgical revascularization, although they have been used as destination therapy for patients with end-stage cardiomyopathy and no alternative therapeutic options. Device-related complications and irreversible organ failure remain their major limitations. Surgically implanted LVADs remove blood through a cannula placed at the LV apex and return blood to the ascending aorta.

Percutaneous LVADs are currently available and can be placed in the cardiac catheterization. The TandemHeart removes blood from the left atrium using a cannula placed through the femoral vein and into the left atrium via transseptal puncture. Blood is then returned to a systemic artery, usually the femoral, with retrograde perfusion of the abdominal and thoracic aorta. Another percutaneous device, the Impella, is a novel intravascular microaxial blood pump, which can be introduced via the femoral artery and placed across the aortic valve in to the left ventricle to unload the left ventricle and provide a short-term mechanical support for the failing heart. The extracorporeal life support (ECLS) involves extracorporeal circulation of blood through a membrane oxygenator, which relieves both the right side and left side of the heart and the lungs of part of their workload. Randomized trials are needed for a more complete assessment of the role of different circulatory support strategies in cardiogenic shock.

19. **What are the mortality and morbidity rates of cardiogenic shock?**
In the modern era, the mortality rate of cardiogenic shock is around 50% (i.e., much lower than the historic figures of 80% and 90%). In the SHOCK trial, the 3- and 6-year survival rates among patients in the early revascularization group were 41% and 33%, respectively, with persistence of treatment benefits for up to 6 years. Importantly, 83% of 1-year survivors in the SHOCK trial were in New York Heart Association (NYHA) classes I or II and many of them enjoyed an acceptable quality of life at 6-year follow-up. Therefore, cardiogenic shock should be regarded as a very serious but treatable (and possibly preventable) condition that, when treated aggressively and in a timely manner, carries a reasonable chance for full recovery.

BIBLIOGRAPHY, SUGGESTED READINGS, AND WEBSITES

1. Menon V, Hochman JS: Treatment and Prognosis of Cardiogenic Shock Complicating Acute Myocardial Infarction: http://www.utdol.com
2. Sharma S, Zevitz M: Cardiogenic Shock: http://www.emedicine.com

3. Antman EM, Anbe DT, Armstrong PW, et al: ACC/AHA guidelines for the management of patients with ST-elevation myocardial infarction, *Circulation* 110(9):e82-e292, 2004.

4. Antman EM, Hand M, Armstrong PW, et al: 2007 focused update of the ACC/AHA 2004 Guidelines for the Management of Patients With ST-Elevation Myocardial Infarction, *Circulation* 117(2):296-329, 2008.

5. Anderson JL, Adams CD, Antman EM, et al: ACC/AHA 2007 guidelines for the management of patients with unstable angina/non–ST-elevation myocardial infarction, *J Am Coll Cardiol* 50(7):e1-e157, 2007.

6. Hochman JS, Sleeper LA, Webb JG, et al: Early revascularization and long-term survival in cardiogenic shock complicating acute myocardial infarction, *JAMA* 295(21):2511-2515, 2006.

7. Hochman JS, Sleeper LA, Webb JG, et al: Early revascularization in acute myocardial infarction complicated by cardiogenic shock. SHOCK Investigators. Should we emergently revascularize occluded coronaries for cardiogenic shock, *N Engl J Med* 341(9):625-634, 1999.

CHAPTER 20

PERCUTANEOUS CORONARY INTERVENTION

Gustavo A. Cardenas, MD and Cindy L. Grines, MD, FACC

Coronary angioplasty, also known as *percutaneous transluminal coronary angioplasty* (PTCA), was first developed and performed in humans in 1977 by Andreas Gruentzig. With advances in technology and development of different balloon types, the procedure progressed to being used in very complex lesions. Since the late 1990s, most angioplasties also involve stent implantation, and with this the nomenclature has changed from PTCA to percutaneous coronary intervention (PCI).

1. **Which patients with chronic stable angina may benefit from PCI?**
   The goals of treatment in patients with stable angina are to improve symptoms, prevent major adverse outcomes, and slow or prevent progression of disease. This is usually accomplished with medical therapy. However, a select group of patients benefit from revascularization (coronary artery bypass grafting [CABG] or PCI). Based on currently available evidence, PCI usually improves symptoms and prolongs exercise duration but probably does not lower mortality in patients with stable angina.

   The largest study comparing medical therapy with PCI (COURAGE) showed that the addition of PCI with bare metal stenting, compared with optimal medical therapy alone, reduced angina but did not reduce long-term rates of death, nonfatal acute myocardial infarction (AMI), and hospitalization for acute coronary syndromes (except in patients with a large area of ischemic and stress testing). However, it should be noted that all patients underwent cardiac catheterization before randomization, and patients who were thought to definitely benefit from revascularization were excluded from randomization (more than 90% of screened patients were excluded).

   Numerous trials have compared PCI with CABG in patients with chronic stable angina. Compared with CABG (based on available studies), PCI provides avoidance of thoracotomy, surgical complications (stroke, dementia, transfusions, prolonged convalescence, pneumonia), shorter convalescence time, and similar survival rates (except in patients with diabetes) but more recurrent symptoms and repeat revascularization. The disadvantages of PCI have been related to early restenosis and the inability to revascularize arteries that are totally occluded or diffusely diseased. Generally speaking, the greater the extent of coronary atherosclerosis, the more compelling the choice of CABG, especially in presence of left ventricular (LV) dysfunction or diabetes.

   In general, patients with chronic stable angina (or in some cases silent ischemia) in whom PCI should be considered include patients:
   - With significant lesion(s) in more than one coronary arteries, a high likelihood of technical success, and a low risk of complications (no need to demonstrate ischemia on noninvasive testing)
   - Who have saphenous vein graft stenoses, who are poor candidates for reoperative surgery
   - With significant left main coronary artery disease (CAD), who are not eligible for CABG
   - With silent ischemia and significant lesion(s) with a high likelihood of success and a low risk of complications. The target vessels must subtend a moderate to large area of viable myocardium or be associated with a moderate to severe degree of ischemia on noninvasive testing.
   - With recurrent stenosis after PCI with a large area of viable myocardium or high-risk criteria on noninvasive testing

2. **Which patients with UA/NSTEMI (NSTE-ACS) should undergo a strategy of early cardiac catheterization and revascularization?**

   According to the 2007 unstable angina/non–ST-segment-elevation myocardial infarction (UA/NSTEMI) guidelines from the American College of Cardiology/American Heart Association (ACC/AHA), an early invasive PCI strategy (i.e., diagnostic angiography with intent to perform revascularization) is indicated for non–ST-segment-elevation acute coronary syndrome (NSTE-ACS) patients who have clinical characteristics indicative of high risk. Such risk factors include the following:

   - Recurrent angina or ischemia at rest or with low-level activities
   - Elevated cardiac biomarkers (troponin T or I)
   - New or presumably new ST-segment depression
   - Congestive heart failure, new or worsening mitral regurgitation, or hypotension
   - High-risk findings from noninvasive testing
   - Reduced LV function (left ventricular ejection fraction [LVEF] less than 40%)
   - Hemodynamic instability (hypotension)
   - Sustained ventricular tachycardia
   - PCI within last 6 months or prior CABG
   - High-risk score as per risk assessment tools (e.g., TIMI, GRACE)

   Initially stabilized patients without the above risk factors (e.g., low-risk patients) may be treated with an initial conservative (or *selective invasive*) strategy.

3. **What are the contraindications to PCI and the predictors of adverse outcomes?**

   The only absolute contraindication to PCI is lack of any vascular access or actively severe bleeding, which precludes the use of anticoagulation and antiplatelet agents. Relative contraindications include the following:

   - Bleeding diathesis or other conditions that predispose to bleeding during antiplatelet therapy
   - Severe renal insufficiency
   - Sepsis
   - Poor patient compliance with medications
   - A terminal condition that indicates short life expectancy
   - Other indications for open heart surgery
   - Anatomic features of poor success
   - Failure of previous PCI

   Patients generally should not undergo PCI if the following conditions are present:

   - There is only a very small area of myocardium at risk.
   - There is no objective evidence of ischemia (unless patient has clear anginal symptoms and has not had a stress test).
   - There is a low likelihood of technical success.
   - The patient has left main coronary artery disease and is a candidate for CABG.
   - There is insignificant stenosis (less than 50% luminal narrowing).

   Clinical predictors of poor outcomes include older age, an unstable condition (acute coronary syndrome [ACS], acute myocardial infarction (MI), decompensated congestive heart failure, cardiogenic shock), LV dysfunction, multivessel coronary disease, diabetes mellitus, renal insufficiency, small body size, and peripheral artery disease.

   Angiographic predictors of poor outcomes include the presence of thrombus, degenerated bypass graft, unprotected left main disease, long lesions (more than 20 mm), excessive tortuosity of proximal segment, extremely angulated lesions (more than 90 degrees), a bifurcation lesion with involvement of major side branches, or chronic total occlusion.

4. **What are the major complications related to PCI?**

The incidence of major complications has constantly decreased over the last two decades as a result of the use of activated clotting time to measure degree of anticoagulation, better antithrombotic and antiplatelet agents, advanced device technology, more skilled operators, and superior PCI strategies. These factors have particularly lowered the incidence of MI and the need for emergent CABG. Major complications include the following:

- Death (incidence 0.4%–1% overall mortality; 5%–7% for patients with ST-segment-elevation myocardial infarction [STEMI])
- MI (0.4%–4.9%)
- Stroke
- The need to perform emergency CABG (0.4%)

Minor complications include transient ischemic attack (TIA), access site complications, renal insufficiency, and adverse reactions to contrast agents.

5. **What are other complications associated with PCI?**

- **Ischemic complications:** The ACC/AHA guidelines recommend measuring creatine kinase, myocardial bound (CK-MB), and troponin I or T in all patients who have signs or symptoms suggestive of MI during or after PCI and in those who undergo complicated procedures. They also consider it reasonable to routinely measure cardiac biomarkers (CK-MB or troponin I or T) in all patients undergoing PCI 8 to 12 hours after the procedure.
- **Abrupt vessel closure:** This is the most common cause of major adverse cardiac event after PCI. It typically occurs within 6 hours of the procedure. Its most common causes are uncovered intimal dissection, thrombus, vessel spasm, or side-branch occlusion. The incidence has decreased to less than 1% related to the routine use of stents and 2b/3a inhibitors. Abrupt vessel closure may also be due to stent thrombosis.
- **Stent thrombosis:** This may occur in the first 24 hours after stent deployment (acute stent thrombosis); in the first month after implantation (subacute stent thrombosis); between 1 to 12 months after implantation (late stent thrombosis); or even more than 1 year after implantation, most notably after drug-eluting stent (DES) implantation (very late stent thrombosis). The primary factors contributing to stent thrombosis are inadequate stent deployment, unrecognized dissection impairing blood flow, and noncompliance with antiplatelet therapy. Stent thrombosis is a potentially catastrophic event, associated with up to a 50% mortality rate.
- **Coronary perforation:** This occurs very infrequently in patients undergoing PTCA or stenting (0.1%–1.14%) and mostly is due to wire perforation. It is slightly more common when atheroablative devices (e.g., rotablation, laser) are used. Most patients are diagnosed during the procedure with visualization of contrast extravasation, but some cases manifest only several hours later as a result of a very slow bleed. In the catheterization laboratory, treatment consists of balloon tamponade of the leak, reversal of anticoagulation, and pericardiocentesis if hemodynamic compromise occurs (a transthoracic echocardiogram should be obtained). For large perforations, covered stents, coils, or surgical repair may be required. When it manifests hours after the PCI procedure, the main treatment is to achieve hemodynamic stabilization and perform pericardiocentesis.
- **Slow-flow and no-flow:** *Slow-flow* is the term applied when contrast injection of the coronary artery reveals slow flow and clearing of the contrast down the coronary artery; *no-flow* is the more extreme form, when the contrast does not appear to flow down the coronary artery at all. These entities are caused by distal embolization and microvascular plugging, impairing epicardial blood flow. These are often seen in degenerated vein graft interventions and can be prevented with the use of intragraft distal protection devices, which trap (or *catch*) and allow removal of embolic debris before it reaches the distal vascular bed. It can also be treated with distal intravascular administration of vasodilators such as adenosine, nitroprusside, and verapamil.

- **Bleeding complications:** Bleeding is a complication of increasing concern with the use of potent antithrombin and antiplatelet agents. It has been determined that major hemorrhage is an independent predictor of early and late mortality in patients undergoing elective or urgent PCI. In addition, accumulating data suggest a possible direct link between blood transfusion and poor outcomes. Proinflammatory and prothrombotic effects of red blood cell transfusion have been demonstrated. Use of a restrictive transfusion policy has been associated with improved outcomes.
- **Access site complications:** Potential complications of vascular access include retroperitoneal bleed, pseudoaneurysm, arteriovenous fistula, arterial dissection, thrombosis, distal artery embolization, groin hematoma, infection/abscess, and femoral neuropathy. Risk factors for access site complications include older age, female gender, morbid obesity or low body weight, hypertension, low platelet count, peripheral artery disease, larger sheath size, prolonged sheath time, intraaortic balloon pump use, concomitant venous sheath, over-anticoagulation, thrombolytic therapy use, and repeat intervention. Patients with a femoral puncture site above the most inferior border of the inferior epigastric artery are at an increased risk for retroperitoneal bleeding. Conversely, development of pseudoaneurysm and arteriovenous fistula are associated with a puncture site at or below the level of the femoral bifurcation.

Several arteriotomy closure devices have emerged as alternatives to mechanical compression to quickly achieve vascular hemostasis. These devices are categorized based on the principle mechanism of hemostasis, which includes biodegradable plug, suture, staples, or ultrasound. Although arteriotomy closure devices offer advantages over mechanical compression (shorter time to hemostasis and patient ambulation, high rate of patient satisfaction, and greater cost effectiveness), no study has been able to show a clear-cut reduction in vascular complications with these devices.

6. **What are some treatment options for various vascular complications?**
   - **Pseudoaneurysm:** If small, observation is recommended. If larger, perform ultrasound-guided compression, thrombin injection, or surgical repair.
   - **Arteriovenous fistula:** If small, observe because most close spontaneously or remain stable. If large or significant shunting is present, options include ultrasound-guided compression, covered stent, or surgical repair.
   - **Dissection:** If there is no effect on blood flow, a conservative approach is indicated. In the presence of flow impairment (distal limb ischemia), angioplasty, stenting, and surgical repair are the treatment options.
   - **Retroperitoneal bleeding:** This should always be suspected with unexplained hypotension, marked decrease in hematocrit, flank/abdominal or back pain, and high arterial sticks. Treatment includes intravascular volume replacement, reversal of anticoagulation, blood transfusion, and occasionally vasopressor agents and monitoring in the intensive care unit. Endovascular management with covered stents, prolonged balloon inflation, or surgical repair are also options but rarely necessary.
   - **Contrast nephropathy:** Contrast-induced nephropathy (CIN) has been associated with increased mortality and morbidity. Several predisposing factors for CIN have been identified, including chronic renal insufficiency (the risk of contrast-induced nephropathy is directly proportional to the severity of preexisting renal insufficiency), diabetes, congestive heart failure, intravascular volume depletion, multiple myeloma, and the use of a large volume of contrast. The most widely accepted measure to prevent CIN consists of assuring adequate hydration with half-normal saline (such as 1 ml/kg/hr for 12 hours before and after procedure). Other measures have shown either only modest benefits or conflicting results or have shown significant benefit in small trials but have not yet been reproduced in larger trials. Such measures include *N*-acetyl-cysteine (Mucomyst, often given as 600 mg

orally twice a day [PO BID] the day before and day of procedure), Isosmolar contrast material, intravenous (IV) sodium bicarbonate, and hemofiltration.

- **Restenosis after PCI:** Restenosis is the process by which the treated lesion in a coronary artery recurs over time (1–6 months). The process is driven by the following:
  - ○ Neointimal hyperplasia caused by smooth muscle cell proliferation and extracellular matrix production
  - ○ Vessel elastic recoil after balloon inflation and vessel negative remodeling over time

Restenosis occurs more commonly in patients with diabetes, renal insufficiency, ostial, bifurcation or saphenous vein graft locations, small vessels, and long lesions.

Angiographic restenosis after balloon PTCA occurs in approximately 40% of patients at 6 months, and 20% to 30% of patients require clinically driven repeat target lesion revascularization within the first year.

Coronary stents prevent vessel elastic recoil and negative remodeling and significantly reduce both angiographic and clinical restenosis rates. The main factor leading to restenosis in coronary arteries treated with bare metal stents (BMS) is thus neointimal hyperplasia as a result of smooth muscle cell proliferation and extracellular matrix production.

Angiographic restenosis with bare metal stents is approximately 20%, and the rate of target lesion revascularization is 10% to 15%. Similar to PTCA, restenosis after BMS typically occurs within the first 6 months.

DES are metal stents coated with a polymer that contains antirestenotic (antiproliferative) medication, which is slowly released over a period of weeks. Restenosis after DES ranges from 5% to 10%, depending on the type of DES, stent size, length, lesion morphology, and presence of diabetes. Compared with BMS, drug-eluting stents significantly reduce the rates of target lesion revascularization (approximately 6.2% versus 16.6%), without any effect on all-cause mortality.

7. **What are the recommendations regarding antiplatelet therapy after PCI?**
   Higher doses of aspirin (162 mg to 325 mg daily) should be given in the following situations:
   - For at least 1 month after implantation of a BMS
   - 3 months after implantation of a sirolimus-eluting stent (SES)
   - 6 months after implantation of a paclitaxel-eluting stent (PES)

   After this period, low-dose (75–162 mg) aspirin should be given indefinitely for patients with coronary artery disease (CAD).

   Clopidogrel, 75 mg daily, should be given for a minimum of 1 month after implantation of a BMS and for 12 months after implantation of a DES because of concerns about delayed endothelialization and late-stent thrombosis with drug-eluting stents. Several investigations have explored various loading doses of clopidogrel. Consistent findings are that, compared with a 300-mg loading dose, doses of either 600 or 900 mg achieve earlier (2 hours versus 6–10 hours) and greater degrees of platelet inhibition with less variability among patients. Fewer patients may demonstrate *resistance* or nonresponsiveness to clopidogrel following the 600-mg dose.

8. **What steps should be taken to prevent premature discontinuation of dual antiplatelet therapy?**
   Although stent thrombosis most commonly occurs in the first month after stent implantation, numerous cases of *late*-stent thrombosis (1 month to 1 year) or even *very late* stent thrombosis (after 1 year) have been reported, particularly in patients who have been treated with DES.

   Premature discontinuation of antiplatelet therapy markedly increases the risk of stent thrombosis, with its catastrophic consequences (MI or death). Factors contributing to premature cessation of thienopyridine therapy include drug cost, inadequate patient and health care provider understanding about the importance of continuing therapy, and requests to discontinue therapy before noncardiac procedures.

   To eliminate premature discontinuation of thienopyridine therapy, the following recommendations should be followed:

- Patients should be clearly educated about the rationale for not stopping antiplatelet therapy and the potential consequences of stopping such therapy. They should be instructed to call their cardiologists if bleeding develops or another physician advised them to stop antiplatelet therapy.
- Health care providers who perform invasive or surgical procedures and are concerned about periprocedural bleeding must be made aware of the potentially catastrophic risks of premature discontinuation of thienopyridine therapy. Such professionals who perform these procedures should contact the patient's cardiologist to discuss optimal patient management strategy.
- Elective procedures for which there is significant risk of perioperative bleeding should be deferred until patients have completed an appropriate course of thienopyridine therapy (12 months after DES implantation if they are not at high risk of bleeding and a minimum of 1 month for bare metal stent implantation).
- For patients treated with DES who are to undergo procedures that mandate discontinuation of thienopyridine therapy, aspirin should be continued if at all possible and the thienopyridine restarted as soon as possible after the procedure.

9. **What should be the management of a patient with a drug-eluting stent who requires urgent noncardiac surgery?**

If at all possible, elective surgery should be avoided until the patient has received a minimum of 1 year of dual antiplatelet therapy after DES. Aspirin should not be discontinued in the perioperative period unless a significant bleeding situation arises (and continuation of clopidogrel is also preferred). Use of heparin or short-acting GP2b/3a inhibitors is not routinely recommended in patients being withdrawn from clopidogrel because of lack of evidence and concern for rebound platelet hyperactivity, especially in absence of ASA, with or without clopidogrel treatment.

Surgery should be performed in an institution with 24-hour catheterization laboratory availability in case of stent thrombosis. Thrombolysis is not very effective because stent thrombosis is mainly a platelet-mediated event.

BIBLIOGRAPHY, SUGGESTED READINGS, AND WEBSITES

1. Boden WE, O'Rourke RA, Teo KK, et al: Optimal medical therapy with or without PCI for stable coronary disease, *N Engl J Med* 356:1503-1516, 2007.

2. Grines CL, Bonow RO, Casey DE, et al: Prevention of premature discontinuation of dual antiplatelet therapy in patients with coronary artery stents, *J Am Coll Cardiol* 49:734-739, 2007.

3. Keeley EC, Boura JA, Grines CL: Comparison of primary and facilitated percutaneous coronary interventions for ST-elevation myocardial infarction: quantitative review of randomised trials, *Lancet* 367(9510):579-588, 2006.

4. King SB, Smith SC, Hirshfeld JW, et al: 2007 Focused Update of the ACC/AHA/SCAI 2005 guideline update for percutaneous coronary intervention, *Circulation* 117:261-295, 2008.

5. Levine GN, Kern MJ, Berger PB, et al: For the American Heart Association Diagnostic and Interventional Cardiac Catheterization Committee: management of patients undergoing percutaneous coronary revascularization, *Ann Intern Med* 139:123-136, 2003.

6. Smith SC, Feldman TE, Hirshfeld JW, et al: ACC/AHA/SCAI 2005 guideline update for percutaneous coronary intervention, *J Am Coll Cardiol* 47:1-121, 2006.

CHAPTER 21

CORONARY ARTERY BYPASS SURGERY

Joseph Huh, MD, Faisal Bakaeen, MD, Danny Chu, MD, FACS, and Matthew J. Wall, Jr., MD, FACS

1. **What are the indications for coronary artery bypass grafting (CABG)?**

   In asymptomatic patients, class I indications for CABG include significant left main stenosis, left main equivalent, and three-vessel disease. In symptomatic patients with documented ischemia, class I indications also include two-vessel disease involving the proximal left anterior descending (LAD) artery and one- or two-vessel disease not involving the LAD if a large area of myocardium is at risk. CABG should be considered as an option in proximal LAD disease and becomes a class I indication if a large area of the anterior myocardium is at jeopardy. Primary surgical revascularization should be considered after myocardial infarction (MI) in patients not suitable for percutaneous coronary intervention (PCI), patients who have failed PCI, or patients with ongoing ischemia or symptoms. After a transmural infarct, mechanical complications such as a postinfarction ventricular septal defect (VSD), acute mitral regurgitation (MR) as a result of papillary rupture, and free-wall pseudoaneurysm should be considered.

2. **How does CABG compare with medical management for coronary artery disease?**

   Three early prospective randomized trials comparing CABG with medical therapy were conducted in the late 1970s and were reported in the early 1980s. The Veterans' Affairs (VA) cooperative trial, European Coronary Surgery Study (ECSS), and Coronary Artery Surgery Study (CASS) showed long-term superiority of surgery over medical therapy in patients with left main (LM) disease, disease involving the LAD artery, and multivessel disease.

3. **How does CABG compare with stents?**

   The Arterial Revascularization Therapies Study (ARTS) was the largest trial comparing CABG with bare metal stents in patients with (1) ejection fraction (EF) greater than 30% and (2) where there was consensus between surgeon and cardiologist that the disease was suitable for both therapies. The study showed improved event-free survival in the CABG group at 1, 2 and 5 years. Drug-eluting stents (DES) have minimized the problem of restenosis in selected patients, but there is limited data directly comparing DES with CABG today. In one real-world outcomes study from the New York state cardiovascular registry databases, CABG did show improved survival at 3 years compared with DES for patients with double- and triple-vessel disease. ARTS II randomized patients to DES or CABG. The primary composite outcomes at one year were similar.

4. **Who benefits most from CABG?**

   The decision for surgery is made based on the comprehensive evaluation of the patient. Although their coronary anatomy may be suitable for bypass, patients' comorbidities need to be considered in the overall risk-benefit analysis. Preoperative presence of renal insufficiency, peripheral vascular disease, recent myocardial infarction, recent stroke, emergency operation, and cardiogenic shock have been identified as factors that increase mortality. Anatomic considerations that favor recommendation for CABG include presence of LM, proximal LAD, multivessel disease, and presence of lesions not amenable to stenting. Diabetes and low ejection fractions also favor surgical revascularization in operable patients.

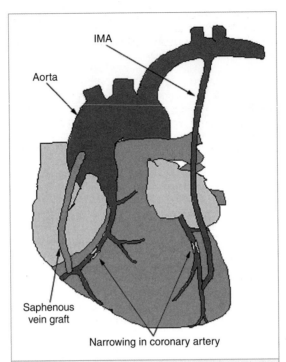

Figure 21-1. Coronary artery bypass grafting. Illustration demonstrates the left internal mammary artery (IMA) anastomosed to the left anterior descending artery (LAD) and a saphenous vein graft anastomosed from the proximal ascending aorta to the right coronary artery. (Modified with permission from Heart Bypass, Irish Heart Foundation. http://www.irishheart.ie/iopen24/defaultarticle.php?cArticlePath=62.)

5. **What are the differences between on-pump and off-pump CABG?**
   In the United States, currently approximately 80% of CABG operations are performed on cardiopulmonary bypass (CPB), whereas 20% are performed off pump. Surgeons have debated the merits of off-pump verses on-pump bypass for many years, but demonstrating differences in hard endpoints such as mortality and stroke have been elusive. Off-pump bypass avoids the CPB and thus should lessen the side effects of the extracorporeal circulation such as activation of inflammatory mediators, coagulopathy, and increased risk of embolic events. In fact, the literature shows equivalency in stroke, renal failure, and perioperative death. In studies, slightly shorter lengths of hospital stay and lower blood usage have been noted for the off-pump group. On-pump bypass surgery produces a heart that is motionless and bloodless, thus allowing precise and exact anastomosis. The cardiopulmonary bypass allows maintenance of hemodynamic stability and aids in complete revascularization. Off-pump revascularization on a beating heart is technically more demanding, and long-term patency of the grafts has been questioned. In experienced centers, patency rates of the bypass grafts performed on pump versus off pump should not differ.

6. **Why is heparin required for cardiopulmonary bypass?**
   The CPB circuit is thrombogenic, and systemic anticoagulation is required to prevent clotting and embolization. The standard agent is heparin (300 U/kg) with activated clotting times

measured to greater than 480 seconds. In patients with previously documented heparin-induced thrombocytopenia, direct thrombin inhibitors have been used. Heparin is used in off-pump CABG at partial dose. After termination of CPB and decannulation, heparin-related anticoagulation is reversed with protamine.

7. **How is cardioplegia administered?**
   Cardioplegia is used on CPB to induce an arrest of the heart. Components of cardioplegia solution are varied in different institutions but include potassium to achieve diastolic arrest. A cross-clamp is applied to the ascending aorta, and the cardioplegia is administered into the aortic root in an antegrade fashion via the coronary ostia. Retrograde cardioplegia is used routinely in many institutions by infusion into the coronary sinus with backward filling of the cardiac veins. Most commonly, cold cardioplegia at $4°$ C is administered intermittently in 15- to 20-minute intervals. Blood can be mixed to the crystalloid component of cardioplegia in a 4:1 mix to provide oxygenated blood to the myocardium and to buffer the pH of the tissue.

8. **How is the myocardium protected during cardiac arrest during bypass surgery?**
   Myocardial ischemia occurs when the aortic cross-clamp is applied, at which time the coronary arteries are not perfusing. Strategies to protect the heart during this time include cooling the heart, unloading the ventricle, and arresting the heart. Systemic cooling of the heart and the body is accomplished with the cardiopulmonary bypass machine. Direct cooling of the heart is also accomplished with cold cardioplegia and topical ice solution. Unloading the ventricles is accomplished by the cardiopulmonary bypass, which empties the heart. The greatest decrease in oxygen demand occurs with the diastolic arrest of the heart using cardioplegia.

9. **Why should the internal mammary artery be used for bypass?**
   Use of the internal mammary artery (IMA) was first described by Kolessov in 1967 (Figure 1), but its impact on survival wasn't noted until the mid-1980s. IMA anastomosed to the LAD artery has an approximately 90% patency at 10 years and offers an advantage in both survival and freedom from reoperation.
   The right IMA, radial artery, gastroepiploic artery, and inferior epigastric arteries have also been used as bypass conduits, and some surgeons have favored all-arterial strategies using only arterial grafts for bypass grafting. However, these other arterial grafts have not duplicated the success of the left IMA to the LAD. The radial artery has been recently evaluated with angiography in several randomized trials and has shown an incremental benefit over saphenous vein graft (SVG) at 1 year. It is hoped that the improvement in patency would be greater at 5 years, and this is the subject of ongoing investigations.

10. **What is the long-term patency of the saphenous vein?**
    Saphenous vein is readily available and relatively easy to procure, provides multiple graft segments, and is the most common bypass graft used other than the IMA. The major limitation of the SVG is its long-term patency. Early attrition of up to 15% can occur by 1 year, with 10-year patency traditionally cited at 60%. Early patency has been shown to be improved by use of aspirin postoperatively. SVG can be harvested using a single long leg incision, multiple short incisions with intervening skin islands, or endoscopic techniques. Early patency has been felt to be equivalent both clinically and angiographically between open and endoscopic techniques.

11. **What complications can occur following CABG?**
    Operative mortality is currently less than 2% overall and less than 1% in low-risk patients. Sentinel complications include stroke, MI, renal failure, pulmonary insufficiency, and mediastinitis. The incidence of each is approximately 1% to 5% and varies with age and preoperative comorbidities of the patient. Atrial fibrillation is the most common complication after cardiothoracic surgery, with an incidence of 20% to 40%.

12. **How is postoperative atrial fibrillation managed?**

    Postoperative atrial fibrillation is usually self-limited and resolves over time as the inflammatory state of the heart improves. The peak incidence is 2 to 4 days after surgery, and the rhythm may persist for 6 to 8 weeks. Incidence increases with age, duration of CPB, presence of chronic obstructive pulmonary disease (COPD), and preexisting heart failure, among other risk factors. Use of beta-blockers postoperatively is the standard of care and helps in atrial fibrillation prophylaxis. Goals of therapy are to rate control and convert if possible. A short duration of anticoagulation may be necessary if the conversion can not be accomplished or the patient shows intermittent tendencies.

13. **Who is at risk for mediastinitis?**

    Mediastinitis is a deep surgical site infection following sternotomy. The infection involves the sternal bone and underlying heart and mediastinum. The organism most commonly recovered is staphylococcal but gram-negative organisms can also be found. The incidence of mediastinitis has been 1% to 4% in the literature, but a recent Society of Thoracic Surgeons (STS) database has shown an incidence less than 1%. Incidence increases with diabetes, morbid obesity, bilateral mammary harvesting, and COPD. Perioperative prophylactic antibiotics, proper skin preparation and clipping, and active control of hyperglycemia in the postoperative setting are important ways to decrease the incidence.

14. **What causes strokes during coronary bypass?**

    Incidence of stroke (type I neurologic deficit) in the perioperative period after cardiac surgery is 1% to 6% and varies with age. Risk of stroke is dependent on the atherosclerotic burden in the brain, aorta, and carotid arteries. Atherosclerotic plaques in the ascending aorta can be the source of atheroemboli during cannulation, cross-clamping, or manipulation of the ascending aorta. Other microemboli include fat and air that can arise during extracorporeal circulation. Alternatively, regional hypoperfusion can occur in the brain as a result of intracranial and extracranial vascular lesions because of significant fluctuations in the blood pressure during on-pump or off-pump surgery.

15. **What is type II neurologic deficit?**

    Type II neurologic deficit is a neurocognitive change after CABG, and its true incidence remains controversial. Changes in intellectual abilities, memory, and mood are more subjective and difficult to evaluate. Reported incidence ranges widely from 2% to 50%. Studies have shown decreases in neurocognitive functioning after CABG, but in small series similar declines over time have been noted in on-pump, off-pump, PCI, and CAD control patients not undergoing intervention.

16. **How should clopidogril be managed preoperatively?**

    Clopidogril increases blood usage during cardiac surgery and increases the risk of reoperation after surgery for mediastinal bleeding. The current recommendation is to avoid clopidogril for 5 days before CABG unless emergent revascularization is needed for ongoing ischemia and the need for revascularization exceeds the risk of bleeding.

17. **What is important in the follow-up of CABG patients?**

    Secondary prevention and control of atherosclerotic risk factors are important in maintaining long-term success of the operation. Use of statins, beta-blockers, and angiotensin-converting enzyme (ACE) inhibitors in low-EF patients are currently the standards of care. In addition, control of hypertension and diabetes and smoking cessation are critical in long-term outcomes.

18. **What is the incidence of recurrent disease requiring redo-CABG?**

    Reoperation may be required because of progression of native coronary disease or failure of previous grafts. The incidence of reoperation has been approximately 10% by 10 years, but aggressive secondary prevention and the successes of PCI may decrease the need for reoperation. Reoperation for bypass is technically more challenging. Complexities of redo bypass surgery include potential injury to the heart and the patent left IMA during sternal reentry, scarring of the mediastinum, presence of graft disease that may embolize, difficulty with myocardial protection, and lack of suitable conduits.

BIBLIOGRAPHY, SUGGESTED READINGS, AND WEBSITES

1. Collins P, Webb CM, Chong CF, et al: Radial artery versus saphenous vein patency randomized trial: five-year angiographic follow-up, *Circulation* 117:2859-2864, 2008.

2. Eagle KA, Guyton RA, et al: ACC/AHA 2004 Guideline update for coronary artery bypass graft surgery: a report of the American College of Cardiology/American Heart Association Task Force on Practice Guidelines (Committee to Update the 1999 Guidelines for Coronary Artery Bypass Graft Surgery), *J Am Coll Cardiol* 44(5):e213-e310, 2004.

3. Goldman S, Zadin K, Moritz T, et al: Long-term patency of saphenous vein and left internal mammary artery grafts after coronary artery bypass surgery: results from a Department of Veterans Affairs cooperative study, *J Am Coll Cardiol* 44:2149-2156, 2004.

4. Hannan EL, Wu C, Walford G, et al: Drug-eluting stents vs. coronary artery bypass grafting in multivessel coronary disease, *N Engl J Med* 358:331-334, 2008.

5. McKhann GM, Grega MA, Borowicz LM Jr, et al: Is there cognitive decline 1 year after CABG? Comparison with surgical and nonsurgical controls, *Neurology* 65:991-999, 2005.

6. Smith SC Jr, Allen J, Blair SN, et al: AHA/ACC Guidelines for secondary prevention for patients with coronary and other atherosclerotic vascular disease: 2006 update, *Circulation* 113:2363-2372, 2006.

7. Sellke FW, DiMaio JM, Caplan LR, et al: Comparing on-pump and off-pump coronary artery bypass grafting: numerous studies but few conclusions: a scientific statement from the American Heart Association Council on Cardiovascular Surgery and Anesthesia in collaboration with the Interdisciplinary Working Group on Quality of Care Outcomes Research, *Circulation* 111:2858-2864, 2005.

IV. CONGESTIVE HEART FAILURE, MYOCARDITIS, AND CARDIOMYOPATHIES

HEART FAILURE: EVALUATION AND LONG-TERM MANAGEMENT

Kumudha Ramasubbu, MD, FACC, Biykem Bozkurt, MD, FACC, and Glenn N. Levine, MD, FACC, FAHA

This chapter deals specifically with the evaluation and long-term management of patients with heart failure caused by depressed ejection fraction. The management of patients with heart failure with preserved ejection fraction *(diastolic dysfunction)* is discussed in Chapter 26. The management of patients with acute decompensated heart failure is discussed in Chapter 23. Specific discussions of the evaluation and management of myocarditis, dilated cardiomyopathy, hypertrophic cardiomyopathy, and restrictive/infiltrative cardiomyopathy, as well as consideration with cardiac transplantation, are discussed in other dedicated chapters in this section of the book. The roles of pacemakers and implantable cardioverter defibrillators in patients with heart failure are discussed in this chapter, as well as in the chapters on pacemakers (Chapter 41) and implantable cardioverter defibrillators (Chapter 42).

1. **What are the most common causes of heart failure?**
   Ischemic heart disease, hypertension, idiopathic dilated cardiomyopathy, valvular heart disease, and chronic alcohol abuse are relatively common causes of heart failure. Less common causes include myocarditis and viral cardiomyopathy, postpartum cardiomyopathy, tachycardia-mediated heart failure, hypothyroidism, infiltrative disorders, high-output states (thyrotoxicosis, beriberi, systemic arterovenous shunting, chronic anemia), genetic cardiomyopathies, muscular dystrophies, and cardiotoxins other than alcohol such as chemotherapeutic agents (e.g., adriamycin) or illicit drugs such as cocaine. Chagas' disease should be considered in patients who have lived in South America.

2. **Initial assessment of the patient with heart failure should include what elements?**
   - Evaluation of heart failure symptoms and functional capacity (dyspnea on exertion, orthopnea, paroxysmal nocturnal dyspnea [PND], fatigue, and lower extremity edema)
   - Evaluation of presence of diabetes; hypertension; smoking; prior cardiac disease; family history of cardiac disease; history of heart murmur, congenital heart disease, or rheumatic fever; sleep disturbances (obstructive sleep apnea [OSA]); thyroid disease history; exposure to parasites; exposure to cardiotoxins; mediastinal irradiation; and past or current use of alcohol and illicit drugs
   - Physical examination, including heart rate and rhythm; blood pressure and orthostatic blood pressure changes; measurements of weight, height, and body mass index; overall volume status; jugular venous distension; carotid upstroke and presence/absence of bruits; lung examination for rales or effusions; cardiac examination for systolic or diastolic murmurs; displaced PMI; presence of left ventricular heave; intensity of S2; presence of S3 or S4; liver size; presence of ascites; presence of renal bruits; presence of abdominal aortic aneurysm; peripheral edema; and peripheral pulses
   - Laboratory tests, including complete blood cell count (CBC), creatinine and blood urea nitrogen (BUN), serum electrolytes, B-type natriuretic peptide (BNP), fasting blood glucose, lipid profile, liver function tests, thyroid-stimulating hormone (TSH), and urine analysis (UA); screening for hemochromatosis, human immunodeficiency virus (HIV), pheochromocytoma, amyloidosis, or rheumatologic diseases reasonable in selected patients, particularly if there is clinical suspicion for testing

- 12-lead electrocardiogram (ECG), assessing for rhythm, conduction abnormalities, QRS voltage and duration, QT duration, chamber enlargement, presence of ST/T changes, and Q waves
- Chest radiograph
- Transthoracic echocardiogram
- Consideration of ischemia workup; depending on patient's age, history, symptoms, and electrocardiogram, this may be no workup, stress testing, or cardiac catheterization
- Endomyocardial biopsy not part of routine workup but can be considered in highly specific circumstances (see later)

3. **How are heart failure symptoms classified?**
Symptoms are most commonly classified using the New York Heart Association (NYHA) classification system:
- **Class I:** No limitation; ordinary physical activity does not cause excess fatigue, shortness of breath, or palpitations.
- **Class II:** Slight limitation of physical activity; ordinary physical activity results in fatigue, shortness of breath, palpitations, or angina.
- **Class III:** Marked limitation of physical activity; ordinary activity will lead to symptoms.
- **Class IV:** Inability to carry on any physical activity without discomfort; symptoms of congestive heart failure are present even at rest; increased discomfort is experienced with any physical activity.

4. **What is the stage system for classifying heart failure?**
In 2001 the American College of Cardiology/American Heart Association (ACC/AHA) introduced a system to categorize the stages of heart failure. This system is somewhat different in focus than the previous NYHA classification system and was intended in part to emphasize the prevention of the development of symptomatic heart failure:
- **Stage A:** Patient at high risk for developing heart failure but without structural heart disease or symptoms of heart failure. Includes patients with hypertension, coronary artery disease (CAD), obesity, diabetes, history of drug or alcohol abuse, history of rheumatic fever, family history of cardiomyopathy, and treatment with cardiotoxins
- **Stage B:** Patient with structural heart disease but without signs or symptoms of heart failure. Includes patients with previous myocardial infarction (MI), left ventricular (LV) remodeling including left ventricular hypertrophy (LVH) and low ejection fraction, and asymptomatic valvular disease.
- **Stage C:** Patient with structural heart disease with prior or current symptoms of heart failure
- **Stage D:** Patient with refractory heart failure requiring specialized interventions

5. **Which patients with heart failure should be considered for endomyocardial biopsy (EMB)?**
In 2007 the American College of Cardiology/American Heart Association/European College of Cardiology (ACC/AHA/ECC) issued a scientific statement on the role of EMB. Most patients who are seen for heart failure should not be referred for EMB. Biopsy results are often nonspecific or unrevealing, and in most cases there is no specific therapy based on biopsy results that have been shown to improve prognosis. However, in certain clinical scenarios EMB should be performed (class I recommendation) or can be considered and is considered reasonable (class IIa recommendation). As given in that document, these include the following:
- New-onset heart failure of less than 2 weeks duration associated with a normal-sized or dilated left ventricle and hemodynamic compromise (class I; level of evidence B)

- New-onset heart failure of 2 weeks' to 3 months' duration associated with a dilated left ventricle and new ventricular arrhythmias, second- or third- degree heart block, or failure to respond to usual care within 1 to 2 weeks (class I; level of evidence B)
- Heart failure of more than 3 months duration associated with a dilated left ventricle and new ventricular arrhythmias, second- or third-degree heart block, or failure to respond to usual care within 1 to 2 weeks (class IIa; level of evidence C)
- Heart failure associated with a dilated cardiomyopathy of any duration associated with suspected allergic reaction or eosinophilia (class IIa; level of evidence C)
- Heart failure associated with suspected anthracycline cardiomyopathy (class IIa; level of evidence C)
- Heart failure with unexplained restrictive cardiomyopathy (class IIa; level of evidence C)

6. **What are the general treatments for patients with heart failure?**
   - Diuretics are indicated for volume overload. Starting doses of furosemide are often 20 to 40 mg once or twice a day, but higher doses will be required in patients with significant renal dysfunction. The dose should be uptitrated to a maximum of up to 600 mg daily. *Failure of therapy* is often the result of inadequate diuretic dosing. Torsemide is more expensive than furosemide but has superior absorption and longer duration of action. Bumentanide is approximately 40 times more potent milligram-for-milligram than furosemide and can also be used in patients who are unresponsive or poorly responsive to furosemide. Synergistic diuretics that act on the distal portion of the tubule (thiaizides, such as metolazone, or potassium-sparing agents) are often added in those who fail to respond to high-dose loop diuretics alone.
   - Inhibition of the renin-angiotensin-aldosterone system should be initiated. Angiotensin-converting enzyme (ACE) inhibitors are first-line agents in those with depressed ejection fraction because they have been convincingly shown to improve symptoms, decrease hospitalizations, and reduce mortality. Angiotensin II receptor blockers (ARBs) are used in those who are ACE-inhibitor intolerant because of persistent cough. ARBs may also be considered *in addition* to ACE inhibitors in select patients (this latter decision is best left to a heart failure specialist). The aldosterone antagonists spironolactone or eplerenone can be considered as additional therapy in carefully selected patients with preserved renal function already on standard heart failure therapies. These drugs are discussed in greater detail in the chapter on ACE inhibitors, ARBs, and other vasodilators (Chapter 24).
   - Hydralazine and isosorbide are used in patients who are unable to tolerate both ACE inhibitors and ARBs because of renal failure. Hydralazine and isosorbide can also be considered *in addition* to an ACE inhibitor or ARB in select patients (this latter decision is best left to a heart failure specialist). These drugs are discussed in greater detail in the chapter on ACE inhibitors, ARBs, and other vasodilators (Chapter 24).
   - Beta-blockers, such as metoprolol succinate (Toprol XL), carvedilol (Coreg), and bisoprolol, have been shown to decrease mortality in appropriately selected patients. These agents should not be initiated in patients with acutely decompensated heart failure and should be initiated in euvolemic patients on stable background heart failure therapy including ACE inhibitors or ARBs.
   - Implantable cardioverter defibrillators (ICDs) are considered for primary prevention in patients whose ejection fractions remain less than 30% to 35% despite optimal medical therapy and who have an expected good-quality life expectancy of at least 1 year. Given numerous different study designs, the exact ejection fraction and duration of therapy applicable for each patient are rather complex (see question 15) and consultation with an electrophysiologist is recommended.

- Biventricular pacing for resynchronization therapy. Biventricular pacing (BiV) or cardiac resynchronization therapy (CRT) should be considered for patients in sinus rhythm with NYHA class III-IV symptoms, left ventricular ejection fraction (LVEF) less than 35%, and QRS greater than 120 msec. Consultation with an electrophysiologist is recommended.

TABLE 22-1. ELEMENTS OF LONG-TERM MANAGEMENT OF PATIENTS WITH CONGESTIVE HEART FAILURE CAUSED BY LEFT VENTRICULAR SYSTOLIC DYSFUNCTION

Treatment/Intervention	Recommendation (Level of Evidence)
Diuretics for fluid retention	Class I (LOE: C)
Salt restriction	Class I (LOE: C)
ACE inhibitors	Class I (LOE: A)
Angiotensin II receptor blockers (ARBs) In ACE inhibitor–intolerant patients	Class I (LOE: A)
ARBs in persistently symptomatic patients with reduced LVEF already being treated with conventional therapy	Class IIb (LOE: C)
Hydralizine + isosorbide in patients ACE inhibitor and ARB intolerant	Class IIb (LOE: C)
Hydralizine + isosorbide in patients already on ACE inhibitor and beta-blocker with persistent symptoms	Class IIa (LOE: A)
Beta-blockers	Class I (LOE: A)
Digoxin in patients with heart failure symptoms. Generally used in those with continued symptoms or hospitalizations despite good therapy with diuretics and ACE inhibitors	Class IIa (LOE: B)
Aldosterone antagonists in patients with moderate to severe symptoms who can carefully be monitored for renal function and potassium level and with baseline creatinine < 2–2.5 mg/dl and potassium < 5 mEq/L	Class I (LOE: B)
Exercise training in ambulatory patients	Class I (LOE: B)
ICD for *secondary prevention* (history of cardiac arrest, ventricular fibrillation, or hemodynamically destabilizing ventricular tachycardia)	Class I (LOE: A)
ICD for *primary prevention* for LVEF < 30%–35% and symptomatic heart failure (see text)	Class I–IIa (LOE: A–B)
Cardiac resynchronization therapy for patients in sinus rhythm with class III-IV symptoms despite medical therapy, LVEF < 35%, and QRS >120 msec (see text)	Class I (LOE: A)

ICD, Implantable cardioverter defibrillator; *LVEF,* left ventricular ejection fraction.

Modified from Hunt SA, Abraham WT, Chin MH, et al: American College of Cardiology/American Heart Association's 2005 updated guidelines for the diagnosis and management of chronic heart failure in the adult, *J Am Coll Cardiol* 46(6):e1-82, 2005.

7. **What approach should be taken if a patient treated with an ACE inhibitor develops a cough?**
   Nonproductive cough related to ACE inhibitors occurs in 5% to 10% of white patients of European descent and in up to 50% of Chinese patients. The cough is believed related to kinin potentiation. The cough usually develops within the first months of therapy and disappears within 1 to 2 weeks of discontinuation of therapy. ACC/AHA guidelines suggest one should first make sure the cough is related to treatment and not another condition. The guidelines state that the demonstration that the cough disappears after drug withdrawal and recurs after rechallenge with another ACE inhibitor strongly suggests that ACE inhibition is the cause of the cough. They emphasize that patients should be *rechallenged*, because many will not redevelop a cough, suggesting the initial development of cough was coincidental and may have been related to heart failure. Patients who do have ACE inhibitor–related cough and cannot tolerate symptoms should be treated with an ARB.

8. **Can all patients with heart failure safely be started on an aldosterone antagonist?**
   No. Aldosterone antagonists should not be started in men with creatinine more than 2.5 mg/dl or women with creatinine more than 2 mg/dl, patients with potassium more than 5 mEq/L, those in whom monitoring for hyperkalemia and renal function is not anticipated to be feasible, and those not already on other diuretics.

9. **How should patients be treated with beta-blockers?**
   Certain beta-blockers have been convincingly shown to decrease mortality in patients with depressed ejection fraction and symptoms of heart failure, and thus it is a class I indication to treat such patients with beta-blockers, with an attempt to reach target doses. The beta-blockers shown to decrease mortality, their starting doses, and their target doses are given in Table 22-2. Recommendations from the Heart Failure Society of America and other organizations include the following:
   - Patients should not be initiated on beta-blocker therapy if in acute decompensated heart failure.
   - Beta-blocker therapy should only be initiated when patients are euvolemic, on a good maintenance dose of diuretics (if indicated), and receiving ACE inhibitors or ARBs.
   - Beta blockers should be initiated at low doses, uptitrated gradually (in at least 2-week intervals), and titrated to target doses shown to be effective in clinical trials (see Table 22-2). Practitioners should aim to achieve target doses in 8 to 12 weeks from initiation of therapy and to maintain patients at maximal tolerated doses.
   - If patient symptoms worsen during initiation or dose titration, the dose of diuretics or other concomitant vasoactive medications should be adjusted and titration to target dose should be continued after the patient's symptoms return to baseline.
   - If uptitration continues to be difficult, the titration interval can be prolonged, the target dose may have to be reduced, or the patient should be referred to a heart failure specialist.
   - If an acute exacerbation of chronic heart failure occurs, therapy should be maintained if possible; the dose can be reduced if necessary, but abrupt discontinuation should be avoided. If the dose is reduced (or discontinued), the beta-blocker (and prior dose) should be gradually reinstated before discharge if possible.

10. **Should patients with heart failure be treated with NSAIDs?**
    No. According to the ACC/AHA guidelines, nonsteroidal antiinflammatory drugs (NSAIDs) can cause sodium retention and peripheral vasoconstriction and can attenuate the efficacy and enhance the toxicity of diuretics and ACE inhibitors. The European Society of Cardiology also cautions against the use of NSAIDs.

TABLE 22-2. INITIAL AND TARGET DOSES FOR COMMONLY USED DRUGS FOR PATIENTS WITH DEPRESSED SYSTOLIC EJECTION FRACTION AND CONGESTIVE HEART FAILURE

Drug	Initial Daily Doses	Target/Maximum Doses
ACE Inhibitors		
Captopril	6.25 mg TID	50 mg TID
Enalapril	2.5 mg BID	10–20 mg BID
Lisinopril	2.5–5 mg qD	20–40 mg qD
Perindolpril	2 mg qD	8–16 mg qD
Ramipril	1.25–2.5 mg qD	10 mg qD
Trandolapril	1 mg qD	4 mg qD
Angiotensin Receptor Blockers (ARBs)		
Candesartan	4–8 mg qD	32 mg qD
Valsartan	20–40 mg BID	160 mg BID
Aldosterone Antagonists		
Spironolactone	12.5–25 mg qD	25 mg qD
Eplerenone	25 mg qD	50 mg qD
Beta–Blockers		
Bisoprolol	1.25 mg qD	10 mg qD
Carvedilol*	3.125 mg BID	25 mg BID (50 mg BID if > 85 kg)
Metoprolol succinate	12.5–25 mg qD	200 mg qD
Loop Diuretics		
Bumentanide	0.5–1.0 mg qD–BID	Max. daily dose 10 mg
Furosemide	20–40 mg qD–BID	Max. daily dose 600 mg
Torsemide	10–20 mg qD	Max. daily dose 200 mg
Thiazide Diuretics		
Chlorthiazide	250–500 mg qD–BID	Max. daily dose 1000 mg
Chlorthalidone	12.5–25 mg qD	Max. daily dose 100 mg
Hydrochlorothiazide	25 mg qD–BID	Max. daily dose 200 mg
Metolazone	2.5 mg qD	Max. daily dose 20 mg
Potassium-Sparing Diuretics		
Amiloride	5 mg qD	Max. daily dose 20 mg
Eplerinone	25 mg qD	50 mg qD
Spironolactone	12.5–25 mg qD	Max. daily dose 50 mg
Triamterene	50–75 mg BID	Max. daily dose 200 mg

BID, Twice a day; *qD,* once a day
*Extended-release carvedilol is now available, although this preparation not specifically tested in heart failure.

Modified from Hunt SA, Abraham WT, Chin MH, et al: American College of Cardiology/American Heart Association's 2005 updated guidelines for the diagnosis and management of chronic heart failure in the adult, *J Am Coll Cardiol* 46(6):e1-e82, 2005.

11. **Is dietary restriction of sodium recommended in patients with symptomatic heart failure?**
Yes. In general, patients should restrict themselves to 2 to 3 g sodium daily, and less than 2 g daily in moderate to severe cases of heart failure.

12. **Is fluid restriction recommended in all patients with heart failure?**
Not necessarily. Expert opinion differs, although some believe fluid restriction generally is not necessary unless the patient (a) is hyponatremic (sodium less than 130 mEq/L) or (b) fluid retention is difficult to control despite high doses of diuretics and sodium restriction. In such cases, patients are generally restricted to less than 2 L/day.

13. **Should patients with congestive heart failure be told to use salt substitutes instead of salt?**
In some cases, the answer is no. Many salt substitutes contain potassium chloride in place of sodium chloride. This could lead to potential hyperkalemia in patients on potassium-sparing diuretics, ACE inhibitors or ARBs, or aldosterone antagonists and those with chronic kidney disease (or those with the potential to develop acute renal failure). Patients who are permitted to use salt substitutes need to be cautioned about potassium issues.

14. **What are the current criteria for consideration of cardiac resynchronization therapy (CRT) with biventricular pacing?**
Patients who should be considered for referral of CRT are those who meet the following criteria:
- Presence of sinus rhythm
- Class III-IV symptoms despite good medical therapy
- LVEF less than 35%
- QRS more than 120 msec (especially if left bundle branch block morphology present)

15. **Which patients with heart failure should be considered for an ICD?**
In the 2008 American College of Cardiology/American Heart Association/Heart Rhythm Society (ACC/AHA/HRS) guidelines on device-based therapy, the writing group stated that they believed guidelines for ICD implantation should reflect the ICD trials that were conducted. Thus, there are many very specific indications for ICD placement, based on symptom class, ischemic or nonischemic causes of heart failure, and ejection fraction. Because ejection fraction may improve significantly after MI (as a result of myocardial salvage and myocardial stunning) and with optimal medical therapy (including ACE inhibitors/ARBs and beta-blockers), patients being considered for ICD implantation for primary prevention should be optimally treated and have their ejection fraction reassessed on optimal medical therapy. ICD should only be considered in patients with a reasonable expectation of survival with an acceptable functional status for at least 1 year. Class I recommendations for ICD include the following:
- Secondary prevention (cardiac arrest survivors of ventricular tachycardia/ventricular fibrillation [VT/VF], hemodynamically unstable sustained VT)
- Structural heart disease and sustained VT, whether hemodynamically stable or unstable
- Syncope of undetermined origin with hemodynamically significant sustained VT or VF induced at electrophysiologic study
- LVEF less than 35% at least 40 days after MI and NYHA functional class II-III
- LVEF less than 30% at least 40 days after MI and NYHA functional class I
- LVEF less than 35% despite medical therapy in patient with nonischemic cardiomyopathy and NYHA functional class II-III
- Nonsustained VT caused by prior MI, LVEF less than 40%, and inducible VF or sustained VT at electrophysiologic study

The 2005 European Society of Cardiology guidelines for the diagnosis and treatment of CHF distill their recommendations into three concise points:

- ICD therapy is recommended to improve survival in patients who have survived cardiac arrest or who have sustained VT, which is either poorly tolerated or associated with reduced systolic LV function (class I; level of evidence A).
- ICD implantation is reasonable in selected patients with LVEF less than 30% to 35%, not within 40 days of an MI, on optimal background therapy including ACE inhibitor, ARB, beta-blocker, and an aldosterone antagonist, where appropriate, to reduce sudden death (class I; level of evidence A).
- ICD implantation in combination with biventricular pacing can be considered in patients who remain symptomatic with severe heart failure, NYHA class III-IV, with LVEF 35% or less and QRS 120 msec or more to improve mortality or morbidity (class IIa; level of evidence B).

BIBLIOGRAPHY, SUGGESTED READINGS, AND WEBSITES

1. Arnold JMO: Heart Failure: http://www.merck.com/mmpe
2. Heart Failure Society of America: http://www.hfsa.org
3. Zevitz ME: Heart Failure: http://www.emedicine.com
4. Cooper LT, Baughman KL, Feldman AM, et al: The role of endomyocardial biopsy in the management of cardiovascular disease: a scientific statement from the American Heart Association, the American College of Cardiology, and the European Society of Cardiology. Endorsed by the Heart Failure Society of America and the Heart Failure Association of the European Society of Cardiology, *J Am Coll Cardiol* 50(19):1914-1931, 2007.
5. Epstein AE, DiMarco JP, Ellenbogen KA, et al: ACC/AHA/HRS 2008 guidelines for device-based therapy of cardiac rhythm abnormalities: a report of the American College of Cardiology/American Heart Association Task Force on Practice Guidelines (Writing Committee to Revise the ACC/AHA/NASPE 2002 Guideline Update for Implantation of Cardiac Pacemakers and Antiarrhythmia Devices) developed in collaboration with the American Association for Thoracic Surgery and Society of Thoracic Surgeons, *J Am Coll Cardiol* 51(21):e1-e62, 2008.
6. Heart Failure Society of America: Heart failure in patients with left ventricular systolic dysfunction, *J Card Fail* 12(1):e38-e57, 2006.
7. Hunt SA, Abraham WT, Chin MH, et al: ACC/AHA 2005 guideline update for the diagnosis and management of chronic heart failure in the adult: a report of the American College of Cardiology/American Heart Association Task Force on Practice Guidelines (Writing Committee to Update the 2001 Guidelines for the Evaluation and Management of Heart Failure), *J Am Coll Cardiol* 46(6):e1-e82, 2005.
8. Mann DL: Management of heart failure patients with reduced ejection fraction. In Libby P, Bonow R, Mann D, et al, editors: *Braunwald's heart disease: a textbook of cardiovascular medicine*, ed 8, Philadelphia, 2008, Saunders.
9. Swedberg K, Cleland J, Dargie H, et al: Guidelines for the diagnosis and treatment of chronic heart failure: executive summary (update 2005): the Task Force for the Diagnosis and Treatment of Chronic Heart Failure of the European Society of Cardiology, *Eur Heart J* 26(11):1115-1140, 2005.

CHAPTER 23

ACUTE DECOMPENSATED HEART FAILURE

G. Michael Felker, MD, MHS, FACC

1. **What is acute decompensated heart failure? Isn't it just a worsening of chronic heart failure?**

   Acute decompensated heart failure (ADHF) is a clinical syndrome of worsening signs or symptoms of heart failure requiring hospitalization or other unscheduled medical care. For many years, ADHF was viewed as simply an exacerbation of chronic heart failure as a result of volume overload, with little implications beyond a short-term need to intensify diuretic therapy (a similar paradigm to exacerbations of chronic asthma). The last decade has seen an explosion of research into the epidemiology, pathophysiology, outcomes, and treatment of ADHF. Multiple lines of evidence now support the concept that ADHF is a unique clinical syndrome with its own epidemiology and underlying mechanisms and a need for specific therapies. ADHF is not just a worsening of chronic heart failure (HF) any more than an acute myocardial infarction (MI) is just a worsening of chronic angina.

   Outcomes data from a variety of studies now support the concept that hospitalization for ADHF can often signal a dramatic change in the natural history of the heart failure syndrome. Rates of rehospitalization or death are as high as 50% within 6 months of the initial ADHF event, which is a much higher event rate than is seen with acute MI.

2. **Are there clinically important subcategories of ADHF?**

   There is great interest in developing a framework for understanding ADHF that would assist in stratifying patients, guiding therapy, and developing new treatments, similar to the basic framework developed for acute coronary syndromes (i.e., ST-segment-elevation myocardial infarction [STEMI], non–ST-segment-elevation myocardial infarction [NSTEMI], and unstable angina). Although this area is rapidly evolving, a few general clinical *phenotypes* of ADHF have emerged.

   - **Hypertensive acute heart failure:** Data from large registries such as ADHERE and OPTIMIZE have shown that a substantial portion of ADHF patients are hypertensive on initial presentation to the emergency department. Such patients often have relatively little volume overload and preserved or only mildly reduced ventricular function and are more likely to be older and female. Symptoms often develop quickly (minutes to hours), and many such patients have little or no history of chronic heart failure. Hypertensive urgency with acute pulmonary edema represents an extreme form of this phenotype.
   - **Decompensated heart failure:** This describes patients with a background of significant chronic heart failure, who develops symptoms of volume overload and congestion over a period of days to weeks. These patients typically have significant left ventricular dysfunction and chronic heart failure at baseline. Although specific triggers are poorly understood, episodes are often triggered by noncompliance with diet or medical therapy.
   - **Cardiogenic shock/advanced heart failure:** Although patients with advanced forms of heart failure are often seen in tertiary care centers, they are relatively uncommon in the broader population (probably fewer than 10% of ADHF hospitalizations). These patients often present with so called *low-output* symptoms that may make diagnosis challenging, including confusion, fatigue, abdominal pain, or anorexia. Hypotension (systolic blood pressure [SBP] less than 90 mm Hg) and significant end-organ dysfunction (especially renal dysfunction) are common features. Many of these patients have concomitant evidence of significant right ventricular dysfunction, with ascites or generalized anasarca.

3. **What is the role of biomarkers like brain natriuretic peptides (BNPs) in the diagnosis of ADHF?**
Although the clinical symptoms (dyspnea, paroxysmal noctural dyspnea [PND], orthopnea, fatigue) and signs (elevated jugular venous pressure, pulmonary rales, edema) of ADHF are well known, the diagnosis can often be challenging in patients presenting to acute care settings. This is especially true in the elderly and patients with significant comorbid conditions such as chronic obstructive pulmonary disease (COPD). The development of natriuretic peptides as a diagnostic tool has been a major advance in ADHF diagnosis. The clinically available natriuretic peptides for ADHF diagnosis include BNP and its biologically inert amino-terminal fragment, N-terminal pro-B type natriuretic peptide (NTproBNP). Despite some subtle differences between these two biomarkers, they provide similar diagnostic information when used in patients presenting to the emergency department with unexplained dyspnea, although the range of values is significantly different (in general, NTproBNP levels are approximately 5 to 10 times greater than BNP levels in the same patient). The landmark Breathing Not Properly Study measured BNP levels in 1586 patients presenting to the emergency department with unexplained dyspnea. In this study, treating physicians were blinded to BNP values and a panel of cardiologists adjudicated whether hospitalizations were due to ADHF or other causes (based on all clinical data other than the BNP values). As shown in Figure 23-1, a cutoff of 100 pg/ml of BNP had a positive predictive value of 79% and a negative predictive value of 89% for the diagnosis of ADHF. The area under the receiver operating curve (ROC) was 0.91, suggesting a very high degree of accuracy for establishing the diagnosis of ADHF. Subsequent studies have demonstrated similar findings for NTproBNP, although optimal diagnostic cutoffs are different (450 pg/ml for patients younger than 50 years and 900 pg/ml for patients older than 50 years). The use of natriuretic peptide has now become standard of care in the diagnosis of patients with dyspnea presenting to acute care settings.

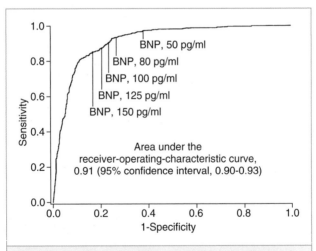

Figure 23-1. Receiver operator curve for use of BNP in making diagnosis of ADHF in patients with acute unexplained dyspnea. (Adapted from Maisel AS, Krishnaswamy P, Nowak RM, et al: Rapid measurement of B-type natriuretic peptide in the emergency diagnosis of heart failure. *N Engl J Med.* 2002; 347(3):161-167.)

4. **What features suggest patients who are particularly high risk?**
Analysis of large datasets from both clinical trials and registries of ADHF patients have identified a few features that consistently suggest a high risk of short-term morbidity and mortality in patients hospitalized with ADHF (Box 23-1). Across studies, the most consistent of these are blood urea

---

BOX 23-1. HIGH-RISK FEATURES IN PATIENTS HOSPITALIZED WITH ADHF

- Lower systolic blood pressure
- Elevated blood urea nitrogen (BUN)
- Hyponatremia
- History of prior heart failure hospitalization
- Elevated BNP or NTproBNP
- Elevated troponin T or I

---

nitrogen (BUN), systolic blood pressure, and hyponatremia. Interestingly, BUN has consistently proved to be a stronger predictor of outcomes than creatinine (Fig. 23-2). One potential explanation of this finding is that BUN may integrate both renal function and hemodynamic information. Unlike the situation in many other cardiovascular conditions, *higher* blood pressure has consistently been associated with *lower* risk. Hyponatremia appears to be associated with lower output and greater neurohormonal activation, and risk appears to be increased with even mild forms of hyponatremia. A variety of biomarkers also appear to have strong prognostic implications in ADHF, in particular the natriuretic peptides (BNP or NTproBNP) and troponin.

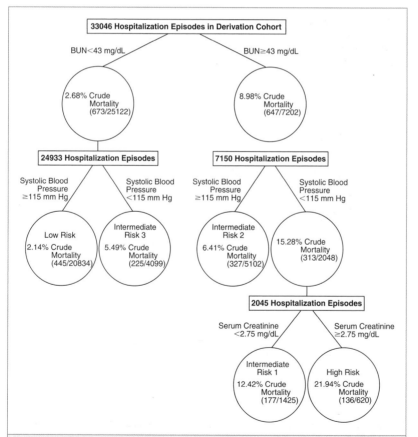

Figure 23-2. Predictors of in-hospital mortality in the ADHERE database. (Reprinted with permission from Fonarow GC, Adams KF Jr, Abraham WT, et al. Risk stratification for in-hospital mortality in acutely decompensated heart failure: classification and regression tree analysis. *JAMA* 293:576, 2005.)

5. **What are the goals of therapy in ADHF?**

Specific therapies for ADHF should be assessed in the context of the overall goals of therapy. A summary of suggested goals of therapy based on current guidelines from the Heart Failure Society of America (HFSA) and European Society of Cardiology (ESC) are shown in Box 23-2.

BOX 23-2. TREATMENT GOALS FOR ADHF HOSPITALIZATION

- Improve symptoms of congestion
- Optimize volume status
- Identify and address triggers for decompensation
- Optimize chronic oral therapy
- Minimize side effects
- Identify patients who might benefit from revascularization
- Educate patients concerning medications and disease management

---

6. **How should we give diuretics in ADHF?**

Because most episodes of ADHF are associated with some degree of congestion or volume overload, intravenous loop diuretics remain a cornerstone of ADHF therapy. Because many symptoms in ADHF (in particular dyspnea) appear to be closely related to elevated ventricular filling pressures, reduction of filing pressures in order to improve acute symptoms is a major goal of therapy. Recently, however, observational data from a variety of sources have led to questions about the appropriate use of diuretics in patients with ADHF. Studies of patients with both chronic heart failure and ADHF have shown that higher diuretic use is associated with a higher incidence of adverse events (especially worsening renal function) and mortality. Interpreting this type of data is highly problematic because of the issue of confounding by indication (i.e., patients who need higher diuretic doses are typically sicker, and thus it is impossible to determine if higher doses of diuretics are simply a marker of greater disease severity or whether they directly contribute to worsening outcomes). Controversy also exists regarding whether continuous infusion (as opposed to intermittent bolus administration) may be a safer and more efficacious way of administering intravenous (IV) diuretics in ADHF. An ongoing National Institutes of Health (NIH)–sponsored randomized clinical trial (the Diuretic Optimization Strategies Evaluation [DOSE]) is attempting to define the best way to use IV diuretics in ADHF. Until more data are available, using the lowest dose of IV diuretics that will effectively result in symptom improvement and clinical decongestion appears the most prudent approach.

7. **What about vasodilators such as nesiritide?**

Nesiritide, a recombinant form of human BNP, is a vasodilator with similar hemodynamic effects to other parenteral vasodilators such as nitroglycerin and sodium nitroprusside. Nesiritide was approved for ADHF therapy based on its ability to speed the resolution of symptoms in patients with ADHF in the Vasodilation in the Management of Acute Congestive Heart Failure (VMAC) study. Subsequently, several retrospective meta-analysis have suggested the possibility that nesiritide therapy could be associated with adverse effects on renal function or even increased mortality. This led to substantial controversy about the appropriate role of nesiritide in ADHF management. At present, a large international study, the ASCEND-HF study, is ongoing to provide definitive evidence about the safety and efficacy of nesiritide with regard to relief of symptoms and harder endpoints like rehospitalization and mortality. Until data from ASCEND-HF is available, current guidelines suggest that vasodilators may be considered to speed resolution of symptoms or in patients who are refractory to initial therapy. Any ADHF patient treated with IV vasodilators should be monitored carefully for the development of hypotension.

8. **What is the role of inotropes like dobutamine or milrinone in patients with ADHF?**

   Inotropic drugs, which increase cardiac contractility, are theoretically appealing as a therapy for ADHF. Despite this theoretical appeal, however, available data clearly demonstrate that such agents are not indicated for the vast majority of ADHF patients. In the OPTIME-CHF study, a large randomized trial of IV milrinone therapy in ADHF, randomization to milrinone did not shorten length of stay or improve other clinical outcomes and was associated with significantly higher rates of arrhythmias and hypotension than was placebo. These data suggest that the routine use of inotropes is not indicated in ADHF management. Importantly, OPTIME-CHF specifically excluded patients with shock or other apparent indications for inotropes. As noted earlier, the vast majority of ADHF patients do not have evidence of end-organ hypoperfusion or shock. In the subset of patients with cardiogenic shock or severe end-organ dysfunction, inotropic therapy may still be indicated as a method of achieving short-term stabilization until more definitive long-term therapy (such are revascularization, cardiac transplantation, or mechanical cardiac support) can be employed.

9. **What is the role for invasive hemodynamic monitoring in patients with ADHF?**

   The routine use of invasive hemodynamic monitoring (such as with pulmonary artery catheters) is not indicated in patients with ADHF. This recommendation is based primarily on the results of the ESCAPE study, which demonstrated no advantage in terms of days alive and free from hospitalization when patients hospitalized with advanced heart failure were randomized to pulmonary artery catheter guided therapy vs. usual care. Invasive hemodynamic monitoring may be indicated to guide therapy in selected patients who are refractory to initial therapy, particularly those with hypotension or worsening renal function.

10. **What is cardiorenal syndrome in ADHF?**

    Worsening renal function during hospitalization for ADHF represents a major clinical challenge. Often termed *cardiorenal syndrome* (CRS), this clinical syndrome is characterized by persistent volume overload accompanied by worsening of renal function. Development of CRS, as defined by an increase in serum creatinine of 0.3 mg/dl or more from admission, occurs in as many as one third of patients hospitalized with ADHF. Development of CRS is associated with higher mortality and increased length of stay in patients with ADHF. Although the underlying mechanisms of CRS remain ill defined, data suggest that higher diuretic doses, preexisting renal disease, and diabetes mellitus are associated with an increased risk. The optimal therapeutic strategy for patients with ADHF and CRS remains unknown. A variety of clinical approaches (hemodynamically guided therapy, inotropes, temporarily holding diuretics, etc.) have all been used with varying results, and there are no large outcomes studies to guide management of these challenging patients. Ultrafiltration therapy, which results in the removal of both free water and sodium, is currently being studied as an approach to CRS in an NIH-sponsored, randomized clinical trial.

11. **How should we determine when to discharge patients?**

    The decision of when to discharge a patient with ADHF from the hospital is often based on clinical judgment rather than objective criteria. Criteria that should be met before consideration of hospital discharge have been published in the HFSA guidelines (Box 23-3). Most patients should have follow-up scheduled with 7 to 10 days of discharge, and high-risk patients should be considered for earlier follow-up (by phone or in person) or referral to a comprehensive disease management program. Early adjustment of diuretics may be required as patients transition from the hospital environment (with IV diuretics and controlled low-sodium diet) to home.

BOX 23-3. CRITERIA FOR HOSPITAL DISCHARGE IN ADHF

- Exacerbating factors addressed
- Near optimal volume status achieved
- Transitioned from IV to oral therapy (consider 24 hours of stability on oral therapy for high-risk patients)
- Education of patient and family
- Near optimal chronic heart failure therapy achieved
- Follow-up appointment scheduled in 7 to 10 days (earlier if high risk)

BIBLIOGRAPHY, SUGGESTED READINGS, AND WEBSITES

1. Adams KF, Lindenfeld J, Arnold JM, et al: HFSA 2006 comprehensive heart failure practice guideline, *J Card Fail* 12:1-119, 2006.

2. Cotter G, Felker GM, Adams KF, et al: The pathophysiology of acute heart failure–is it all about fluid accumulation? *Am Heart J* 155(1):9 18, 2008.

3. ESCAPE Investigators and ESCAPE Study Coordinators: Evaluation Study of Congestive Heart Failure and Pulmonary Artery Catheterization Effectiveness: the ESCAPE trial, *JAMA* 294(13):1625-1633, 2005.

4. Fonarow GC, Adams KF Jr, Abraham WT, et al for the ADHERE Scientific Advisory Committee: Risk stratification for in-hospital mortality in acutely decompensated heart failure: classification and regression tree analysis, *JAMA* 293(5):572-580, 2005.

5. Forman DE, Butler J, Wang Y, et al: Incidence, predictors at admission, and impact of worsening renal function among patients hospitalized with heart failure, *J Am Coll Cardiol* 43(1):61-67, 2004.

6. Gheorghiade M, Zannad F, Sopko G, et al: Acute heart failure syndromes: current state and framework for future research, *Circulation* 112(25):3958-3968, 2005.

7. Hasselblad V, Stough WG, Shah MR, et al: Relation between dose of loop diuretics and outcomes in a heart failure population: results of the ESCAPE trial, *Eur J Heart Fail* 9(10):1064-1069, 2007.

8. Maisel AS, Krishnaswamy P, Nowak RM, et al: Rapid measurement of B-type natriuretic peptide in the emergency diagnosis of heart failure, *N Engl J Med* 347(3):161-167, 2002.

9. Nieminen MS, Bohm M, Cowie MR, et al: Executive summary of the guidelines on the diagnosis and treatment of acute heart failure: the Task Force on Acute Heart Failure of the European Society of Cardiology, *Eur Heart J* 26(4):384-416, 2005.

10. Sackner-Bernstein JD, Kowalski M, Fox M, et al: Short-term risk of death after treatment with nesiritide for decompensated heart failure: a pooled analysis of randomized controlled trials, *JAMA* 293(15):1900-1905, 2005.

CHAPTER 24

INHIBITORS OF THE RENIN-ANGIOTENSIN–ALDOSTERONE SYSTEM

Kumudha Ramasubbu, MD, FACC and Anita Deswal, MD, MPH

1. **What is the rationale for blocking the renin-angiotensin-aldosterone system in heart failure?**

   Activation of the renin-angiotensin-aldosterone system (RAAS) plays a critical role in the pathogenesis of heart failure. The deleterious effects of renin-angiotensin system activation in heart failure are mediated primarily through increased levels of the neurohormone angiotensin (AT) II. Angiotensin II is a potent vasoconstrictor; it causes sodium retention (via aldosterone and renal vasoconstriction) and fluid retention (via antidiuretic hormone). At the cellular level, angiotensin II promotes migration, proliferation, and hypertrophy, thus producing numerous adverse effects resulting in remodeling of the left ventricle and alterations in the vasculature.

   Angiotensin-converting enzyme (ACE) inhibitors exert their effects mainly by inhibiting the production of angiotensin II (Fig. 24-1). Initially, the hemodynamic effects of ACE inhibitors were thought to be central to their role in heart failure. Studies with the ACE inhibitor captopril demonstrated an acute decrease in peripheral vascular resistance, resulting in an increase in cardiac output and lowering of left ventricular (LV) filling pressures in patients with heart failure

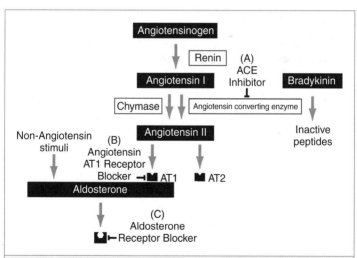

Figure 24-1. The renin-angiotensin system can be inhibited at various levels. **A,** Angiotensin-converting enzyme (ACE) inhibitors block ACE, the enzyme that converts angiotensin I to angiotensin II, thereby reducing the angiotensin II available to stimulate the angiotensin receptors. **B,** Angiotensin receptor blockers selectively block the binding of angiotensin II to the AT_1 receptor thereby blocking the effect of angiotensin II on endorgans. **C,** Aldosterone receptor blockers block the aldosterone receptor in the distal renal tubules, thereby decreasing sodium chloride absorption, potassium excretion, and water retention. (Reprinted from Kazi D, Deswal A: Heart failure clinics: role and optimal dosing of angiotensin-converting enzyme inhibitor therapy, *Cardio Clin* 2008; 26(1):1-14.)

and LV systolic dysfunction. These effects were sustained with long-term ACE inhibition. It has since been recognized that the beneficial effects of ACE inhibitors on the neurohormonal milieu in heart failure and LV remodeling may be more important for their efficacy in patients with heart failure. Most recently, there has been increasing recognition that the antiatherogenic, antiinflammatory, antiproliferative, and antithrombotic properties of ACE inhibitors are likely to contribute to their protective effects, noted in patients with and without heart failure. Thus, ACE inhibition attenuates many of the key hemodynamic, mechanical, and functional disturbances crucial to the pathophysiology of heart failure.

The use of ACE inhibitors does not lead to complete suppression of angiotensin II levels in patients with heart failure, and levels of angiotensin II gradually increase despite chronic ACE inhibitor therapy. Various pathways have been proposed to explain this *escape* from ACE inhibition. First, the competitive inhibition of ACE results in an increase in renin and angiotensin I, which may overcome the blockade of this enzyme. Second, angiotensin I is converted to angiotensin II through alternative, non-ACE enzymatic pathways using chymase, kallikrein, cathepsin G, and tonin. On the premise of such observations, angiotensin receptor blockers (ARBs) were developed to enable a more complete inhibition of angiotensin II activity by directly blocking the AT_1 receptor.

Short-term therapy with ACE inhibitors and ARBs can lower aldosterone levels, but the suppression is not sustained, again because of nonangiotensin stimuli for the production of aldosterone. Moreover, aldosterone independently appears to have adverse effects on structure and function of the heart (myocardial fibrosis) which can lead to adverse left ventricular remodeling. Therefore, the use of aldosterone antagosists (spironolactone and eplerenone) has also been investigated in patients with chronic heart failure.

2. **What antagonists of the renin-angiotensin-aldosterone system are available and how do they exert their effects (see Fig. 24-1)?**
ACE inhibitors inhibit ACE, thus blocking the conversion of angiotensin I to angiotensin II. ACE is predominantly found in the pulmonary and to a lesser extent in the renal endothelium. By decreasing the production of angiotensin II, ACE inhibitors attenuate sympathetic tone, decrease arterial vasoconstriction, and attenuate myocardial hypertrophy. Because angiotensin II stimulates aldosterone production, circulating levels of aldosterone are reduced. This results in a decrease in sodium chloride absorption, potassium excretion in the distal tubules, and water retention. Through a decrease in antidiuretic hormone (ADH) production, ACE inhibitors also decrease water absorption in the collecting ducts.

The currently recommended ACE inhibitors for heart failure, with their respective goal dosages, are shown in Table 24-1.

TABLE 24-1. CURRENTLY RECOMMENDED ACE INHIBITORS FOR HEART FAILURE WITH THEIR RESPECTIVE GOAL DOSAGES

ACE Inhibitors	Initial Daily Dose(s)	Maximum Daily Dose(s)
Captopril	6.25 mg 3 times	50 mg 3 times
Enalapril	2.5 mg twice	10–20 mg twice
Lisinopril	2.5–5 mg once	20–40 mg once
Fosinopril	5–10 mg once	40 mg once
Perindopril	2 mg once	8–16 mg once
Quinapril	5 mg twice	20 mg twice
Ramipril	1.25–2.5 mg once	10 mg once
Trandolapril	1 mg once	4 mg once

ARBs selectively block the binding of angiotensin II to the AT_1 receptor, thereby blocking the effect of angiotensin II on endorgans. This results in attenuation of sympathetic tone, decrease in arterial vasoconstriction, and attenuation of myocardial hypertrophy. Because angiotensin II stimulates aldosterone production, circulating levels of aldosterone are reduced. This results in a decrease in sodium chloride absorption, potassium excretion in the distal tubules, and water retention.

The currently recommended ARBs for heart failure, with their respective goal dosages, are shown in Table 24-2.

TABLE 24-2. CURRENTLY RECOMMENDED ARBs FOR HEART FAILURE WITH THEIR RESPECTIVE GOAL DOSAGES

Angiotensin Receptor Blockers	Initial Daily Dose(s)	Maximum Daily Dose(s)
Candesartan	4–8 mg once	32 mg once
Valsartan	20–40 mg twice	160 mg twice
Losartan*	25–50 mg once	50–100 mg once

*While trials using candesartan and valsartan showed equivalent efficacy compared with ACE inhibitors, the ELITE II trial comparing losartan with captopril showed a trend toward improved outcomes with captopril. Thus, candesartan and valsartan are the recommended ARBs for patients with chronic heart failure caused by LV systolic dysfunction.

Aldosterone receptor blockers block the mineralocorticoid receptor in the distal renal tubules, thereby decreasing sodium chloride absorption, potassium excretion, and water retention. In addition, they block the direct deleterious effects of aldosterone on the myocardium and may thus decrease myocardial fibrosis and its consequences.

The currently recommended aldosterone antagonists for heart failure, with their respective goal dosages, are shown in Table 23-3.

TABLE 24-3. CURRENTLY RECOMMENDED ALDOSTERONE ANTAGONISITS FOR HEART FAILURE WITH THEIR RESPECTIVE GOAL DOSAGES

Aldosterone Antagonists	Initial Daily Dose(s)	Maximum Daily Dose(s)
Spironolactone	12.5–25 mg once	25 mg once
Eplerenone	25 mg once	50 mg once

Renin inhibitors directly block the renin receptor. Because renin, which catalyzes the first step of the RAAS cascade, is inhibited, more downstream products of the RAAS will be affected than is the case with ARBs and ACE inhibitors, which may result in a more wide-ranging inhibition of the RAAS. The renin inhibitor aliskiren has been investigated for the treatment of hypertension. So far, clinical trials evaluating aliskiren in patients with hypertension have demonstrated modest blood pressure reductions with good tolerability. The role for renin inhibitors in heart failure patients is unclear at the time of this writing. Although a more comprehensive blockade of the RAAS may be beneficial in heart failure, it is unknown if this may potentially worsen outcomes as a result of complete inhibition of a compensatory system. Ongoing trials are investigating the use of aliskerin in heart failure at the time of this writing.

3. **What are the indications for using ACE inhibitors in heart failure?**

Symptomatic Systolic Heart Failure

The body of evidence supporting the use of ACE inhibitors in heart failure is enormous, with ACE inhibitors having been evaluated in clinical trials of more than 7,000 patients with symptomatic heart failure. In patients with symptomatic heart failure (New York Heart Association [NYHA] functional class II-IV) and LV systolic dysfunction (defined as a left ventricular ejection fraction of 40% or less in most trials), ACE inhibitors showed a significant reduction in mortality (which chiefly was due to a reduction in deaths attributable to progressive heart failure). Apart from their benefit on mortality, a number of trials have also shown that ACE inhibitors improve symptoms and exercise capacity in patients with heart failure and reduce hospitalizations for heart failure. In addition, significant reductions in myocardial infarction and nonsignificant reductions in strokes and other thromboembolic events were seen. Moreover, ACE inhibitors have been shown to have a beneficial effect on reverse remodeling of the left ventricle.

Asymptomatic LV Systolic Dysfunction

Unlike other heart failure medications, ACE inhibitors have been shown to be beneficial in patients with asymptomatic LV systolic dysfunction (i.e., left ventricular ejection fraction 40% or less) and in preventing heart failure development in patients at risk. Thus, ACE inhibitors should be used in patients at risk of developing heart failure (stage A) and in patients with asymptomatic LV systolic dysfunction (stage B).

Heart Failure with Preserved Ejection Fraction

Thus far only one large clinical trial has assessed the role of ACE inhibitors in patients with heart failure and preserved ejection fraction. The Perindopril for Elderly People with Chronic Heart Failure (PEP-CHF) study was a randomized double-blind trial, comparing placebo with perindopril in patients 70 years and older with a diagnosis of heart failure and preserved LV systolic function (left ventricular ejection fraction 40% or greater). Although the primary endpoint did not demonstrate benefit with the use of perindopril over placebo, perindopril-treated patients showed improved symptoms, better exercise capacity, and fewer hospitalizations for heart failure in the first year. The effect of perindopril on long-term morbidity and mortality remains uncertain because this study was underpowered to determine this. For further information on heart failure with preserved ejection fraction, see Chapter 26.

Post–Myocardial Infarction LV Dysfunction

Three long-term trials demonstrated benefit of the ACE inhibitors captopril, ramipril, and trandolapril in patients with LV systolic dysfunction or heart failure after an acute myocardial infarction (MI). The use of ACE inhibitor therapy, begun within 3 to 16 days after an acute MI and continued long term, was associated with an overall reduction in mortality, recurrent MI, hospitalization for heart failure, and development of heart failure.

4. **What is the efficacy of ARBs compared with ACE inhibitors in patients with chronic heart failure?**

Trials comparing the efficacy of ARBs with ACE inhibitors in chronic heart failure revealed that treatment with ARB was equivalent to ACE inhibition (trials using valsartan and candesartan); however, a trend toward improved outcomes was noted with ACE inhibitors in a trial using the ARB losartan.

In view of the vast experience with the ACE inhibitors as compared with ARBs, ACE inhibitors continue to be the recommended agents of choice for patients with heart failure and depressed LV systolic function. That said, ARBs—specifically, candesartan and valsartan—confer significant benefit on mortality and morbidity in patients with heart failure who are intolerant of ACE inhibitors and therefore offer a good alternative strategy in these patients. Candesartan and valsartan are the recommended ARBs for patients with heart failure who are intolerant of ACE inhibitors.

5. **When should ARBs be added to ACE inhibitors in patients with chronic heart failure?**
    Theoretically, the more complete angiotensin II inhibition using a combination of ACE inhibitors and ARBs in patients with heart failure may translate into improved clinical outcomes.
    Two large clinical trials in patients with heart failure, the Val-HeFT and the CHARM-Added trial, evaluated the impact on morbidity and mortality of adding ARBs to ACE inhibitors. Both trials suggest that adding an ARB to an ACE inhibitor leads to a reduction in heart failure hospitalizations, although combination therapy had no impact on mortality. Thus, the current Heart Failure Society guidelines recommend the addition of ARBs to ACE inhibitors in patients who meet the following conditions:
    - Continue to have symptoms of heart failure despite receiving target doses of ACE inhibitors and beta-blockers
    - Are taking ACE inhibitors but are unable to tolerate beta-blockers and have persistent symptoms, if there are no contraindications

6. **List indications for ARB use in chronic systolic heart failure.**
    In patients with heart failure, the clinical efficacy of ARBs and ACE inhibitors is comparable. However, as a result of the extensive experience in efficacy and safety with ACE inhibitors, they remain the first choice. ARBs are considered good alternatives in patients intolerant of ACE inhibitors.
    Indications for ARBs include the following:
    - Patients who are intolerant of ACE inhibitors because of angioedema or intractable cough can take ARBs.
    - ARBs can be added to an ACE inhibitor if the patient still has symptomatic heart failure or uncontrolled hypertension and there are no contraindications.

7. **List the indications and recommended dosing of aldosterone antagonists in heart failure.**
    Indications include the following:
    - Chronic NYHA class III-IV heart failure and left ventricular ejection fraction 35% or less; already receiving standard therapy for heart failure, including ACE inhibitors, beta-blockers, and diuretics (Randomized Aldactone Evaluation Study [RALES] trial)
    - Post-MI LV dysfunction (ejection fraction less than 40%) and heart failure; already receiving standard therapy, including ACE inhibitors and beta-blockers (Eplerenone Post-Acute Myocardial Infarction Heart Failure Efficacy and Survival Study [EPHESUS] trial)
    Dosing is as follows:
    - **Spironolactone:** 12.5 mg daily, increased to 25 mg daily
    - **Eplerenone:** 25 mg daily, increased to 50 mg daily

8. **Describe common adverse effects of ACE inhibitors, ARBs, and aldosterone antagonists.**
    Common adverse effects include the following:
    - **ACE inhibitors:** hypotension, worsening renal function, hyperkalemia, cough, angioedema
    - **ARBs:** hypotension, worsening renal function, hyperkalemia
    ARBs are as likely as ACE inhibitors to produce hypotension, worsening renal function, and hyperkalemia. Otherwise, ARBs are better tolerated than ACE inhibitors. The incidence of cough is much lower in ARBs (approximately 1%) compared with ACE inhibitors (approximately 10%). The incidence of angioedema with ACE inhibitors is rare (less than 1%; more common in African Americans) and even more rare with ARBs. However, because there have been case

reports of patients developing angioedema on ARBs, the guidelines advise that ARBs may be considered in patients who have had angioedema while taking an ACE inhibitor, albeit with extreme caution. Practically, if a patient develops angioedema while taking an ACE inhibitor, an ARB is generally not initiated.

- **Aldosterone antagonists:** hyperkalemia; renal dysfunction may be aggravated
Gynecomastia and other antiandrogen effects can occur with spironolactone and are not generally seen with eplerenone.

9. **What are the indications and dosing of nitrates/hydralazine in patients with chronic heart failure?**
The vasodilator combination of isordil/hydralazine (I/H) has been shown to produce modest benefit in patients with heart failure compared with placebo. The combination has, however, been shown to be less effective than ACE inhibitors. The recent A-Heft trial, which was limited to African-American patients with class III-IV heart failure, showed that the addition of I/H to standard therapy with ACE inhibitor or a beta-blocker conferred significant morbidity and mortality benefit.

Taking all the evidence together, the I/H combination is indicated in the following patients:
- Those who cannot take an ACE inhibitor or ARB because of renal insufficiency or hyperkalemia
- Those who are hypertensive/symptomatic despite taking ACE inhibitor, ARB, and beta-blockers

Dosages are as follows:
- Hydralazine: start at 37.5 mg three times a day and increase to a goal of 75 mg three times a day
- Isosorbide dinitrate: start at 20 mg three times a day and increase to a goal of 40 mg three times a day

10. **How do you initiate and maintain ACE inhibitors, ARBs, and aldosterone antagonists in patients with chronic heart failure?**
ACE inhibitors and ARBs should be initiated at low doses (starting doses shown in Tables 24-1 and 24-2), followed by gradual increments as tolerated. Titration is generally achieved by doubling doses, with an attempt to reach goal doses that have been shown to reduce the risk of cardiovascular events in clinical trials. If these target doses cannot be reached or are poorly tolerated, the highest tolerated dose should be used.

Blood pressure, renal function, and potassium should be evaluated within 1 to 2 weeks after initiation and followed closely after changes in dose.

Patients with systolic blood pressure below 80 to 90 mm Hg, low serum sodium, diabetes mellitus, or impaired renal function or those taking potassium supplements should be monitored closely.

Initiation or uptitration of ACE inhibitor and ARB should not be performed or should be very carefully monitored in patients with creatinine 3 mg/dl or higher and potassium 5.5 mEq/L or higher.

Other caveats when using ACE inhibitors and ARBs include the following:
- Fluid retention can blunt the therapeutic effects of ACE inhibitors. Fluid depletion can potentiate the adverse effects of ACE inhibitors. Thus, patients should be given appropriate doses of diuretics to achieve a euvolemic status.
- Abrupt withdrawal of an ACE inhibitor can lead to clinical deterioration and should be avoided in the absence of life-threatening complications (e.g., angioedema).
- Use of an ACE inhibitor or ARB may minimize or eliminate the need for long-term potassium supplementation.
- Nonsteroidal antiinflammatory drugs (NSAIDs) can block the favorable effects and enhance the adverse effects of ACE inhibitors in patients with heart failure. Thus, NSAIDs should be avoided in heart failure patients.

When treating with aldosterone receptor blockers, spironolactone should be initiated at a dose of 12.5 to 25 mg daily, or occasionally on alternate days, with a goal dose of 25 mg daily. Eplerenone should be initiated at a dose of 25 mg per day, increasing to 50 mg daily.

Aldosterone blockers should be avoided when the serum creatinine is greater than 2.5 mg/d (or creatinine clearance is less than 30 ml/min) or serum potassium is greater than 5 mEq/L or when the patient is being treated with other potassium-sparing diuretics.

Potassium levels and renal function should be rechecked within 3 to 7 days after initiation of an aldosterone antagonist. Subsequent monitoring should be dictated by the renal function and fluid status but should be performed at least monthly for the first 3 months and every 3 months thereafter.

Potassium supplementation is generally stopped after starting aldosterone antagonists, and patients should be counseled to avoid high potassium–containing foods. However, some patients may still require potassium supplementation. In such patients, decreasing the potassium supplements by half at the time of initiation of aldosterone blockers may be considered with close monitoring of serum potassium.

Patients should avoid using NSAIDs and cyclo-oxygenase-2 (COX-2) inhibitors, which can lead to worsening renal function and hyperkalemia.

The addition or an increase in dosage of ACE inhibitors or ARBs should prompt closer laboratory monitoring.

The dose of the aldosterone antagonist may need to be reduced or stopped completely while loop diuretic therapy is reduced or stopped.

Potassium levels in excess of 5.5 mEq/L should generally lead to discontinuation or dose reduction of the ACE inhibitor, ARB, and aldosterone antagonist unless the patient has been receiving potassium supplementation, which should first be stopped and potassium levels be rechecked.

The development of progressively worsening renal function should also prompt consideration of reducing the dose or stopping the ACE inhibitor, ARB, or aldosterone antagonist once other causes of worsening renal insufficiency have been ruled out.

In view of the potential risk for hyperkalemia, the triple combination of ACE inhibitors, ARBs, and an aldosterone antagonist should be avoided.

11. **ACE inhibitor therapy for LV systolic dysfunction has been shown to reduce morbidity and mortality in which New York Heart Association symptom classes groups?**

NYHA classes I to IV. ACE inhibitor therapy is the only medical therapy that has been shown in clinical trials to reduce morbidity and mortality in all symptom classes of patients with LV systolic dysfunction, from asymptomatic (NYHA class I) to severely symptomatic (NYHA class IV).

BIBLIOGRAPHY, SUGGESTED READINGS, AND WEBSITES

1. Celebi M: Cardiomyopathy, Dilated: http://www.emedicine.com
2. Colucci WS: ACE Inhibitors in Heart Failure Due to Systolic Dysfunction: Therapeutic Use: http://www.utdol.com
3. Colucci WS, Pfeffer MA: Angiotensin II Receptor Blockers in Heart Failure Due to Systolic Dysfunction: Therapeutic Use: http://www.utdol.com
4. Heart Failure (Congestive Heart Failure): http://www.merck.com/mmpe
5. Rose BD, Colucci WS: Renal Effects of ACE Inhibitors in Heart Failure: http://www.utdol.com
6. Zevitz ME: Heart Failure: http://www.emedicine.com
7. Deswal A, Yao D: Aldosterone receptor blockers in heart failure, *Curr Treat Options Cardiovasc Med* 6:327-334, 2004.
8. Heart Failure Society of America: HFSA 2006 comprehensive heart failure practice guideline, *J Card Fail* 12(1): e1-e122, 2006.

9. Hunt SA: ACC/AHA 2005 guideline update for the diagnosis and management of chronic heart failure in the adult: a report of the American College of Cardiology/American Heart Association Task Force on Practice Guidelines (Writing Committee to Update the 2001 Guidelines for the Evaluation and Management of Heart Failure), *J Am Coll Cardiol* 46:1-82, 2005.

10. Kazi D, Deswal A: Role and optimal dosing of angiotensin-converting enzyme inhibitors in heart failure, *Cardiol Clin* 26:1-14, 2008.

11. Ramasubbu K, Mann DL, Deswal A: Anti-angiotensin therapy: new perspectives, *Cardiol Clin* 25(4): 573-580, 2007.

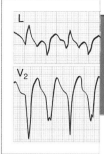

Figure 25-2. Bidirection[al]
toxicity. (Adapted from [...]
arrhythmias, ed 2, St. L[...]

9. **How is digoxin toxicity tre[...]**
It depends on the clinical severit[...]
Activated charcoal may enhance[...]
6 hours of ingestion. Drugs tha[...]
discontinued (except amiodaror[...]
(intravenous [IV] replacement t[...]
but judgment is needed in the [...]
may respond to atropine or to [...]
response or side effects); if no [...]
should be avoided. Patients with[...]
to atropine. Lidocaine and pher[...]
potentially life-threatening brad[...]
Dialysis has no role because of [...]

10. **What are the indications [...]**
The indications for Digibind in[...]
hemodynamic instability caus[...]
setting of acute ingestion, reg[...]
than 10 ng/ml or the ingestion[...]
findings. Digibind is an antibo[...]
creating a concentration gradi[...]
Na^+-K^+ ATPase is relieved K^+[...]
hypokalemia; potassium levels[...]
digoxin-digibind complex is 1[...]
concentration rises significant[...]
bloodstream bound to the an[...]
To use Digibind, follow the [...]
- First, estimate the total b[...]
  - For acute digoxin inge[...]
  - For toxicity during ch[...]
    (in kg) × 5.6[†]]/1000
- Second, calculate the dig[...]
  - Number of digibind vi[...]

---

*Oral bioavailability of digoxin
†Volume of distribution of digoxin in th[...]
‡Binding capacity of Digibind (0.6 mg [...]

CHAPTER 25

DIGOXIN AND OTHER POSITIVE INOTROPIC AGENTS

Jacobo Alejandro Vazquez, MD and Biykem Bozkurt, MD, FACC

1. **What are the positive inotropic agents available for clinical use?**
There are three different classes:
- Cardiac glycosides, like digoxin (most commonly used) and digitoxin
- Beta-agonists (or sympathomimetics), which include dopamine, dobutamine, epinephrine, norepinephrine, and isoproterenol
- Inodilators or inhibitors of the phosphodiesterase III, such as milrinone and amrinone

2. **What are the pharmacokinetic characteristics of the cardiac glycosides?**
The oral bioavailability of digoxin is 60%, and its half-life is 32 to 48 hours. Protein binding is 25% for digoxin and 93% for digitoxin. Digoxin has an onset of action of 0.5 to 2 hours when given orally and 5 to 30 minutes when given intravenously; peak action for digoxin occurs in 6 to 8 hours (orally) and 1 to 4 hours (intravenously). Digoxin is excreted primarily through the kidneys (50%–70%), whereas digitoxin is cleared 70% through the liver.

3. **What is the mechanism of action of the cardiac glycosides?**
They are inhibitors of the Na^+-K^+ ATPase pump in the sarcolemic membrane of the myocyte and other cells. This inhibition causes intracellular accumulation of Na^+, which makes the Na^+-Ca^{++} pump extrude less Ca^{++}, causing Ca^{++} to accumulate inside the cell. This effect results in increased force of contraction. Cardiac glycosides also have effects in the central nervous system, enhancing parasympathetic and reducing sympathetic outputs to the heart, through carotid sinus baroreflex sensitization. This is the mechanism that underlies the reduction in sinus node activity and slowing in atrioventricular (AV) conduction, which makes digoxin the only agent with a positive inotropic-bradycardic effect and is the basis for its use in the control of some supraventricular arrhythmias.

4. **Is there scientific evidence for the use of digoxin?**
The Digitalis Investigation Group (DIG) trial was a multicenter, randomized, double-blinded, placebo-controlled study of 6801 symptomatic patients with heart failure and ejection fraction (EF) less than 45% who were in sinus rhythm. Mean follow-up was 37 months. Patients already receiving digoxin were allowed into the trial and randomized to digoxin or placebo without a washout period. About 95% of patients in both groups received angiotensin-converting enzyme (ACE) inhibitors; beta-blockers were not in use for heart failure at the time. The primary outcome was total mortality. Digoxin did not improve total mortality (34.8% versus 35.1% in the placebo group, p = 0.80) or deaths from cardiovascular causes (29.9% versus 29.5, p = 0.78). Hospitalizations as a result of worsening heart failure (a secondary endpoint) were significantly reduced by digoxin (26.8% versus 34.7% in the placebo group, risk ratio 0.72, p < 0.001). Hospitalizations for suspected digoxin toxicity were higher in the digoxin group (2% versus 0.9%, p < 0.001). In an ancillary, parallel trial in patients with EF greater than 45% and sinus rhythm, the findings were consistent with the results of the main trial. Whether these results hold with contemporary heart failure treatment that includes beta-blockers, aldosterone-receptor blockers, and resynchronization therapy is not known.

5. **Within the therapeutic range, is there any relevance in the serum concentration of digoxin?**
A posthoc analysis of the DIG trial found that in *men* with symptomatic heart failure, sinus rhythm, and EF less than 45%, higher blood concentrations of digoxin were associated

with higher all-cause morta
and 1.2 ng/ml or more, 48
0.5 to 0.8 ng/ml had a 6.3
compared with patients re

6. **What are some of the**
    - Quinidine, verapamil,
      may double digoxin l
      combination with any
    - Tetracyline, erythrom
      cholestyramine and l
    - Thyroxine and albute
    - Cyclosporine and par
      can increase serum (

7. **What are the clinical**
    Digoxin has a narrow safe
    therapeutic and toxic leve
    vomiting, anorexia, diarrh
    halos around lights and o
    toxicity may occur within
    patients, in patients with
    min), and when combine
    levels should be measure

8. **What are the electroc**
    Digoxin toxicity can resul
    conduction abnormalities
    - Sinus bradycardia
    - Sinus arrest
    - First- and second-d
    - AV junctional escap
    - Paroxysmal atrial ta
    - Bidirectional ventric
    - Premature ventricu
    - Bigeminy
    - Regularized atrial fi
    These arrhythmias res
    intracellular Ca^{++} levels
    increased automaticity (
    excessive vagal effects
    and blocks are more co

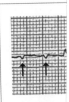

Figure 25-1. S
tachycardias. S
QRS complexe
for the presenc

CHAPTER 26

HEART FAILURE WITH PRESERVED EJECTION FRACTION

John S. Nguyen, MD and Anita Deswal, MD, MPH

1. **What is diastolic dysfunction?**
    Diastolic dysfunction occurs when there is an abnormality in the mechanical function of the myocardium during the diastolic phase of the cardiac cycle. This mechanical abnormality can occur with or without systolic dysfunction, as well as with or without the clinical syndrome of heart failure (HF). Diastolic dysfunction may include decreased left ventricular (LV) compliance, delayed or incomplete LV relaxation, and impaired LV filling.

2. **What is diastolic heart failure?**
    Whereas diastolic dysfunction describes abnormalities in mechanical function, diastolic heart failure is a clinical syndrome characterized by the signs and symptoms of HF, a preserved left ventricular ejection fraction (LVEF; 45%–50% or more), and evidence of diastolic dysfunction. Earlier studies of patients with HF with preserved LVEF uniformly referred to this condition as *diastolic heart failure,* based on the premise that diastolic dysfunction was the sole mechanism for this syndrome. However, more recent studies suggest that a number of other abnormalities, both cardiac and noncardiac, may play an important role in the pathophysiology of HF with normal or near normal ejection fraction. Therefore, current clinical management guidelines and other studies often refer to this clinical syndrome as *heart failure with preserved ejection fraction* (HF-PEF).

3. **What is the prevalence of heart failure with preserved ejection fraction?**
    Approximately 5 million Americans currently have a diagnosis of HF, and more than half a million new cases of HF are diagnosed annually. Epidemiologic studies of various HF cohorts have documented a prevalence of HF-PEF ranging from 40% to 71% (average approximately 50%). In addition, the prevalence of this condition is increasing as the population ages and is higher in women.

4. **What is the morbidity and mortality associated with HF-PEF compared with heart failure with reduced ejection fraction?**
    Compared with age-matched controls without HF, patients with HF-PEF have a significantly higher mortality. However, studies examining the risk of death in patients with HF-PEF compared with patients with HF caused by reduced ejection fraction, commonly known as systolic HF, have shown either similar mortality or a somewhat lower mortality in patients with HF-PEF. The differing results are likely based on different populations studied—that is, community-based cohorts versus hospitalized cohorts, as well as the age of the patients. Once hospitalized for HF, mortality in patients with HF-PEF may be as high as 22% to 29% at 1 year and approximately 65% at 5 years. Although survival has significantly improved over time for patients with systolic HF, there has been no similar improvement in survival for HF-PEF patients. The morbidity of HF-PEF and systolic HF is comparable, with similar high rates of hospitalizations for decompensated HF in both groups.

5. **Which patients are at the highest risk for developing HF-PEF?**

As mentioned earlier, gender and age are important risk factors for the development of HF-PEF. Patients with HF-PEF are generally elderly and are predominantly women (60%–70%). Reasons for the female predominance in HF-PEF are not entirely clear but may be related to the fact that women have a greater tendency for the left ventricle to hypertrophy in response to load and lesser predisposition for the ventricle to dilate. Hypertension is the most common cardiac condition associated with HF-PEF. Hypertensive heart disease results in LV hypertrophy with resultant decreased LV compliance and impaired relaxation. Acute myocardial ischemia results in diastolic dysfunction, although its role in chronic diastolic dysfunction and chronic HF remains unclear. Valvular heart diseases, including regurgitatant and stenotic aortic and mitral valve disease, can also result in the development of HF-PEF. Other recognized risk factors associated with HF-PEF include obesity, diabetes mellitus, and renal insufficiency. Onset of atrial fibrillation with rapid ventricular response may precipitate decompensation of HF-PEF, and the presence of diastolic dysfunction in general is a risk factor for the development of this arrhythmia as well.

6. **What are proposed pathophysiologic mechanisms of HF-PEF?**

Diastolic dysfunction has been thought to be the major mechanism contributing to HF-PEF, with abnormalities in active LV relaxation and abnormalities of LV passive diastolic stiffness. LV relaxation is an active, energy-dependent process that may begin during the ejection phase of systole and continue throughout diastole. Animal studies and various models have shown that impaired LV relaxation can contribute to elevated mean LV diastolic filling pressures in HF-PEF when the heart rate is increased (as during exercise or uncontrolled atrial fibrillation). On the other hand, LV stiffness consists of the passive viscoelastic properties that contribute to returning the ventricular myocardium to its resting force and length. These viscoelastic properties are dependent on both intracellular and extracellular structures. The greater the stiffness of the LV myocardium, for any given change in LV volume during diastolic filling, the higher the corresponding filling pressures. In other words, when comparing left ventricle with normal diastolic function with that of a left ventricle with diastolic dysfunction, for any given left ventricle volume during diastole, LV pressure will be higher in the ventricle with diastolic dysfunction compared with normal. The net result of these processes is that LV diastolic pressures and left atrial pressures become elevated either at rest or during exercise, with resultant elevation of pulmonary capillary wedge pressure and pulmonary vascular congestion.

Clinically, this manifests as dyspnea at rest or with exertion, paroxysmal nocturnal dyspnea, and orthopnea. Furthermore, these stiffer hearts have an inability to increase end-diastolic volume and stroke volume via the Frank-Starling mechanism despite significantly elevated LV filling pressure. The resultant decrease in augmentation of cardiac output, which normally occurs with exercise, results in reduced exercise tolerance and fatigue.

In addition to diastolic dysfunction, a number of additional factors are now thought to contribute to the development of HF-PEF. For example, increased arterial vascular stiffness along with LV systolic stiffness may increase systolic blood pressure sensitivity to circulating intravascular volume and may predispose to rapid-onset pulmonary edema. Neurohormonal activation may result in increased venous vascular tone, which in turn may result in a shift of the blood volume to the central circulation. Concurrent atrial dysfunction may result in further elevation in left atrial pressures and pulmonary vascular congestion. In the elderly, chronotropic incompetence with exercise is more commonly seen and may contribute to further limitation in exercise cardiac output with resultant exertional fatigue.

7. **What factors may precipitate decompensated HF-PEF?**

In patients with underlying diastolic dysfunction, acute decompensation of HF-PEF may often be contributed to by uncontrolled hypertension, atrial fibrillation, or flutter, especially with rapid ventricular rates, myocardial ischemia, medication noncompliance (especially diuretics and antihypertensives), dietary indiscretion (e.g., high-sodium foods), anemia, and infection.

8. **How is the diagnosis of HF-PEF made?**
The clinical diagnosis of HF-PEF depends on the presence of signs and symptoms of HF and documentation of normal or near-normal LVEF by echohocardiography, radionuclide ventriculography, or contrast ventriculography.

9. **What common tests are useful in the diagnosis of HF-PEF, and what do they often reveal?**
   - Chest radiographs may demonstrate cardiomegaly as a result of hypertrophy, pulmonary venous congestion, pulmonary edema, or pleural effusions.
   - The electrocardiogram (ECG) may demonstrate hypertrophy, ischemia, or arrhythmia.
   - Echocardiography can be used to assess ventricular function; atrial and ventricular size; hypertrophy; diastolic function and filling pressures (see Question 11); wall motion abnormalities; and pericardial, valvular, or myocardial disease. By definition, the LVEF is normal or near normal. Echocardiography often demonstrates left ventricular hypertrophy, increased left ventricular mass, enlarged left atrium, diastolic dysfunction, and pulmonary hypertension.
   - Routine laboratory analysis can help identify renal failure or anemia as factors associated with decompensation, electrolyte abnormalities such as hyponatremia seen with HF, and transaminase or bilirubin elevation due to hepatic congestion.
   - Studies have shown that brain natriuretic peptide (BNP) and N-terminal (NT) pro-BNP levels are elevated in HF-PEF patients compared with persons without HF. However, BNP and NT-proBNP levels in HF-PEF patients are usually lower compared with systolic HF patients. Of note, increased BNP levels may identify patients with elevation of the LV diastolic pressure but may not be clinically useful in individual patients to predict preserved versus reduced LVEF. Also, it should be kept in mind that BNP levels increase with age and are higher in women, both of which are common features of HF-PEF.
   - Other tests, such as stress testing and coronary angiography, can identify coronary artery disease as a contributor.

10. **What is the clinical approach to further evaluate patients with HF-PEF?**
   - A diagnostic algorithm, based on the 2006 Heart Failure Society of America Heart Failure Practice Guidelines, provides a systematic approach for the clinical workup and classification of HF-PEF (Fig. 26-1). This framework addresses the common clinical conditions presenting as HF-PEF, including hypertensive heart disease, familial hypertrophic cardiomyopathy, ischemic HF, valvular heart disease, infiltrative (restrictive) cardiomyopathy, pericardial constriction, high-cardiac-output state, and right ventricular dysfunction.

11. **What tests are available to evaluate diastolic function?**
Cardiac catheterization with a high-fidelity pressure manometer allows for precise intracardiac pressure measurements. This information can be used to estimate the rate of LV relaxation by calculation of indices such as peak instantaneous LV pressure decline (-dP/dt max) and the time constant of LV relaxation, tau (τ). Estimation of LV myocardial stiffness requires simultaneous assessment of LV volume and pressure to evaluate the end-diastolic pressure-volume relationship. However, these measurements are invasive and cannot be made on a routine basis. Therefore, noninvasive markers of diastolic dysfunction are more commonly used in clinical practice.

Echocardiography with Doppler examination offers a noninvasive method of evaluating diastolic function. In addition to the Doppler criteria for diastolic dysfunction, enlargement of the left atrium on two-dimensional (2D) echocardiography suggests the presence of significant

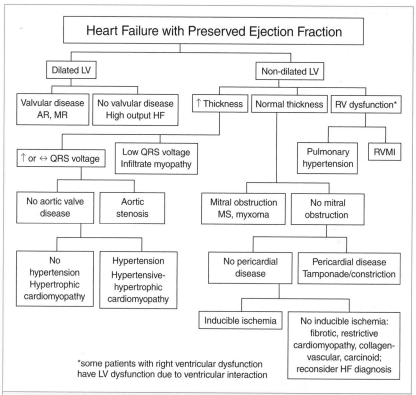

Figure 26-1. Diagnostic considerations in patients with heart failure with preserved ejection fraction. *LV,* Left ventricle; *HF,* heart failure; *RV,* right ventricle; *AR,* aortic regurgitation; *MR,* mitral regurgitation; *MS,* mitral stenosis. (From J Card Fail, 12, Adams KF, et al: *Executive summary: HFSA 2006 comprehensive heart failure practice guideline,* 2006, pp. 10-38.)

diastolic dysfunction. The degree of left atrial (LA) enlargement estimated either by LA diameter or more accurately by LA volume is a marker of the severity and duration of diastolic dysfunction.

Doppler measurements of mitral and pulmonary venous flow, as well as Doppler tissue imaging (DTI), allow for determination of ventricular and atrial filling patterns and estimation of LV diastolic filling pressures. The normal transmitral filling pattern consists of early rapid filling (E wave) and atrial contraction (A wave). The contribution of each of these stages of diastole is expressed as the E/A ratio. Mitral annular tissue Doppler velocities (which measure tissue velocities rather than the conventional Doppler, which measures blood flow velocities) are relatively independent of preload conditions. As such the early diastolic filling annular tissue velocity (E'a marker of LV relaxation and correlates well with hemodynamic catheter-derived values of tau (τ). The ratio of the transmitral early filling velocity to the annular DTI early filling velocity (E/E') has been shown to accurately estimate mean left atrial pressure. Using these various echocardiographic parameters, the severity of diastolic dysfunction and of elevated left ventricular diastolic pressures can be assessed. These issues are also discussed in Chapter 6 on echocardiography.

Nuclear imaging is another less commonly used noninvasive modality for evaluating diastolic dysfunction. Certain diastolic parameters such as peak filling rate (PFR) and time to peak rate (TTPR) can be calculated using this modality.

12. **How do you treat acutely decompensated HF-PEF?**
The cornerstones of treatment of acutely decompensated HF-PEF are blood pressure control, volume management with diuresis, and treatment of exacerbating factors.
    Systemic blood pressure control is of paramount importance because blood pressure directly affects LV diastolic pressure and thus LA pressures. The goal of blood pressure control should be a systolic blood pressure less than 140/90 and possibly even less than 130/80 mm Hg.
    Volume management in the inpatient setting often requires use of intravenous diuretics. Loop diuretics (e.g., furosemide) are the primary diuretic of choice but may be combined with thiazide diuretics for additional effect. Although treatment of pulmonary vascular congestion with diuresis is a primary goal of therapy, rapid or aggressive diuresis in some of these patients who have a combination of severe LV hypertrophy and small LV volume may result in the development of hypotension and renal insufficiency. While a patient is undergoing diuresis, it is imperative to monitor electrolytes (particularly potassium, sodium, and magnesium), renal function (serum blood urea nitrogen [BUN] and creatinine), and clinical response (daily weights, meticulous fluid balance, blood pressure) and perform physical examinations (jugular venous distension, lung examination, and peripheral edema) in order to adjust diuretic doses appropriately. Patients with renal failure and volume overload who are refractory to diuretics may require urgent dialysis.
    Evaluation and treatment of exacerbating factors form a crucial part of the treatment of acutely decompensated HF-PEF. Uncontrolled atrial arrhythmias such as atrial fibrillation or atrial flutter can be detrimental in HF-PEF. The combination of the loss of atrial contraction to LV diastolic filling and shortened diastolic filling time with tachycardia can cause marked elevation of mean left atrial pressure and result in pulmonary edema. In the setting of acute-onset atrial fibrillation or flutter, direct current cardioversion with restoration of sinus rhythm may be beneficial. Alternatively, rate control alone with beta-blockers, nondihydropyridine calcium channel blockers (verapamil or diltiazem), or digoxin, with a target heart rate less than 70 to 80 beats/min at rest, will also improve symptoms. In addition, management of other factors such as myocardial ischemia, anemia, medical noncompliance, and infections is key.

13. **How do you treat patients with chronic HF-PEF?**
Nonpharmacologic therapy for HF-PEF is the same as therapy for HF with reduced ejection fraction. This includes daily home monitoring of weight, compliance with medical treatment, dietary sodium restriction (2–3 g sodium daily), and close medical follow-up. Because ischemia is a significant risk factor for the development of HF-PEF, evaluation and treatment for ischemic heart disease and inducible ischemia is recommended.
    Aggressive management of hypertension is strongly recommended. Diuretic therapy with either a loop diuretic or a thiazide diuretic is recommended in patients with clinical findings of volume overload. Excessive diuresis should be avoided because this may lead to symptomatic orthostatic hypotension and worsening renal function. The use of an angiotensin-converting enzyme (ACE) inhibitors or angiotension-receptor blockers (ARBs) should be considered in patients with HF-PEF, particularly in patients with evidence of atherosclerotic cardiac or peripheral vascular disease or diabetes. If the patient displays ACE inhibitor intolerance, in the form of cough or angioedema, an ARB should be considered. Recent randomized clinical trials suggest that ACE inhibitors or ARBs may lead to a modest reduction in HF hospitalizations for patients with HF-PEF, although these agents were not shown to confer any benefit on survival in this elderly HF-PEF patient population with significant comorbidities.
    Although there have been no large-scale trials specifically addressing the benefits of beta-blockers in HF-PEF, many patients with HF-PEF have other comorbidites that may benefit from beta-blocker therapy. As such, beta-blockers should be considered in patients with a history of prior myocardial infarction, hypertension, or atrial fibrillation (for adequate rate control).
    Similarly, large controlled trials evaluating the efficacy of calcium channel blockers in HF-PEF are lacking. In patients with atrial fibrillation in whom the ventricular rate is not adequately controlled by beta-blockers or for patients in whom beta-blockers are not tolerated, the addition

of diltiazem or verapamil may be considered. In patients with hypertension, the calcium channel blocker amlodipine is a reasonable therapeutic option. In addition, several studies have shown the benefit of verapamil and diltiazem in symptom-limiting angina.

Digoxin is not recommended for treatment of patients with HF-PEF in sinus rhythm but may be used for rate control in patients with HF-PEF and atrial fibrillation in addition to beta-blockers or calcium channel blockers or as an alternative in patients intolerant of these agents.

In patients with atrial fibrillation or atrial flutter who remain significantly symptomatic despite adequate rate control, it is reasonable to consider restoration and maintenance of sinus rhythm, often with antiarrhythmic agents such as amiodarone. Several limited studies suggest that catheter ablation of atrial fibrillation by pulmonary veins isolation may provide symptomatic improvement in patients with HF. Clinical trials in patients with atrial fibrillation have not shown benefit of the an overall rhythm control strategy for all patients over rate control strategy, including one clinical trial targeting patients with HF with reduced ejection fraction. However, no trials have specifically targeted patients with HF-PEF and atrial fibrillation, and the decision to purse a rhythm control strategy in such patients will need to be individualized. Of note, the general recommendations regarding anticoagulation for atrial fibrillation are applicable to this patient population with HF-PEF.

BIBLIOGRAPHY, SUGGESTED READINGS, AND WEBSITES

1. Adams KF, Lindenfeld J, Arnold JMO, et al: Executive summary: HFSA 2006 comprehensive heart failure practice guideline, *J Card Fail* 12:10-38, 2006.
2. Cleland JGF, Tenderar M, Adamus J, et al: The Perindopril in Elderly People with Chronic Heart Failure (PEP-CHF) study, *Eur Heart J* 27:2338-2345, 2006.
3. Hoit BD: Left ventricular diastolic function, *Crit Care Med* 35:S340-347, 2007.
4. Hunt SA, Abraham WT, Chin MH, et al: ACC/AHA 2005 Guideline update for the diagnosis and management of chronic heart failure in the adult: a report of the American College of Cardiology/American Heart Association Task Force on Practice Guidelines (Writing Committee to Update the 2001 Guidelines for the Evaluation and Management of Heart Failure), *J Am Coll Cardiol* 46:e1-e82, 2005.
5. Kass DA, Bronzwaer JG, Paulus WJ: What mechanisms underlie diastolic dysfunction in heart failure? *Circ Res* 94:1533-1542, 2004.
6. Paulus WJ, Tschöpe C, Sanderson JE, et al: How to diagnose diastolic heart failure: a consensus statement on the diagnosis of heart failure with normal left ventricular ejection fraction by the Heart Failure and Echocardiography Associations of the European Society of Cardiology, *Eur Heart J* 28:2539-2550, 2007.
7. Redfield MM: Heart failure with normal ejection fraction. In Libby P, Bonow RO, Mann DL, et al: *Braunwald's heart disease: a textbook of cardiovascular medicine*, Philadelphia, 2007, Saunders.
8. Yusuf S, Pfeffer MA, Swedberg K, et al: Effects of candesartan in patients with chronic heart failure and preserved left-ventricular ejection fraction: the CHARM-Preserved Trial, *Lancet* 362:777-781, 2003.
9. Zile MR, Brutsaert DL: New concepts in diastolic dysfunction and diastolic heart failure: Part I: Diagnosis, prognosism and measurement of diastolic function, *Circulation* 105:1387-1393, 2002.

CHAPTER 27

MYOCARDITIS

Rudy M. Haddad, MD and Biykem Bozkurt, MD, FACC

1. **What is myocarditis?**
   Simply stated, myocarditis is inflammation of cardiac muscle. However, myocarditis has a wide spectrum of clinical presentations and causes that make the consensus on diagnosis and universal classification scheme difficult. In an attempt to incorporate the clinical presentation and histopathologic findings into diagnosis, we will classify mycarditis into four categories: acute myocarditis, fulminant myocarditis, giant cell myocarditis, and chronic active myocarditis. This classification incorporates the chronicity and severity of disease, as well as potential specific treatment strategies. This is particularly important for giant cell myocarditis, which requires early endomyocardial biopsy and consideration for immunosuppressive therapy as well as cardiac transplantation.

2. **What is the pathophysiology of myocarditis?**
   The pathophysiology of myocarditis has been best studied in viral models. A three-phase model has been proposed to characterize the progression of myocarditis. First, direct viral entry and proliferation leads directly to cell damage. The second phase is characterized by the overwhelming immune response with activation of innate and acquired immunity. The final phase is characterized by viral modification of cytoskeleton and matrix metalloproteinase release after the initial complex immune response and may lead to cardiac remodeling and ultimately affect cardiac structure and function. Histologically, fibrosis replaces the earlier acute inflammatory response seen in the earlier phases. Disease may be local or diffuse and may affect any of the four heart chambers.

3. **Who gets myocarditis?**
   It is important to realize that anyone can get myocarditis. However, certain groups of patients may be at increased risk. This includes immunocompromised patients such as children (neonates) and patients after transplantation, who may be at increased risk for certain strains of viral myocarditis. Previous reports have suggested that younger patients may have a bimodal presentation with more acute symptoms and older patients with more chronic symptoms. An emerging population of human immunodeficiency virus (HIV)–associated myocarditis and a geographic distribution reflect endemic infectious causes as leading culprits of myocarditis in specific areas of the world.

4. **What are the causes of myocarditis?**
   Mycoarditis is most commonly caused by a viral infection. However, other infections (bacterial, fungal, protozoal, parasitic), cardiac toxins, hypersensitivity reactions, and systemic disease (usually autoimmune) have been implicated as causes of myocarditis (Table 27-1).

5. **Which viral infections are commonly associated with myocarditis?**
   Viral infection is the most common cause of myocarditis in developed countries.
   - Enteroviruses, including the Coxsackie viruses, are the most commonly associated viral species. The Coxsackie virus may have a myocardial affinity because of its easy entrance into the myocardial cell through the coxsackie-adenoviral-receptor (CAR), which triggers the host immune response.

TABLE 27-1. CAUSES OF MYOCARDITIS

Viral	**Parasitic**
Adenovirus	Schistosomiasis
Enterovirus	**Toxins**
Cytamegalovirus	Anthrocylines
Hepatitis C virus	Cocaine
Influenza	Cyclophospamide
Human immunodeficiency virus (HIV)	5-Flurouracil
Herpes virus	Lithium
Epstein-Barr virus	Quinidine
Poliomyelitis	Theophylline
Varicella	**Hypersensitivity**
Respiratory syncytial virus	Carbamazepine
Bacterial	Chloramphenicol
Streptococcal species	Isoniazid
Borrelia burgdorferi	Methyldopa
Clostridium perfingens	Penicillins
Diphteria	Sulfonamides
Mycoplasma species	Tricyclic antidepressants
Tropheryma whippeli	**Autoimmune**
Chlamydia pneumonia	Giant cell myocarditis
Fungal	Churg-Strauss syndrome
Aspergillus	Shögren syndrome
Candida	Inflammatory bowel disease
Coccidioides	Celiac disease
Cryptococcus	Sarcoidosis
Histoplasma	Systemic lupus erythematosus
Blastomycosis	Takayasu arteritis
Mucormycosis	Wegener granulomatosis
Protozoal	
Trypanosoma cruzi	

Modified From Libby P, Bonow R, Mann D, et al: *Braunwald's heart disease: a textbook of cardiovascular medicine,* ed 8, Philadelphia, 2008, Saunders.

- Cytomegalovirus is commonly associated with posttransplantation myocarditis.
- HIV is now increasing in prevalence as an cause of myocarditis as highly active retroviral therapy has increased survival in these patients. Cardiac involvement related to HIV disease is as high as 70% in some reports. It may be difficult to determine the exact cause of cardiac dysfunction because symptoms may be from an autoimmune or inflammatory

response to HIV; the HIV infection itself; or coexisting opportunistic infections, side effects of antiretroviral treatment, or a combination of these causes.

- Influenza may lead to myocarditis and is associated with massive hemorrhagic pulmonary edema. Preexisting cardiac disease increases morbidity and mortality.
- Hepatitis C virus is also implicated in myocarditis.

Other viral causes of myocarditis include adenovirus, parvovirus B19, poliomyelitis, varicella, variola, arbovirus, respiratory syncytial virus (RSV), herpes simplex virus (HSV), yellow fever virus, rabies, and Epstein Barr virus (EBV).

6. What are infectious causes of myocarditis other than viral infections?

Bacterial

- Streptococcal infection (β-hemolytic streptococcus) may lead to myocarditis with conduction abnormalities, including sudden cardiac death as part of the syndrome of acute rheumatic fever.
- Spirochetes, including *Borrelia burgdorferi* (Lyme disease), *Rickettsia rickettsii* (Rocky Mountain spotted fever), *Ehrlichia,* and *Babesia* species, may have cardiac involvement. Patients with Lyme disease may present with characteristic rash, neurologic, and joint complaints and with atrioventricular (AV) nodal block as a common cardiac symptom. AV nodal block may range from first to third degree and require prolonged temporary pacemaker. Symptoms may improve with antibiotics, and a permanent pacemaker may be avoided in some cases.
- *Clostridium perfingens* releases a toxin that leads to myocyte damage with gas bubbles in the myocardium. Abscess formation may occur with rupture into the pericardium causing purulent pericarditis.
- Diphtheria may lead to myocardial damage in up to 50% of infected patients. A toxin released by the bacteria inhibits protein synthesis and leads to cell damage. The toxin has a high affinity for the conducting system, and AV nodal block may occur, requiring temporary or a permanent pacemaker. Antitoxin should be given for treatment immediately and before antibiotics.
- *Mycobacterium tuberculosis* more commonly affects the pericardium but may cause myocarditis. Multiple conduction system abnormalities may be noted, including ventricular tachycardia, AV nodal block, atrial fibrillation, or sudden cardiac death.
- *Tropheryma whippeli* is associated with myocardial and valvular inflammation and fibrosis leading to left ventricular (LV) dysfunction, conduction system abnormalities, and valvular dysfunction. The cardiac symptoms caused by this organism may be seen in combination with the other symptoms of Whipple's disease.

Protozoal

- Chagas' disease is one of the most common causes of dilated cardiomyopathy worldwide, with a high incidence in patients from Central and South America. Caused by *Trypanosoma cruzi,* patients with Chagas' cardiomyopathy usually present with heart failure, conduction system disease, and even death. Treatment with standard heart failure agents should be used, and antiparasitic agents may be effective early in the infection. Efforts to prevent the disease should be the first-line approach to management of Chagas' disease.

7. What is giant cell myocarditis?

This uncommon but often fulminant form of myocardtis is characterized by multinucleated giant cells and myocyte destruction. Patients with giant cell myocarditis usually have deteriorating left ventricular function and ventricular arrhythmias with rapid progression to death. Endomyocardial biopsy should be considered early in these patients, with consideration of immunosuppressive therapy. These patients have a poor prognosis, and heart transplantation may be the only alternative for survival.

8. **What are the clinical presentations of myocarditis?**
Patients with myocarditis may have a wide spectrum of symptoms that may reflect the various etiologic agents associated with myocarditis, as well as the local or diffuse area of disease affecting any of the heart chambers or conduction system. Patients may be asymptomatic with abnormality being detected incidentally on electrocardiogram (ECG) or echocardiogram; may have a viral syndrome with fever, muscle aches, or symptoms of upper respiratory tract infection; or may have heart failure and dilated cardiomyopathy with hemodynamic collapse (cardiogenic shock), sometimes rapidly progressing to death. Symptoms of LV failure may include generalized fatigue, dyspnea, orthopnea, or paroxysmal nocturnal dyspnea. Patients may have symptoms of right-sided heart failure, including elevated jugular venous pressure, ascites, or lower extremity edema. Some patients may present with a viral prodrome including fever, rash, and arthralgia. Younger patients may have chest pain mimicking acute myocardial infarction. Other common clinical presentations are related to cardiac conductions system disease. These include sinus tachycardia, atrial fibrillation, any level of AV block, ventricular tachycardia, ventricular fibrillation, and even sudden cardiac death.

9. **What are common physical examination findings in patients with myocarditis?**
Common physical examination findings include signs of fluid retention (elevated jugular venous pressure, pulmonary rales, ascites, peripheral edema). S3 or S4 gallops may be present when there is cardiac failure. If there is significant right or left ventricular dilation or elevated filling pressures, auscultation may reveal murmurs of tricuspid or mitral insufficiency. A pericardial friction rub may be heard in some patients with myopericarditis.

10. **What laboratory tests should we order?**
Cardiac-specific biomarkers such as troponin I or T are usually elevated in patients with myocarditis, especially during the acute phase. Troponin I or T are more likely to be elevated than creatine kinase–myocardial bound (CK-MB), especially in patients with biopsy-proven myocarditis. Persistent elevation of troponin levels may suggest ongoing myocyte necrosis. Some cytokine levels such as interleukin-10 (IL-10) have been associated with poorer prognosis in small case series. Other serum tests such as complement levels, erythrocyte sedimentation rate (ESR), C-reactive protein (CRP), aspirate aminotransferase (AST), alanine aminotransferase (ALT), lactate dehydrogenase (LDH), or even antiviral antibody levels may be elevated but are usually nonspecific.

11. **List the diagnostic tools available to make the diagnosis of myocarditis.**
Historically, clinicians and researchers relied on a histopathologic categorization of myocarditis, outlined by the Dallas criteria. Dallas criteria require inflammatory infiltrate and associated myocyte necrosis or damage not characteristic of an ischemic event. However, it has been recognized that focal myocarditis may be missed by myocardial biopsy because of heterogeneous involvement of the myocardium, right ventricular sampling may not yield the pathology in the left ventricle, biopsy findings did not correlate with prognosis except in the setting of giant cell myocarditis, and treatment guided according to biopsy results failed to demonstrate any clinical benefit. This prompted development of newer, more practical, less invasive, and potentially higher yield diagnostic strategies incorporating clinical history, physical examination, laboratory tests, chest radiograph, ECG, echocardiogram, indium-111 antimyosin scintigraphy, and cardiac magnetic resonance imaging (CMRI).

12. **What abnormalities will be seen on an ECG?**
A vast range of abnormalities may potentially be seen on an ECG. These usually reflect the area of cardiac involvement and are generally nonspecific. They range from sinus tachycardia, loss

TABLE 27-2. EXPANDED CRITERIA FOR THE DIAGNOSIS OF MYOCARDITIS

Suspicious for myocarditis = 2 positive categories

Compatible with myocarditis = 3 positive categories

High probability of being myocarditis = all 4 categories positive
(Any matching feature in category = positive for category)

Category I: Clinical Symptoms

Clinical heart failure

Fever

Viral prodrome

Fatigue

Dyspnea on exertion

Chest pain

Palpitations

Presyncope or syncope

Category II: Evidence of Cardiac Structural/Functional Perturbation *in the Absence of* Regional Coronary Ischemia

Echocardiography evidence

Regional wall motion abnormalitites

Cardiac dilation

Regional cardiac hypertrophy

Troponin release

High sensitivity (>0.1 ng/ml)

Positive indium 111 antimyosin scintigraphy

and

Normal coronary angiography *or*

Absence of reversible ischemia by coronary distribution on perfusion scan

Category III: Cardiac Magnetic Resonance Imaging

Increased myocardial T_2 signal on inversion recovery sequence

Delayed contrast enhancement following gadolinium DTPA intusion

Category IV: Myocardial Biopsy—Pathological or Molecular Analysis

Pathology findings compatible with Dallas criteria

Presence of viral genome by polymerase chain reation or in situ hybridization

From Libby P, Bonow R, Mann D, et al: *Braunwald's heart disease: a textbook of cardiovascular medicine,* ed 8, Philadelphia, 2008, Saunders.

of R-wave progression, development of Q waves, T-wave inversion, and frank ST elevation to varying arrhythmias, including atrial fibrillation, AV node block, and ventricular tachycardia or fibrillation.

13. **What findings may we see on echocardiogram?**

Two-dimensional echocardiographic findings of myocarditis are usually not specific. Ventricular dilation or regional hypertrophy may be noted. Regional wall motion abnormalities in the absence of matching regional coronary artery disease may be suggestive of myocarditis. There may be signs of increased wall thickness and edema that may reflect severity and acuity of the myocarditis. Some studies suggest that echocardiography may help differentiate fulminant from acute myocarditis with fulminant myocarditis having less ventricular dilation but increased hypertrophy or wall edema. Acute myocarditis may result in diastolic dysfunction and restrictive filling patterns. Signs of right ventricular (RV) failure on echocardiogram may predict a worse prognosis and a higher incidence of need for cardiac transplantation. Echocardiography may also be used to follow a patient's clinical course and response to treatment.

14. **What is the role of CMRI in diagnosing myocarditis?**

CMRI is a new and evolving diagnostic tool that has been found to be useful in the evaluation of patients with suspected myocarditis. CMRI allows for visualization of the entire myocardium with focal inflammation leading to characteristic T2-weighted images and gadolinium-enhanced T1 images identifying areas of myocardial injury. Studies have shown that diffuse or heterogeneous involvement in the lateral wall, subepicardial, or mid-myocardial regions or combined enhancement is highly suggestive of myocarditis. Other investigations have proven that CMRI may be very useful in guiding diagnostic myocardial biopsy in suspected areas of myocardial necrosis.

15. **Should we do a myocardial biopsy on our patient suspected to have myocarditis?**

In the past, endomyocardial biopsy (EMB) was required to confirm the diagnosis of myocarditis, with the Dallas criteria being developed in an attempt to standardize the histopathologic diagnosis. Newer strategies now incorporate clinical presentation and cardiovascular imaging, such as CMRI together with EMB, in an attempt to establish the diagnosis of myocarditis. Several factors may contribute to the insensitivity of using EMB alone. First, as mentioned earlier, the myocarditic involvement may be patchy and biopsy may miss affected areas of the myocardium. Secondly, some reports suggest that inconsistencies in interpretation of biopsy results may exist when examined by multiple pathologists. Finally, newer evidence has suggested that CMRI shows that disease is often located in the lateral wall of the LV, which may be difficult to biopsy. This has led to recommendations from the American Heart Association/ American College of Cardiology/European Society of Cardiology (AHA/ACC/ESC) in the 2007 scientific statement on the role of EMB suggesting that biopsies should be taken in multiple areas of the RV, with at least 5 to 10 samples being sent for interpretation. The current ACC/AHA guidelines for treatment of heart failure consider EMB a class IIb recommendation. The 2007 AHA/ACC/ESC scientific statement on the role of EMB outlined 14 clinical scenarios in which EMB may be considered and focus on unexplained progressive cardiomyopathy not responsive to standard therapy and cardiomyopathy associated with significant conduction system disease. Current recommendations for EMB are based on the idea that the clinical scenario suggests a likely high yield of the biopsy and that, if positive, potentially effective treatment is available.

It is important to remember that this procedure is not without risk. These include risk of venous access (bleeding, infection, hematoma, pneumothorax) and of biopsy itself (ventricular perforation with cardiac tamponade, cardiac conduction abnormalities, arrythmias). Careful consideration to the clinical presentation and expected yield of the biopsy should be given when considering biopsy in individual patients.

16. **How is myocarditis treated?**
    Supportive care is a mainstay in the treatment of myocarditis and the subsequent heart failure that may develop. When hemodynamic compromise occurs, the use of vasopressors, intraaortic balloon pump (IABP), and even a ventricular assist device (VAD) may need to be considered. Patients with resulting heart failure from myocarditis should be treated like other patients with heart failure, following the ACC/AHA/ESC and Canadian Cardiovascular Society (CCS) guidelines for treatment of patients with heart failure. This may include such things as intravenous vasodilators, angiotensin-converting enzyme (ACE) inhibitors, and beta-blockers when clinically indicated. Patients with arrhythmias should be treated with standard therapy, including the potential need for pacemaker or defibrillator. Heart transplantation must be considered in patients who do not recover after standard therapy. In the past, a general belief existed that immunosuppressive therapy should be useful in the treatment of myocarditis. However, clinical trials have not confirmed this. In the Myocarditis Treatment Trial, patients with biopsy-proven lymphocytic myocarditis were randomized to either (a) placebo, (b) prednisolone plus cyclosporine, or (c) prednisolone plus azathioprine. Patients in all groups were treated with standard heart failure treatment. Significant improvement was seen in left ventricular ejection fraction (LVEF) in both placebo and treatment groups, with no statistically significant difference in LVEF or mortality at the end of the trial. On the basis of this and other small trials, current recommendations do not include routine treatment with immunosuppressive agents for postviral or lymphocytic myocarditis. However, in patients with giant cell, autoimmune, or hypersensitivity myocarditis and in those with deteriorating hemodynamic compromise, immunosuppressive treatment may be considered (Fig. 27-1).

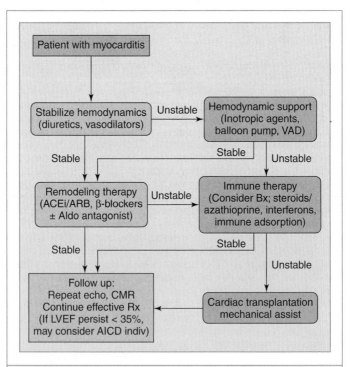

Figure 27-1. Treatment algorithm for myocarditis. (From Libby P, Bonow R, Mann D, et al: *Braunwald's heart disease: a textbook of cardiovascular medicine*, ed 8, Philadelphia, 2008, Saunders.)

17. What is the prognosis of myocarditis?

Prognosis depends on the initial presentation of symptoms, with those having minimal cardiac compromise usually having good prognosis with limited long-term complications and those with more severe cardiac dysfunction having a worse outcome. Predictors of death or need for heart transplantation include syncope, bundle branch block, left ventricular enlargement (LVEDD greater than 7 cm), or low LVEF (less than 30%). The type of the myocarditis may also predict overall prognosis, with giant cell myocarditis having one of the worst prognoses at a median survival of 6 months.

BIBLIOGRAPHY, SUGGESTED READINGS, AND WEBSITES

1. Abdel-Aty H, Boye P, Zargrosek, et al: Diagnostic performance of cardiovascular magnetic resonance in patients with suspected acute myocarditis: comparison of different approaches, *J Am Coll Cardiol* 45:1815, 2005.

2. Baughman KL: Diagnosis of myocarditis: death of Dallas criteria, *Circulation* 113:593, 2006.

3. Cooper LT, Baughman KL, Feldman Am, et al: The role of endomyocardial biopsy in the management of cardiovascular disease: a scientific statement from the American Heart Association, the American College of Cardiology, and the European Society of Cardiology, *Circulation* 116:2216, 2007.

4. Hagar J, Rahimtoola SH: Chagas' heart disease, *Curr Prob Cardiol* 20:825, 1995.

5. Hunt SA: ACC/AHA 2005 guideline update for the diagnosis and management of chronic heart failure in the adult: a report of the American College of Cardiology/American Heart Association Task Force on Practice Guidelines (Writing Committee to Update the 2001 Guidelines for the Evaluation and Management of Heart Failure), *J Am Coll Cardiol* 46:e1, 2005.

6. Kuhl U, Pauschinger M, Seeberg B, et al: Viral persistence in the myocardium is associated with progressive cardiac dysfunction, *Circulation* 112:1965, 2005.

7. Libby P, Bonow R, Mann D, et al: *Braunwald's heart disease: a textbook of cardiovascular medicine*, ed 8, Philadelphia, 2008, Saunders.

8. Liu PP, Yan AT: Cardiovascular magnetic resonance for the diagnosis of acute myocarditis: prospects for detecting myocardial inflammation, *J Am Coll Cardiol* 45:1823, 2005.

9. Magnani JW, Dec GW: Myocarditis: current trends in diagnosis and treatment, *Circulation* 113:876, 2006.

10. Mahrholdt H, Wagner A, Deluigi CC, et al: Presentation, patterns of myocardial damage, and clinical course of viral myocarditis, *Circulation* 114:1581, 2006.

11. Mason JW, O'Connell JB, Herskowitz A, et al: A clinical trial of immunosuppressive therapy for myocarditis. The Myocarditis Treatment Trial Investigators, *N Engl J Med* 333:269, 1995.

12. McCarthy RE, Boehmer JP, Hruban RH, et al: Long-term outcome of fulminant myocarditis as compared with acute (nonfulminant) myocarditis, *N Engl J Med* 342:690, 2000.

13. Skouri HN, Dec GW, Friedrich MG, et al: Noninvasive imaging in myocarditis, *J Am Coll Cardiol* 48:2085, 2006.

14. Zipes DP, Camm AJ, Borggrefe M, et al: ACC/AHA/ESC 2006 guidelines for management of patients with ventricular arrhythmias and the prevention of sudden cardiac death: executive summary. A report of the American College of Cardiology/American Heart Association Task Force and the European Society of Cardiology Committee for Practice Guidelines (Writing Committee to Develop Guidelines for Management of Patients with Ventricular Arrhythmias and the Prevention of Sudden Cardiac Death), *J Am Coll Cardiol* 48:1064, 2006.

CHAPTER 28

DILATED CARDIOMYOPATHY

Amandeep Dhaliwal, MD and Biykem Bozkurt, MD, FACC

1. **What is the definition of dilated cardiomyopathy?**
   Dilated cardiomyopathy (DCM) refers to a spectrum of heterogeneous myocardial disorders characterized by ventricular dilation and depressed myocardial contractility in the absence of abnormal loading conditions (e.g., hypertension or valvular heart disease) or ischemic heart disease sufficient to cause global systolic impairment. Thus, DCM can be envisioned as the final common pathway for myriad cardiac disorders that either damage the heart muscle or, alternatively, disrupt the ability of the myocardium to generate force and subsequently cause chamber dilation.

   In practice and clinical trials, DCM is used interchangeably with nonischemic cardiomyopathy (NICM), although the latter includes systolic heart failure (HF) related to hypertension or valvular disease.

2. **How prevalent is dilated cardiomyopathy?**
   The incidence of DCM is 5 to 8 per 100 000 persons, whereas the prevalence is 36 per 100,000. DCM accounts for 10,000 deaths annually and represents approximately 30% to 40% of HF cases (as defined by NICM). African Americans are three times more likely to develop DCM than Caucasians and more likely to die from DCM compared with age-matched Caucasians.

3. **How does dilated cardiomyopathy present?**
   The presenting features of DCM are typical of HF and include symptoms of left ventricular (LV) failure, including progressive exertional dyspnea, fatigue, weakness, diminished exercise capacity, orthopnea, paroxysmal nocturnal dyspnea, and nocturnal cough. Abdominal distension, right upper quadrant abdominal pain, early satiety, postprandial fullness, and nausea are seen with the development of right-sided heart failure. In advanced heart failure, cardiac cachexia may develop. Approximately 4% to 13% of the patients with DCM will present with asymptomatic LV dysfunction and LV dilation.

4. **What kind of diagnostic studies should be carried out for DCM?**
   The diagnostic evaluation is similar to those with ischemic heart failure and should include routine assessment of serum electrolytes, liver function tests, complete blood cell count, cardiac enzymes, serum brain natriuretic peptide (BNP), chest radiograph, electrocardiogram, and assessment of LV function by echocardiography or radionuclide imaging.

   Echocardiography typically shows four-chamber dilation, wall thinning, global hypokinesis, and left ventricular ejection fraction (LVEF) less than 35% to 40%. LV apical thrombi can be identified in up to 40% of patients with DCM. Tricuspid and mitral regurgitation may be present as a result of annular dilation and altered LV geometry. Doppler mitral inflow patterns may reveal elevated filling pressures.

   Multigated radionuclide angiocardiography (MUGA) may be used to assess LV systolic function in those with poor echocardiographic windows. Compared with echo assessment of LV ejection fraction, multigated radionuclide angiocardiography may have less interobserver and intertest variability. Thallium-201 myocardial scintigraphy is not a reliable technique for differentiating patients with ischemic cardiomyopathy (ICM) from those with DCM, as patients with DCM may have both reversible and fixed perfusion abnormalities related to the presence of myocardial fibrosis.

Cardiac catheterization may be performed if symptoms suggestive of ischemia are present or if coronary artery disease is strongly suspected. Catheterization in DCM generally shows normal coronary arteries or mild, nonobstructive, isolated atherosclerotic lesions that are insufficient to explain the extent of cardiomyopathy.

Endomyocardial biopsy may be performed if and only if a specific diagnosis is suspected in which specific therapy may be efficacious upon establishment of diagnosis.

5. **What is the natural history of dilated cardiomyopathy?**
    The natural history depends on the underlying cause (Fig. 28-1). Generally, symptomatic patients have a 25% mortality at 1 year and 50% mortality at 5 years. The prognosis in those with asymtomatic LV dysfunction is less clear. Pump failure accounts for approximately 70% of deaths, whereas sudden cardiac death accounts for approximately 30%.

    Approximately 25% of symptomatic DCM patients will improve spontaneously. Idiopathic DCM has a lower total mortality compared with ICM, although the risk of sudden death may be higher.

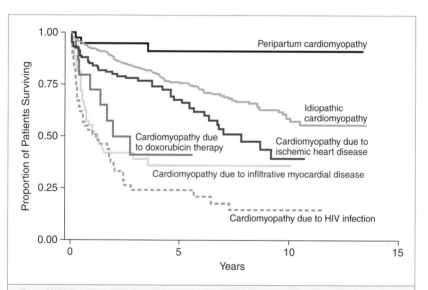

Figure 28-1. Variable survival in patients with dilated cardiomyopathy depending on underlying etiological basis. *HIV,* Human immunodeficiency virus. (From Felker GM, et al: Underlying causes and long-term survival in patients with initially unexplained cardiomyopathy, *N Engl J Med* 342:1077-1084, 2000.)

6. **What are the prognostic features of dilated cardiomyopathy?**
    Many of the prognostic features are similar to those in ischemic cardiomyopathy, including age, LVEF, New York Heart Association (NYHA) class, lack of heart rate variability, elevated levels of neurohormones, and elevated markers of myocardial cell death. However, certain causes of DCM carry a more favorable prognosis and are potentially reversible—for example, cardiomyopathy associated with alcohol, trastuzumab, or tachycardia. Other causes, such as anthracyclines or human immunodeficiency virus (HIV), have a worse prognosis.

7. **What are the common causes of dilated cardiomyopathy?**

The term *nonischemic cardiomyopathy* may include cardiomyopathies commonly caused by hypertension or valvular heart disease, which are not conventionally accepted under the definition of DCM. Causes for DCM include toxic (alcohol, cocaine, pharmaceuticals such as anthracycline antibiotics, transtuzumab), infection (such as Coxsackie virus, HIV, *Trypanosoma cruzi*), inflammatory (such as collagen vascular disease, hypersensitivity myocarditis), nutritional (such as thiamine deficiency), pregnancy, endocrine (such as diabetes, hyperthyroidism), tachycardia, or familial.

8. **What are the features of alcohol-induced cardiomyopathy?**

Alcohol-induced cardiomyopathy is said to occur when cardiomyopathy is noted in a heavy drinker in the absence of other causes (i.e., by exclusion). Alcoholic patients consuming more than 90 g of alcohol a day (approximately 7–8 standard drinks per day) for more than 5 years are at risk for this entity. Symptoms may develop with continued drinking. Approximately 20% of subjects with excessive drinking may demonstrate clinical HF. The typical patient is a man 30 to 55 years old who has been a heavy alcohol consumer for 10 years. Women may be more susceptible to the cardiodepressive effects of alcohol. Death rates are higher in African Americans (versus Caucasians). Abstinence may partially or completely reverse the cardiomyopathy. Overall prognosis remains poor, with a mortality of 40% to 50% at 3 to 6 years without abstinence.

9. **What are the features of cocaine-induced cardiomyopathy?**

Approximately 4% to 18% of cocaine users have depressed LV function. Cardiac catheterization reveals normal or mildly diseased coronary arteries insufficient to explain extent of myocardial dysfunction. Abstinence may lead to reversal.

10. **What are the features of chemotherapy-induced cardiomyopathy?**

Anthracyclines and trastuzumab are among the more prominent chemotherapeutic agents associated with cardiomyopathy. Three major types of anthracycline cardiotoxicity are distinguished: acute, chronic, and late onset, which differ considerably in clinical picture and prognosis. Cardiac failure is rare with acute toxicity. Chronic cardiotoxicity is observed in 0.4% to 23% several weeks or months after chemotherapy. Such anthracycline-induced cardiomyopathy carries a 27% to 61% mortality rate despite aggressive medical treatment. Late cardiotoxicity occurs years after chemotherapy at 5% at 10 years and presents as HF, arrhythmia, or conduction abnormalities. The primary risk factor for cardiomyopathy is cumulative dose administered. Toxicity is rare with cumulative doses below 400 mg/m^2 (less than 3%). Other risk factors include extremes of age and coexisting cardiac disease. Elevated cardiac troponin and brain natriuretic peptide after chemotherapy may allow identification of patients who may develop cardiac toxicity. Anthracyclines should *not* be administered to patients with a baseline LVEF of 30% or less. LV function should be assessed repeatedly before each subsequent dose (or if the initial ejection fraction [EF] is more than 50%, after a cumulative dose of 350–500 mg/m^2), and treatment stopped if EF declines by 10% or more or to a value less than 30% (or less than 50% if EF was normal at baseline). Reversibility has been documented anecdotally. The most effective protection is dexrazoxane (an iron chelator), with a twofold to threefold decrease in the risk of cardiomyopathy.

Trastuzumab is a monoclonal antibody that selectively binds human epidermal growth factor receptor-2 (HER2), which is expressed in 25% of breast cancer. In earlier trials in advanced breast cancer, trastuzumab was associated with the development of HF in up to 27% of patients. The majority of these patients, however, had received significant cumulative doses of anthracyclines or had preexisting cardiac disease. Risk factors for development of trastuzumab-associated HF include increasing age, lower LVEF, and higher anthracycline dose. Trastuzumab-associated HF responds better to standard therapy than anthracycline-induced HF, with complete recovery usually seen within 6 months of discontinuing trastuzumab.

11. **What are the features of HIV-related cardiomyopathy?**
    HIV-related cardiomyopathy accounts for up to 4% of DCM. The incidence is higher among patients with a CD4 count less than 400 cells/mm^3. Cardiomyopathy confers a poor prognosis in these patients. Mortality is four times higher compared with other causes of DCM. Most patients have evidence of myocarditis on biopsy.
    Highly active antiretroviral therapy (HAART) should be considered in the appropriate clinical setting. Retrospective data suggest that the incidence of HIV-related cardiomyopathy has decreased with the use of HAART. Some concerns exist about an increased risk of artherosclerosis with protease inhibitor-based HAART. For a further discussion, see Chapter 69 on cardiac manifestations of HIV/AIDS.

12. **What are the associations between collagen vascular disease and dilated cardiomyopathyies?**
    In systemic lupus erythematosus (SLE), global LV dysfunction has been reported in 5% of patients, segmental LV wall motion abnormalities in 4% of patients, and right ventricular enlargement in 4% of patients, but DCM is rare. In rheumatoid arthritis, symptomatic cardiac disease, including myocarditis, develops in 8% of patients. Progressive systemic sclerosis can rarely lead to heart failure through myocardial fibrosis, arrhythmia, or intermittent vascular spasm. For a further discussion, see Chapter 68 on cardiac manifestations of connective tissue disorders and vasculidities.

13. **What is peripartum cardiomyopathy?**
    Peripartum cardiomyopathy (PPCM) is the development of symptomatic HF in the last trimester of pregnancy or within 6 months of parturition. Other causes of DCM must be excluded in such patients before making the PPCM diagnosis. PPCM occurs in 1 per 2289 to 4000 live births. Risk factors may include older age, multiparity, African-American race, multiple gestation, toxemia, chronic hypertension, and use of tocolytics. In recent case series, up to 50% of PPCM developed with the first two pregnancies. Fifty percent of women recover baseline cardiac function within 6 months. Even though the prognosis in subsequent pregnancies is better if cardiac function recovers, 21% of these patients will develop HF symptoms. The prognosis in subsequent pregnancies is poorer if cardiac function remains abnormal—37% deliver prematurely and 19% die.

14. **What are the features of tachycardia-induced cardiomyopathy?**
    Sustained elevated ventricular rates have been shown to cause changes in LV geometry and dilation. This entity should be considered in patients with no other explanation for LV dysfunction and a concomitant tachyarrhythmia. Hyperthyroid-induced sinus tachycardia or atrial fibrillation should be excluded in such patients. Treatment involves restoration of normal sinus rhythm or control of ventricular rate, with which there is typically resolution in as early as 4 to 6 weeks.

15. **What are the features of nutritional causes of dilated cardiomyopathy?**
    Thiamine deficiency causes cardiovascular beriberi, in which the circulation is hyperkinetic and DCM results. Treatment for beriberi should consist of administration of thiamine along with standard HF therapy. DCM may occur with chronic alcoholism and with anorexia nervosa.

16. **What are the features of cardiomyopathy caused by iron overload?**
    Iron-overload cardiomyopathy occurs as a result of increased cardiac iron deposition, commonly in disorders such as hereditary hemochromatosis and β-thalassemia major. Extra-cardiac manifestations typically precede symptomatic HF. Initially the hemodynamic profile represents a restrictive pattern. As cardiomyopathy advances, DCM ensues. The diagnosis of iron overload is suggested by elevated serum ferritin and a ratio of iron to total iron-binding capacity greater than 50%. The most definitive test for calculation of iron stores is measurement of iron concentration by liver biopsy.

The mainstays of therapy are phlebotomy (in hereditary hemochromatosis) and chelation therapy (in secondary iron overload related to blood transfusions, prophylactically after transfusion of 20–30 units of red blood cells (RBCs) or when serum ferritin is more than 2500 ng/ml). Early diagnosis and treatment before tissue damage has occurred is essential, because life span seems to be normal in treated patients but markedly shortened in those who are not.

17. **What are the pharmacologic treatments to be used in DCM?**
Similar to therapy for chronic stable HF, standard medical therapy with beta-blockers and angiotensin-converting enzyme (ACE) inhibitors (or angiotensin-receptor blockers) is indicated per current guidelines from the American College of Cardiology/American Heart Association (ACC\AHA). Intake of salt should be restricted. Depending on the circumstances, low-dose digoxin, spironolactone, or a combination of isosorbide dinitrate-hydralazine may be added in *symptomatic* HF. However, use of spironolactone should entail judicious adjustment of potassium supplements and close laboratory follow-up. Diuretics should be used to manage volume overload symptoms.

Antiarrhythmic therapy is reserved for individualized treatment of symptomatic arrhythmias, especially for suppression of ventricular arrhythmias after an implantable cardioverter defibrillator (ICD). Recent data suggest that use of such agents in HF patients with atrial fibrillation for maintaining sinus rhythm may not be better than rate control.

Patients with refractory heart failure symptoms may require chronic inotrope therapy.

18. **What are the device treatments to be used in DCM?**
Defibrillators are indicated for secondary prevention in survivors of ventricular fibrillation (VF) or hemodynamically significant ventricular tachycardia (VT); in patients with structural heart disease or unexplained syncope with hemodynamically significant VF or VT on electrophysiologic study; and in patients with NICM who have an LVEF 35% or lower and who are in NYHA functional class II-III.

Recent trials of cardiac resynchronization therapy (with or without concomitant defibrillator) have shown a 50% decrease in all-cause mortality versus placebo among subjects with NICM or DCM. In addition to the mortality benefit, resynchronization improves quality of life. Thus, resynchronization therapy, with or without defibrillator, should be offered to patients who have an LVEF 35% or less, a QRS duration 0.12 or more, and sinus rhythm who continue to have NYHA functional class III or IV despite optimal recommended medical therapy.

19. **Should DCM patients be anticoagulated?**
Patients with dilated cardiomyopathy have multiple risk factors that predispose to thromboembolic events—with the incidence ranging from 0.8 to 2.5 per 100 patient-years. Pooled data from small-randomized controlled clinical trials and current guidelines do not support routine anticoagulation in heart failure with sinus rhythm. The ongoing (at the time of this writing) WARCEF study (warfarin versus aspirin in reduced cardiac ejection fraction) may provide further evidence for the optimal use of antithrombotic therapy in heart failure. Available data do support the use of anticoagulants in the presence of atrial fibrillation, previous stroke or other thromboembolic events, or visible protruding or mobile thrombus on echocardiography.

20. **What is the role of exercise therapy?**
Exercise training should be considered in stable patients. Training has been shown to decrease symptoms, improve exercise tolerance, and improve quality of life beyond pharmacologic treatment. Long-term outcomes, however, are not entirely known, although small studies have shown reduction in mortality or readmission for heart failure. The Heart Failure and a Controlled Trial Investigating Outcomes of Exercise Training (HF-ACTION) trial failed to demonstrate a reduction in all-cause mortality or all-cause hospitalization in patients randomized to a structured exercise program when compared to "usual care", although secondary analysis did suggest some benefit.

BIBLIOGRAPHY, SUGGESTED READINGS, AND WEBSITES

1. Arnold JMO: Heart Failure: http://www.merck.com/mmpe

2. Heart Failure Society of America: http://www.hfsa.org

3. Wigner M, Morgan JP: Causes of Dilated Cardiomyopathy: http://www.utdol.com

4. Zevitz ME: Heart Failure: http://www.emedicine.com

5. ACC/AHA 2005 guideline update for the diagnosis and management of chronic heart failure in the adult, *J Am Coll Cardiol* 46:1–82, 2005.

6. Cooper LT, Baughman KL, Feldman AM, et al: The role of endomyocardial biopsy in the management of cardiovascular disease: a scientific statement from the American Heart Association, the American College of Cardiology, and the European Society of Cardiology. Endorsed by the Heart Failure Society of America and the Heart Failure Association of the European Society of Cardiology, *J Am Coll Cardiol* 50(19):1914-1931, 2007.

7. Dries D, Exner D, Gersh B, et al: Racial differences in the outcome of left ventricular dysfunction, *N Engl J Med* 340:609-616, 1999.

8. Epstein AE, DiMarco JP, Ellenbogen KA, et al: ACC/AHA/HRS 2008 Guidelines for Device-Based Therapy of Cardiac Rhythm Abnormalities: a report of the American College of Cardiology/American Heart Association Task Force on Practice Guidelines (Writing Committee to Revise the ACC/AHA/NASPE 2002 Guideline Update for Implantation of Cardiac Pacemakers and Antiarrhythmia Devices) developed in collaboration with the American Association for Thoracic Surgery and Society of Thoracic Surgeons, *J Am Coll Cardiol* 51(21):e1-e62, 2008.

9. Heart Failure Society of America. Heart failure in patients with left ventricular systolic dysfunction, *J Card Fail* 12(1):e38-e57, 2006.

10. ICD/CRT-D systematic review, *JAMA* 292:2874-2879, 2004.

11. Koniaris L, Goldhaber S: Anticoagulation in dilated cardiomyopathy, *J Am Coll Cardiol* 31:745-748, 1998.

12. Mann DL: Management of heart failure patients with reduced ejection fraction. In Libby P, Bonow R, Mann D, et al, editors: *Braunwald's heart disease: a textbook of cardiovascular medicine*, ed 8, Philadelphia, 2008, Saunders.

13. Piano M: Alcoholic cardiomyopathy: incidence, clinical characteristics, and pathophysiology, *Chest* 121: 1638-1650, 2002.

14. Report of the 1995 World Health Organization/International Society and Federation of Cardiology Task Force on the Definition and Classification of Cardiomyopathies, *Circulation* 93:841-842, 1996.

15. Saxon L, De Marco T: Arrhythmias associated with dilated cardiomyopathy, *Card Electrophysiol Rev* 6:18-25, 2002.

16. Sliwa K, Fett J, Elkayam U: Peripartum cardiomyopathy, *Lancet* 368:687-693, 2006.

17. Swedberg K, Cleland J, Dargie H, et al: Guidelines for the diagnosis and treatment of chronic heart failure: executive summary (update 2005): The Task Force for the Diagnosis and Treatment of Chronic Heart Failure of the European Society of Cardiology, *Eur Heart J* 26(11):1115-1140, 2005.

CHAPTER 29

HYPERTROPHIC CARDIOMYOPATHY

David Yao, MD and Kumudha Ramasubbu, MD, FACC

1. **What is hypertrophic cardiomyopathy?**

   Hypertrophic cardiomyopathy (HCM) is a primary disorder of the cardiac muscle characterized by inappropriate myocardial hypertrophy of a nondilated left ventricle (LV) in the absence of a cardiovascular or systemic disease (i.e., aortic stenosis or systemic hypertension). Historically, HCM has been known by a confusing array of names, such as idiopathic hypertrophic subaortic stenosis (IHSS), muscular subaortic stenosis, and hypertrophic obstructive cardiomyopathy (HOCM). Presently, *hypertrophic cardiomyopathy* is the preferred term because only a small percentage of patients actually have left ventricular outflow tract (LVOT) obstruction.

2. **What is the prevalence of HCM?**

   The reported prevalence of HCM from epidemiologic studies is about 1:500 in the general population (0.2%). HCM affects men and women equally and occurs in many races and countries.

3. **What are the genetic mutations that cause HCM, and how are they transmitted?**

   Thus far, more than 400 mutations in 11 genes have been identified that can cause HCM. These genes encode for cardiac sarcomere proteins that serve contractile, structural, and regulatory functions. They are cardiac troponin T, cardiac troponin I, myosin regulatory light chain, myosin essential light chain, cardiac myosin binding protein C, alpha- and beta-cardiac myosin heavy chain, cardiac alpha actin, alpha tropomyosin, titin, and muscle LIM protein (MLP). Mutations in cardiac myosin binding protein C and beta-cardiac myosin heavy chain are the most common and account for 82% of all mutations. HCM is inherited as an autosomal dominant trait; therefore, patients with HCM have a 50% chance of transmitting the disease to each of their offspring.

4. **Who should be screened for HCM?**

   First-degree relatives of patients with HCM should be screened, and screening is performed primarily with history, physical examination, 12-lead electrocardiogram (ECG), and two-dimensional echocardiography. Traditionally, screening was performed on a 12- to 18-month basis, usually beginning by age 12 until age 18 to 21. However, it is now recognized that development of the HCM phenotype uncommonly can occur later in adulthood. Therefore, the current recommendation is to extend clinical surveillance into adulthood at about 5-year intervals or to undergo genetic testing (Table 29-1).

5. **What are the histologic characteristics of HCM?**

   The histology of HCM is characterized by hypertrophy of cardiac myocytes and myocardial fiber disarray. The abnormal myocytes contain bizarre-shaped nuclei and are arranged in disorganized patterns. The volume of the interstitial collagen matrix is greatly increased, and the arrangement of the matrix components is also disorganized. Myocardial disarray is seen in substantial portions of hypertrophied and nonhypertrophied LV myocardium. Almost all HCM patients have some degree of disarray, and in the majority at least 5% of the myocardium is involved.

TABLE 29-1. CLINICAL SCREENING STRATEGIES FOR DETECTION OF HCM IN FAMILIES*

<12 yrs old
Optional unless:

Malignant family history of premature HCM death or other adverse complications

Competitive athlete in an intense training program

Onset of symptoms

Other clinical suspicion of early LV hypertrophy

12 to 18–21 yrs old
Every 12–18 months

>18–21 yrs old
Probably approximately every 5 years or more frequent intervals with a family history of late-onset HCM and/or malignant clinical course

---

*In the absence of laboratory-based genetic testing.

From Maron BJ, Seidman JG, Seidman CE: Proposal for contemporary screening strategies in families with hypertrophic cardiomyopathy, *J Am Coll Cardiol* 44:2129, 2004.

---

6. **What are the common types of HCM?**
   The distribution and severity of LV hypertrophy in patients with HCM can vary greatly. Even first-degree relatives, with the same genetic mutation, usually show different patterns of hypertrophy. Various patterns of LV hypertrophy have been reported. The most common site of hypertrophy is the anterior interventricular septum, which is seen in more than 80% of HCM patients and is known as asymmetrical septal hypertrophy (ASH). Concentric LV hypertrophy, with maximal thickening at the level of the papillary muscles, is seen in 8% to 10%. A variant with primary involvement of the apex (apical HCM) is common in Japan and rare in the U.S. (less than 2%) and is characterized by spadelike deformity of the LV.

7. **What are the most common symptoms in patients with HCM?**
   Most patients with HCM have no or only minor symptoms and often are diagnosed during family screening. The most common symptoms are as follows:
   - Dyspnea
     - Present in more than 90% of symptomatic patients
     - Caused mainly by LV diastolic dysfunction with impaired filling caused by abnormal relaxation and increased chamber stiffness
     - Also caused by dynamic LV outflow tract obstruction leading to elevated intraventricular pressures.
   - Angina pectoris
     - May occur in both obstructive and nonobstructive HCM
     - Caused by a mismatch of supply and demand in myocardial perfusion
     - Several mechanisms have been proposed, including increased muscle mass and wall stress, decreased coronary perfusion pressure secondary to LV outflow obstruction, elevated diastolic filling pressures, systolic compression of large intramural coronary arteries, inadequate capillary density, impaired vasodilatory reserve, and abnormally narrowed small intramural coronary arteries

■ Syncope and presyncope
  o Caused by inadequate cardiac output with exertion (as a result of LVOT obstruction) or as a result of cardiac arrhythmia
  o Identifies patients at risk for sudden death

8. **How is HCM differentiated from athlete's heart?**
Long-term athletic training can lead to cardiac hypertrophy, known as *athlete's heart*. This clinically benign physiologic condition must be differentiated from HCM, because HCM is the most common cause of sudden death in competitive athletes. Clinical parameters that support the diagnosis of HCM instead of athlete's heart are asymmetric hypertrophy greater than 16 mm, LV end-diastolic dimension less than 45 mm, enlarged left atrium, impaired LV relaxation on Doppler mitral valve inflow parameters and tissue Doppler echocardiography, absent response to deconditioning (e.g., hypertrophy does not regress with absence of exercise), family history of HCM, and sacromeric protein mutation identified by genetic testing. These parameters are summarized in Table 29-2.

TABLE 29-2. CLINICAL PARAMETERS USED TO DISTINGUISH HCM FROM ATHLETE'S HEART

Parameters	HCM	Athlete's heart
LV wall thickness	> 16 mm	< 16 mm
Pattern of hypertrophy	Asymmetric, symmetric or apical	Symmetric
LV end-diastolic dimension	< 45 mm	> 55 mm
Left atrium size	Enlarged	Normal
LV diastolic filling pattern	Impaired relaxation	Normal
Response to deconditioning	None	LV wall thickness decreases
ECG findings	Very high QRS voltage; Q waves; deep negative T waves	Criteria for LVH but without unusual features
Family history of HCM	Present	Absent
Sacromeric protein mutation	Present	Absent

LVH, Left ventricular hypertrophy.

Modified from Elliott PM, McKenna WJ: *Diagnosis and evaluation of hypertrophic cardiomyopathy*, www.UpToDate.com, accessed February 2008.

9. **Describe the classic murmur of obstructive HCM and bedside maneuvers that differentiate it from other cardiac abnormalities.**
The classic murmur of obstructive HCM is a harsh crescendo–decrescendo systolic murmur and is heard best between the left sternal border and apex. It often radiates to the axilla and base but not into the neck vessels. A variety of provocative maneuvers can augment or suppress the murmur to help differentiate it from other systolic murmurs.
  Maneuvers that increase intracardiac blood volume or decrease contractility typically lead to a decrease in murmur intensity, and maneuvers that decrease intracardiac blood volume or increase contractility lead to an increase in murmur intensity (Table 29-3).

TABLE 29-3. EFFECT OF BEDSIDE MANEUVERS ON SYSTOLIC MURMURS

Maneuver	HCM	AS	MR	VSD
Valsalva	↑	↓	↓	↓
Handgrip	↓	↓	↑	↑
Squatting	↓	↑	↑	↑
Amyl nitrite	↑	↑	↓	↓
Leg raise	↓	↑	↑	↑

AS, Aortic stenosis; *MR*, mitral regurgitation; *VSD*, ventricular septal defect.

10. **How does the carotid pulse in obstructive HCM differ from that in valvular aortic stenosis?**

    In patients with obstructive HCM, the carotid pulse has an initial brisk rise, followed by midsystolic decline as a result of LVOT obstruction, then a second rise *(pulsus bisferiens)*. In contrast, as a result of the fixed obstruction in aortic stenosis, the carotid upstroke is diminished in amplitude and delayed *(pulsus parvus and tardus)*.

11. **What noninvasive studies are helpful in making the diagnosis of HCM?**

    ECG is abnormal in the majority of patients with HCM; however, no changes are pathognomonic for HCM. The common abnormalities are ST-segment and T-wave changes, voltage criteria for left ventricular hypertrophy (LVH), prominent Q waves in the inferior (II, III, aVF) or precordial (V2-V6) leads, left axis deviation, and left atrial enlargement. Apical HCM, seen predominantly in Japanese patients, is characterized by giant negative T waves in the precordial leads.

    Echocardiography is the primary and preferred diagnostic modality for HCM. The cardinal feature is LVH with diastolic wall thickness 15 mm or greater. Other findings include a septal-to-posterior wall ratio 1.3 or more, small LV cavity, reduced septal motion and thickening, normal or increased motion of the posterior wall, systolic anterior motion of the mitral leaflets, mitral regurgitation, partial midsystolic closure of aortic valve with coarse fluttering of the leaflets in late systole, and diastolic dysfunction. In the setting of LVOT obstruction, a resting LVOT gradient can be detected. A significant gradient is defined as a resting gradient more than 30 mm Hg and a provocable gradient more than 50 mm Hg. The LVOT Doppler signal in HCM is typically late peaking and is referred to as *dagger shaped*.

    Magnetic resonance imaging (MRI) is becoming a valuable tool to complement echocardiographic findings. It offers high-resolution images, three-dimensional imaging, and tissue characterization. MRI is especially useful to detect LVH in areas that may be difficult to assess by echocardiography or if the technical quality of echocardiographic images is inadequate.

12. **What is systolic anterior motion and what causes it?**

    Systolic anterior motion (SAM) is the abnormal anterior displacement of the anterior mitral leaflet toward the septum during mid-systole. Several mechanisms have been proposed for SAM:
    - The anterior mitral leaflet is drawn toward the septum by a Venturi effect produced by the lower pressure in the LVOT that occurs as blood is ejected at a high velocity.
    - The anterior mitral leaflet is pulled against the septum by contraction of abnormally inserted and oriented papillary muscles.

    This typically results in eccentric mitral regurgitation directed posteriorly. Because SAM worsens during the course of systole, the mitral regurgitation also becomes more prominent during mid- to late systole.

13. **Describe the mechanism of LVOT obstruction in HCM.**
    Obstruction in HCM is produced by SAM of the anterior mitral leaflet and mid-systolic contact with the hypertrophic ventricular septum. The magnitude of the subaortic gradient is directly related to the duration of contact between the mitral leaflet and the septum. The subaortic gradient is often dynamic and responds to provocative maneuvers in the same manner as the systolic murmur (see question 9 and Table 29-3).

14. **What are the characteristic hemodynamic findings during cardiac catheterization in obstructive HCM?**
    Cardiac catheterization is not required for the diagnosis of HCM, and the diagnosis is usually made using noninvasive tests. Cardiac catheterization is generally reserved for assessment of coronary artery disease and evaluation before surgical procedures such as myectomy and mitral valve replacement. The typical findings during cardiac catheterization are subaortic or mid-ventricular outflow gradient on catheter pullback, spike-and-dome pattern of aortic pressure tracing, elevated left atrial and LV end-diastolic pressures, elevated pulmonary capillary wedge pressure, increased V wave on wedge tracing (as a result of mitral regurgitation), and elevated pulmonary arterial pressure.

15. **What is the Brockenbrough-Braunwald sign?**
    Normally, following a premature ventricular contraction (PVC), with the subsequent sinus beat there is an increased contractility and stroke volume, leading to an increase in the systolic blood pressure and thus an increase in the pulse pressure (the difference between systolic and diastolic pressure). However, in patients with HCM, the increased contractility after a PVC results in increased LVOT obstruction, leading to a decrease in stroke volume and systolic pressure and thus a decrease in pulse pressure. This phenomenon is known as the Brockenbrough-Braunwald sign.

16. **What are the risk factors for sudden cardiac death in patients with HCM?**
    Sudden cardiac death (SCD) is the most devastating consequence of HCM and is often the initial clinical manifestation in asymptomatic individuals. The most common cause of SCD in HCM patients is ventricular tachyarrhythmias. Seven major risk factors for SCD have been identified: prior cardiac arrest or sustained ventricular tachycardia (VT), family history of SCD, unexplained syncope, hypotensive blood pressure response to exercise, nonsustained VT on ambulatory (Holter) monitoring, identification of a high-risk mutant gene and massive LVH with wall thickness 30 mm or greater.

17. **What medications should generally be avoided in patients with obstructive HCM?**
    Medications that decrease preload and afterload and increase contractility will worsen LVOT obstruction and therefore should be avoided.
    - **Preload reducing** agents are diuretics and nitroglycerin. Diuretics may be used cautiously in patients with persistent heart failure symptoms and volume overload.
    - **Afterload reducing** agents include dihydropyridine calcium channel blockers (CCB), nitroglycerin, angiotensin-converting enzyme (ACE) inhibitors, and angiotensin II receptor blockers.
    - **Increased contractility** is produced by medications such as digoxin, dobutamine, and phosphodiesterase inhibitors (milrinone).

18. **What are the pharmacologic therapies for patients with HCM?**
    Pharmacologic therapy is primarily used to alleviate symptoms of heart failure, angina, and syncope in HCM patients. Routine pharmacologic therapy is not recommended in asymptomatic patients.
    - **Beta-blockers** are generally considered first-line therapy for HCM. The beneficial effects of beta-blockers are mediated by the negative chronotropic property, which increases ventricular diastolic filling time, and by the negative inotropic property.
    - **Nondihydropyridine calcium channel blockers (CCB)** are an alternative to beta-blockers in the treatment of HCM. Verapamil has been the most widely used CCB and improves symptoms by

increasing LV relaxation and diastolic filling and by decreasing LV contractility. However, because of its vasodilatory effect, verapamil should be avoided in patients with marked outflow obstruction. Diltiazem has been used less often but may improve LV diastolic function. Dihydropyridine CCBs should be avoided in patients with HCM because of their predominantly vasodilatory properties, which can result in worsening of the LVOT obstruction.

- **Disopyramide** is a class IA antiarrhythmic drug with potent negative inotropic effect that is used when beta-blockers and CCB have failed to improve symptoms. Disopyramide is used in combination with a beta-blocker because it may accelerate AV nodal conduction.

19. **What nonpharmacologic treatments are available to patients with HCM?**
    - **Septal myectomy** surgery has been the gold standard for more than 45 years for patients with severe symptoms that are refractory to medical therapy. Septal myectomy, known as the Morrow procedure, uses a transaortic approach to resect a small amount of muscle from the proximal septum. It is associated with persistent and long-lasting improvement in symptoms and exercise capacity.
    - **Alcohol septal ablation** has gained tremendous popularity in recent years as a new treatment modality for HCM. The procedure is performed by injecting 1 to 3 ml of 96% to 98% ethanol into a septal perforator branch of the left anterior descending coronary artery to create a limited myocardial infarction in the proximal septum. This scarring leads to progressive thinning and hypokinesis of the septum, increases LVOT diameter, improves mitral valve function, and ultimately reduces LVOT obstruction. The procedure-related mortality rate is 1% to 2%, which is similar to that of surgery.
    - **Dual-chamber pacing** was promoted to be an alternative to myectomy to improve symptoms and reduce LVOT obstruction in the early 1990s. However, subsequent randomized studies have shown that subjectively perceived symptomatic improvement was not accompanied by objective evidence of improved exercise capacity and may be due to a placebo effect. Dual-chamber pacing has a limited role in the contemporary management of HCM, mainly in the subgroup of elderly patients who are not candidates for myectomy or alcohol septal ablation (ASA).

20. **What are the indications for an implantable cardioverter defibrillator in HCM?**
    An implantable cardioverter defibrillator (ICD) is the preferred therapy for prevention of SCD in HCM patients. The recommended indications are as follows:
    - ICD can be used for secondary prevention in survivors of cardiac arrest or sustained VT.
    - ICD is indicated for high-risk patients, defined as having two or more of the major risk factors for SCD (see Question 16).
    - In patients with one major risk factor, care needs to be individualized. The decision to implant an ICD should take into account the age of the patient, strength of the risk factor, the level of risk acceptable to the patient and family, and the potential complications.
    - ICD can be used in patients with end-stage HCM, characterized by LV systolic dysfunction, LV wall thinning, and chamber dilation.

21. **What is the natural history of HCM?**
    The clinical course of patients with HCM is variable. Clinical manifestation can present at any age, from birth to age 90 or older. Many patients remain asymptomatic or mildly symptomatic for many years and achieve normal life expectancy. Others develop progressive symptoms of heart failure with exertional dyspnea and functional limitation despite medical therapy. Increase in LVH is predominately seen in adolescents and young adults. In older adults, LV wall thickness generally remains stable. Approximately 10% to 15% of patients will progress to end-stage HCM as described earlier. Atrial fibrillation occurs in 10% to 20% of HCM patients and may lead to clinical deterioration. The annual mortality rate in patients with HCM is about 1% in adults and 2% in children.

BIBLIOGRAPHY, SUGGESTED READINGS, AND WEBSITES

1. Elliot PM, McKenna WJ: Diagnosis and Evaluation of Hypertrophic Cardiomyopathy: http://www.utdol.com

2. Hypertrophic Cardiomyopathy: http://www.maerck.com/mmpe

3. Sarcomere Protein Gene Mutation Database: http://genepath.med.harvard.edu/~seidman/cg3

4. Zevitz ME: Cardiomyopathy, Hypertrophic: http://www.emedicine.com

5. Fatkin D, Seidman JG, Seidman CE: Hypertrophic cardiomyopathy. *Cardiovascular medicine*, ed 3, 2007.

6. Kimmelstiel CD, Maron BJ: Role of percutaneous septal ablation in hypertrophic obstructive cardiomyopathy, *Circulation* 109(4):452-456, 2004.

7. Maron BJ, Dearani JA, Ommen SR, et al: The case for surgery in obstructive hypertrophic cardiomyopathy, *J Am Coll Cardiol* 44(10):2044-53, 2004.

8. Maron BJ: Hypertrophic cardiomyopathy: a systematic review, *JAMA* 287(10):1308-1320, 2002.

9. Maron BJ: Hypertrophic cardiomyopathy. In *Braunwald's heart disease*, ed 8, 2008.

10. Maron BJ, Pelliccia A: The heart of trained athletes: cardiac remodeling and the risks of sports, including sudden death, *Circulation* 114:1633-1644, 2006.

11. Maron BJ, Seidman JG, Seidman CE: Proposal for contemporary screening strategies in families with hypertrophic cardiomyopathy, *J Am Coll Cardiol* 44:2125-2132, 2004.

12. Ommen SR, Maron BJ, Olivotto I, et al: Long-term effects of surgical septal myectomy on survival in patients with obstructive hypertrophic cardiomyopathy, *J Am Coll Cardiol* 46(3):470-476, 2005.

13. Richard P, Charron P, Carrier L, et al: Hypertrophic cardiomyopathy: distribution of disease genes, spectrum of mutations, and implications for a molecular diagnosis strategy. *Circulation* 107(17):2227-2232, 2003.

14. Sherrid MV, Barac I, McKenna WJ, et al: Multicenter study of the efficacy and safety of disopyramide in obstructive hypertrophic cardiomyopathy, *J Am Coll Cardiol* 45(8):1251-1258, 2005.

15. Maron BJ, McKenna WJ, Danielson GK, et al: American College of Cardiology/European Society of Cardiology clinical expert consensus document of hypertrophic cardiomyopathy, *J Am Coll Cardiol* 42:1687-1713, 2003.

CHAPTER 30

RESTRICTIVE CARDIOMYOPATHY

Glenn N. Levine, MD, FACC, FAHA

1. **What is the basic physiologic problem in restrictive cardiomyopathy?**
   The basic physiologic problem in restrictive cardiomyopathy is increased *stiffness* of the ventricular walls, causing impaired diastolic filling of the ventricles and leading to heart failure. Systolic function is usually preserved (at least in the early stages of disease, although it may become severely impaired in the later stages of amyloidosis).

2. **What are the main causes of restrictive cardiomyopathy?**
   Approximately half the cases of restrictive cardiomyopathy have an identifiable cause. The most common identifiable cause is myocardial infiltration in patient with amyloidosis. Other infiltrative diseases include sarcoidosis, Gaucher's disease, and Hurler's disease. Storage diseases include hemochromatosis, glycogen storage disease, and Fabry's disease. Endomyocardial involvement from endomyocardial fibrosis, radiation, and anthracycline treatment can also lead to restrictive cardiomyopathy. Although restrictive cardiomyopathy is a rather uncommon cause of heart failure in North America and Europe, it is a common cause of heart failure and death in tropical regions, including parts of Africa, Central and South America, India, and other parts of Asia (where the incidence of endomyocardial fibrosis is relatively high). Causes of restrictive cardiomyopathy are summarized in Table 30-1.

3. **What are the usual echocardiographic findings in restrictive cardiomyopathy?**
   Echocardiography usually demonstrates normal or near-normal systolic function, ventricles of normal or decreased volumes, biatrial enlargement, normal or only minimally increased ventricular wall thickness, and impaired ventricular filling *(diastolic dysfunction)*. As discussed in question 4, these findings may be different in later stages of amyloidosis and certain other conditions.

4. **How does amyloidosis affect the heart?**
   As with other organs, in amyloidosis there may be protein deposition in myocardial tissue. The term *amyloidosis* was reportedly coined by Virchow and means "starchlike." The myocardium is found to be firm, rubbery, and noncompliant. This protein deposition leads to restrictive physiology, as well as eventual systolic heart dysfunction and possible conduction abnormalities. Patients are thus struck with a double whammy of restrictive cardiomyopathy and systolic dysfunction. They are often extremely fluid sensitive, walking a fine line between volume overload and inadequate preload. They often manifest orthostatic hypotension and may develop additional conduction-related disorders. The prognosis is generally extremely poor.

5. **How is cardiac amyloidosis diagnosed?**
   If the patient is not otherwise known to have amyloidosis, cardiac amyloidosis may be suggested by symptoms and signs of heart failure, an echocardiogram that demonstrates impaired filling and often thickened ventricular walls, a "sparkling" pattern on echocardiography (Fig. 30-1), and the finding of thickened ventricular walls yet low voltage on the electrocardiogram. The diagnosis is usually confirmed, if necessary, by biopsy.

TABLE 30-1. CLASSIFICATION OF TYPES OF RESTRICTIVE CARDIOMYOPATHY ACCORDING TO CAUSE
Infiltrative
Amyloidosis
Sarcoidosis
Gaucher's disease
Hurler's disease
Fatty infiltration
Storage Disease
Hemochromatosis
Fabry's disease
Glycogen storage disease
Endomyocardial
Endomyocardial fibrosis
Radiation
Hypereosinophilic syndrome (Löffler's endocarditis)
Carcinoid syndrome
Myocardial Noninfiltrative
Idiopathic cardiomyopathy
Familial cardiomyopathy
Hypertrophic cardiomyopathy
Scleroderma

Modified from Kushwaha S, Fallon JT, Fuster V: Restrictive cardiomyopathy, *N Engl J Med* 336-267, 1997.

6. **What are the main cardiac manifestations of sarcoidosis?**
   Sarcoidosis can lead to noncaseating granulomas infiltrating the myocardium and leading to fibrosis and scar formation. Infiltration may be patchy throughout the myocardium. Infiltration can lead to congestive heart failure, heart block and syncope (as a result of infiltration of the conduction system), and ventricular arrhythmias (including syncope and sudden death). Pulmonary involvement may lead to pulmonary hypertension and its associated effects on right-sided heart function.

7. **Is endomyocardial biopsy useful in cases of suspected restrictive cardiomyopathy?**
   Endomyocardial biopsy is considered *reasonable* in the setting of heart failure associated with unexplained restrictive cardiomyopathy (it is a class IIa, level of evidence C, recommendation in the scientific statement on endomyocardial biopsy by the American College of Cardiology/American Heart Association/European Society of Cardiology [ACC/AHA/ESC]). Endomyocardial biopsy may reveal specific disorders, such as amyloidosis or hemochromatosis, or myocardial fibrosis and myocyte hypertrophy consistent with idiopathic restrictive cardiomyopathy. Endomyocardial biopsy should not be performed if computed tomography (CT) or magnetic resonance imaging (MRI) suggests the patient instead has pericardial constriction or if other less invasive tests and studies can identify a specific cause of the restrictive cardiomyopathy.

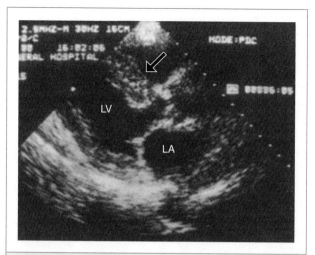

Figure 30-1. Echocardiogram demonstrating the *sparkling* pattern that can be seen in patients with cardiac amyloidosis. This sparkling pattern is best seen in this picture in the thickened ventricular septum. (Modified from Levine RA: Echocardiographic assessment of the cardiomyopathies. In Weyman AE: *Principles and practice of echocardiography*, ed 2, Philadelphia, 1994, Lea & Febiger, p. 810.)

8. **Is cardiac CT or cardiac MRI useful in cases of possible restrictive cardiomyopathy?**

   Both cardiac CT and cardiac MRI can be useful in cases of restrictive cardiomyopathy. Both imaging modalities can demonstrate a thickened pericardium, which may suggest constrictive pericarditis as the actual cause of the patient's ailment. Cardiac MRI, with the use of delayed hyperenhancement in many cases, may demonstrate findings suggestive of sarcoidosis, eosinophilic endomyocardial disease, amyloidosis, and other causes of restrictive cardiomyopathy. Cardiac MRI can also be used to make the diagnosis of cardiac hemochromatosis. In some cases, MRI may also be used to guide endomyocardial biopsy and to assess the likelihood of obtaining diagnostic biopsy samples.

9. **What are hypereosinophilic syndrome (HES) and Loeffler's disease?**

   HES and Loeffler's disease are similar (and possibly the same) diseases characterized by persistent marked eosinophilia, absence of a primary cause of eosinophilia (e.g., parasitic or allergic disease), and eosinophil-mediated end-organ damage. The most common cardiac manifestation of HES is endomyocardial fibrosis, which was first described in the 1930s by Loeffler. Secondary thrombosis may contribute to ventricular cavity obliteration, and thus these conditions are sometimes referred to as "restrictive obliterative cardiomyopathies" (Fig. 30-2). The reader should be aware that there is a confusing and variable use of the terms *HES*, *Loeffler's disease*, *Loeffler's endomyocardial fibrosis*, and *endomyocardial fibrosis* throughout the literature, with some authorities believing the syndromes are related and others treating them as distinct entities.

10. **What is Gaucher's disease?**

    Gaucher's disease is a disease in which there is deficiency of the enzyme β-glucocerebrosidase, resulting in the accumulation of cerebroside in the heart and other organs.

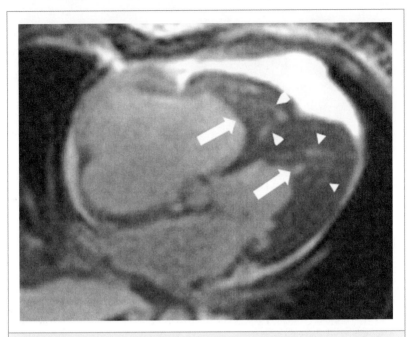

Figure 30-2. Cardiac MRI demonstrating endomyocardial fibrosis and intracardiac thrombus, partially obliterating the left and right ventricles. The *long arrows* point to ventricular thrombus; the *arrow heads* demonstrate areas of endomyocardial fibrosis. (Modified from Salanitri GC, et al: Endomyocardial fibrosis and intracardiac thrombus occurring in idiopathic hypereosinophilic syndrome. *Am J Roentgenol* 184:1432-1433, 2005.)

11. **How does Hurler's syndrome affect the heart?**
    Hurler's syndrome leads to the deposition of mucopolysaccharides in the myocardium, cardiac valves, and coronary arteries.

BIBLIOGRAPHY, SUGGESTED READINGS, AND WEBSITES

1. Ammash NM, Tajik AJ: Idiopathic Restrictive Cardiomyopathy: http://www.utdol.com
2. Arnold JMO: Restrictive Cardiomyopathy: http://www.merck.com/mmhe
3. Cooper LT: Definition and Classification of the Cardiomyopathies: http://www.utdol.com
4. Goswami VJ: Cardiomyopathy, Restrictive: http://www.emedicine.com
5. Cooper LT, Baughman K, Feldman AM, et al: AHA/ACC/ESC joint scientific statement: the role of endomyocardial biopsy in the management of cardiovascular disease, *Circulation* 116:2216-2233, 2007.
6. Hare JM: The dilated, restrictive, and infiltrative cardiomyopathies. In Libby P, Bonow RO, Mann DL, et al, editors: *Braunwald's heart disease: a textbook of cardiovascular medicine*, ed 8, Philadelphia, 2008, Saunders.
7. Kushwaha SS, Fallon JT, Foster V: Restrictive cardiomyopathy. *N Engl M Med* 335:267-276, 1997.

CHAPTER 31

CARDIAC TRANSPLANTATION

Kaity Lin, MD and Kumudha Ramasubbu, MD, FACC

1. **List the common indications for heart transplantation.**

   Approximately 2000 to 2200 hearts are currently transplanted in the United States each year. Dr. Christiaan Barnard performed the first human allograft transplant in 1967. The most common indications for transplant are nonischemic cardiomyopathy (46%) and coronary artery disease (40%). Specific indications for transplant include the following:

   - Severe heart failure (New York Heart Association [NYHA] class III or IV) requiring continuous inotropic therapy or poor short-term prognosis despite maximal medical therapy
   - Restrictive or hypertrophic cardiomyopathy with NYHA class III or IV symptoms
   - Refractory angina despite medical therapy, not amenable to revascularization, with poor short-term prognosis
   - Recurrent or refractory ventricular arrhythmias, despite medical or device therapy
   - Complex congenital heart disease with progressive ventricular failure not amenable to surgical or percutaneous repair
   - Hypoplastic left-sided heart syndrome
   - Unresectable low-grade tumors confined to the myocardium, without evidence of metastasis

2. **What baseline evaluations are obtained in the pretransplant workup?**

   Pretransplant evaluation serves the purpose of assessing a patient's severity of heart failure, mortality benefit from surgery, comorbidities, and potential contraindications to surgery. Factors that are assessed include the following:

   - **History, physical, and psychosocial evaluation**
   - **Heart failure (HF) severity:** Cardiopulmonary exercise test with respiratory exchange ratio, echocardiogram (echo), right-sided heart catheter with vasodilator challenge (if indicated), and electrocardiogram (ECG)
   - **Immunocompatibility:** ABO and human leukocyte antigen (HLA) typing, panel-reactive antibody (PRA)/flow
   - **Infections:** Hepatitis B and C, human immunodeficiency virus (HIV), syphilis, tuberculosis (purified protein derivative [PPD]; check titers for immunoglobulin (Ig) G for herpes simplex virus (HSV), cytomegalovirus (CMV), toxoplasma, Epstein Barr virus (EBV), and varicella
   - **Organ function:** Basic metabolic panel, complete blood cell count, liver function tests, prothombin time/international normalized ratio (PT/INR), urinalysis, glomerular filtration rate, urine protein, pulmonary function test with arterial blood gas, posteroanterior (PA) lateral chest radiograph (CXR), abdominal ultrasound, carotid Doppler, ankle-brachial index (ABI), dual-energy x-ray absorptiometry (DEXA), dental examination, and ophthalmologic examination if patient has diabetes mellitus (DM).
   - **Vaccination history:** Influenza, pneumococcal, and hepatitis B
   - **Preventive and age-appropriate screening:** Colonoscopy, mammography, gynecologic/Papanicolaou examination, and prostate evaluation

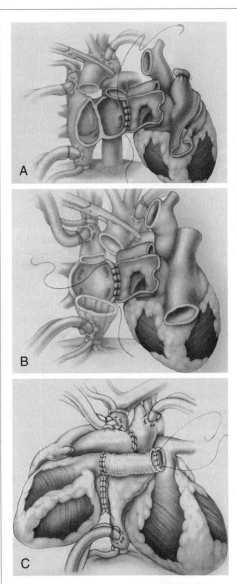

Figure 31-1. Methods of heart transplantation. **A,** Orthotopic biatrial approach in which the donor atrial cuff is anastomosed to the recipient left atrium and right atrium, followed by aortic and pulmonary artery anastomosis. **B,** Orthotopic bicaval approach, in which the donor left atrial cuff is anastomosed to the recipient left atrium, followed by inferior vena cava, superior vena cava, aortic, and pulmonary artery anastomoses. **C,** Heterotopic heart transplantation, in which the recipient's heart is left in the mediastinum and the donor heart is attached *parallel* to the recipient heart. (From Kirklin J, Young J, McGiffin D, et al: *Heart transplantation,* Philadelphia, 2002, Churchill Livingstone.)

3. **What are contraindications to heart transplantation?**

   Contraindications include any noncardiac conditions that may decrease a patient's survival and increase risk of rejection or infection. Contraindications include the following:

   - Systemic illness limiting survival despite heart transplant (e.g., malignancies, acquired immunodeficiency syndrome [AIDS] with CD4 count less than 200 cells/mm3, sarcoidosis, systemic lupus erythematosus)
   - Systemic illness with high probability of recurrence in the transplanted heart
   - Fixed pulmonary hypertension (HTN) (pulmonary vascular resistance greater than 5 Wood units, transpulmonary gradient more than 15 mm Hg) unresponsive to pulmonary vasodilators
   - Age older than 65 years (program dependent)
   - Severe peripheral vascular or cerebrovascular disease not amenable to surgical or percutaneous therapy
   - DM with end-organ damage
   - Uncorrected abdominal aortic aneurysm greater than 4 to 6 cm
   - Systemic infection that may be worsened by immunosuppression (HIV, hepatitis B, CMV)
   - Active infection or malignancy
   - Morbid obesity (body mass index cutoff is program dependent)
   - Nonreversible renal insufficiency (creatinine clearance less than 40–50 ml/min)
   - Nonreversible hepatic dysfunction (liver cirrhosis, bilirubin more than 2.5 mg/dl, transaminases more than twice normal)
   - Severe pulmonary dysfunction (forced vital capacity [FVC] and forced expiratory volume [FEV1] less than 40% of predicted)
   - Psychosocial impairment (e.g., polysubstance abuse, psychiatric instability, noncompliance, lack of social support system)

4. **Define allotransplantation versus xenotransplantation and orthotopic versus heterotopic transplantation.**

   - **Allotransplantation** involves transplantation of cells, tissue, or organs between *same* species, whereas *xenotransplantation* involves *different* species.
   - In **orthotopic heart transplant**, the donor heart is transplanted in place of the recipient's heart. Two anastomotic approaches are used (Figure 31-1):
     - **Biatrial approach:** The donor atrial cuff is anastomosed to the recipient left atrium, and then right atrium, followed by aortic and pulmonary artery anastomosis.
     - **Bicaval approach:** The donor left atrial cuff is anastomosed to the recipient left atrium, followed by inferior vena cava, superior vena cava, aortic, and pulmonary artery anastomosis. This approach may be associated with improved atrial function, lower incidence of atrial arrhythmias, sinus node dysfunction, and tricuspid insufficiency.
   - **Heterotopic heart transplantation:** The recipient's heart is left in the mediastinum, and the donor heart is attached *parallel* to the recipient heart. In this procedure the donor/recipient left atrial cuff is anastomosed, followed by superior vena cava, aortic, and pulmonary artery anastomosis via Dacron graft. The procedure is considered in the following situations:
     - Donor/recipient body size mismatch
     - Recipient pulmonary artery systolic pressure greater than 60 mm Hg
     - Suboptimal donor heart systolic function

5. **What is the estimated graft survival 3 months, 1 year, 3 years, 5 years, and 10 years after transplant? What are the common causes of death?**

   Based on the 2007 U.S. Organ Procurement and Transplantation Network (OPTN) and Scientific Registry of Transplant Recipients (SRTR) report, graft survival approximates 95% at 1 month, 88% at 1 year, 73% at 5 years, and 50% at 10 years after transplantation. The major causes of post-transplant death include the following:

- **Less than 30 days:** graft failure, multiorgan failure, infection
- **Less than 1 year:** infection, graft failure, acute allograft rejection
- **More than 5 years:** allograft vasculopathy, late graft failure, malignancies, infection

6. **What is cardiac allograft vasculopathy (CAV)? Describe its pathophysiology, incidence, risk factors, and outcome.**

Also known as transplant vasculopathy or transplant coronary artery disease (CAD), CAV is the progressive narrowing of the coronary arteries of the transplanted heart. Angiographic incidence of CAV is approximately 30% at 5 years and 50% at 10 years. CAV is associated with a significantly increased risk of death. After the first post-transplant year, CAV is the second most common cause of death (after malignancy).

In CAV, diffuse, concentric proliferation of the intimal smooth muscle cells typically involves the entire length of the coronary artery, whereas conventional atherosclerosis results from fibrofatty plaque producing concentric or eccentric focal lesions.

The cause of CAV remains unclear, but both immunologic (cellular/humoral rejection, histocompatibility leukocyte antigen [HLA mismatch]) and nonimmunologic (CMV infection, hypercholesterolemia, older age/male donors, younger recipients, history of CAD, DM and insulin resistance) factors have been implicated.

Note that cardiac transplant recipients can also develop conventional atherosclerosis through two main mechanisms:
- *Progression* of preexisting donor CAD
- *De novo* development as a result of transplant-related HTN, DM, and dyslipidemia

7. **How do patients with transplant vasculopathy clinically present? What invasive and noninvasive tests are used to assist in the diagnosis of transplant vasculopathy?**

Because transplanted hearts are denervated, cardiac transplant recipients typically do not present with angina when they develop transplant vasculopathy. Clinical manifestations include silent myocardial infarctions, symptoms of heart failure, syncope, sudden cardiac death, and arrhythmias.
- **Coronary angiography:** Most centers have adopted surveillance angiographies for early diagnosis of CAV. However, CAV is often diffuse and concentric in its distribution and may be underestimated by angiography. To improve detection and sensitivity, intravascular ultrasound and quantitative coronary angiography are used as adjunctive modalities.
- **Noninvasive stress testing:** Dobutamine stress echo or myocardial perfusion imaging can be used to diagnose CAV but have a lower sensitivity when compared with angiography. To avoid contrast-induced nephropathy, noninvasive stress testing is used in patients with renal insufficiency.

8. **List infections that are encountered early and late after cardiac transplantation.**
- **Early (less than 1 month):** The most common early infections include donor transmitted pathogens, nosocomial infections related to surgery or invasive procedures (mediastinitis, wound/line/urinary tract infections, ventilator associated pneumonia), and early virus reactivation (typically herpes simplex virus, human herpesvirus-6).
- **Intermediate (1-6 months):** With continued immunosuppressive use, patients are predisposed to opportunistic infections, including bacterial (mycobacteria, *Listeria, Nocardia*), viral (cytomegalovirus [CMV], Epstein Barr virus [EBV], varicella zoster immunoglobulin [VZV], adenovirus, papovavirus), fungal (*Aspergillus,* pneumocystitis, *Cryptococcus*), and protozoal (strongyloides, toxoplasma). Suspect tuberculosis (TB) if the patient has prior exposure to *Mycobacterium tuberculosis* and a history of positive PPD.
- **Late (more than 6 months):** Most patients have stable graft function by this time; therefore, the immunosuppressive regimen is reduced and the risk for opportunisitic

infection decreases. Typically encountered infections include common viral and bacterial respiratory pathogens; however, some patients may develop chronic or recurrent opportunistic infections (e.g., CMV-related superinfection, EBV-associated lymphoproliferative disease).

9. **What type of malignancies are encountered after transplant? List incidence, time course, and prognosis.**
   - Malignancy risk in cardiac transplant recipients approaches 1% to 4% per year and is 10 to 100 times higher when compared with age-matched controls. Malignancy is the major cause of late death in heart transplant recipients and is thought to be a result of chronic immunosuppression.
   - The most common malignancy encountered is skin cancer. Squamous cell carcinoma is more prevalent in transplant patients compared with basal cell cancer, which is more prevalent in the general population.
   - The second most common malignancy found in cardiac transplant recipients is post-transplant lymphoproliferative disorder (PTLD). PTLD can be associated with primary or reactivated EBV infection, which leads to abnormal proliferation of lymphoid cells and can involve gastrointestinal, pulmonary, and central nervous systems; PTLD usually presents as non-Hodgkin's lymphoma (predominately B-cell type). Risk of PTLD varies with allograft type, immunosuppression, EBV immunity before transplant, and previous CMV infection.

10. **Describe potential arrhythmias encountered after transplantation.**
    The donor heart is disconnected from sympathetic and parasympathetic innervation; therefore, the resting heart rate is higher than normal (90–110 beats/min) and atropine has no effect on the denervated heart. Early post-transplant arrhythmia can be a result of surgical trauma to the sinoatrial (SA) or atrioventricular (AV) nodes, prolonged ischemic time, surgical suture lines, and rejection. Late-occurring arrhythmias may suggest rejection or the presence of post-transplant vasculopathy.
    - **Sinus node dysfunction** occurs in up to 50% of cardiac transplant recipients. Treatment of sinus bradycardia includes temporary pacing and intravenous (isoproterenol or dobutamine) or oral (theophylline or terbutaline) therapy in the immediate postoperative period; however, severe persistent bradycardia may require permanent pacemaker placement (up to 15% patients). Sinus node dysfunction early after transplant does not appear to affect mortality but has been associated with increased morbidity.
    - **AV nodal block** is rarely encountered; its occurrence may indicate the presence of transplant vasculopathy and has been associated with increased mortality.
    - **Atrial arrhythmias:** Transient atrial arrhythmias, especially *premature atrial contractions* (PACs) are common in the early postoperative period; their clinical significance remains unclear, but frequent occurrences should prompt evaluation for rejection. *Atrial fibrillation* or *flutter* can occur in up to 25% of cardiac transplant recipients; late occurrence warrants evaluation for rejection. Treatment includes rate control with beta-blockers, calcium channel blockers, cardioversion, overdrive pacing, and treatment for rejection. Atrial flutter can be treated with radiofrequency ablation.
    - **Ventricular arrhythmias:** *Premature ventricular contractions* (PVCs) are not uncommon early after cardiac transplantation, and their clinical significance is unknown. However, nonsustained ventricular tachycardia (more than three consecutive PVCs) has been associated with rejection and transplant vasculopathy. *Sustained ventricular tachycardia* and *ventricular fibrillation* are associated with poor prognosis and indicate severe transplant vasculopathy or high-grade rejection. Treatment includes correcting electrolyte abnormalities, intravenous amiodarone or lidocaine, defibrillation, and prompt evaluation for rejection and transplant vasculopathy.

11. **Describe typical maintenance immunosuppression therapy.**
    The goal of maintenance immunosuppression is to suppress the recipient immune system from rejecting the transplanted heart while balancing sufficient immunosuppression with potential risk for infection/malignancy. This *triple therapy* regimen consists of the following:
    - **Calcineurin inhibitors:** cyclosporine or tacrolimus
    - **Antimetabolites** or **cell cycle modulators:** mycophenolate mofetil (MMF) or azathioprine
    - **Corticosteroids**

12. **What are common medical conditions encountered in post-transplant patients?**
    - **Hypertension** (attributed to sympathetic stimulation, neurohormonal activation, renal vasoconstriction by calcineurin inhibitors, and mineralocorticoid effect of steroids)
    - **Renal impairment** (pretransplant low cardiac output, ischemic injury during transplantation, and calcineurin-related renal arteriolar vasoconstriction and tubulointerstitial fibrosis)
    - **Dyslipidemia** (weight gain, corticosteroid and cyclosporine use)
    - **Diabetes** (corticosteroid use)
    - **Osteoporosis** (corticosteroid use)
    - **Gout** (hyperuricemia from decreased uric acid clearance with cyclosporine use)

    Calcineurin inhibitor use can also result in *rhabdomyolysis* when used concurrently with HMG-CoA reductase inhibitors (statins), because calcineurin inhibitors can inhibit metabolism of certain statins (lovastatin, simvastatin, cerivastatin, and atorvastatin). Fluvastatin, pravastatin, and rosuvastatin are less likely to be involved in this type of interaction.

13. **What are the clinical signs and symptoms associated with acute cardiac transplant rejection (allograft rejection)?**
    Approximately 40% to 70% of cardiac transplant recipients experience rejection within the first year after transplant.

    The majority of patients are asymptomatic early in the course of rejection; therefore, routine biopsies are necessary to assist in the diagnosis of rejection. Acute allograft rejection is the leading cause of death in the first year after transplant; this emphasizes the importance of early diagnosis and treatment.

    The clinical presentation of rejection can be variable. Patients may have nonspecific constitutional symptoms such as fever, malaise, fatigue, myalgias, and joint pain and flulike symptoms. Signs and symptoms of left ventricular (LV) and right ventricular (RV) dysfunction include severe fatigue, loss of energy, listlessness, weight gain, sudden onset of dyspnea, syncope/presyncope, orthopnea/paroxysmal nocturnal dyspnea, and abdominal bloating/nausea/vomiting. Physical examination can reveal elevated jugular venous pulse, peripheral edema, hepatomegaly, S3 or S4 gallop, and lower than usual blood pressure. Signs of cardiac irritation may include sinus tachycardia, bradycardia, arrhythmias, pericardial friction rub, or new pericardial effusion by echo.

    Echocardiographic findings can suggest rejection, although endomyocardial biopsy (EMB) remains the gold standard for the diagnosis of allograft rejection. However, rejection is a clinically diagnosed event, and even if biopsies do not support rejection, treatment can still be initiated on the basis of symptoms.

    Treatment depends on the type of rejection but for acute cellular rejection may include high-dose corticosteroids and antilymphocyte antibodies (ATG or OKT3) and for acute humoral rejection may include plasmapheresis, intravenous immunoglobulins, rituximab, antilymphocyte antibodies (ATG or OKT3), intravenous heparin, TOR inhibitors, cyclophosphamide, or photopheresis.

BIBLIOGRAPHY, SUGGESTED READINGS, AND WEBSITES

1. Collaborative Transplant Study: http://www.ctstransplant.org

2. International Society for Heart and Lung Transplantation: http://www.ishlt.org

3. The *Journal of Heart and Lung Transplantation*: http://www.jhltonline.org

4. United Network for Organ Sharing: http://www.unos.org

5. Department of Health and Human Services, *2007 U.S. Organ Procurement and Transplantation Network (OPTN) and the Scientific Registry of Transplant Recipients (SRTR) annual report: transplant data 1997-2006.* http://www.ustransplant.org/annual_reports/current/

6. Eisen HJ: Immunosuppression on the horizon, *Heart Fail Clin* 3(1):43-49, 2007.

7. Jessup M, Banner N, Brozena S, et al: Optimal pharmacologic and non-pharmacologic management of cardiac transplant candidates: approaches to be considered prior to transplant evaluation: International Society for Heart and Lung Transplantation guidelines for the care of cardiac transplant candidates—2006, *J Heart Lung Transplant* 25(9):1003-1023, 2006.

8. Kirklin J, Young J, McGiffin D, et al: *Heart transplantation*, Philadelphia, 2002, Churchill Livingstone.

9. Kobashigawa JA: Contemporary concepts in noncellular rejection, *Heart Fail Clin* 3(1):11-15, 2007.

10. Sipahi I, Starling RC: Cardiac allograft vasculopathy: an update, *Heart Fail Clin* 3(1):87-95, 2007.

11. Steinman TI, Becker BN, Frost AE, et al: Guidelines for the referral and management of patients eligible for solid organ transplantation, *Transplantation* 71(9):1189-1204, 2001.

12. Stewart S, Winters GL, Fishbein MC, et al: Revision of the 1990 working formulation for the standardization of nomenclature in the diagnosis of heart rejection, *J Heart Lung Transplant* 24(11):1710-1720, 2005.

13. Taylor DO, Edwards LB, Boucek MM, et al: Registry of the International Society of Heart and Lung Transplantation: twenty-fourth official adult heart transplant report—2007, *J Heart Lung Transplant* 26:769, 2007.

V. VALVULAR HEART DISEASE AND ENDOCARDITIS

CHAPTER 32

AORTIC VALVE DISEASE

Blase A. Carabello, MD, FACC

1. **What is the most common cause of aortic stenosis in developed countries today, and what is the current thinking about its pathogenesis?**
   Although rheumatic fever was once the most common cause of aortic stenosis (AS), today calcific disease of either bicuspid or tricuspid AS is the leading cause. Once considered a degenerative disease, it is now clear that calcific AS is an inflammatory process with many similarities to atherosclerosis. A normal aortic valve, and aortic stenosis as a result of congenital bicuspid aortic valve, rheumatic aortic stenosis, and calcific aortic stenosis, are shown in Fig. 32-1.

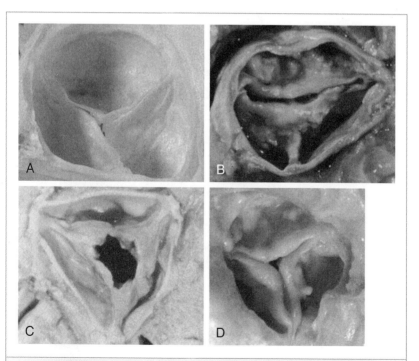

Figure 32-1. Normal and stenotic aortic valves. **A,** Normal aortic valve. **B,** Congenital bicuspid aortic stenosis. A false raphe is present at 6 o'clock. **C,** Rheumatic aortic stenosis. The commissures are fused with a fixed central orifice. **D,** Calcific degenerative aortic stenosis. (From Libby P, Bonow RO, Mann DL, et al: *Braunwald's heart disease: a textbook of cardiovascular medicine,* ed 8, Philadelphia, 2008, Saunders.)

2. **What is the pathophysiology of AS, and what effect does it have on the left ventricle?**
AS exerts a pressure overload on the left ventricle (LV). Normally, pressure in the LV and aorta are similar during systole, as the normal aortic valve permits free flow of blood from LV to aorta. However, in aortic stenosis the stenotic valve forces the LV to generate higher pressure to drive blood through the stenosis, causing a pressure difference (gradient) from LV to aorta. The LV compensates for this pressure overload by increasing its mass (left ventricular hypertrophy [LVH]). The ways in which the transvalvular gradient are measured and quantified are shown in Fig. 32-2.

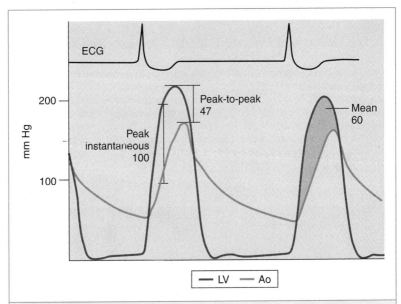

Figure 32-2. Various methods of describing an aortic transvalvular gradient. The figure shows representative pressure tracings measured during cardiac catheterization in a patient with aortic stenosis. One pressure transducer is placed in the left ventricle and a second pressure transducer is positioned in the ascending aorta. The peak-to-peak gradient (47 mm Hg) is the difference between the maximal pressure in the aorta (Ao) and the maximal left ventricle (LV) pressure. The peak instantaneous gradient (100 mm Hg) is the maximal pressure difference between the Ao and LV when the pressures are measured in the same moment (usually during early systole). The mean gradient *(shaded area)* is the integral of the pressure difference between the LV and Ao during systole (60 mm Hg). *ECG,* Electrocardiogram. (From Bashore TM: *Invasive cardiology: principles and techniques,* Philadelphia, 1990, BC Decker, p. 258.)

3. **How is left ventricular hypertrophy compensatory?**
The Law of Laplace states that systolic wall stress is equal to:

$$(\text{pressure}(p) \times \text{radius}(r))/2 \times \text{thickness}(h), \text{ or } \sigma = p \times r/2h$$

As the pressure term in the numerator increases, it is offset by an increase in thickness in the denominator, thus normalizing afterload. Because afterload is a key determinant of ejection, LVH helps to maintain ejection fraction and cardiac output.

4. **Are there downsides to LVH?**
Yes. Although LVH is initially compensatory, as it progresses it takes on pathologic characteristics, leading to morbidity and mortality.

5. **What are the classic symptoms of AS, and why are they important?**
The classic symptoms of AS are angina and syncope and those of heart failure (dyspnea, orthopnea, paroxysmal nocturnal dyspnea, edema, etc.) Their importance is graphically

displayed in Figure 32-3. In the absence of symptoms, survival is nearly the same as in an unaffected population. However, at the onset of symptoms there is a dramatic demarcation such that mortality increases to 2% per month, so that three quarters of all AS patients are dead within 3 years of symptom onset unless proper therapy is instituted.

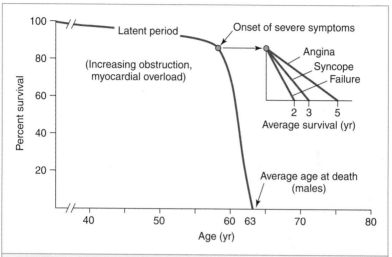

Figure 32-3. The natural history of medically treated aortic stenosis. Once symptoms develop in a patient with aortic stenosis, the average survival with "medical" treatment (e.g., no curative surgery) is only 2 to 5 years. (From Townsend C, Evers BM, Beauchamp RD, et al: *Sabiston textbook of surgery*, ed 18, Philadelphia, 2008, Saunders.)

6. **What are findings of AS on physical examination?**
   AS is usually recognized by the presence of a harsh systolic ejection murmur that radiates to the neck. In mild disease the murmur peaks in intensity early in systole, peaking progressively later as severity of disease increases. The carotid upstrokes become delayed in timing and reduced in volume because the stenotic valve steals energy from the flow of blood as it passes the valve. The apical beat is forceful. Palpation of this strong apical beat with one examining hand while the other hand palpates the weakened delayed carotid upstroke is dynamic proof of the obstruction that exists between the LV and the systemic circulation. Because the severely stenotic aortic valve barely opens, there is little valve movement upon closing. Thus, the A2 component of S2 is lost, rendering a soft single second sound. An S4 is usually present in patients in sinus rhythm, reflecting impaired filling of the thickened, noncompliant LV.

7. **How is echocardiography used to assess the patient with AS?**
   Currently, echocardiography is the central tool in diagnosing the presence and severity of AS. In severe AS the aortic valve is calcified and has limited mobility. The amount of LVH and the presence or absence of LV dysfunction can be established. Because

$$flow = area \times velocity$$

as the valve area decreases, velocity of flow must increase for flow to remain constant (Fig. 32-4). This increase in blood velocity at the valve orifice is detected by Doppler ultrasound. The severity of AS is assessed using the factors given in Table 32-1. In general, if a patient has the symptoms of AS and assessment indicates severe disease, then the symptoms are attributed to AS. However, it must be emphasized that the benchmarks listed here are only guidelines to severity and some patients are exceptions to them.

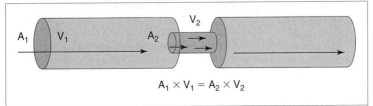

Figure 32-4. Determination of aortic valve area using the continuity equation. For blood flow $(A_1 \times V_1)$ to remain constant when it reaches a stenosis (A_2), velocity must increase to V_2. Determination of the increased velocity V_2 by Doppler ultrasound permits calculation of both the aortic valve gradient and solution of the equation for A_2. *A*, Area; *V*, velocity. (From Townsend C, Evers BM, Beauchamp RD, et al: *Sabiston textbook of surgery*, ed 18, Philadelphia, 2008, Saunders.)

TABLE 32-1. ECHOCARDIOGRAPHIC CRITERIA FOR THE DEGREE OF AORTIC STENOSIS

	Mild	Moderate	Severe
Peak jet velocity (msec)	<3.0	3.0–4.0	>4.0
Mean gradient (mm Hg)	<25	25–40	>40
Aortic valve area (cm^2)	>1.5	1.0–1.5	<1.0
Valve area index (cm^2/m^2)			<0.6
Outflow track velocity-to-aortic valve velocity			<0.25

Modified from Bonow RO, Carabello BA, Chatterjee K, et al: ACC/AHA 2006 guidelines for the management of patients with valvular heart disease, *J Amer Coll Cardiol* 48:e1-e148, 2006.

8. **What other tests are useful in assessing AS?**
   As noted earlier, the presence or absence of symptoms is a key determinant of outcome, yet in some patients an accurate history may be difficult to obtain. In such cases more objective evidence of cardiac compromise, such as exercise intolerance, may be helpful. Although exercise stress testing should *never* be performed in symptomatic AS patients, stress testing may be very helpful in establishing more objective evidence of symptomatic status when the history is unclear. As many as one third of AS patients may become symptomatic for the first time during stress testing. This phenomenon probably indicates a previous denial of symptoms or a lifestyle altered to avoid symptoms. Such stress testing, if undertaken, should only be done with careful physician supervision.
   Natriuretic peptides may also be useful in assessing the effects of AS on the heart. Brain natriuretic peptide (BNP) is released from the myocardium when sarcomere stretch increases to provide preload reserve. As such, increasing BNP indicates cardiac decompensation. Increasing BNP in AS patients is considered an ominous finding, although there is no agreement about what BNP level indicates the need for aortic valve replacement (AVR).

9. **What is the therapy for AS?**
   Because AS has many similarities to atherosclerosis, many have hypothesized that effective treatments for coronary disease might be able to retard the progression of AS. Although observational studies of the use of statins in AS have suggested those drugs might be effective, prospective trials have been as yet inconclusive.

No effective medical therapy is effective in the chronic treatment of this disease. The mainstay of therapy for this mechanical problem is mechanical relief of the obstruction in the form of aortic valve replacement. Currently this is performed during open heart surgery. However, percutaneous delivery of substitute aortic valves is currently in the developmental stage in the United States and is commercially available in Europe. This nonsurgical approach is likely to have an important role in AS treatment in the near future.

10. **What are the class I indications for aortic valve replacement?**
According to the American College of Cardiology/American Heart Association (ACC/AHA) guidelines, AVR is indicated in the following situations:
- Symptomatic patients with severe AS
- Severe AS with left ventricular systolic dysfunction (LV ejection fraction [LVEF] less than 50%)
- Severe AS in patients undergoing coronary artery bypass grafting, other heart valve surgery, or thoracic aortic surgery (if AS is instead moderate, then AVR in these situations is considered a class IIa indication, *reasonable*)

11. **What is the outcome after AVR?**
Survival of patients after AVR is dramatically improved compared with those who received medical therapy.

12. **What are the causes of aortic regurgitation?**
Abnormalities of either the aortic root or of the aortic valve leaflets can cause aortic regurgitation (AR). Common root abnormalities that cause AR include Marfan syndrome, annuloaortic ectasia, and aortic dissection. Leaflet causes include infective endocarditis, rheumatic heart disease, collagen vascular diseases, and previous use of anorectic drugs.

13. **What is the pathophysiology of aortic regurgitation?**
The incompetent aortic valve allows ejected blood to return to the LV during diastole. This regurgitant volume is lost from the effective cardiac output. In turn, the LV must pump extra blood to make up for this loss; thus, AR constitutes an LV volume overload. Compensation comes from an increase in LV volume (eccentric hypertrophy). The larger LV can pump more blood to compensate for that lost to AR. Because all the stroke volume is pumped into the aorta during systole (while some leaks back into the LV during diastole), pulse pressure, which is dependent on stoke volume, widens as systolic pressure increases and diastolic pressure decreases. Thus, AR imparts not only a volume overload on the LV but also a pressure overload. Because of this second load, LV thickness in AR patients is slightly greater than normal. Increased wall thickness and the increased diastolic LV volume lead to increased LV diastolic filling pressure.

14. **What are the symptoms of aortic regurgitation?**
Dyspnea and fatigue are the main symptoms of AR. Occasionally patients experience angina because reduced diastolic aortic pressure reduces coronary filling pressure, impairing coronary blood flow. Reduced diastolic systemic pressure may also cause syncope or presyncope.

15. **What are the findings of AR on physical examination?**
Chronic AR produces myriad physical findings because of the large stroke volume pumped by the LV. The pulse pressure is wide. The dynamic LV apical beat is displaced downward and to the left and is often visible several feet away from the patient. A diastolic blowing murmur is present and is heard best along the left sternal border with the patient sitting upward and leaning forward. A second murmur (Austin Flint) thought to be due to vibration of the mitral valve caused by the impinging AR is a low-pitched diastolic rumble heard toward the LV apex.
The widened pulse pressure and high total stroke volume cause several physical signs of AR:
- The head may bob with each heartbeat (de Musset's sign).
- Auscultation of the femoral artery may produce a sound similar to a pistol shot (pistol shot pulse).

- If the bell of the stethoscope is compressed over the femoral artery, a to-and-fro bruit (Duroziez sign) may be heard.
- Compression of the nailbed may demonstrate systolic plethora and diastolic blanching of the nail bed (Quincke's pulse).

16. **How is the diagnosis of AR confirmed?**
    Although a chest radiograph is helpful in evaluating heart size and pulmonary congestion, echocardiography remains the mainstay of diagnosis. Cardiac size and function are evaluated using this technique. Often the anatomic abnormality responsible for the patient's AR can be established. As shown in Figure 32-5, Doppler interrogation of the valve reveals the jet of blood leaking across the valve in diastole. Table 32-2 displays current criteria for establishing the severity of AR.

17. **How is AR managed?**
    Patients with severe AR should been seen at least once a year or more often to evaluate symptomatic status and to perform repeat echocardiograms to assess LV size and function.
    AVR is indicated (ACC/AHA and European Society of Cardiology [ESC] class I recommendations) for the following patients:

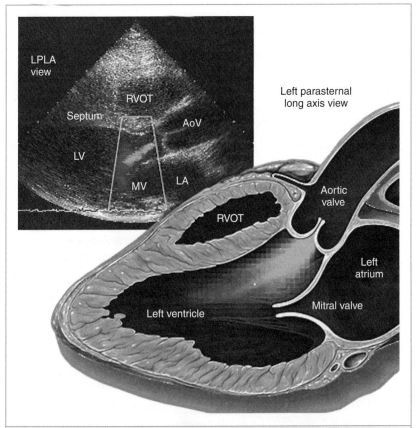

Figure 32-5. Aortic regurgitation. Left parasternal long-axis view of the heart, demonstrating aortic regurgitation seen on Doppler echocardiogram, along with the corresponding anatomic illustration. In actuality, the regurgitant jet is displayed in color, reflecting the direction of blood flow. (From Yale Atlas of Echocardiography. http://www.med.yale.edu/intmed/cardio/echo_atlas/entities/aortic_regurgitation.html. Accessed August 30, 2008.)

TABLE 32-2. CARDIAC CATHETERIZATION AND ECHOCARDIOGRAPHIC CRITERIA FOR THE DEGREE OF AORTIC REGURGITATION

	Mild	Moderate	Severe
Angiographic grade	1+	2+	3–4+
Color Doppler central jet width	<25% LVOT		>65% LVOT
Doppler vena contracta width	<0.3 cm	0.3–0.6 cm	>0.6 cm
Regurgitant volume (ml/beat)	30 ml	30–59 ml	$\geq$60 ml
Regurgitant fraction	<30%	30–49%	$\geq$50%
Regurgitant orifice area	<0.10 cm^2	0.10–0.29 cm^2	$\geq$0.30 cm^2
LV size			Increased
Pressure ½ time			<250 msec

LVOT, Left ventricular outflow tract.

Modified from Bonow RO, Carabello BA, Chatterjee K, et al: ACC/AHA 2006 guidelines for the management of patients with valvular heart disease, *J Amer Coll Cardiol* 48:e1-e148, 2006.

- Symptomatic patients with severe AR, irrespective of LV systolic function
- Asymptomatic patients with chronic severe and LV systolic dysfunction (LVEF 50% or less)
- Patients with chronic severe AR who are undergoing coronary artery bypass grafting (CABG), other heart valve surgery, or thoracic aortic surgery

AVR is considered reasonable (ACC/AHA and ESC class IIa recommendation) for asymptomatic patients with severe AR with normal LV systolic function (LVEF more than 50%) but with severe LV dilation (end-diastolic dimension greater than 70–75 mm or end-systolic dimension greater than 50–55 mm).

As with AS, there is no proven medical therapy for AR, although vasodilator therapy can be considered in patients with severe AR who are not surgical candidates.

18. **Is the presentation of acute AR different from that of chronic AR?**
    Yes, dramatically. In chronic AR there has been no time for LV dilation so that the increased forward stroke volume and widened pulse pressure that drive the dynamic examination of a patient with chronic AR are absent. Thus the examination of a patient with severe acute AR may be misleadingly bland, belying a potentially fatal condition. Acute AR occurs most commonly in the patient with infective endocarditis. When such patients develop evidence of heart failure, AR should be suspected even if there is only a faint murmur or no murmur at all.

BIBLIOGRAPHY, SUGGESTED READINGS, AND WEBSITES

1. Gaasch WH: Course and Management of Chronic Aortic Regurgitation in Adults: http://www.utdol.com
2. Hilkert RJ: Aortic Regurgitation: http://www.emedicine.com
3. Otto CM: Pathophysiology and Clinical Features of Valvular Aortic Stenosis in Adults: http://www.utdol.com
4. Talano JV: Aortic Stenosis: http://www.emedicine.com
5. Bekeredjian R, Grayburn PA: Valvular heart disease: aortic regurgitation, *Circulation* 112(1):125-134, 2005.
6. Bonow RO, Carabello BA, Chatterjee K, et al: ACC/AHA 2006 guidelines for the management of patients with valvular heart disease, *J Am Coll Cardiol* 48:e1-e148, 2006.

7. Carabello BA: Clinical practice. Aortic stenosis, *N Engl J Med* 346(9):677-682, 2002.
8. Carabello BA: Evaluation and management of patients with aortic stenosis, *Circulation* 105(15):1746-1750, 2002.
9. Enriquez-Sarano M, Tajik AJ: Clinical practice. Aortic regurgitation, *N Engl J Med* 351(15):1539-1546, 2004.
10. Vahanian A, Baumgartner H, Bax J, et al: Guidelines on the management of valvular heart disease: the Task Force on the Management of Valvular Heart Disease of the European Society of Cardiology, *Eur Heart J* 28(2):230-268, 2007.

CHAPTER 33

MITRAL STENOSIS, MITRAL REGURGITATION, AND MITRAL VALVE PROLAPSE

Blase A. Carabello, MD, FACC

1. **What is the usual cause of mitral stenosis?**
   Almost all cases of mitral stenosis (MS) stem from previous episodes of rheumatic fever. Most cases of rheumatic heart disease are seen in patients who emigrate from areas of the world where rheumatic fever is still common, including the Middle East, Asia, and South Africa. Although the rate of rheumatic fever is similar in men and women, MS is three times more common in women than in men.

2. **What is the pathophysiology of MS?**
   MS inhibits the normal free flow of blood from left atrium (LA) to left ventricle (LV) in diastole. Normally, diastolic left atrial and left ventricular pressures equalize shortly after mitral valve opening. In mitral stenosis, the stenotic valve impedes left atrial emptying, inducing a diastolic gradient between LA and LV (Fig. 33-1). Elevated LA pressure is referred to the lungs, where it causes pulmonary congestion. Simultaneously, impaired LA emptying reduces LV filling, limiting cardiac output. Thus, the combination of increased LA pressure and decreased cardiac output produce the syndrome of heart failure. Because increased LA pressure increases pulmonary pressure, the right ventricle becomes pressure overloaded, eventually leading to right ventricular (RV) failure.

3. **What are the typical symptoms of MS?**
   Patients with mild disease are likely to be asymptomatic. As MS worsens, dyspnea appears, as does orthopnea and paroxysmal nocturnal dyspnea. If RV failure ensues, it may be accompanied by edema and ascites. During exercise, sudden increases in LA pressure and pulmonary venous pressure may cause rupture of anastamoses between pulmonary and systemic veins, leading to hemoptysis.

4. **What are the signs of MS at physical examination?**
   The gradient across the mitral valve holds the valve open throughout diastole, so that when it closes, S1 may be quite loud. The murmur of MS is a soft diastolic rumble heard near the apex. The murmur is often preceded by an opening snap, caused by sudden opening of the stiffened mitral valve from higher than normal atrial pressure. If pulmonary hypertension has developed, P2 is increased in intensity. If RV failure has occurred, elevated neck veins, ascites, and edema are likely to be present.

5. **How is the diagnosis made?**
   The chest radiograph used to be at the forefront of diagnosis and still can be helpful today. It demonstrates an enlarged left atrium, seen as a double shadow along the right-sided heart border. Thickened lymphatics from high pulmonary venous pressure are seen as Kerley's lines. The pulmonary artery is usually enlarged.
   Today, however, the echocardiogram is key to the diagnosis because it images the mitral valve so well. The valve is thickened and takes on a *hockey stick* appearance (Fig. 33-2). The left

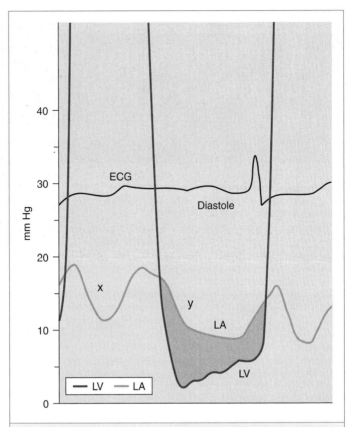

Figure 33-1. Pressure gradient in a patient with mitral stenosis. The pressure in the left atrium (LA) exceeds the pressure in the left ventricle (LV) during diastole, producing a diastolic pressure gradient *(shaded area).* (Modified from Bashore TM: *Invasive cardiology: principles and techniques,* Philadelphia, 1990, BC Decker, p. 264.)

atrium is almost always enlarged. Valve area can be determined from direct visualization and planimetry of the mitral orifice, from Doppler assessment of the transvalvular gradient, and from measuring the delay in LA emptying. Pulmonary pressure, left ventricular function, and right ventricular function are also evaluated. In general, the main criteria for severe mitral stenosis are as follows:

- Mean gradient more than 10 mm Hg
- Valve area less than 1.0 cm^2
- Pulmonary arterial (PA) systolic pressure greater than 50 mm Hg

The severity of MS is estimated using the criteria given in Table 33-1.

6. **Is there effective medical management for MS?**
   Yes. Patients with mild symptoms and normal pulmonary artery pressure can be treated with diuretics to lower left atrial pressure and relieve pulmonary congestion. The combination of LA enlargement and continued inflammation from a smoldering rheumatic process predisposes patients with MS to develop atrial fibrillation (AF). AF with rapid heart rate affects the MS patient gravely because it diminishes transit time for blood flow from LA to LV, further increasing LA pressure and diminishing cardiac output. Rate control with beta-blockers, calcium

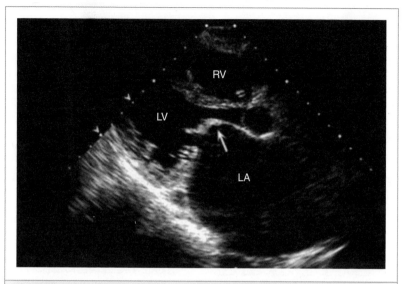

Figure 33-2. Two-dimensional echocardiogram of the parasternal long-axis view during diastole of a patient with mitral stenosis. The mitral valve leaflets are thickened and have the typical *hockey-stick* appearance *(arrow)*. Note also that the left atrium (LA) is enlarged. *LV,* Left ventricle; *RV,* right ventricle. (Modified from Libby P, Bonow RO, Mann DL, et al: *Braunwald's heart disease: a textbook of cardiovascular medicine,* ed 8, Philadelphia, 2008, Saunders.)

TABLE 33-1. ECHOCARDIOGRAPHIC CRITERIA FOR THE ASSESSMENT OF THE SEVERITY OF MITRAL STENOSIS

	Mild	Moderate	Severe
Mean gradient	<5 mm Hg	5–10 mm Hg	>10 mm Hg
PA systolic	<30 mm Hg	30–50 mm Hg	>50 mm Hg
Valve area	>1.5 cm^2	1.0–1.5 cm^2	<1.0 cm^2

Modified from Bonow RO, Carabello BA, Chatterjee K, et al: ACC/AHA 2006 guidelines for the management of patients with valvular heart disease. *J Amer Coll Cardiol* 48:e1-e148, 2006.

channel blockers, or digoxin is imperative. If these agents fail to control heart, cardioversion is indicated. Once AF has developed in the MS patient, the risk of stroke approaches 10% per year. Thus, anticoagulation to an international normalized ratio (INR) of 2.5 to 3.5 is mandatory unless a grave contraindication exists.

7. **What is the definitive management for severe MS?**
   If symptoms cannot be controlled easily medically or if asymptomatic pulmonary hypertension develops, this mechanical lesion must be treated by mechanical relief of the stenosis, because both conditions worsen MS prognosis. In most cases, mitral balloon valvotomy is the preferred therapy. In this procedure, a balloon is passed percutaneously from the femoral vein across the atrial septum (by needle puncture) through the mitral valve, where it is inflated

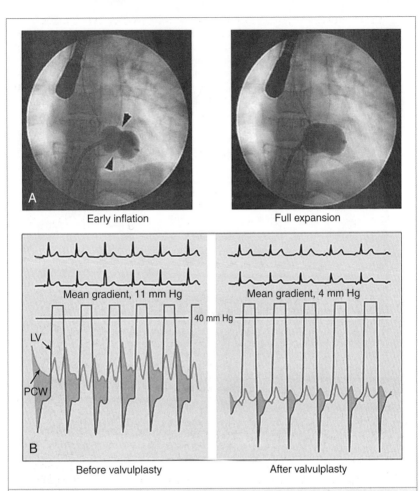

Figure 33-3. Percutaneous balloon mitral valvotomy (BMV) for mitral stenosis using the Inoue technique. **A,** The catheter is advanced into the left atrium via the transseptal technique and guided antegrade across the mitral orifice. As the balloon is inflated, its distal portion expands first and is pulled back so that it fits snugly against the orifice. With further inflation, the proximal portion of the balloon expands to center the balloon within the stenotic orifice *(left)*. Further inflation expands the central *waist* portion of the balloon *(right)*, resulting in commissural splitting and enlargement of the orifice. **B,** Successful BMV results in significant increase in mitral valve area, as reflected by reduction in the diastolic pressure gradient between left ventricle (LV) and pulmonary capillary wedge (PCW) pressure, as indicated by the *shaded area*. (From Delabays A, Goy JJ: Images in clinical medicine: Percutaneous mitral valvuloplasty, *N Engl J Med* 345:e4, 2001.)

(Fig. 33-3). Balloon inflation ruptures the adhesions at the commissures caused by the rheumatic process, allowing as much as doubling of the mitral valve area and normalizing cardiac output, left atrial pressure, and pulmonary artery pressure, in turn relieving symptoms.

Criteria have been established to determine whether balloon valvotomy should be performed or the patient referred for surgery. These four criteria are valve mobility, subvalvular thickening, leaflet thickening, and degree of valvular calcification. In addition to these characteristics, the degree of mitral regurgitation is assessed, because balloon valvotomy can worsen the degree of mitral regurgitation.

Class I indications for percutaneous mitral balloon valvotomy include the following:

- Symptomatic (New York Heart Association [NYHA] class II–IV) patients with moderate-severe MS with favorable valve characteristics, in the absence of left atrial thrombus or moderate to severe mitral regurgitation (MR) (class I; level of evidence A)
- Asymptomatic patients with moderate-severe MS and pulmonary hypertension (PA systolic pressure greater than 50 mm Hg at rest or more than 60 mm Hg with exercise) and valve morphology favorable for balloon valvotomy, in the absence of left atrial thrombus or moderate to severe MR (class I; level of evidence C)

8. **What are the causes of mitral regurgitation (MR)?**
   There are two broad categories of MR, primary and secondary. In primary MR, disease of the mitral valve causes it to leak, imparting a volume overload on the LV. In secondary MR, disease of the LV causes wall motion abnormalities, ventricular dilation, and annular dilation, rendering the mitral valve incompetent. The most common causes of primary MR include myxomatous degeneration and mitral valve prolapse, infective endocarditis, rheumatic heart disease, and collagen vascular disease. Causes of secondary MR include coronary artery disease and subsequent myocardial infarction and dilated cardiomyopathy.

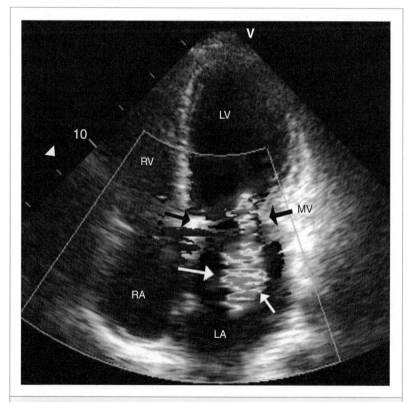

Figure 33-4. Mitral regurgitation. Apical four-chamber view with color Doppler revealing severe mitral regurgitation *(white arrows)*. *Black arrows* point to the mitral valve. Note that in actuality, the regurgitant jet is displayed in color, corresponding to the flow of blood. *MV,* Mitral valve; *LA,* left atrium; *LV,* left ventricle; *RA,* right atrium; *RV,* right ventricle. (Courtesy Hisham Dokainish.)

9. **How does primary MR affect the left ventricle?**
   MR imparts a volume overload on the left ventricle (LV) because the LV must pump additional volume to compensate for that lost to regurgitation. In some way, MR causes sarcomeres to lengthen, increasing end-diastolic volume, enabling the LV to increase its total stroke volume.

10. **What are the other effects of primary MR on the heart and lungs?**
    MR also causes volume overload on the LA, increasing LA pressure. Increased LA pressure leads to pulmonary congestion and the symptoms of dyspnea, orthopnea, and paroxysmal nocturnal dyspnea. Eventually MR may also lead to pulmonary hypertension, right ventricular pressure overload, and right ventricular failure. LA enlargement also predisposes the patient to atrial fibrillation.

11. **What are the clues to MR on physical examination?**
    The typical murmur of MR is holosystolic, radiating to the axilla. It may be accompanied by a systolic apical thrill; the apical beat is displaced downward and to the left, indicating LV enlargement. In severe MR, an S3 is usually heard. Here the S3 may not indicate heart failure but rather is caused by the increased LA volume emptying into the LV at higher than normal pressure.

12. **How is the diagnosis of MR confirmed?**
    Although both the chest radiograph and the electrocardiogram (ECG) may indicate LV enlargement, as with other valvular heart diseases, echocardiography is the diagnostic modality of choice. It demonstrates LA and LV size and volume, allows assessment of LV function and pulmonary artery pressure, and can reliably quantify the amount of MR present.
    Echocardiographic findings suggestive of severe mitral regurgitation include enlarged left atrium or left ventricle, the color Doppler mitral regurgitation jet occupying a large proportion (more than 40%) of the left atrium, a regurgitant volume 60 ml or more, a regurgitant fraction 50% or greater, a regurgitant orifice 0.40 cm^2 or greater, and a Doppler vena contracta width 0.7 cm or larger.
    Severity of MR is established using the criteria in Table 33-2.

TABLE 33-2. ANGIOGRAPHIC AND ECHOCARDIOGRAPHIC CRITERIA FOR THE ASSESSMENT OF THE SEVERITY OF MITRAL REGURGITATION

	Mild	Moderate	Severe
Angiographic grade	1+	2+	3-4+
Color Doppler jet area	Small central jet (< 4 cm^2 or <20% LA area)		Vena contracta width > 0.7 cm with large central MR jet (area > 40% LA), any wall-impinging jet, or any swirling in LA
Doppler vena contracta width	<0.3 cm	0.3-0.69 cm	≥0.7 cm
Regurgitant volume	<30 ml	30-59 ml	≥60 ml
Regurgitant fraction	<30%	30-49%	≥50%
Regurgitant orifice	<0.20 cm^2	0.2-0.39 cm^2	≥0.40 cm^2
Chamber size			Enlarged LA or LV

Modified from Bonow RO, Carabello BA, Chatterjee K, et al: ACC/AHA 2006 guidelines for the management of patients with valvular heart disease. *J Amer Coll Cardiol* 48:e1-e148, 2006.

13. **Are there effective medical therapies for chronic primary MR?**
    No. The asymptomatic patient will not benefit from medical therapy, and once symptoms develop, MR should be treated surgically. It should be noted that some patients with MR also have systemic hypertension, which should be treated in the same manner in which hypertension is routinely treated.

14. **What is the definitive therapy for primary MR, and when should it be employed?**
    As with all primary valve disease, MR is a mechanical problem requiring a mechanical solution. Here, however, the therapy for MR departs from that of other valve lesions. Unlike the aortic valve, the mitral valve serves to do more than just direct forward cardiac flow. The mitral valve is also an integral part of the LV, coordinating LV contraction and maintaining LV shape. When the valve is destroyed at the time of surgery, there is a precipitous fall in LV function postoperatively, which does not occur when the valve apparatus is conserved. Further, operative mortality is lower with valve repair than with valve replacement. Thus, every attempt should be made to repair rather than replace the valve at the time of surgery.
    Because the onset of symptoms worsens prognosis for patients with MR, mitral valve repair should be performed at that time. However, some patients fail to develop symptoms even though LV dysfunction has ensued. To guard against permanent LV dysfunction, mitral surgery should be performed before ejection fraction falls to 60% or less or before the LV can no longer contract to an end-systolic dimension of 40 mm. The onset of atrial fibrillation or pulmonary hypertension is also an indication for surgery. It should be noted that not all mitral valves can be repaired. In such cases, mitral valve replacement is performed.
    Class 1 indications for mitral valve repair or replacement include the following:
    - Symptomatic acute severe MR
    - Development or presence of NYHA class II–IV symptoms in patients with chronic severe MR in the absence of severe LV dysfunction (ejection fraction less than 30% or end-systolic dimension greater than 55 mm)
    - Asymptomatic patients with chronic severe MR and mild-moderate LV dysfunction (ejection fraction of 30%–60% or end-systolic dimension 40 mm or more)

15. **How is secondary MR managed?**
    This area is one of substantial uncertainty. In virtually all cases of secondary MR there is also severe LV dysfunction and heart failure. As such, standard therapy for heart failure is indicated. When mitral surgery should be undertaken is unclear, but it is usually reserved for those patients who have failed medical therapy for heart failure.

16. **What is mitral valve prolapse?**
    Mitral valve prolapse (MVP) is the condition in which there is systolic billowing of one or both mitral leaflets into the left atrium (Fig. 33-5), with or without resulting mitral regurgitation. It is usually diagnosed by echocardiography according to established criteria (valve prolapse of 2 mm or more above the mitral annulus, as seen in the parasternal long-axis view). Its prevalence is 1%–2.5%.

17. **What is the classic auscultatory finding in mitral valve prolapse?**
    The classic finding is a mid-systolic click and late systolic murmur, although the click may actually vary somewhat within systole, depending on changes in left ventricular dimension. There may actually be multiple clicks. The clicks are believed to result from the sudden tensing of the mitral valve apparatus as the leaflets prolapse into the left atrium during systole.

18. **What is the natural history of asymptomatic mitral valve prolapse?**
    The course of patients with MVP can range from benign, with a normal life expectancy, to worsening mitral regurgitation and progressive left atrial dilation and left ventricular dysfunction and congestive heart failure.

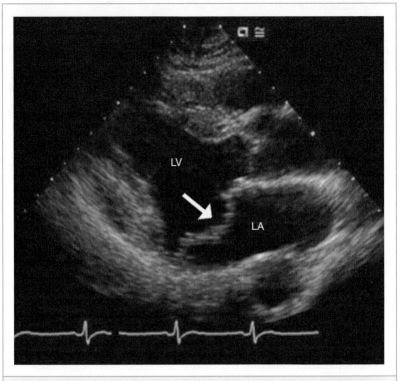

Figure 33-5. Mitral valve prolapse. The mitral leaflets *prolapse* across the plain of the mitral valve, into the left atrium *(arrow)*. *LA,* Left atrium; *LV,* left ventricle. (Modified from Libby P, Bonow RO, Mann DL, et al: *Braunwald's heart disease: a textbook of cardiovascular medicine,* ed 8, Philadelphia, 2008, Saunders.)

BIBLIOGRAPHY, SUGGESTED READINGS, AND WEBSITES

1. Gaasch WH: Overview of the Management of Chronic Mitral Regurgitation: http://www.utdol.com
2. Hanson I, Afonso LC: Mitral Regurgitation: http://www.emedicine.com
3. Nachimuthu S, Balasundaram K, Salazar HP: Mitral Stenosis: http://www.emedicine.com
4. Otto CM: Pathophysiology and Clinical Features of Mitral Stenosis: http://www.utdol.com
5. Bonow RO, Carabello BA, Chatterjee K, et al: ACC/AHA 2006 guidelines for the management of patients with valvular heart disease, *J Amer Coll Cardiol* 48:e1-e148, 2006.
6. Carabello BA: Modern management of mitral stenosis, *Circulation* 112(3):432-437, 2005.
7. Carabello BA: The current therapy for mitral regurgitation, *J Am Coll Cardiol* 52(5):319-326, 2008.
8. Carabello BA: The pathophysiology of mitral regurgitation, *J Heart Valve Dis* 9(5):600-608, 2000.
9. Vahanian A, Baumgartner H, Bax J, et al: Guidelines on the management of valvular heart disease: the Task Force on the Management of Valvular Heart Disease of the European Society of Cardiology, *Eur Heart J* 28(2): 230-268, 2007.

CHAPTER 34

PROSTHETIC HEART VALVES

Stephan M. Hergert, MD and Ann F. Bolger, MD, FACC, FAHA

Heart valve diseases are common and may result from congenital, inflammatory, infectious, or degenerative causes. The decisions regarding how to surgically correct these valvular problems, how to follow the patients after surgery, and what problems to anticipate are addressed in this chapter.

1. **What are important considerations in the preoperative evaluation and planning of patients who are to undergo valve repair/replacement?**
   Patients who are advised to have valve surgery require careful preoperative planning and assessment. Cardiac catheterization to rule out coronary artery obstructions that might require bypass is advised in adults more than 40 years old. Dental evaluation to identify abscesses or other potential sources of postoperative valvular infection is advisable. Carotid ultrasound to exclude significant stenosis in patients with bruits or neurologic symptoms is often requested. Visualization of the aorta to assess atherosclerosis at potential cannulation sites and root dimensions may occasionally be required before valve replacement.

2. **What types of prosthetic valves are used for valve replacement, and which ones are most commonly used in current practice?**
   Representative bioprosthesic and mechanical heart valves are shown in Fig. 34-1 and discussed here.

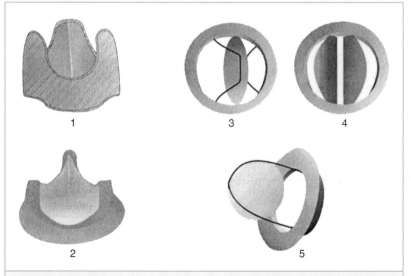

Figure 34-1. Bioprosthetic and mechanical heart valves. **(1)** Biologic nonstented and **(2)** stented valves; **(3)** mechanical single tilting disc, **(4)** bileaflet, and **(5)** ball-in-cage valves.

- Stentless bioprosthesis is a bovine or porcine heart valve implanted without a frame. In the aortic position the aortic root is used to attach the valve. The major advantage is that the implanted valve can be larger because no space is required for a supporting frame. Data suggest that left ventricular function is better protected with nonstented compared with stented valves. Anticoagulation is recommended for the first three months after implantation.
- A stented bioprosthesis has a wire frame that provides the structure for the biologic material. The biologic material is usually bovine or porcine pericardium, which is specially treated to reduce antigenicity. Anticoagulation is recommended for the first 3 months after implantation.
- A single tilting disc mechanical valve opens with a minor and major orifice. The disc material is polycarbonate. The first successful valve was the Bjork-Shiley valve, introduced in 1969. These valves are rarely if ever used in current practice.
- A bileaflet mechanical valve has two semicircular discs. The disc material is polycarbonate. The first bileaflet valve was introduced in 1977 by St. Jude Medical. Bileaflet valves are the most common mechanical heart valves used in current practice.
- The ball-in-cage model is an older type of valve that is still encountered in some patients today. The Starr Edwards mechanical valve prosthesis was introduced by Professor Albert Starr in 1961. It was the first mechanical heart valve. Some patients still have functioning Starr Edwards prostheses after more than 30 years. The main drawback of this valve is its high-pressure gradient and the nonphysiologic streaming of flow through the valve. For these reasons, as well as the need for higher degrees of anticoagulation, the valve is no longer used in clinical practice.

3. **What is a heterograft and what is a homograft/allograft, and what is a Ross procedure?**
A heterograft is a biologic valve derived from an animal. A homograft/allograft is a heart valve taken from a cadaveric human donor. Homografts have the advantage of natural configuration and the fact that they include a portion of the aortic root that can be incorporated in the valve replacement procedure if necessary (e.g., aortic root abscess). Careful matching of homograft size to the patient is critical to the performance and durability of the valve.

The Ross procedure uses the patient's own pulmonic valve to replace their aortic valve. The pulmonic valve is then replaced with a bioprosthesis. Advantages are a lack of antigenicity and the potential for growth of the valve over time, as required by children.

4. **How does one choose between bioprosthetic and mechanical valves?**
A bioprosthesis is preferred in older patients and in patients in whom lifetime anticoagulation poses important risks. This includes persons with high trauma risk, clotting disorders, and gastrointestinal problems with the potential for bleeding and persons who may not be able to comply with required anticoagulant medication and follow-up testing. The major disadvantage of biologic prostheses is primary valve failure as a result of leaflet degeneration, which limits their functional life span. Mechanical heart valves, which have greater durability than bioprosthetic valves, are usually preferred in patients younger than 65 years without contraindications to long-term anticoagulation.

5. **How does one anticoagulate patients with prosthetic valves, and what are the risks for thromboembolic or hemorrhagic events?**
In general, patients with mechanical valves in the aortic position should maintain an international normalized ratio (INR) between 2 and 3. For bileaflet Medtronic Hall valves, or for patients with additional thrombotic risk factors such as atrial fibrillation, left ventricular dysfunction, or hypercoagulable state, the recommended INR is between 2.5 and 3.5. In very high risk patients, and if aspirin or clopidogrel cannot be used, an INR between 3.5 and 4.5 may be indicated.

In the mitral position the recommended INR is between 2.5 and 3.5 for all mechanical valve types. In very high risk patients with additional prothrombotic risk factors, and if aspirin or clopidogrel cannot be used, an INR between 3.5 and 4.5 may be indicated.

Biologic valves have a much lower thromboembolic risk than mechanical valves. With biologic valves, warfarin is recommended for the first 3 months because of a higher risk for thromboembolic events during this time when endothelialization of the prosthesis is incomplete. This risk is highest in the first few days after implantation, and therefore unfractionated heparin (UFH) can be initiated within the first 24 to 48 hours, keeping the activated partial thromboplastin time (aPTT) between 55 and 70. Warfarin can then be started and continued until an INR between 2 and 3 is achieved. Unless other prothrombotic risk factors are present, anticoagulation can be discontinued after 3 months.

Oral anticocagulation issues are also discussed in Chapter 36 on oral anticoagulation with warfarin. Guidelines on anticoagulation of prosthetic heart valves have been published by both the American College of Cardiology/American Heart Association (ACC/AHA) and the American College of Chest Physicians (ACCP).

6. **How does one handle anticoagulation issues in patients with mechanical valve prostheses before elective surgery or invasive procedures?**
   When coumadin must be discontinued for elective procedures, the patient can be treated with UFH (target aPTT 55–70 seconds) while the INR decreases. Low-molecular weight-heparin (LMWH) is not *approved* for protection against thromboembolism from mechanical valve prostheses; although a recent American College of Chest Physicians practice guidelines does discuss LMWH use for bridging patients off and back on warfarin. Vitamin K administration can create a hypercoagulable state, which increases the risk of thromboembolism, and should not be used to accelerate the normalization of the INR.

7. **How are anticoagulation issues managed in patients with mechanical heart valves who become pregnant?**
   Female patients who anticipate pregnancy may initially opt for valve prostheses that avoid the need for anticoagulation. For patients with mechanical prostheses, anticoagulation must be continued during pregnancy, but the risk of adverse fetal effects from coumadin mandates a different anticoagulation strategy. The ACCP's Conference on Antithrombotic and Thrombolytic Therapy recommends one of the following three regimens:
   - Treatment with LMWH or UFH between weeks 6 and 12 and close to term; warfarin during the rest of the pregnancy
   - Treatment with UFH throughout the whole pregnancy (subcutaneous UFH 17500–20000 U twice a day; aPTT between 55 and 70 by 6 hours after injection)
   - Weight-adjusted subcutaneous LMWH twice a day throughout the whole pregnancy (plasma level of anti Xa 0.7–1.2 U/ml by 4–6 hours after injection)

   Concerns about the efficacy of subcutaneous UFH or LMWH in patients with mechanical valve prosthesis persist; the pros and cons of each regimen needs to be discussed carefully.

8. **How does one prevent, diagnose, or treat prosthetic valve endocarditis?**
   Endocarditis on a prosthetic valve is a potentially catastrophic event that may require repeat surgery to cure the infection. Such infections may originate on the prosthetic sewing ring and rapidly extend into perivalvular tissues. The risk of endocarditis is approximately the same for mechanical and biologic valve prostheses, although some studies have suggested slightly higher risks for biologic valves. All patients with prosthetic heart valves should receive endocarditis prophylaxis for procedures likely to create bacteremia with an endocarditis-causing organisms; the American Heart Association published new prophylaxis guidelines in 2007. Generally, prophylaxis should be administered 2 hours before the procedure in a single dose. For dental procedures in non–penicillin-allergic adults, amoxicillin, 2 g orally, is recommended. Alternative agents and pediatric doses are presented in the guidelines. See also Chapter 35 on endocarditis and endocarditis prophylaxis.

Before any antibiotic administration, blood cultures should be obtained on any patient with a prosthetic valve and a fever. Two positive blood cultures or a majority of positive blood cultures constitute a major criterion for the diagnosis of endocarditis. Demonstration of a vegetation, perivalvular abscess, or new regurgitation or valvular destruction is a second major criterion in the diagnosis. Because artificial valves often create artifacts that complicate imaging the valve, transesophageal echocardiography is almost always required to adequately assess prosthetic heart valves for endocarditis and to rule out perivalvular extension of infection.

In cases of mechanical heart valve endocarditis, early surgery and re-replacement is often required, especially in the presence of perivalvular extension of infection, and may improve patient survival. Attempted medical treatment of prosthetic valve endocarditis requires at least 4 to 6 weeks of antibiotic therapy.

9. **How does one use echocardiography to follow patients after heart valve surgery?**
All prosthetic valves are stenotic compared with natural valves because of the extra space required for their sewing ring. As a result, the transvalvular flow velocity is expected to be higher than normal across prostheses; each valve type and size has an expected range of velocities and pressure gradients defined by the manufacturer. Flow patterns at closure are also valve specific; mechanical prostheses normally have multiple regurgitation jets (an exception to this being the ball-in-cage prosthesis).

In evaluating prosthetic valves, it is important to know the valve type and size. The forward flow across the valve is measured with Doppler and used to calculate the peak and mean gradients for comparison to normal values. The gradients will increase with higher heart rate and with increased flow volume. Unexplained increases in valve gradients may indicate obstruction from endocarditis, thrombosis, leaflet calcification, or tissue overgrowth.

During phases when the valve is closed, spectral and color Doppler are used to look for valvular insufficiency. The closure volume of mechanical valves can be seen as multiple (up to seven) jets of regurgitation from the leaflet coapture and hinge points. With biologic prostheses, transvalvular insufficiency jets indicate valve dysfunction.

Eccentric regurgitation in any type of prosthesis may result from paravalvular leaks caused by sutural dehiscence with or without endocarditis.

Other echocardiographic clues to prosthetic valve dysfunction are progressive chamber enlargement, abnormal pulmonary vein flow patterns (for mitral regurgitation), diastolic reversal of aortic flow (aortic prosthetic regurgitation), and pulmonary hypertension (as estimated from the tricuspid insufficiency jet).

10. **What can cause recurrent symptoms when the prosthetic valve appears normal?**
A mitral prosthesis that extends into the left ventricle (high profile) may crowd the outflow tract and cause signs and symptoms of outflow obstruction. This can also be seen after mitral valve repair, where redundant components of the native valve oppose the septum in systole. Intraventricular pressure gradients in the outflow tract can be identified with Doppler echocardiography. Low-profile valves have largely addressed this problem.

All prostheses are smaller than the natural valves that they replace because of the space required for their sewing ring. Undersized valves relative to patient requirements can result in relative valvular stenosis. This can be investigated with Doppler studies.

11. **What about magnetic resonance imaging (MRI) after valve replacement?**
According to a recent AHA scientific statement, the majority of prosthetic heart valves that have been tested have been labeled as *MR safe*; the remainder of heart valves and rings that have been tested have been labeled as *MR conditional*. On the basis of various studies and findings, the presence of a prosthetic heart valve that has been formally evaluated for MR safety should not be considered a contraindication to an MR examination at 3 Tesla or less (and possibly even 4.7 Tesla in some cases) any time after implantation. In cases where there is any doubt as to the safety of MRI scanning of a specific valve, the safety of the study should be discussed with an MRI specialist.

BIBLIOGRAPHY, SUGGESTED READINGS, AND WEBSITES

1. Aurigemma GP, Gaasch WH: Routine Management of Patients with Prosthetic Heart Valves: http://www.utdol.com

2. Ali A, Halstead JC, Cafferty F, et al: Are stentless valves superior to modern stented valves? A prospective randomized trial, *Circulation* 114(1 Suppl):1535-1540, 2006.

3. Bates SM, Greer IA, Hirsh J, et al: Use of antithrombotic agents during pregnancy: the Seventh ACCP Conference on Antithrombotic and Thrombolytic Therapy, *Chest* 126(3 Suppl):627S-644S, 2004.

4. Bonow RO, Carabello B, Chatterjee K, et al: ACC/AHA 2006 guidelines for the management of patients with valvular heart disease: executive summary, *Circulation* 114(5): e84-e231, 2006.

5. Edwards MB, Taylor KM, Shellock FG, et al: Prosthetic heart valves: evaluation of magnetic field interactions, heating, and artifacts at 1.5 T, *J Magn Reson Imaging* 12(2):363-369, 2000.

6. Elkayam U, Bitar F: Valvular heart disease and pregnancy: part II: prosthetic valves, *J Am Coll Cardiol* 46(3): 403-410, 2005.

7. Gott VL, Alejo DE, Cameron DE: Mechanical heart valves: 50 years of evolution, *Ann Thorac Surg* 76(6): S2230-S2239, 2003.

8. Hammermeister K, Sethi GK, Henderson WG, et al: Outcomes 15 years after valve replacement with a mechanical versus a bioprosthetic valve: final report of the Veterans Affairs randomized trial, *J Am Coll Cardiol* 36(4):1152-1158, 2000.

9. Kovacs MJ, Kearon C, Rodger M, et al: Single-arm study of bridging therapy with low-molecular-weight heparin for patients at risk of arterial embolism who require temporary interruption of warfarin, *Circulation* 110(12): 1658-1663, 2004.

10. Kulik A, Bédard P, Lam B-K, et al: Mechanical versus bioprosthetic valve replacement in middle-aged patients, *Eur J Cardiothorac Surg* 30(3):485-491, 2006.

11. Levine GN, Arai A, Bleumke D, et al: Safety of MRI/MRA in patients with cardiovascular devices; a scientific statement: statement by the AHA Council on Clinical Cardiology, *Circulation* 116:2878-2921, 2007.

12. Mohty D, Orszulak TA, Schaff HV, et al: Very long-term survival and durability of mitral valve repair for mitral valve prolapse, *Circulation* 104(12 Suppl 1):11-I7, 2001.

13. Stein PD, Alpert JS, Bussey HI, et al: Antithrombotic therapy in patients with mechanical and biological prosthetic heart valves, *Chest* 119(Suppl 1):220S-227S, 2001.

14. Wilson W, Taubert KA, Gewitz M, et al: Prevention of infective endocarditis: guidelines from the American Heart Association, *J Am Dent Assoc* 138(6):739-745, 747-60, 2007.

15. Dokeuketis JD, Berger PB, Dunn AS, et al. The perioperative management of antithrombotic therapy: American College of Chest Physicians evidence-based clinical practice guidelines (8th edition). *Chest* 2008;133:299S-339S.

CHAPTER 35

ENDOCARDITIS AND ENDOCARDITIS PROPHYLAXIS

Glenn N. Levine, MD, FACC, FAHA

1. **What are believed to be the first steps in the development of infective endocarditis?**

   Infective endocarditis (IE) is believed to occur only after one first develops what is termed nonbacterial thrombotic endocarditis (NBTE). According to the most recent American Heart Association (AHA) statement on endocarditis, it is believed that turbulent blood flow produced by certain types of congenital or acquired heart disease traumatizes the endothelium. This turbulent blood flow may be the result of flow from a high- to a low-pressure chamber or across a narrowed orifice. This trauma of the endothelium then creates a predisposition for deposition of platelets and fibrin on the surface of the endothelium, resulting in what is called NBTE. If bacteremia (or fungemia) occurs, the organisms may then colonize this site, resulting in infective endocarditis.

2. **How often does routine tooth brushing and flossing cause transient bacteremia?**

   Transient bacteremia occurs 20% to 68% of the time with routine tooth brushing and flossing. It occurs 20% to 40% of the time with use of wooden toothpicks, and 7% to 71% of the time with chewing food. This is part of the rationale of the latest AHA guidelines deemphasizing antibiotic prophylaxis during certain dental and other procedures—namely, that the vast majority of the time bacteremia is due to daily activities and not to the occasional or rare dental or other procedure. The emphasis now is more on maintaining good oral hygiene and access to routine dental care.

3. **True or false: Prospective randomized placebo-controlled trials have demonstrated that antibiotic prophylaxis before a dental or other procedure reduces the risk of infective endocarditis?**

   False. Despite the fact that for 50 years antibiotic prophylaxis has been recommended, there has never been a prospective randomized placebo-controlled trial to support this recommendation. In fact, the data on whether antibiotic prophylaxis even significantly affects bacteremia is contradictory, with some studies showing some reduction and others showing no reduction.

4. **What are the four conditions identified as having the highest risk of adverse outcome from endocarditis for which prophylaxis with dental procedures is still recommended?**

   - Prosthetic cardiac valve
   - Previous infective endocarditis
   - Certain cases of congenital heart disease (CHD), such as:
     - Unrepaired cyanotic CHD
     - Repaired CHD with prosthetic material or devices during the first 6 months after the procedure
     - Repaired CHD with residual defects
   - Cardiac transplantation recipients who develop cardiac valvulopathy

5. **In the new AHA guidelines, for those patients with conditions listed in Question 4, which dental procedures carry a recommendation of endocarditis prophylaxis?**

The guidelines emphasize that *all dental procedures* that involve the manipulation of gingival tissue or the periapical region of teeth or perforation of the oral mucosa should receive endocarditis prophylaxis. Procedures that do not require prophylaxis include routine anesthetic injections through noninfected tissue, dental radiographs, placement of removable prosthodontic or orthodontic appliances, bleeding from trauma to the lips or oral mucosa, and select other procedures and manipulations. The guidelines emphasize that prophylaxis for the former mentioned procedures "may be reasonable for these patients," although "its effectiveness is unknown" (and this prophylaxis recommendation is given a class IIb recommendation, with level of evidence C). New changes in the AHA guidelines on infective endocarditis are summarized in Box 35-1.

BOX 35-1. SUMMARY OF THE MAJOR CHANGES IN THE UPDATED AMERICAN HEART ASSOCIATION'S SCIENTIFIC STATEMENT ON INFECTIVE ENDOCARDITIS PROPHYLAXIS

- Bacteremia resulting from daily activities is much more likely to cause infective endocarditis (IE) than bacteremia associated with a dental procedure.
- Only an extremely small number of cases of IE might be prevented by antibiotic prophylaxis even if prophylaxis is 100% effective.
- Antibiotic prophylaxis is not recommended based solely on an increased lifetime risk of acquisition of IE.
- Recommendations for IE prophylaxis are limited to only the four conditions identified as having the highest risk of adverse outcome from endocarditis (see text).
- Antibiotic prophylaxis is no longer recommended for any other form of congenital heart disease, except for the conditions listed in the text.
- Antibiotic prophylaxis is recommended for all dental procedures that involve manipulation of gingival tissues or periapical region of teeth or perforation of oral mucosa only for patients with underlying cardiac conditions associated with the highest risk of adverse outcome from IE (see text).
- Antibiotic prophylaxis is recommended for procedures on respiratory tract or infected skin, skin structures, or musculoskeletal tissue only for patients with underlying cardiac conditions associated with the highest risk of adverse outcome from IE (see text).
- Antibiotic prophylaxis solely to prevent IE is not recommended for GU or GI tract procedures.

Modified from Wilson W, Taubert KA, Gewitz M, et al: Prevention of infective endocarditis guidelines from the American Heart Association. *Circulation* 2007; 116(15):1736-1754.

---

6. **For those patients with conditions for which antibiotic prophylaxis is recommended, undergoing dental procedures for which prophylaxis is recommended, what regimens are recommended?**

Antibiotic treatment should be administered as a single dose before the procedure, with antimicrobial therapy directed against Viridians group streptococci. Amoxicillin (2 g orally [PO]), administered 30 to 60 minutes before the procedure, is the first-line recommendation. Those unable to take oral medication can be treated with ampicillin (2 g intramuscularly [IM] or intravenously [IV]) or cefazoline or ceftriaxone (1 g IM or IV). For those allergic to the penicillins or ampicillin, potential agents to use include cephalexin, clindamycin, azithromycin, clarithromycin, cefazolin, and ceftriaxone.

7. **For what other procedures may prophylaxis be considered in patients with high-risk lesions?**
   The new AHA guidelines deemphasize prophylaxis for most other procedures. Antibiotic prophylaxis solely to prevent IE is not recommended for genitourinary (GU) or gastrointestinal (GI) tract procedures. Among those procedures where prophylaxis may be considered (class IIb, level of evidence C) are:
   - Invasive procedures of the respiratory tract that involve incision or biopsy of the respiratory mucosa (e.g., tonsillectomy, adenoidectomy)
   - Bronchoscopy with incision of the respiratory tract mucosa (but not otherwise for bronchoscopy)
   - Invasive respiratory tract procedures to treat an established infection (e.g., drainage or an abscess or empyema)
   - Surgical procedures that involve infected skin, skin structures, or musculoskeletal tissue

8. **Do the European Society of Cardiology's (ESC's) guidelines on endocarditis prophylaxis differ from the American Heart Association's guidelines?**
   Yes. As of this writing, the ESC guidelines were last updated in 2004 and recommend endocarditis prophylaxis for *traditional* indications, including acquired valvular heart disease, mitral valve prolapse (MVP) with valvular regurgitation, and hypertrophic cardiomyopathy (in addition to the conditions discussed earlier in the latest American Heart Association [AHA] guidelines). The procedures for which prophylaxis are recommended are also broader than the current AHA guidelines.

9. **Is endocarditis prophylaxis recommended in patients treated with coronary stents, pacemakers, or defibrillators, or those who have undergone coronary artery bypass grafting (CABG) (without valve replacement)?**
   No.

10. **Is endocarditis prophylaxis indicated for cardiac catheterization, stent implantation, pacemaker or defibrillator implantation, or transesophageal echocardiography?**
    No. Note, however, that some electrophysiologists will pretreat or post-treat patients undergoing pacemaker/defibrillator with antibiotics to prevent local infection (but not endocarditis).

11. **What factors (discussed in detail in the ESC guidelines on endocarditis) should raise the suspicion for endocarditis?**
    - Bacteremia/sepsis of unknown cause
    - Fever
    - Constitutional symptoms, such as unexplained malaise, weakness, arthralgias, and weight loss
    - Hematuria, glomerulonephritis, and suspected renal infarction
    - Embolic event of unknown origin
    - New heart murmur (primarily regurgitant murmurs)
    - Unexplained new atrioventricular (AV) nodal conduction abnormality (prolonged PR interval, heart block)
    - Multifocal or rapid changing pulmonic infiltrates
    - Peripheral abscesses
    - Cutaneous lesions (Osler's nodes, Janeway's lesions)
    - Ophthalmic manifestations (Roth's spots)

12. **When should cardiac echo be obtained in cases of suspected endocarditis?**
    As soon as possible. Transthoracic echocardiography (TTE) has a sensitivity of 60% to 75% in the detection of native valve endocarditis. It can detect 70% of vegetations larger than 6 mm but only 25% of vegetations less than 5 mm. In cases where the clinical suspicion of

endocarditis is low, a good-quality TTE is usually adequate. In cases where the suspicion of endocarditis is higher, a negative TTE should be followed by transesophageal echocardiography (TEE), which has a sensitivity of 88% to 100% and a specificity of 91% to 100% for native valves. TTE is not considered a sensitive test for prosthetic valve endocarditis, and a TEE is routinely obtained in such cases. TEE is also considerably more sensitive for detecting myocardial abscesses. Figure 35-1 demonstrates a mitral valve vegetation visualized by TEE.

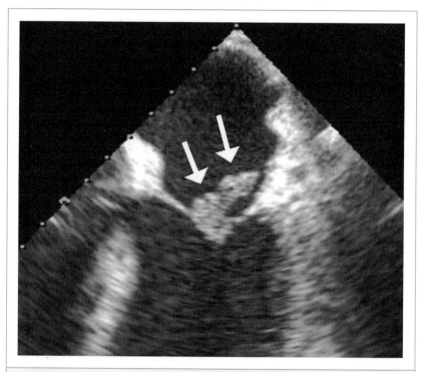

Figure 35-1. A vegetation on the mitral valve as visualized by transesophageal echo. (Courtesy Dr. Kumudha Ramasubbu.)

13. **What is the procedure for obtaining blood cultures in cases of suspected endocarditis?**
   Three separate sets of blood cultures should be obtained, each at least 1 hour apart from the others (different authorities differ on the exact timing recommendations, but this is a reasonable ballpark figure). For what is called *subacute* infective endocarditis, some experts recommend the cultures be drawn over a period of 24 hours. These blood cultures should not be obtained from intravenous lines (although some may recommend additional blood cultures be obtained from indwelling lines). At least 5 ml, and ideally 10 ml, of blood should be added to each culture bottle. In patients treated for a short period with antibiotics, one should wait, if possible, for at least 3 days after antibiotic discontinuation before obtaining new blood cultures.

14. **What is the most common overall organism reported to cause endocarditis?**
   Staphylococcus aureus, followed by Viridians group streptococci and then enterococci and coagulase-native staphylococci.

15. **What is the most common organism causing subacute native valve endocarditis?**
Streptococcus viridians.

16. **What is the most common organism causing endocarditis in intravenous drug abusers (IVDA)?**
Staphylococcus aureus.

17. **What is the most common organism causing early prosthetic valve endocarditis?**
Staphylococcus infection, particularly *S. epidermidis* and *S. aureus.*

18. **What is the most common cause of *culture-negative* endocarditis?**
The most common cause of culture-negative endocarditis is prior use of antibiotics. Other causes include fastidious organisms (HACEK group, *Legionella, Chlamydia, Brucella,* certain fungal infections, etc.) and noninfectious causes.

19. **What is the *Duke criteria* for the diagnosis of endocarditis?**
The Duke criteria is a set of criteria proposed for the *definite* and *possible* diagnosis of infective endocarditis, published In 1994 (see Bibliography), based on both pathologic and clinical criteria. These criteria were a modification of previously proposed criteria (the *Von Reyn criteria*). These criteria were then themselves slightly modified in 2000, with the criteria incorporating the value of transesophageal echo, special recognition of *Coxiella burnetti,* and several other issues (see Bibliography). These revisions became known as the "modified Duke criteria" and are presented in Boxes 35-2 and 35-3.

BOX 35-2. THE *MODIFIED* DUKE CRITERIA DEFINITIONS OF DEFINITE, POSSIBLE, AND REJECTED ENDOCARDITIS

Definite Infective Endocarditis
- Pathologic criteria
  1. Microorganisms demonstrated by culture or histologic examination of a vegetation, a vegetation that has embolized, or an intracardiac abscess specimen; or
  2. Pathologic lesions; vegetation or intracardiac abscess confirmed by histologic examination showing active endocarditis
- Clinical criteria
  1. Two major criteria; or
  2. One major criterion and three minor criteria; or
  3. Five minor criteria

Possible Infective Endocarditis
  1. One major criterion and one minor criterion; or
  2. Three minor criteria

Rejected
  1. Firm alternate diagnosis explaining evidence of infective endocarditis; or
  2. Resolution of infection endocarditis syndrome with antibiotic therapy for less than or equal to 4 days; or
  3. No pathologic evidence of infective endocarditis at surgery or autopsy, with antibiotic therapy for less than or equal to 4 days; or
  4. Does not meet criteria for possible infective endocarditis, as above

Modified from Li JS, Sexton DJ, Mick N, et al: Proposed modifications to the Duke criteria for the diagnosis of infective endocarditis, *Clin Infect Dis* 30(4):633-638, 2000.

BOX 35-3. THE *MODIFIED* DUKE CRITERIA FOR THE DIAGNOSIS OF ENDOCARDITIS

Major Criteria
- Blood culture positive for IE
- Typical microorganisms consistent with IE from two separate blood cultures:
- Viridans streptococci; *Streptococcus bovis,* HACEK group *(Haemophilus, Actinobacillus, Cardiobacterium, Eikenella, Kingella), Staphylococcus aureus;* or
  - ○ Community-acquired enterococci, in the absence of a primary focus; or
- Microorganisms consistent with IE from persistently positive blood cultures, defined as follows:
- At least two positive blood cultures of blood samples drawn more than 12 hours apart; or
- All of three or a majority of four or more separate cultures of blood (with first and last sample drawn at least 1 hour apart)
  - ○ Single positive blood culture for *Coxiella burnetii* or antiphase I IgG antibody titer greater than 1:800
- Evidence of endocardial involvement
- Echocardiogram positive for IE (TEE recommended in patients with prosthetic valves, rated at least "possible IE" by clinical criteria, or complicated IE [paravalvular abscess]; TTE as first test in other patients), defined as follows:
  - ○ Oscillating intracardiac mass on valve or supporting structures, in the path of regurgitant jets, or on implanted material in the absence of an alternative anatomic explanation; or
  - ○ Abscess; or
  - ○ New partial dehiscence of prosthetic valve
- New valvular regurgitation (worsening or changing or preexisting murmur not sufficient)

Minor Criteria
- Predisposition, predisposing heart condition or injection drug use
- Fever, temperature more than 38° C
- Vascular phenomena, major arterial emboli, septic pulmonary infarcts, mycotic aneurysm, intracranial hemorrhage, conjunctival hemorrhages, and Janeway's lesions
- Immunologic phenomena: glomerulonephritis, Olser's nodes, Roth's spots, and rheumatoid factor
- Microbiologic evidence: positive blood culture but does not meet a major criterion as noted above (excluding single positive cultures for coagulase-negative staphylococci and organisms that do not cause endocarditis) or serologic evidence of active infection with organism consistent with IE
- Echocardiographic minor criteria eliminated

Modified from Li JS, Sexton DJ, Mick N, et al: Proposed modifications to the Duke criteria for the diagnosis of infective endocarditis, *Clin Infect Dis* 30(4):633-638, 2000.

20. **What are among the complications of endocarditis?**
    - Valve destruction and development of regurgitant lesions (aortic insufficiency [AI] or mitral regurgitation [MR])
    - Abscess formation
    - AV node heart block (as a result of abscess formation and extension to the area of the AV node/bundle of His)
    - Prosthetic valve dehiscence and perivalvular leaks
    - Peripheral embolization (brain, kidneys, spleen, lungs, etc.)

21. **What are generally accepted indications for surgery in patients with active IE?**
   Decisions regarding surgery will depend both on the indications for surgery and the patient's overall status and risks of surgery. Recommendations vary among the American College of Cardiology [ACC]/AHA guidelines on valvular disease, the ESC guidelines on infective endocarditis, and other experts who have weighed in on the topic. Although each patient requires careful individualized decisions, the following are generally considered to be indications for surgery in appropriate candidates:
   - Acute AI or MR leading to congestive heart failure
   - Cardiac abscess formation/perivalvular extension
   - Persistence of infection despite adequate antibiotic treatment
   - Recurrent peripheral emboli
   - Cerebral emboli
   - Infection caused by microorganisms with a poor response to antibiotic treatment (e.g., fungi)
   - Prosthetic valve endocarditis, particularly if hemodynamic compromise exists
   - Mitral kissing infection—when cardiac echo demonstrates a large vegetation on the aortic valve that *kisses* the anterior mitral leaflet
   - Large (more than 10 mm) mobile vegetations (given as an indication by some, but not all experts and expert organizations)

22. **Are patients with mechanical prosthetic heart valves more likely to develop endocarditis than those with bioprosthetic heart valves?**
   No. The incidence for patients with both types of prosthetic heart valves is approximately 1% per year of follow-up.

23. **What are Osler nodes?**
   Osler nodes are small, tender red-purple nodules. They most commonly occur in the fingers, hands, toes, and feet. They may be caused by circulating immunocomplexes.

24. **What are Janeway lesions?**
   Janeway lesions are irregular macules located on the hands and feet. As opposed to Osler nodes, they are painless.

25. **What is marantic endocarditis?**
   Marantic endocarditis is the term previously used to for what is now referred to as nonbacterial thrombotic endocarditis. The term reportedly derived from the Greek *marantikos,* meaning "wasting away." The vegetations in NBTE are sterile and believed to be composed of platelets and fibrin. The finding of such sterile vegetations occurs in the setting of chronic wasting diseases, chronic infections (e.g., tuberculosis [TB], osteomyelitis), certain cancers, and disseminated intravascular coagulation. These often large vegetations may embolize to the brain, the coronary arteries, and the periphery.

26. **What is Libman-Sacks endocarditis?**
   Libman-Sacks endocarditis is a form of nonbacterial thrombotic endocarditis seen in patients with systemic lupus erythematosus (SLE). Described in 1924, the vegetations most commonly occur on the mitral valve, although they can affect all four cardiac valves. The lesions are due to accumulations of immune complexes, fibrin, and mononuclear cells. Most lesions do not cause symptoms, although valvular regurgitation or stenosis can occasionally occur because of the lesions. Embolization of the lesions is rare.

BIBLIOGRAPHY, SUGGESTED READINGS, AND WEBSITES

1. Marill KA: Endocarditis: http://www.emedicine.com
2. Pelletier LL: Infective Endocarditis: http://www.merck.com/mmpe/index.html
3. Pelletier LL: Noninfective Endocarditis: http://www.merck.com/mmpe/index.html
4. Ren X: Libman-Sacks Endocarditis: http://www.emedicine.com
5. Sexton DJ: Infective Endocarditis: http://www.utdol.com
6. Bonow RO, Carabello BA, Kanu C, et al: ACC/AHA 2006 guidelines for the management of patients with valvular heart disease, *Circulation* 114(5):84-231, 2006.
7. Durack DT, Lukes AS, Bright DK: New criteria for diagnosis of infective endocarditis: utilization of specific echocardiographic findings. Duke Endocarditis Service, *Am J Med* 96(3):200-209, 1994.
8. Horstkotte D, Follath F, Gutschik E, et al: Guidelines on prevention, diagnosis and treatment of infective endocarditis executive summary; the task force on infective endocarditis of the European society of cardiology, *Eur Heart J.* 25(3):267-276, 2004.
9. Li JS, Sexton DJ, Mick N, et al: Proposed modifications to the Duke criteria for the diagnosis of infective endocarditis, *Clin Infect Dis* 30(4):633-638, 2000.
10. Mylonakis E, Calderwood SB: Infective endocarditis in adults, *N Engl J Med* 345:1318-1330, 2001.
11. Wilson W, Taubert KA, Gewitz M, et al: Prevention of infective endocarditis: guidelines from the American Heart Association, *Circulation* 116(15):1736-1754, 2007.

CHAPTER 36

ORAL ANTICOAGULATION: WARFARIN

Michael B. Bottorff, PharmD, FCCP, CLS and Bradley E. Hein, PharmD

1. **How does warfarin work?**
   Warfarin (and related coumarin compounds) inhibit the activity of hepatic vitamin K-2,3 epoxide, which is used to recycle the *active* form of vitamin K, vitamin K hydroquinone. Without sufficient vitamin K hydroquinone, clotting factors II, VII, IX and X fail to be carboxylated, leaving them in an inactive state. The onset of warfarin anticoagulation is gradual and related to the elimination half-lives of the already synthesized active forms of these pro-coagulation factors. In addition to inhibiting the formation of active factors II, VII, IX and X, warfarin also inhibits the vitamin K-dependent formation of two coagulation inhibitors, proteins C and S, which may temporarily create a relative pro-coagulant state until full anticoagulation is achieved. Warfarin is a racemic mixture of S and R isomers. The S isomer has more inhibitory activity and is metabolized by cytochrome P450 2C9, which is the major source of drug interactions with warfarin.

2. **What are the clinical situations in which warfarin is used and at what intensity?**
   The intensity of anticoagulation depends primarily on the indication for anticoagulation. These are given in Table 36-1.

TABLE 36-1. INDICATIONS FOR ANTICOAGULATION AND RECOMMENDED INR INTENSITY		
Indication	**Class and Source of Recommendation**	**INR Intensity**
Stroke prevention in atrial fibrillation	Class Ia recommendation from ACC/AHA/ESC 2006 guidelines for management of patients with atrial fibrillation	2.0–3.0
Post-MI	Class IIb recommendation from ACC/AHA 2007 guidelines for management of patients with unstable angina/ non–ST-elevation myocardial infarction	With 75–81 mg aspirin, 2.0–2.5 Without aspirin, 2.5–3.5
DVT/PE	Grade 1A from ACCP 2008 recommendations on antithrombotic therapy for venous thromboembolic disease	Transient or reversible factor Target 2.5 (range 2.0–3.0) for 3 months Unprovoked DVT Target 2.5 (range 2.0–3.0) for at least 3 months Repeat unprovoked DVT Target 2.5 (range 2.0–3.0) long-term treatment

(Continued)

TABLE 36-1. INDICATIONS FOR ANTICOAGULATION AND RECOMMENDED INR INTENSITY (CONTINUED)		
Indication	Class and Source of Recommendation	INR Intensity
Mechanical heart valves	Grade 1B recommendation from ACCP 2008 recommendations on valvular and structural heart disease	Bileaflet mechanical valve in aortic position Target 2.5, range 2.0–3.0 Tilting-disk or bileaflet mechanical valve in mitral position Target 3.0, range 2.5–3.5 Caged-ball or caged-disk, any position Target 3.0, range 2.5–3.5 Bioprosthetic valve in mitral position Target 2.5, range 2.0–3.0 for first 3 months Bioprosthetic valve in aortic position ASA, not warfarin, indicated
Reduced left ventricular ejection fraction	Class IIb recommendation from ACC/AHA 2005 guideline update for the diagnosis and management of chronic heart failure in adults	Usefulness of anticoagulation has not been established in the absence of atrial fibrillation or previous thromboembolic events.
Left ventricular thrombus	Class IIa recommendation from 2006 AHA/ASA guidelines for the prevention of stroke in patients with ischemic stroke or transient ischemic attack	INR 2.0–3.0 for at least 3 months and up to 1 year

ACC, American College of Cardiology; *ACCP*, American College of Chest Physicians; *AHA*, American Heart Association; *ASA*, aspirin (acetylsalicylic acid); *DVT*, deep vein thrombosis; *ESC*, European Society of Cardiology; *INR*, international normalized ratio; *MI*, myocardial infarction; *PE*, pulmonary embolism.

3. **What is the role of warfarin in preventing transient ischemic attack/stroke in a patient with a history of ischemic stroke?**
For most patients with ischemic stroke, the underlying pathophysiology is similar to that of acute coronary syndromes—that is, atherothrombosis. Therefore, antiplatelet drugs either alone or in combination have been slightly superior to warfarin in comparative trials for stroke prevention. In addition, despite no clinical advantage, the warfarin patients experience much more major and minor bleeding. Thus, warfarin has no role in the treatment of ischemic stroke (class Ia recommendation for antiplatelet therapy rather than oral anticoagulation).

4. **How should unfractionated heparin (UFH), low-molecular-weight heparin (LMWH), or fondaparinux and warfarin be overlapped for acute treatment of venous thromboembolism?**
Regardless of the parental agent chosen for initial anticoagulation, warfarin should be initiated on day 1 of treatment. Choice of dose must be individualized based on patient-specific

factors (age, concurrent medications, nutrition status, comorbidities). However, for most patients, 5 mg daily is an adequate starting dose. For younger, healthier patients, consideration may be given for initiating warfarin at 10 mg daily. UFH, LMWH, or fondaparinux should be overlapped with warfarin for a minimum of 4 to 5 days and until the international normalized ratio (INR) is therapeutic (more than 2.5 for 1 day or more than 2 for 2 consecutive days).

5. **What is the role of pharmacogenomics in warfarin dosing?**
   Warfarin dosing is challenging, in part, because of the varied response and the wide range of doses required to achieve a therapeutic INR in an individual patient. Contributors to this variability are polymorphisms in the cytochrome P450 (CYP) 2C9 metabolizing enzyme responsible for the majority of warfarin metabolism and in the target enzyme for warfarin, vitamin K epoxide reductase. Patients with either or both of these genetic polymorphisms tend to be more sensitive to warfarin and require lower doses. As genetic testing for these polymorphisms becomes less expensive and more accessible, pharmacogenetic dose selection may allow for a shorter time to a therapeutic INR and reduced bleeding complications.

6. **How should warfarin be managed in patients who need surgery?**
   For patients who need INR normalized before surgery, warfarin should be stopped 5 days before the surgery. Depending on the reason for anticoagulation, bridging may be necessary. The most common indications for bridging therapy are patients with mechanical valves and recent deep vein thrombosis/pulmonary embolism (DVT/PE). These patients should receive full-dose LMWH during the bridging period. The last dose of LMWH should be given no later than 24 hours before the procedure. LMWH should be resumed 24 to 72 hours after the procedure, depending on bleeding and thrombotic risks of the patient. Warfarin should be restarted 24 hours after the procedure, with risk somewhat mitigated by delayed onset of effect. The reader should be aware that, as with many drugs, although LMWH is not *approved* for bridging, it is often used for this purpose. Different practitioners will have different *thresholds* of confidence for the use of LMWH as a bridging agent. The most caution in exercising decisions regarding outpatient LMWH bridging versus inpatient intravenous UFH bridging should be in patients with mechanical mitral valves (as the low pressure gradient between the left atrium and left ventricle during diastole may increase the risks of thrombosis compared with mechanical valves in the aortic position). A recently published American College of Chest Physicians guideline discusses bridging and the role of LMWH (see bibliography).
   For patients who need urgent surgery, it is recommended to give low dose (2.5–5 mg) oral or intravenous vitamin K. Fresh frozen plasma or other similar agents will give a more rapid (albeit temporary) reversal of anticoagulation therapy and can be combined with vitamin K.
   Relatively minor surgeries, such as dental and dermatologic procedures, do not generally require the discontinuation of warfarin. Typically, any excess in bleeding can be managed with local hemostatic agents.

7. **What are some of the common drug interactions with warfarin?**
   Because of its complex metabolism and relatively narrow therapeutic index, drug interactions involving warfarin are both common and clinically significant. The majority of the interactions occur at the level of CYP metabolism, although other mechanisms may be possible. Table 36-2 lists some of the more common interactions.
   For interactions listed as the causation being probable or highly probable, the strength of the clinical evidence is sufficient to expect a change in INR, requiring either adjusting the warfarin dose up or down by 25% to 50% in anticipation of the resulting change in INR or frequent INR monitoring to determine the dose adjustment necessary.
   Foods and supplements may also alter the INR. Foods that increase the INR include fish oil, mango, grapefruit juice, and cranberry juice. Foods and supplements that reduce the INR include high vitamin K–content food, enteral feeds, soy milk, ginseng, and sushi containing seaweed.

VI.

ATF

Jose

1. **How c**
Atrial fi
accoun
age for
As mar
to have

2. **What**
Hypert
dysfun
heart d
withou
have *Ic*
and m

3. **What**
AF may
tachyc:
during
electro
activat
and A\

4. **What**
Availat
reentra
atrial ii
sympa
inflam

5. **Whicl**
In the
metop
diltiaze
cautio
dysfun
recom

6. **How**
Sever:
least f
the Ch

TABLE 36-2. MEDICATION INTERACTIONS THAT INCREASE AND DECREASE INR*

Causation	Antiinfective	Cardiovascular	Antiinflammatory	CNS
Interactions That Reduce INR				
Highly probable	Ciprofloxacin Cotrimoxazole Erythromycin Fluconazole Isoniazid Metronidazole Miconazole oral gel Miconazole vaginal suppositories Voriconazole	Amiodarone Diltiazem Fenofibrate Propafenone Propranolol	Piroxicam	Alcohol (if with liver disease) Citalopram Sertraline
Probable	Amoxicillin/ clavulanate Azithromycin Clarithromycin Itraconazole Levofloxacin Ritonavir Tetracycline	Aspirin Fluvastatin Quinidine Simvastatin	Acetaminophen Aspirin Celecoxib Dextropropoxyphene Interferon Tramadol	Disulfiram Fluvoxamine Phenytoin (later, reduction in INR)
Interactions That Increase INR				
Highly Probable	Griseofulvin Nafcillin Ribavirin Rifampin	Cholestyramine		Barbiturates Carbamazepine
Probable	Dicloxacillin/ Ritonavir	Bosentan	Azathioprine	Chlordiazepoxide

CNS, Central nervous system.

*Only interactions that are considered to be *highly probable* or *probable*, for which the strength of the clinical evidence is sufficient to expect a change in INR, requiring either adjusting the warfarin dose up or down by 25% to 50% in anticipation of the resulting change in INR or frequent INR monitoring to determine the dose adjustment necessary, are given in this table. Many other drugs fall under the categories of *possible* interactions.

Modified from Holbrook AM, Pereira JA, Labiris R, et al: Systematic overview of warfarin and its drug and food interactions, *Arch Int Med* 165:1095-1106, 2005.

risk stratified according to the presence of moderate risk factors (1 point) and high risk factors (2 points). The use of appropriate anticoagulation is then decided according to the sum of points as outlined in Table 37-1.

13. WI
    Dir
    Dru
    age
    dir
    var
    he

BIBLIOG

1. Ande
   unsta
2. Anse
   of Ch
3. Douk
   Colle
4. Fuste
   fibrill
5. Garci
   Antic
6. Holb
   Arch
7. Hunt
   chro
8. Kear
   133:
9. Sacc
   trans
10. Sale
11. Scor
    patie
12. Dok
    Colle
    2999

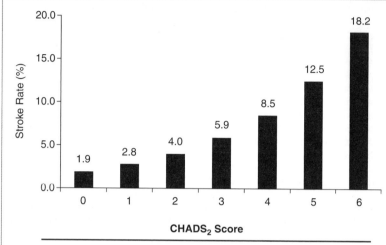

Risk Factors		Score
C	Recent congestive heart failure	1
H	Hypertension	1
A	Age ≥75 yrs	1
D	Diabetes mellitus	1
S$_2$	History of stroke or transient ischemic attack	2

Figure 37-1. CHADS$_2$ stroke risk scheme. The more risk factors, the higher the risk of stroke. (Modified from Rockson SG, Albers GW: Comparing the guidelines: anticoagulation therapy to optimize stroke prevention in patients with atrial fibrillation, *J Am Coll Cardiol* 43:929-935, 2004.)

TABLE 37-1. ACC/AHA/ESC 2006 GUIDELINES: RECOMMENDED THERAPIES ACCORDING TO CHADS$_2$ STROKE RISK

Risk Category	Recommended Therapy
No risk factors	Aspirin, 81–325 mg daily
One moderate risk factor	Aspirin, 81–325 mg daily, or warfarin (INR 2–3, target 2.5) (depending on patient preference)
Any high risk factor or >1 moderate risk factor	Warfarin (INR 2–3, target 2.5)

INR, International normalized ratio.

7. **Why is antithrombotic therapy so important in atrial fibrillation?**
   AF is an independent risk factor for stroke. The rate of ischemic stroke in patients with nonvalvular AF is about 2 to 7 times that of people without AF, and the risk increases dramatically as patients age. Both paroxysmal and chronic AF carry the same risk of thromboembolism. Anticoagulation therapy is essential in patients with AF to reduce the risk of embolic stroke. Aspirin (81 or 325 mg/day) reduces the risk of thromboembolism by approximately 35%. Warfarin reduces the risk by 65%. Full-dose warfarin is also superior to low-dose warfarin (international normalized ratio [INR] 1.2–1.5) with aspirin. The risk of a serious bleeding complication while on warfarin therapy (with an INR goal of 2–3) is 1.3% to 2.5% per year. Although the elderly may have a greater risk of bleeding, they also carry a greater risk of stroke and therefore benefit the most from warfarin therapy.

8. **When should cardioversion be considered to convert a patient from AF to sinus rhythm?**
   Cardioversion (CV) may be achieved by means of drugs or direct-current electrical shocks when the patient has new-onset AF that is less than 48 hours in duration. If the duration is more than 48 hours or unknown, the patient should be anticoagulated 3 weeks before and 4 weeks after CV to prevent thromboembolism. Alternatively, a patient can undergo transesophageal echocardiography to rule out left atrial thrombus and, if negative, proceed with CV while receiving appropriate anticoagulation with heparin. In case of early relapse of AF after CV, repeated direct-current cardioversion attempts may be made after administration of antiarrhythmic medication. Administration of flecainide, dofetilide, propafenone, or ibutilide is recommended for pharmacologic cardioversion of AF.

9. **How do you approach rate vs. rhythm control issues?**
   Two landmark studies, the Atrial Fibrillation Follow-up Investigation of Rhythm Management (AFFIRM) and the Rate Control versus Electrical Cardioversion (RACE) trials, found that treating AF with a rhythm-control strategy involving CV and antiarrhythmic drug (AAD) therapy offers no survival or clinical advantages over a simpler rate-control strategy. However, these studies primarily enrolled older patients (older than age 65 years) with persistent AF who were mildly symptomatic. Moreover, in the AFFIRM study, fewer than two thirds of those in the rhythm control arm were actually able to stay in sinus rhythm. Thus, the results cannot be extrapolated to many subgroups of patients, including younger patients; those with new, first-onset AF who may benefit from early conversion to sinus rhythm; patients with persistent AF who are highly symptomatic; and patients with significant systolic heart failure who have a hemodynamic benefit from the *atrial kick*.

10. **Which AADs are most commonly used to maintain long-term sinus rhythm and prevent AF recurrence?**
    Before initiating any AADs, treatment of precipitating or reversible causes of AF is recommended. The antiarrhythmics most commonly used have been sotalol, amiodarone, propafenone, dofetilide, flecainide, and disopyramide. Quinidine and procainamide are no longer used because of safety concerns. The class Ic (e.g., propafenone) and class III drugs also have a rate control effect when the patient is in AF.

11. **When is catheter ablation of AF indicated, and who is the ideal candidate?**
    Pulmonary vein isolation (PVI) with radiofrequency catheter ablation (RFA) is the most common ablation procedure performed nowadays. PVI appears in the new guidelines as an option for treatment of paroxysmal or persistent AF in patients who have failed one or more courses of an AAD regimen. It is mostly considered as an alternative to chronic amiodarone therapy and generally is not performed as a first-line therapy for AF. Patient selection, optimal catheter positioning, absolute rates of treatment success, and the frequency of complications remain incompletely defined. The ideal candidate for PVI is a person more than 70 years old with paroxysmal AF, who has failed at least one AAD, and who is highly symptomatic. The patient's

left atrial should be less than 5.5 cm with an ejection fraction greater than 40%, without other significant cardiac disease. However, the procedure has shown efficacy in patients with chronic atrial fibrillation, as well as in patients with congestive heart failure. Therefore, indications for catheter ablation of atrial fibrillation are rapidly expanding.

12. **What are potential complications of pulmonary vein isolation?**
A worldwide survey on AF catheter ablation showed an overall incidence of major complications of 6%. Potential complications include bleeding/hematoma at the site of femoral access, periprocedural thromboembolism, cardiac perforation/tamponade, esophageal injury including atrioesophageal fistula, PV stenosis, phrenic nerve injury, and radiation-induced skin injury. Development of reentrant and focal left atrial tachycardias, often more symptomatic than the initial AF, is also commonly seen after the procedure and may be transient.

13. **What is the role of AV nodal ablation followed by permanent pacing in treating AF?**
The guidelines specifically state that AV node ablation followed by permanent pacing should be used only as a fallback treatment rather than a primary strategy because of the risk of long-term right ventricular (RV) pacing. In general, patients most likely to benefit from this strategy are those with symptoms or tachycardia-mediated cardiomyopathy related to rapid ventricular rate during AF that cannot be controlled adequately with antiarrhythmic or negative chronotropic medications. Although the symptomatic benefits of AV nodal ablation are clear, limitations include the persistent need for anticoagulation, loss of AV synchrony, and lifelong pacemaker dependency.

BIBLIOGRAPHY, SUGGESTED READINGS, AND WEBSITES

1. Arnsdorf MF, Podrid PJ: Overview of the Presentation and Management of Atrial Fibrillation: http://www.utdol.com
2. Rosenthal L: Atrial Fibrillation: http://www.emedicine.com
3. Fuster V, Rydén LE, Cannom DS, et al: ACC/AHA/ESC 2006 guidelines for the management of patients with atrial fibrillation: a report of the American College of Cardiology/American Heart Association Task Force on Practice Guidelines and the European Society of Cardiology Committee for Practice Guidelines, *J Am Coll Cardiol* 48:e149-e246, 2006.
4. Gage BF, Waterman AD, et al: Validation of clinical classification schemes for predicting stroke: results from the National Registry of Atrial Fibrillation, *JAMA* 285:2864-2870, 2001.
5. Hsu L-F, Jaïs P, Sanders P, et al: Catheter ablation for atrial fibrillation in congestive heart failure, *N Engl J Med* 351:2373-2383, 2004.
6. Kalman J, Kim Y-H, Klein G, et al: Worldwide survey on the methods, efficacy, and safety of catheter ablation for human atrial fibrillation, *Circulation* 111:1100-1105, 2005.
7. Oral H, Pappone C, Morady F, et al: Circumferential pulmonary-vein ablation for chronic atrial fibrillation, *N Engl J Med* 354:934-941, 2006.
8. Van Gelder IC, Hagens VE, Bosker HA, et al: A comparison of rate control and rhythm control in patients with recurrent persistent atrial fibrillation, *N Engl J Med* 347:1834-1840, 2002.
9. Wolf PA, Abbott RD, Kannel WB: Atrial fibrillation as an independent risk factor for stroke: the Framingham Study, *Stroke* 22:983-988, 1991.
10. Wyse DG, Waldo AL, DiMarco JP, et al: The atrial fibrillation follow-up investigation of rhythm management (AFFIRM Investigators). A comparison of rate control and rhythm with atrial fibrillation, *N Engl J Med* 347:1825-1833, 2002.

CHAPTER 38

SUPRAVENTRICULAR TACHYCARDIA

Glenn N. Levine, MD, FACC, FAHA

1. **What does the term *supraventricular tachycardia (SVT)* mean?**
   By strict definition, a supraventricular tachycardia is any tachycardia whose genesis is not in the ventricles. Thus, the term can encompass atrial fibrillation and flutter, atrial tachycardia and multifocal atrial tachycardia, and reentrant tachycardias. Others will use the terms *SVT* or *paroxysmal SVT* to more specifically refer to the reentrant tachycardias of atrioventricular (AV) nodal reentrant tachycardia (AVNRT) and AV reentrant tachycardia (AVRT), as well as atrial tachycardia and several uncommon supraventricular arrhythmias. For the purposes of this chapter, we will use the term *SVT* to refer to any tachycardia not caused by ventricular tachycardia and the term *paroxysmal SVT* to refer to tachycardias as a result of AVNRT, AVRT, and atrial tachycardia (although the reader should recognize that this is somewhat arbitrary and not universally accepted, and we will not discuss in detail other rare causes of paroxysmal SVT).

2. **What is the most common cause of paroxysmal SVT?**
   AVNRT accounts for 60% to 70% of paroxysmal SVTs, followed by AVRT.

3. **What factors are part of the *generic* workup for supraventricular tachycardia?**
   - History, including type and duration of symptoms (palpitations, lightheadedness, chest pains, dyspnea, presyncope, precipitating factors)
   - Questions regarding the intake of alcohol, caffeine, and illicit drugs
   - Cardiac history (myocardial infarction, valvular disease, cardiac surgery)
   - Physical examination (although often unrevealing)
   - 12-lead electrocardiogram (ECG) (looking for signs of chamber enlargement, preexcitation, etc.)
   - Echocardiogram (often unrevealing because paroxysmal SVT can occur in the absence of structural heart disease, although atrial arrhythmias will often occur in the setting of dilated atria)
   - Laboratory tests (electrolyte abnormalities, hyperthyroidism)

4. **What are the causes of narrow complex regular tachycardias (regular referring to fixed R-R intervals—the time or *distance* between QRS complexes)?**
   - Sinus tachycardia (not really an arrhythmias but still in the differential)
   - Atrial flutter (Fig. 38-1)
   - Atrial tachycardia
   - AVNRT (Fig. 38-2)
   - AVRT
   - Rare causes of narrow complex QRS, especially in adults, that are often difficult to diagnose and are more suited for discussion at the cardiology fellow or attending level, include sinoatrial (SA) nodal reentrant tachycardia and focal junctional tachycardia.

5. **What are the causes of narrow complex irregular tachycardias (tachycardias with irregular R-R intervals)?**
   - Multifocal atrial tachycardia (MAT) (Fig. 38-3)
   - Atrial flutter with "variable conduction"
   - Atrial fibrillation

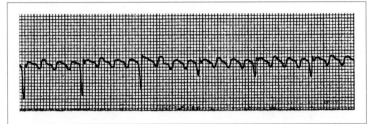

Figure 38-1. Atrial flutter. Note the *saw-tooth*–like flutter waves. Although most commonly there is 2:1 AV nodal conduction, in this case the patient has been treated with verapamil and there is 4:1 AV nodal conduction.

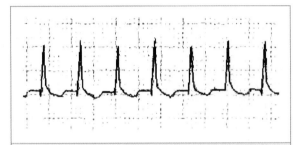

Figure 38-2. AV nodal reentrant tachycardia (AVNRT). No evidence of P waves or atrial activity is present.

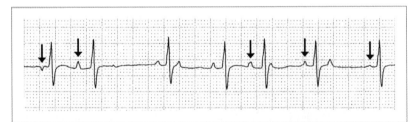

Figure 38-3. Multifocal atrial tachycardia (MAT). Multiple P waves of differing morphology *(arrows)* are present before each QRS complex in this narrow complex irregular tachycardia, making the diagnosis of MAT.

6. **How should one go about figuring out the diagnosis of a narrow complex tachycardia?**
This can be done in two simple steps. First, decide if the rhythm is regular or irregular. Second, look for P waves or atrial activity. Figure 38-4 demonstrates how this simple two-step process will lead to the correct diagnosis.

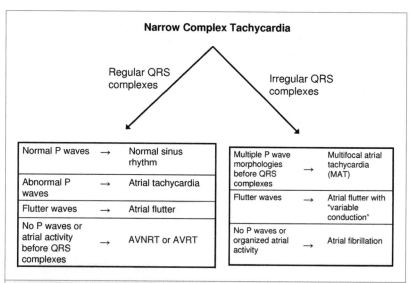

Figure 38-4. Simple algorithm for the diagnosis of narrow complex tachycardias. Step one is to decide if the rhythm is regular or irregular (are the QRS complexes occurring at regular or irregular intervals). Step two is to search for the presence of P waves or organized atrial activity.

7. **What drug is most commonly implicated in cases of drug-induced atrial tachycardia?**
Digoxin. Digoxin toxicity can cause many arrhythmias, including *paroxysmal atrial tachycardia with block*. In paroxysmal atrial tachycardia (PAT) with block, there is atrial tachycardia but also AV nodal block, leading to a slow ventricular response rate (Fig. 38-5). In cases of PAT with block, digoxin toxicity should be suspected.

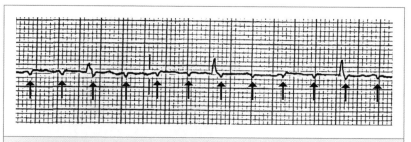

Figure 38-5. Atrial tachycardia with block. The finding of atrial tachycardia with significant AV node block is highly suggestive of digoxin toxicity.

8. **What is the most common ventricular response rate in patients who develop atrial flutter?**
Atrial flutter most commonly occurs at a rate of 300 beats/min, although the rate can be somewhat slower in patients on antiarrhythmic agents that slow ventricular conduction (such as amiodarone) or in cases of massively dilated atria. Most commonly, there is 2:1 AV block, meaning that only

every other atrial impulse is conducted down to the ventricles. Thus, the most common ventricular response rate is 150 beats/min. The finding of a regular narrow complex tachycardia at exactly 150 beats/min should raise suspicion of atrial flutter as the causative arrhythmia.

9. **Which is more common, AVNRT or AVRT?**
AVNRT is more common in the general population. In patients with known preexcitation syndrome (Wolff-Parkinson-White syndrome [WPW]), AVRT, which requires an accessory circuit, is more common. Thus, statistically, the cause of a narrow complex regular tachycardia is more likely to be AVNRT than AVRT, unless the patient has known WPW (or evidence of it on a baseline ECG).

10. **What is the most common cause of atrial tachycardia?**
Atrial tachycardia is most commonly caused by a discrete autonomic focus, although a microreentrant circuit can cause a small percentage of atrial tachycardias. Precipitating factors and causes of atrial tachycardia include:
   - Diseased atrial tissue (fibrosis, inflammation, etc.)
   - Increased sympathetic stimulation (hyperthyroidism, caffeine, etc.)
   - Excessive alcohol consumption
   - Digoxin toxicity
   - Electrolyte abnormalities
   - Hypoxemia

   Although textbooks describe the rate of atrial tachycardia as anywhere between 100 and 220 beats/min, a rate of approximately 160 to 180 beats is most common. AV conduction is usually 1:1 unless the tachycardia is very rapid, in which 2:1 conduction may occur. Because most cases of atrial tachycardia are due to an autonomic focus and not a reentrant pathway, the arrhythmia most commonly does not terminate with cardioversion. Adenosine usually (but not always) will not terminate the arrhythmia, but adenosine administration may be useful in cases in which the cause of regular SVT is unclear (see question 12 below).

11. **What is *concealed conduction*?**
In many patients with preexcitation syndrome (WPW), conduction from the atrium to the ventricle will result in the appearance of a *delta wave* on the 12-lead ECG. However, in some patients with WPW, the accessory bypass tract does not conduct in such an antegrade direction but only in a retrograde direction (*up* from the ventricle to the atrium). No delta wave appears on the baseline ECG because there is no antegrade conduction, but the accessory pathway is capable of retrograde conduction and participating in the genesis of AVRT (impulse travels down the His-Purkinje system, into the ventricle, and then up the accessory pathway into the atrium).

12. **In cases of SVT in which the cause is not clear, what is generally considered first-line drug therapy?**
Adenosine is most commonly administered in cases of SVT of unclear origin. Adenosine will transiently block AV nodal conduction. In patients with atrial flutter or atrial tachycardia, it will slow the ventricular response rate and may allow identification of flutter waves or the abnormal P waves of atrial tachycardia. In cases of AVNRT and AVRT, it may break the arrhythmia by interrupting the reentrant circuit. The dosing is 6 mg, administered quickly through a large-bore intravenous (IV) line, followed if unsuccessful in terminating the arrhythmia by a first dose of 12 mg, followed in term by a second dose of 12 mg. Lower doses of adenosine (such as 3 mg) are recommended by some authorities if adenosine is administered through a central line, and adenosine should be used with caution, if at all, in lower doses, in heart transplant patients.

   Although adenosine is a front-line agent for arrhythmia diagnosis and termination, it is not useful for more sustained ventricular rate control in patients with atrial fibrillation or atrial flutter because of its very short half-life. Patients who do not respond to adenosine can be treated acutely with IV beta-blockers or IV diltiazem or verapamil, both of which have onset of action within minutes and are good AV node blocking agents. Intravenous digoxin is not considered a good choice for acute therapy because its onset of action is approximately 1 hour.

13. **For what arrhythmia should AV nodal blocking agents *not* be administered?**
In rare cases of atrial fibrillation in the setting of an accessory bypass tract (WPW syndrome), some conduction of impulses will occur down the AV node and His-Purkinje system into the ventricle and some conduction down the bypass tract. In such cases, administration of AV nodal blocking agents (adenosine, digoxin, beta-blockers, calcium channel blockers) may lead to increased conduction down the accessory bypass tract, producing an increased ventricular response rate and possibly precipitating ventricular fibrillation.

14. **Do patients with atrial flutter require anticoagulation before cardioversion?**
Previously it was believed that the risk of embolization during cardioversion for atrial flutter was negligible. However, observational studies have reported rates of embolization with cardioversion of atrial flutter ranging between 1.7% to 7%. Although a collective review showed that the rate of embolization with cardioversion for atrial flutter was lower than for that with atrial fibrillation (2.2% versus 5% to 7%), expert consensus is that this rate is sufficient to warrant anticoagulation (and/or transesophageal echocardiogram) similar to that used in patients with atrial fibrillation who are to undergo cardioversion.

15. **Can SVT cause a wide QRS complex tachycardia?**
Yes. SVT occurring in the setting of baseline bundle branch block will produce a wide complex (QRS 120 msec or more) tachycardia. At faster heart rates, patients can also develop what is called *rate-related* bundle branch block. A wide complex SVT rarely can also be caused by AVRT with antedromic conduction.

16. **What is AVRT with antedromic conduction?**
In approximately 90% of cases of AVRT, the reentrant circuit is composed of conduction *down* the AV node and His-Purkinje system, into the ventricle, and then *up* the bypass tract (this is called orthodromic conduction). However, in about 10% of cases of AVRT, the reentrant circuit is composed of conduction from the atrium *down* the bypass tract, into the ventricle, and then *up* the His-Purkinje system and AV node and into the atrium. This is termed *antedromic conduction*. Because ventricular depolarization occurs without the use of the His-Purkinje system and left and right bundle branches, the QRS complexes appear wide.

17. **What factors make the diagnosis of a wide QRS complex more likely to be ventricular tachycardia (VT) than SVT?**
   - **P-wave dissociation** (also called AV dissociation): In P-wave dissociation, the QRS complexes occur at a greater rate than the P waves and there is no fixed relationship between the QRS complexes and the P waves. This finding is highly suggestive of VT. Unfortunately, P-wave dissociation can only be clearly discerned in 30% of cases of VT.
   - **QRS complex width:** In the absence of antiarrhythmic agents or an accessory pathway, a QRS width of more than 140 msec with a right bundle branch block (RBBB) morphology or a QRS width of more than 160 msec with a left bundle branch block (LBBB) morphology favors the diagnosis of VT.
   - **Negative concordance:** Negative concordance is the finding of similar QRS morphologies in all the precordial leads, with QS complexes present. This finding is essentially diagnostic for VT.
   - **Ventricular fusion beats:** Fusion beats are QRS complexes that may be formed from the *fusion* of an impulse originating in the ventricle with an impulse originating in the atria and traveling down the AV node and His-Purkinje system. The finding of fusion beats indicates VT.

   Importantly, the presence of stable hemodynamics and no cardiac symptoms does not distinguish between SVT and VT.

BIBLIOGRAPHY, SUGGESTED READINGS, AND WEBSITES

1. Blomström-Lundqvist C, Scheinman MM, Aliot EM, et al: ACC/AHA/ESC guidelines for the management of patients with supraventricular arrhythmias, *J Am Coll Cardiol* 42(8):1493-1531, 2003.
2. Delacrétaz E: Clinical practice. Supraventricular tachycardia, *N Engl J Med* 354(10):1039-1051, 2006.

CHAPTER 39

VENTRICULAR TACHYCARDIA

Jose L. Baez-Escudero, MD and Miguel Valderrábano, MD

1. **What is the differential diagnosis of a wide complex tachycardia (WCT)?**
   The differential includes the following:
   - Ventricular tachycardia (VT) (monomorphic or polymorphic)
   - Supraventricular tachycardia (SVT) with aberrant conduction or underlying bundle branch block
   - SVT using an accessory pathway (Wolff-Parkinson-White syndrome)
   - Toxicity related (hyperkalemia, digoxin, other drugs; Fig. 39-1)
   - Pacemaker-mediated tachycardia
   - Telemetry artifacts

   Of note, a wide-QRS tachycardia should always be presumed to be VT if the diagnosis is unclear. VT is defined as three or more consecutive QRS complexes arising from the ventricles. Sustained VT is that which causes symptoms or lasts more than 30 seconds.

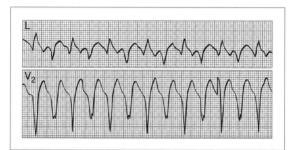

Figure 39-1. Bidirectional ventricular tachycardia in a patient with digitalis toxicity. (Modified from Marriott HJL, Conover MB: *Advanced concepts in arrhythmias,* ed 2, St. Louis, 1989, Mosby.)

2. **What is the pathophysiologic substrate of ventricular tachycardia?**
   It depends on the clinical scenario, but the most common mechanism is reentry, followed by automaticity.

3. **What is the most common underlying heart disease predisposing to VT?**
   Coronary artery disease and coronary ischemia. VT in the setting of acute ischemia and immediately after myocardial infarction (MI) is related to excess ventricular ectopy as a result of increased automaticity (Na-K pump malfunction, increase in intracellular calcium, tissue acidosis, and locally released catecholamines). After completion of an infarct, patients with resultant ischemic cardiomyopathy can suffer from recurrent sustained monomorphic VT. In this case, VT originates in scarred myocardium where islands of infarcted tissue surrounded by strands of functional myocytes provide the substrate for the creation of a reentrant circuit.

4. **Can VT occur in other nonischemic heart diseases?**

Scar-related VT can occur in other nonischemic conditions whenever an inflammatory or infiltrative disorder damages the myocardium. Sarcoidosis or Chagas' disease are typical examples in which VT can occur as a result of such nonischemic scars. Fatty infiltration of the right ventricle leads to areas of unexcitable myocardium that can generate reentrant circuits in patients with arrhythmogenic right ventricular dysplasia. Myocardial scars leading to reentry also occur after surgical correction of congenital heart diseases. Dilated cardiomyopathies can lead to reentry within the diseased conduction system, the so-called bundle-branch reentry, where impulses use the right and left bundles as antegrade and retrograde pathways (less commonly in the opposite direction). Conceivably, any structural heart disease can lead to reentry.

5. **Can VT occur in the absence of structural heart disease?**

VT can occur in the structurally normal heart. Monomorphic VT occurs in two distinct clinical entities in the absence of heart disease. One is outflow tract VT. This condition leads to VT typically during or after exercise or in enhanced catecholamine states. It is thought to be generated by triggered activity in the form of delayed after-depolarizations, typically created in situations of calcium overload. It originates most commonly from the right ventricular outflow tract but occasionally can arise from the left ventricular outflow tract and even the aortic cusps. The second condition is idiopathic fascicular VT (also known as verapamil-sensitive, or Belhassen's, VT). It typically occurs in young healthy individuals with normal hearts and most commonly involves a right bundle branch block (RBBB) and left anterior fascicular block pattern, because it arises from the left posterior fascicle. Both these forms are curable with mapping and ablation.

Primary electrical disorders can also lead to VT. Familial long QT syndromes typically lead to torsades des pointes, as does short QT syndrome. Brugada syndrome leads to primary ventricular fibrillation (Fig. 39-2). Catecholaminergic polymorphic ventricular tachycardia (CPVT) is a mutation of the ryanodine receptor that typically causes exercise-induced bidirectional and polymorphic VT.

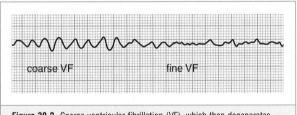

Figure 39-2. Coarse ventricular fibrillation (VF), which then degenerates further into fine ventricular fibrillation. (From Goldberger E: *Treatment of cardiac emergencies,* ed 5, St. Louis, 1990, Mosby.)

6. **What electrocardiogram features favor VT as the cause of a wide complex tachycardia (WCT)?**

VT rhythms have rates between 100 and 280 beats/min and can be monomorphic or polymorphic. Typical electrocardiogram (ECG) clues that favor VT include the following:

- Presence of **fusion beats,** which identify simultaneous depolarization of the ventricle by both the normal conduction system and an ectopic impulse originating in the ventricle.
- **Capture beats,** which are normally conducted sinus beats with a narrow QRS complex that generally occur at a shorter interval than the tachycardia.
- **Atrioventricular (AV) dissociation,** the finding of independent atrial and ventricular activity at differing rates (30% of cases). Look for visible P waves that "march through" (scan and compare ST segments and T waves, look for subtle QRS changes). If there are more QRSs than Ps, it is likely to be VT. If AV dissociation is not obvious, it can be unmasked with carotid sinus massage or administration of adenosine.

- A **QRS width** more than 140 msec (RBBB morphology) or more than 160 msec (left bundle branch block [LBBB] morphology). These suggest VT, especially in the setting of a normal QRS during sinus rhythm.
- Limb lead concordance (identical QRS direction). If QRS is negative in I, II, and III (an extreme leftward or **northwest axis**), this strongly favors VT.
- **Precordial lead concordance** (V1–V6), especially negative concordance. This is highly specific for the diagnosis of VT.
- Certain **QRS morphologic features** also may be helpful. Most aberrant conduction patterns have a precordial rS complex, whereas the absence of rS complexes suggests VT. An atypical right bundle pattern (R > R'), a monophasic or biphasic QRS in lead V1, and a small R wave coupled with a large deep S wave or a Q-S complex in V6 support the diagnosis of VT.
- **Presence of Q waves.** Remember that postinfarction Q waves are preserved in VT. Their presence in WCT is a sign of previous infarction; therefore, VT is more likely.

7. **What is torsade de pointes?**

Torsade de pointes, or *torsades,* is a French term that literally means "twisting of the points." It was first described by Dessertenne in 1966 and refers to a polymorphic intermediate ventricular rhythm between VT and ventricular fibrillation. It has a distinct morphology in which cycles of tachycardia with alternating peaks of QRS amplitude turn about the isoelectric line in a regular pattern (Fig. 39-3). Before the rhythm is triggered, a baseline prolonged QT interval and pathologic U waves are present, reflecting abnormal ventricular repolarization. A short-long-short sequence between the R-R interval (marked bradycardia or preceding pause) occurs before the trigger response. Drugs that prolong the QT (e.g., antiarrhythmics, some antibiotics and antifungals, tricyclic antidepressants) and electrolyte disorders such as hypokalemia and hypomagnesemia are common triggers. When the ECG finding occurs, it should be treated as any life-threatening VT, and immediate efforts must be made to determine the underlying cause of QT lengthening.

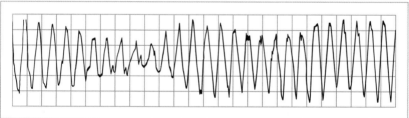

Figure 39-3. Torsades de pointes, in which the QRS axis seems to rotate about the isoelectric point. (Modified from Olgin JE, Zipes DP: Specific arrhythmias: diagnosis and treatment. In Libby P, Bonow R, Mann D, et al: *Braunwald's heart disease: a textbook of cardiovascular medicine,* ed 8, Philadelphia, 2008, Saunders.)

8. **What critical decisions must be made in the management of sustained VT?**

The critical decision in the management of a patient with sustained VT is the urgency with which to treat the rhythm. In a hemodynamically stable and minimally symptomatic patient, treatment should be delayed until a 12-lead ECG can be obtained. The axis and morphology help to make the diagnosis of VT, as well as shed light on the potential mechanism and origin of the rhythm. During the delay, a brief medical history and baseline laboratory values can be obtained (especially serum levels of potassium and magnesium, as well as cardiac biomarkers). Specific attention should be paid to a history of myocardial infarction, systolic heart failure, history of structural heart disease, family history of sudden cardiac death, and potentially proarrhythmic drugs.

9. **What methods are used to terminate sustained VT?**
   With any question of hemodynamic instability, termination should be done immediately with synchronized direct current electrical cardioversion. Hemodynamic instability is defined as hypotension resulting in shock, congestive heart failure, myocardial ischemia (infarction or angina), or signs or symptoms of inadequate cerebral perfusion. It is important to ensure that the energy is delivered in a synchronized fashion before cardioversion. Failure to do so may accelerate the rhythm or induce ventricular fibrillation. If the patient is conscious, adequate intravenous (IV) sedation should always be provided. Termination of hemodynamically stable VT may be attempted medically. Reasonable drugs of choice are IV procainamide (or amjaline in some European countries), lidocaine, and IV amiodarone. If VT is associated with acute ischemia, urgent angiography and revascularization are paramount. IV beta-blockers, followed by IV antiarrhythmics (amiodarone and procainamide), are recommended. For ischemic monomorphic VT, intravenous lidocaine is also a reasonable option. Pace termination (either through transvenous insertion of a temporary pacer or by reprogramming an implantable cardioverter defibrillator [ICD]) can be useful to treat patients with sustained monomorphic VT that is refractory to cardioversion or is recurrent despite the use of the above-mentioned drugs.

10. **Once the acute episode is terminated, what are the next managing strategies?**
    This depends on the clinical situation and on the individual patient. Any potentially reversible cause should be sought and treated aggressively—specifically, ischemia, heart failure, or electrolyte abnormalities. In general, beta-blockers are usually safe and effective and should be administered in most patients in whom concomitant antiarrhythmic drugs are indicated. Amiodarone and sotalol have been the mainstay of preventive therapy, especially in patients with left ventricle (LV) dysfunction. However, the long-term clinical success of medical regimens is low, and amiodarone caries a risk of serious side effects. All patients should be risk stratified for the likelihood of recurrence and subsequent risk of sudden cardiac death. Appropriate consultation with an electrophysiologist should be obtained to assess the need for ICD implantation. (Indications for ICDs are discussed in Chapter 42.) Although cardiac device therapy has revolutionized treatment providing excellent protection from sudden cardiac death, it does not prevent recurrences. Patients with defibrillators may remain symptomatic with palpitations, syncope, and recurrent shocks for VT. Ablation of the reentrant circuits that cause VT also provides a nonpharmacologic option for the reduction of symptoms.

11. **How is catheter ablation of VT performed?**
    VT ablation remains challenging and is offered primarily at experienced centers. Endocardial mapping of VT to identify an optimal region for ablation can be time consuming because of the complexity of the reentry circuits and the existence of certain circuit portions deep into the endocardium. Most ventricular reentry circuits have an exit somewhere along the border zone of the infarct scars. It is near such an exit that sinus rhythm pacing (pace mapping) is expected to produce a QRS morphology similar to that of VT. This approach, combined with modern three-dimensional voltage-mapping technologies that reconstruct and relate electrophysiologic characteristics to specific anatomy, have greatly facilitated the ablation procedure. Ablation can be achieved using traditional radiofrequency or with other technologies like cryoablation or laser. When endocardial circuits are resistant to ablation, the technique of transthoracic pericardial access with epicardial mapping of VT is used. This approach facilitates localization and ablation of deep and epicardial circuits and requires the insertion of a sheath into the pericardial space using a needle and guidewire under fluoroscopic control. If a separate indication for heart surgery is present (e.g., need for surgical revascularization, LV aneurysmectomy, mitral valve repair or replacement), surgical ablation may be considered.

12. **When is catheter ablation used to treat VT?**

Ablation has traditionally been used for secondary prevention after an ICD-terminated VT and as an alternative to chronic antiarrhythmic therapy. It may also be considered as an option for reducing ICD therapies in patients with recurrent appropriate shocks and as an alternative to drug therapy for idiopathic VT. The success rates vary depending on an individual's substrate for the arrhythmia. A patient with a VT arising from the right ventricular outflow tract in a structurally normal heart will likely have a much higher success rate when compared with a patient with a severely reduced ejection fraction from a large anterior wall MI with multiple VT morphologies. The target endpoint of any VT ablation is always lack of inducible VT.

BIBLIOGRAPHY, SUGGESTED READINGS, AND WEBSITES

1. Compton SJ: Ventricular Tachycardia: http://www.emedicine.com

2. Podrid P: Invasive Cardiac Electrophysiology Studies: Tachyarrhythmias: http://www.utdol.com

3. Podril P, Ganz LI: Approach to the Diagnosis and Treatment of Wide QRS Complex Tachycardias: http://www.utdol.com

4. Brugada P, Brugada J, Mont L, et al: A new approach to the differential diagnosis of a regular tachycardia with a wide QRS complex, *Circulation* 83:1649-1659, 1991.

5. Marchlinski FE, Callans DJ, Gottlieb CD, et al: Linear ablation lesions for control of unmappable ventricular tachycardia in patients with ischemic and nonischemic cardiomyopathy, *Circulation* 101:1288-1296, 2000.

6. Reddy VY, Reynolds MR, Neuzil P, et al: Prophylactic catheter ablation for the prevention of defibrillator therapy, *N Engl J Med* 357:2657-2665, 2007.

7. Stevenson W, Friedman P, Kocovic D, et al: Radiofrequency catheter ablation of ventricular tachycardia after myocardial infarction, *Circulation* 98:308-314, 1998.

8. Zipes DP, Camm AJ, Borggrefe M, et al: ACC/AHA/ESC 2006 guidelines for management of patients with ventricular arrhythmias and the prevention of sudden cardiac death: a report of the American College of Cardiology/American Heart Association Task Force and the European Society of Cardiology Committee for Practice Guidelines (Writing Committee to Develop Guidelines for Management of Patients with Ventricular Arrhythmias and the Prevention of Sudden Cardiac Death): developed in collaboration with the European Heart Rhythm Association and the Heart Rhythm Society, *Circulation* 114:e385-e484, 2006.

CHAPTER 40

AMIODARONE AND ANTIARRHYTHMIC DRUGS

Glenn N. Levine, MD, FACC, FAHA

1. **Which antiarrhythmic drug is considered to be *most effective* in maintaining sinus rhythm in patients with recent atrial fibrillation?**
Amiodarone is considered the most effective drug in maintaining sinus rhythm. Although it is not FDA-approved for this indication, it is the most commonly used drug for this purpose. In one study, it has been shown to have a 1-year efficacy rate for maintaining sinus rhythm of greater than 60%, compared with 50% or less for other antiarrhythmic agents. However, because of its side effects and potential for end-organ toxicity, sotalol and dofetilide are preferred as first-line agents in many patients.

2. **What are the main side effects of amiodarone?**
Amiodarone can affect many organ systems, including the heart's conduction system, the lungs, the central nervous system, the gastrointestinal (GI) tract and liver, the thyroid gland, and the eyes. Table 40-1 lists the main side effects of amiodarone, as well as their frequency, diagnosis, and management.

TABLE 40-1. ADVERSE REACTIONS TO AMIODARONE		
Symptoms	Incidence (%)	Diagnosis/Management
Pulmonary toxicity with cough and/or dyspnea, pulmonary fibrosis	2	High-resolution CT scan, decrease in DLCO. Discontinue drug. Consider corticosteroids
Nausea, anorexia, constipation	30	Symptoms may decrease with decrease in dose
AST or ALT elevation >2 times normal	15–30	If hepatitis considered, exclude other causes
Hepatitis and cirrhosis	<3	Consider discontinuation, biopsy, or both
Hypothyroidism	4–22	Thyroid function tests. L-Thyroxine
Hyperthyroidism	2–12	Thyroid function tests. Corticosteroids, PTU or methimazole. May need to discontinue drug
Blue skin discoloration	<10	Reassurance. Decrease in dose

(Continued)

TABLE 40-1. ADVERSE REACTIONS TO AMIODARONE (CONTINUED)

Symptoms	Incidence (%)	Diagnosis/Management
Photosensitivity	25–75	Avoidance of prolonged sun exposure
Central nervous system symptoms (ataxia, parasthesias, peripheral polyneuropathy, impaired memory, tremor, sleep disturbance)	3–30	Often dose dependent; may improve or resolve with dose adjustment
Halo vision, especially at night	<5	Corneal deposits the norm
Optic neuropathy	≤1	Discontinue drug and consult ophthalmology
Photophobia, visual blurring, and microdeposits	>90	
Bradycardia and AV block	5	May need to decrease/discontinue dose or consider pacemaker
Proarrhythmia	<1	May need to discontinue drug
Epididymitis and erectile dysfunction	<1	Pain may resolve spontaneously

AST, Alanine trasaminase; *ALT,* aspartate aminotransferase; *AV,* atrioventricular; *CT,* Computed tomography; *DLCO,* carbon monoxide diffusing capacity; *PTU,* propylthiouracil.

Modified from Goldschlager N, Epstein AE, Naccarelli GV et al: Practice Guidelines Sub-committee, North American Society of Pacing and Electrophysiology (HRS). A practical guide for clinicians who treat patients with amiodarone, *Heart Rhythm* 4(9):1250-1259, 2007.

3. What is the loading dose of amiodarone?
This depends on the situation.
   - For life-threatening VT, such as during a "code blue" a 300-mg loading dose is administered. This can be followed by an additional 150-mg loading dose 3 to 5 minutes after the initial 300-mg dose.
   - For ventricular arrhythmias, the suggested dosing is as follows: an initial "bolus" of 150 mg is given intravenously (IV) over 10 minutes, followed by an infusion of 1 mg/min for 6 hours (total 360 mg), then an infusion of 0.5 mg/min over the next 18 hours (540 mg).
   - Oral "loading doses" of amiodarone are not standardized and vary somewhat physician to physician. Generally, total daily doses of 400 to 800 mg are administered in divided doses (twice a day, three times a day [bid-tid]) for several weeks. Some practitioners will decrease the total daily loading dose after 1 to 2 weeks and administer a lower total dose for 1 to 2 weeks. Maintenance doses for ventricular arrhythmias are usually 200 to 400 mg daily, and maintenance doses for atrial fibrillation are most commonly 200 mg daily (with a range of 100–400 mg daily).

4. Can amiodarone be safely started in a patient with an implantable cardioverter defibrillator (ICD) without any subsequent electrophysiology follow-up?
No. Amiodarone can increase the defibrillation threshold (the minimum energy required to be generated by the ICD to terminate ventricular tachycardia/ventricular fibrillation), and

amiodarone may slow the rate of ventricular tachycardia, so that the ICD may not recognize and treat the arrhythmia if it occurs. Thus, decisions regarding amiodarone initiation or dose titration should be made in consultation with a cardiologist or electrophysiologist.

5. **What baseline and subsequent tests should be routinely obtained in asymptomatic patients started and maintained on amiodarone?**
   - Liver function tests at baseline and every 6 months
   - Thyroid function tests (thyroid-stimulating hormone [TSH], free T4) at baseline and every 6 months
   - Chest radiograph at baseline and then yearly
   - Pulmonary function tests (including carbon monoxide diffusion in the lung [DLCO]) at baseline and subsequently if clinically indicated because of unexplained pulmonary symptoms
   - Electrocardiogram at baseline and then yearly
   - Ophthalmologic evaluation should be obtained at baseline in patients with significant baseline visual abnormalities and subsequently if clinically indicated

6. **What are the most important drug interactions that occur with amiodarone?**
   Amiodarone interacts with numerous drugs. Particularly important are its interactions with digoxin and warfarin, because these drugs are often also used in the treatment of atrial fibrillation. Because amiodarone increases the concentration of digoxin and its effects on the sinoatrial (SA) and atrioventricular (AV) nodes, which are also affected by amiodarone, reducing the dose of digoxin (such as halving the dose) when starting amiodarone is recommended. Because amiodarone increases the concentration and effect on the international normalized ratio (INR) of warfarin, reducing the dose of warfarin (such as halving the dose) when starting amiodarone is recommended, with more closely and more frequently monitored INR levels. Table 40-2 highlights some of the major drug interactions with amiodarone. A more complete list is given in the excellent review article by Vassallo and Trohman, "Prescribing Amiodarone: An Evidence-Based Review of Clinical Indications" (see Bibliography).

TABLE 40-2. SELECTED MAJOR DRUG INTERACTIONS WITH AMIODARONE

Drug	Interactions
Digoxin	Increased concentration and effect with SA and AV node depression/block Increased GI and neurologic toxicity
Warfarin	Increased concentration and effect (raises INR)
Type Ia antiarrhythmics (quinidine, procainamide, disopyrimide)	Increased concentration and effect Increased risk of torsades de pointes/ventricular tachycardia
Diltiazem, verapamil, beta-blockers	Increased bradycardia and AV block, because amiodarone also affects SA and AV nodes
Flecainide	Increased concentration and effect
Phenytoin	Increased concentration and effect
Anesthetic drugs	Hypotension and bradycardia
Cyclosporine	Increased concentration and effect
Simvastatin, atorvastatin	Can promote liver abnormalities

Modified from Goldschlager N, Epstein AE, Naccarelli GV, et al: Practice Guidelines Sub-committee, North American Society of Pacing and Electrophysiology (HRS). A practical guide for clinicians who treat patients with amiodarone, *Heart Rhythm* 4(9):1250-1259, 2007.

7. **What is the loading dose of lidocaine?**
For life-threatening ventricular arrhythmias, the regimen is as follows: 1 to 1.5 mg/kg IV, with subsequent doses of 0.5 to 0.75 mg/kg IV given over 5- to 10-minute intervals, to a maximum total lidocaine dose of 3 mg/kg. The subsequent maintenance dose is 2 to 4 mg/min (most commonly 2 mg/min).

8. **What is "lidocaine toxicity"?**
Lidocaine may cause a variety of central nervous system symptoms, including seizures, visual disturbances, tremors, coma, and confusion. Such symptoms are often referred to as "lidocaine toxicity". The risks of lidocaine toxicity are increased in elderly patients, those with depressed left ventricular function, and those with liver disease. In such patients, a lower maintenance dose (such as 1 mg/min) is sometimes used.

9. **What are the main side effects of sotalol?**
Sotalol (Betapace) is most commonly used in the treatment of atrial fibrillation. Because of its beta-blocking properties, it has many of the same side effects as commonly used beta-blockers. Worsening congestive heart failure can occur. An important side effect is QT-segment prolongation and torsades de pointes. Torsade de pointes occurs in approximately 2% of patients. Therefore, the QT segment should be carefully monitored and patients should be on telemetry during sotalol loading. The incidence of torsade de pointes is reported to be 3.4% to 5.6% for a QT_c interval of 500 to 550 msec and 10.8% for a QT_c interval of more than 550 msec. Different physicians will have different criteria for the amount of QT prolongation they will tolerate, but in general the QT_c should certainly not exceed 550 msec. Because sotalol has significant renal clearance, the dosing interval should be increased in patients with renal insufficiency to decrease the risks of adverse side effects and should not be used if renal function is unstable. Sotalol should not be used in patients with left ventricular hypertrophy (unless they have an ICD).

10. **What are the main side effects of propafenone?**
Propafenone (Rythmol) is a class IC antiarrhythmic that is most commonly used in the treatment of supraventricular arrhythmias. It has structural similarities to propranolol and has many of the same side effects as common beta-blockers.

BIBLIOGRAPHY, SUGGESTED READINGS, AND WEBSITES

1. American Heart Association 2005 Guidelines for CPR and ECC: http://www.americanheart.org
2. Giardina EG: Therapeutic Use of Amiodarone: http://www.utdol.com
3. *Advanced cardiovascular life support provider manual*, Dallas, 2006, American Heart Association.
4. Goldschlager N, Epstein AE, Naccarelli GV, et al: Practice Guidelines Sub-committee, North American Society of Pacing and Electrophysiology (HRS). A practical guide for clinicians who treat patients with amiodarone, *Heart Rhythm* 4(9):1250-1259, 2007.
5. Fuster V, Rydén LE, Cannom DS, et al: ACC/AHA/ESC 2006 guidelines for the management of patients with atrial fibrillation, *Circulation* 114(7):e257-e354, 2006.
6. Vassallo P, Trohman RG: Prescribing amiodarone: an evidence-based review of clinical indications, *JAMA* 298(11):1312-1322, 2007.
7. Zipes DP, Camm AJ, Borggrefe M, et al: ACC/AHA/ESC 2006 guidelines for management of patients with ventricular arrhythmias and the prevention of sudden cardiac death, *J Am Coll Cardiol* 48(5):247-356, 2006.

CHAPTER 41

CARDIAC PACEMAKERS AND RESYNCHRONIZATION THERAPY

Jose L. Baez-Escudero, MD and Miguel Valderrábano, MD

1. **What are the components of a pacing system?**
   Pacing systems consist of a pulse generator and pacing leads, which can be placed in either the atria or the ventricles. Pacemakers provide an electrical stimulus to cause cardiac depolarization during periods when intrinsic cardiac electrical activity is inappropriately slow or absent. The battery most commonly used in permanent pacers has a life span of 5 to 9 years.

2. **What is the accepted pacing nomenclature for the different pacing modalities?**
   The North American Society of Pacing and Electrophysiology and the British Pacing and Electrophysiology Group have developed a code to describe various pacing modes. It usually consists of three letters, but some systems use four or five:
   - Letter 1: chamber that is paced (*A* = atria, *V* = ventricles, *D* = dual chamber)
   - Letter 2: chamber that is sensed (*A* = atria, *V* = ventricles, *D* = dual chamber, *0* = none)
   - Letter 3: response to a sensed event (*I* = pacing inhibited, *T* = pacing triggered, *D* = dual, *0* = none)
   - Letter 4: rate-responsive features (an activity sensor), for example, an accelerometer in the pulse generator that detects bodily movement and increases the pacing rate according to a programmable algorithm (*R* = rate-responsive pacemaker)
   - Letter 5: Antitachycardia features

   A pacemaker in VVI mode denotes that it paces and senses the ventricle and is inhibited by a sensed ventricular event. The DDD mode denotes that both chambers are capable of being sensed and paced.

3. **What is the most important clinical feature that establishes the need for cardiac pacing?**
   The most important clinical feature consists of symptoms clearly associated with bradycardia. Symptomatic bradycardia is the cardinal feature in the placement of a permanent pacemaker in acquired atrioventricular (AV) block in adults. Reversible causes, such as drug toxicity (digoxin, beta-blockers, and calcium channel blockers), electrolyte abnormalities, Lyme disease, transient increases in vagal tone, and sleep apnea syndrome, should be sought, and the offending agents should be discontinued. The clinical manifestations of symptomatic bradycardia include fatigue, lightheadedness, dizziness, presyncope, syncope, manifestations of cerebral ischemia, dyspnea on exertion, decreased exercise tolerance, and congestive heart failure.

4. **What are the three types of acquired AV block?**
   There are three degrees of AV block: first, second, and third (complete). This classification is based on both the electrocardiogram and the anatomic location of the conduction disturbance.

   First-degree block refers to a stable prolongation of the PR interval to more than 200 msec and represents delay in conduction at the level of the AV node. There are no class I indications for pacing in isolated asymptomatic first-degree block.

   Second-degree block is divided into two types. Mobitz type I (Wenckebach) exhibits progressive prolongation of the PR interval before an atrial impulse fails to stimulate the ventricle. Anatomically, this form of block occurs above the bundle of His in the AV node. Type II exhibits

no prolongation of the PR interval before a dropped beat and anatomically occurs at the level of the bundle of His. This rhythm may be associated with a wide QRS complex.

Third-degree or **complete block** defines the absence of AV conduction and refers to complete dissociation of the atrial and ventricular rhythms, with a ventricular rate less than the atrial rate. The width and rate of the ventricular escape rhythm help to identify an anatomic location for the block: narrow QRS is associated with minimal slowing of the rate, generally at the AV node, and wide QRS is associated with considerable slowing of rate at or below the bundle of His. Permanent pacemaker implantation is indicated for third-degree and advanced second-degree AV block at any anatomic level associated with bradycardia with symptoms (including heart failure) or ventricular arrhythmias presumed to be due to AV block.

5. **What is the anatomic location of bifascicular or trifascicular block?**
Bifascicular block is located below the AV node and involves a combination of block at the level of the right bundle with block within one of the fascicles of the left bundle (left anterior or left posterior fascicle).

Trifascicular block refers to the presence of a prolonged PR interval in addition to a bifascicular block. Based on the surface electrocardiogram (ECG), it is impossible to tell whether the prolonged PR interval is due to delay at the AV node (suprahisian) or in the remaining conducting fascicle (infrahisian, hence the term *trifascicular block*). Pacing is indicated when bifascicular or trifascicular block is associated with the following:
  ■ Complete block and symptomatic bradycardia
  ■ Alternating bundle branch block
  ■ Intermittent type II second-degree block with or without related symptoms
  ■ Symptoms suggestive of bradycardia and an HV interval greater than 100 ms on invasive electrophysiology study

6. **When is pacing indicated for asymptomatic bradycardia?**
There are few indications for pacing in patients with bradycardia who are truly asymptomatic:
  ■ Third-degree AV block with documented asystole lasting 3 or more seconds (in sinus rhythm) or escape rates below 40 beats/min in patients while awake
  ■ Third-degree AV block or second-degree AV Mobitz type II block in patients with chronic bifascicular and trifascicular block
  ■ Congenital third-degree AV block with a wide QRS escape rhythm, ventricular dysfunction, or bradycardia markedly inappropriate for age
Potential (class II) indications for pacing in asymptomatic patients include the following:
  ■ Third-degree AV block with faster escape rates in patients who are awake
  ■ Second-degree AV Mobitz type II block in patients without bifascicular or trifascicular block
  ■ The finding on electrophysiologic study of block below or within the bundle of His or an HV interval of 100 msec or longer
When bradycardia, even if extreme, is present only during sleep, pacing is not indicated.

7. **What is *sick sinus syndrome*?**
Sinus node dysfunction (SND), also referred to as *sick sinus syndrome,* is a common cause of bradycardia. Its prevalence has been estimated to be as high as 1 in 600 patients over the age of 65 years, and the syndrome accounts for approximately 50% of pacemaker implantations in the United States. Sinus node dysfunction may be due to replacement of nodal tissue with fibrous tissue at the sinus node itself, or it may be due to extrinsic causes (drugs, electrolyte imbalance, hypothermia, hypothyroidism, increased intracranial pressure, and excessive vagal tone). Abnormal automaticity and conduction in the atrium predispose patients to atrial fibrillation and flutter, and the bradycardia–tachycardia syndrome is a common manifestation of sinus node dysfunction. Therapy to control the ventricular rate during tachycardia by blocking AV conduction with ß-adrenergic blockers, calcium-channel blockers, or digitalis may not be possible, because it may further depress the sinus node. Permanent pacemaker implantation is

indicated for sinus-node dysfunction with documented symptomatic bradycardia, including frequent sinus pauses that produce symptoms. It is also indicated for symptomatic chronotropic incompetence and for symptomatic sinus bradycardia that results from required drug therapy for medical conditions (rate control for atrial tachyarrhythmias, chronic stable angina, systolic heart failure).

8. **Is pacing indicated for neurocardiogenic syncope?**
   Neurocardiogenic syncope occurs when triggering of a neural reflex results in a usually self-limited episode of systemic hypotension characterized by both bradycardia and peripheral vasodilation. Many of these patients have a prominent vasodepressor component to their syndrome, and implantation of a pacemaker may not completely relieve symptoms. Hence, the role of pacing in patients with neurocardiac syncope and confirmed bradycardia is controversial. When bradycardia occurs only in specific situations, patient education, pharmacologic trials, and prevention strategies are indicated before pacing in most patients.

9. **What are the indications for pacing after myocardial infarction (MI)?**
   Indications in this setting do not require the presence of symptoms. The indications in large part are to treat the intraventricular conduction defects that result from infarction. Pacing is indicated in the setting of acute MI for the following:
   - Complete third-degree block or advanced second-degree block that is associated with block in the His-Purkinje system (wide complex ventricular rhythm)
   - Transient advanced (second- or third-degree) AV block with a new bundle branch block. Pacing in the setting of an acute MI may be temporary rather than long-term or permanent.

10. **What are potential complications associated with pacemaker implantation?**
    Complications in the hands of experienced operators are rare (approximately 1% to 2%) and include the following: bleeding, infection, pneumothorax, hemothorax, cardiac arrhythmias, cardiac perforation causing tamponade, diaphragmatic/phrenic nerve pacing, pocket hematoma, coronary sinus trauma, and prolonged radiation exposure. Late complications include erosion of the pacer through the skin (requires pacer replacement, lead extraction, and systemic antibiotics), and lead malfunction (lead fracture, break in lead insulation, or dislodgement).

11. **What is pacemaker syndrome?**
    Historically, *pacemaker syndrome* refers to progressive worsening of symptoms, particularly congestive heart failure, after single-chamber ventricular pacing. This was due to asynchronous ventricular pacing, leading to inappropriately timed atrial contractions, including those occurring during ventricular systole. Dual-chamber pacing and appropriate pacing mode selection prevent the occurance of pacemaker syndrome. Pseudopacemaker syndrome occurs when a patient without a pacemaker has PR prolongation so severe that the P waves are closer to the preceding R waves than to the following ones, leading to atrial contractions during the preceding ventricular systole.

12. **What is Twiddler's syndrome?**
    Twiddler's syndrome is a rare complication of pacemaker implantation caused by repetitive and often unintentional twisting of the generator in the pacemaker pocket, producing lead dislodgement or fracture and subsequent pacemaker failure. It is most commonly observed in patients with behavioral disorders.

13. **What is pacemaker-mediated tachycardia?**
    Pacemaker-mediated tachycardia (PMT) is a form of reentrant tachycardia that can occur in patients who have a dual-chamber pacemaker. If the AV node retrogradely conducts a ventricular-paced beat or a premature ventricular contraction (PVC) back to the atrium and depolarizes the atrium before the next atrial-paced beat, this atrial activation will be sensed by the pacemaker atrial lead and interpreted as an intrinsic atrial depolarization. Consecutively,

the pacemaker will then pace the ventricle after the programmed AV delay and perpetuate the cycle of ventricular pacing–retrograde ventriculo–atrial (VA) conduction–atrial sensing–ventricular pacing (the pacemaker forms the antegrade limb of the circuit, and the AV node is the retrograde limb). Consider PMT in patients with a dual-chamber pacemaker who experience palpitations, rapid heart rates, lightheadedness, syncope, or chest discomfort. It is corrected by programming the pacemaker with a postventricular atrial refractory period (PVARP) so that atrial events occurring shortly after ventricular events are ignored by the pacemaker.

14. **What is cardiac resynchronization therapy?**

Cardiac resynchronization therapy (CRT) refers to simultaneous pacing of both ventricles (biventricular [Bi-V] pacing). The rationale for CRT is based on the observation that the presence of a bundle branch block or other intraventricular conduction delay can worsen systolic heart failure by causing ventricular dyssynchrony, thereby reducing the efficiency of contraction. Pacing of the left ventricle (LV) is achieved either by placing a transvenous lead in the lateral venous system of the heart through the coronary sinus (preferred approach; Fig. 41-1) or by placement of an epicardial LV lead (requires a limited thoracotomy and general anesthesia). The rationale for CRT is that ventricular dyssynchrony can further impair the pump function of a failing ventricle. Potential mechanisms of benefit include improved contractile function (improvement in ejection fraction, increase in cardiac index and blood pressure, decrease in pulmonary capillary wedge pressure) and reverse ventricular remodeling (reductions in LV end-systolic and end-diastolic dimensions, severity of mitral regurgitation, and LV mass).

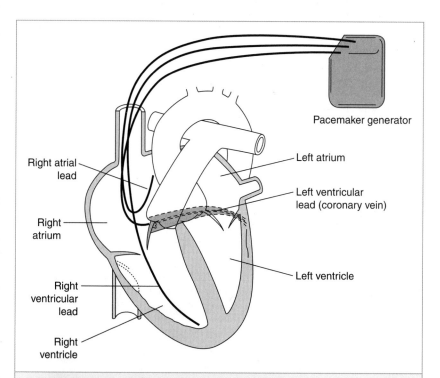

Figure 41-1. Biventricular pacemaker. Note the pacemaker lead in the coronary sinus vein that allows pacing of the left ventricle simultaneously with the right ventricle. Bi-V pacing is used in selected patients with congestive heart failure with left ventricular conduction delays to help *resynchronize* cardiac activation and thereby improve cardiac function. (From Goldberger AL: *Clinical electrocardiography: a simplified approach,* ed 7, Philadelphia, 2006, Mosby.)

15. **When is CRT indicated?**

CRT is indicated in patients with advanced heart failure (usually New York Heart Association [NYHA] class III or IV), severe systolic dysfunction (left ventricular ejection fraction 35% or less), and intraventricular conduction delay (QRS more than 120 msec), who are in sinus rhythm and have been on optimal medical therapy. CRT can be achieved with a device designed only for pacing or can be combined with a defibrillator (many patients who are candidates for an implantable cardioverter defibrillator [ICD] are also candidates for CRT). CRT has been shown not only to improve quality of life and decrease heart failure symptoms (improvement in NYHA class by one class or increased 6-minute walk distance) but also to reduce mortality and improve survival.

16. **Do all patients with dyssynchrony respond to CRT?**

Not all patients who undergo CRT have a clinical response to it. In general, responders have lower mortality, fewer heart failure events, and fewer symptoms than nonresponders. The incidence of nonresponders is about 25% and is similar among patients with ischemic and nonischemic cardiomyopathy.

17. **What are some additional benefits seen in responders to CRT?**

CRT allows patients to tolerate more aggressive medical therapy and neurohormonal blockade, particularly with beta blockers. It also improves diastolic function. CRT reduces frequency of ventricular arrhythmias and ICD therapies among patients previously treated with an ICD who were upgraded to a CRT device. It may also reduce frequency and duration of atrial tachyarrhythmias, including atrial fibrillation.

18. **Can ventricular pacing be deleterious?**

In patients with left ventricular dysfunction, right ventricular pacing alone can lead to intraventricular dyssynchrony, precipitate heart failure, and lead to overall worse outcomes. In such patients, consideration should be given to CRT.

BIBLIOGRAPHY, SUGGESTED READINGS, AND WEBSITES

1. Abraham WT, Fisher WG, Smith AL, et al: Cardiac resynchronization in chronic heart failure, *N Engl J Med* 346:1845, 2002.
2. Bristow MR, Saxon LA, Boehmer J, et al: Cardiac-resynchronization therapy with or without an implantable defibrillator in advanced chronic heart failure, *N Engl J Med* 350:2140, 2004.
3. Ellenbogen KA, Wilkoff BL, Kay GN, et al: *Clinical cardiac pacing, defibrillation and resynchronization therapy*, ed 3, Philadelphia, 2006, Saunders.
4. Epstein AE, DiMarco JP, Ellenbogen KA, et al: ACC/AHA/HRS 2008 guidelines for device-based therapy of cardiac rhythm abnormalities: executive summary: a report of the American College of Cardiology/American Heart Association Task Force on Practice Guidelines (Writing Committee to Revise the ACC/AHA/NASPE 2002 Guideline Update for Implantation of Cardiac Pacemakers and Antiarrhythmia Devices), *J Am Coll Cardiol* 51:2085-2105, 2008.
5. Jarcho JA: Resynchronizing ventricular contraction in heart failure, *N Engl J Med* 352:1594, 2005.

IMPLANTABLE CARDIOVERTER DEFIBRILLATORS

Jose L. Baez-Escudero, MD and Miguel Valderrábano, MD

1. **What are the components of an implantable cardioverter defibrillator (ICD) system?**

   ICDs are composed of a pulse generator (typically implanted in the left pectoral region) and one or more intracardiac leads. Typically the right ventricular lead contains two distal electrodes (tip and ring) that are used to sense local electrical ventricular signals and to pace if necessary. This lead also contains one or two defibrillation coils (one sits in the right ventricle and the other in the superior vena cava) specifically designed to deliver high voltages. Additional leads may include an atrial lead (for pacing, sensing, and arrhythmia discrimination) or a left ventricular lead for cardiac resynchronization. All defibrillators are also capable of pacemaker functions.

2. **How does an ICD deliver shocking energy?**

   ICDs use lithium-vanadium batteries that are reliable energy sources with predictable discharge curves. An ICD is able to deliver a charge larger than its battery voltage because of a system of internal capacitors. These hold a charge and then release it all at once when it is large enough. Shocking energy travels around a circular circuit usually formed between the defibrillator lead coils and the device titanium-housed can.

3. **How does the ICD detect and define a rhythm?**

   The ICD collects intracardiac electrical signals (a process called *sensing*) and then processes them with dedicated software to classify the rhythm (a process called *detection*). The ICD identifies an arrhythmia by counting intervals between successive electrograms sensed by the intracardiac leads. In the ventricular lead, beat-to-beat intervals are counted and assigned into a category, usually called a *zone*. For example, normal sinus rhythm is expected to be slower than approximately 160 beats/min, which corresponds to beat-to-beat intervals longer than 375 msec. Shorter intervals would fall in the ventricular tachycardia (VT) zone and even shorter ones in the ventricular fibrillation (VF) zone. The ICD diagnoses an abnormally fast rhythm when a sufficient number of consecutive beat-to-beat intervals fall into either the VT or VF zone. This rate-based detection scheme can be adjusted to meet the individual patient's needs by programming for different categories and therapies (e.g., antitachycardia pacing as appropriate therapy for slow VT). Also, detection algorithms can take into account onset of tachycardia (abrupt in VT versus gradual in sinus tachycardia), stability (regular in VT versus irregular in atrial fibrillation), the relationship with the atrial activation timings, and even the morphology of the ventricular signal to maximize accuracy of detection and minimize inappropriate therapies. After therapy is delivered, the ICD monitors the following intervals to redetect sinus rate (which means the therapy was successful) or redetect the arrhythmia (which results in additional therapy).

4. **How does ICD therapy improve survival?**

   ICD therapy, compared with conventional or traditional antiarrhythmic drug therapy, has been associated with mortality reductions from 23% to 55%, depending on the risk group participating in each trial, with the improvement in survival due almost exclusively to a reduction in sudden cardiac death (SCD). The trials are subcategorized into two types: *primary prevention* (prophylactic) trials, in which the subjects have not experienced life-threatening sustained VT, VF, or resuscitated cardiac arrest but are at risk; and *secondary prevention* trials, involving subjects who have had an abortive cardiac arrest, a life-threatening VT, or ventricular tachyarrhythmia as the cause of syncope.

5. **What are the key clinical trials that evaluated the benefit of ICD for primary prevention?**
Clinical trials have evaluated the risks and benefits of ICDs in prevention of sudden death and have improved survival in multiple patient populations, including those with prior myocardial infarction (MI) and heart failure caused by either coronary artery disease or nonischemic dilated cardiomyopathy (DCM). Table 42-1 summarizes the important trials that evaluated the mortality benefit of ICDs for primary prevention.

TABLE 42-1. TRIALS THAT EVALUATED THE BENEFIT OF ICD FOR PRIMARY PREVENTION OF SUDDEN CARDIAC DEATH

Trial	# of pts	Age (Yrs)	LVEF (%)	Follow-up (Months)	Control Therapy	Mortality (%) Control	ICD	P
MUSTT (Multicentre Unstable Tachycardia Trial)	704	67 ± 12	30	39	No EP-guided therapy	48	24	.06
MADIT (Multicentre Automatic Defibrillator Implantation Trial)	196	63 ± 9	26	27	Conventional	38.6	15.7	.009
MADIT II (Multicentre Automatic Defibrillator Implantation Trial)	1232	64 ± 10	23	20	Optimal medical therapy	19.8	14.2	.007
DEFINITE (Defibrillators in Non-Ischemic Cardiomyopathy Treatment Evaluation)	458	58	21	29.0±14.4	Optimal medical therapy	14.1	7.9	.08
SCD-HeFT (Sudden Cardiac Death in Heart Failure)	2521	60.1	25	45.5	Optimal medical therapy	36.1	28.9	.007

EP, electrophysiologic.

6. **What are the current class I indications for ICD implantation for primary prevention of SCD?**

Assuming patients are receiving chronic optimal medical therapy and have a reasonable expectation of survival with good functional status for more than 1 year, the following are the current indications for ICD therapy:

- Patients with left ventricular ejection fraction (LVEF) less than 35% as a result of prior MI who are at least 40 days post-MI and are in New York Heart Association (NYHA) functional class II or III.
- Patients with left ventricular (LV) dysfunction as a result of prior MI who are at least 40 days post-MI, have an LVEF less than 30%, and are in NYHA functional class I.
- Patients with nonischemic DCM who have an LVEF 35% or less and who are in NYHA functional class II or III.
- Patients with nonsustained VT as a result of prior MI, LVEF less than 40%, and inducible VF or sustained VT at electrophysiologic study.
- Patients with syncope of undetermined origin with clinically relevant, hemodynamically significant sustained VT or VF induced at electrophysiologic study.
- Patients with structural heart disease and spontaneous sustained VT, whether hemodynamically stable or unstable.

7. **What are the current class I indications for ICD implantation for secondary prevention of SCD?**

Secondary prevention refers to prevention of SCD in those patients who have survived a prior sudden cardiac arrest or sustained VT. Evidence from multiple randomized controlled trials supports the use of ICDs for secondary prevention of SCD regardless of the type of underlying structural heart disease. In patients resuscitated from cardiac arrest, the ICD is associated with clinically and statistically significant reductions in SCD total mortality compared with antiarrhythmic drug therapy in prospective randomized controlled trials. Hence, ICDs are indicated for secondary prevention of SCD in patients who survived VF or hemodynamically unstable VT or experienced VT with syncope and have an LVEF 40% or less, after evaluation to define the cause of the event and to exclude any completely reversible causes.

8. **What other special populations may also benefit from ICD therapy?**

Certain patients with less common forms of cardiomyopathy, as well as patients with inherited conditions who share genetically determined susceptibility to VT and SCD, also benefit from ICD therapy (especially when a history of arrhythmia or syncope is present or for primary prevention in patients with a very strong family history of early mortality). These patients meet class II indications for ICD implantation that are outlined in the current guidelines in detail, including the following:

- Patients with congenital heart disease who are survivors of cardiac arrest after evaluation to define the cause of the event and exclude any reversible causes
- Hyperthrophic cardiomyopathy (HCM) with one or more risk factor for SCD (VF, VT, family history of SCD, unexplained syncope, LV thickness 30 mm or more, abnormal exercise blood pressure [BP]).
- Brugada syndrome with a history of previous cardiac arrest, documented sustained VT, or classic electrocardiogram (ECG) phenotype with unexplained syncope
- Idiopathic VF/VT
- Noncompaction of the left ventricle
- Long- and short-QT syndromes with previous cardiac arrest or unexplained syncope
- Catecholaminergic polymorphic VT
- Arrhythmogenic right ventricular dysplasia/cardiomyopathy
- Infiltrative cardiomyopaties such as sarcoidosis, amyloidosis, Fabry's disease, hemochromatosis, giant cell myocarditis, or Chagas' disease
- Certain muscular dystrophies

9. **What is defibrillator threshold testing?**
   The defibrillation threshold (DFT) is defined as the amount of energy required to reliably defibrillate the heart during an arrhythmia. During implant, the electrophysiologist may elect to perform DFT testing, in which ventricular fibrillation (VF) is induced, detected, and then terminated by the device in a step-down sequence to find the minimal reliable level of energy needed to achieve defibrillation. Defibrillation efficacy traditionally has been performed with successive DFT attempts using approximately 20 J in a device that delivered 25 to 30 J. A safety margin of 10 J was required for the implantation of the earliest defibrillators. Because DFT testing involves inducing potentially fatal VF several times and requires deep conscious sedation, some electrophysiologists forego DFT testing at implant and program the device to the highest output settings. Additionally, an ICD can be potentially tested without inducing VF using upper limit of vulnerability (ULV) testing.

10. **What is antitachycardia pacing?**
    Antitachycardia pacing (ATP) has long been recognized as a way to pace-terminate certain types of arrhythmias, particularly slow monomorphic VT involving a reentry circuit. The idea is to deliver a few seconds of pacing stimuli to the heart at a rate faster than the tachycardia. The basic principle is that in most reentrant circuits there an excitable gap—that is, a time between successive activations when the myocardium is available to respond to excitations. Pacing in a reentrant circuit during the excitable gap introduces new activation wavefronts that collide with the one of the preexisting tachycardia and can terminate it. Advantages offered by ATP include the following:
    - ATP is not painful (sometimes barely noticed by some patients).
    - ATP may reduce battery drainage by terminating the arrhythmia without the need for shocks.
    - It is an easy programmable feature on most ICDs.

    On the other hand, ATP has potential disadvantages. If ineffective, it can delay defibrillation therapies and prolong the time during which the patient is in tachycardia, which may lead to syncope. ATP can also accelerate VT into faster rhythms and even VF.

    For this reason, it is mostly used in patients that remain stable and asymptomatic during episodes of slow VT, generally below 200 beats/min. However, more aggressive ATP programming has been shown to decrease ICD shocks, and newer ICDs incorporate ATP while charging for a shock.

11. **How common are inappropriate shocks in patients with ICDs?**
    Inappropriate shocks occur when a device delivers therapy for a fast supraventricular rhythm or for abnormal sensing in the ventricle. They occur in up to 11% of patients with ICDs and can constitute up to a third of all shock episodes a patient experiences. The most common rhythm triggering an inappropriate shock is atrial fibrillation with rapid ventricular response, followed by other SVTs including sinus tachycardia. Smoking, atrial fibrillation, diastolic hypertension, young age, nonischemic cardiomyopathy, and prior appropriate shocks increase the chance of receiving an inappropriate shock. They are associated with increased mortality in patients with ICDs and have important psychologic effects in this population. ICD programming options currently available should be used to reduce the risk of inappropriate shocks.

BIBLIOGRAPHY, SUGGESTED READINGS, AND WEBSITES

1. Beyerbach DM: Implantable Cardioverter Defibrillators: http://www.emedicine.com
2. General Principles of the Implantable Cardioverter-Defibrillator: http://www.utdol.com
3. Bardy GH, Lee KL, Mark DB, et al: Amiodarone or an implantable cardioverter-defibrillator for congestive heart failure, *N Engl J Med* 352:225-237, 2005.

4. Daubert JP, Zareba W, Cannom DS, et al: Inappropriate implantable cardioverter-defibrillators shocks in the MADIT II study: frequency, mechanisms, predictors, and survival impact, *J Am Coll Cardiol* 51:1357-1365, 2008.

5. DiMarco JP: Implantable cardioverter-defibrillators, *N Engl J Med* 349:1836-1847, 2003.

6. Kadish A, Dyer A, Daubert JP, et al: Prophylactic defibrillator implantation in patients with nonischemic dilated cardiomyopathy, *N Engl J Med* 350:2151-2158, 2004.

7. Epstein AE, DiMarco JP, Ellenbogen KA, et al: ACC/AHA/HRS 2008 guidelines for device-based therapy of cardiac rhythm abnormalities: executive summary: a report of the American College of Cardiology/American Heart Association Task Force on Practice Guidelines (Writing Committee to Revise the ACC/AHA/NASPE 2002 Guideline Update for Implantation of Cardiac Pacemakers and Antiarrhythmia Devices), *J Am Coll Cardiol* 51:2085-2105, 2008.

8. Hohnloser SH, Kuck KH, Dorian P, et al: Prophylactic use of an implantable cardioverter-defibrillator after acute myocardial infarction, *N Engl J Med* 351:2481-2488, 2004.

9. Moss AJ, Zareba W, Hall WJ, et al: Prophylactic implantation of a defibrillator in patients with myocardial infarction and reduced ejection fraction, *N Engl J Med* 346:877-883, 2002.

CHAPTER 43

ADVANCED CARDIAC LIFE SUPPORT

Glenn N. Levine, MD, FACC, FAHA

1. **In patients with respiratory arrest (with a perfusing rhythm), how often are breaths delivered?**
   For respiratory arrest with a perfusion cardiac rhythm, breaths should be delivered every 5 to 6 seconds (10–12 breaths per minute).

2. **What is the most common cause of airway obstruction in the unconscious adult patient?**
   In adults the most common cause of airway obstruction in an unconscious patient is loss of tone in the throat muscles, leading to airway occlusion by the tongue. This may be treated by head tilt–chin lift, jaw thrust, or insertion of an oropharyngeal airway.

3. **How many joules (J) are indicated for the treatment of ventricular fibrillation (VF) or pulseless ventricular tachycardia (VT) when using a biphasic defibrillator?**
   Biphasic defibrillators are now used at many institutions, replacing the older monophasic defibrillators. The amount of joules will often be device specific, ranging from 120 to 200 J. If the appropriate setting is unknown, use 200 J. This is in contrast to the older monophasic defibrillators, in which 360 J are recommended.

4. **In order, what are the preferred routes of drug administration?**
   - Intravenous (IV) is the preferred route of drug administration. The guidelines emphasize that resuscitation attempts should not be delayed by trying to achieve central IV access when peripheral IV access can be easily achieved.
   - When IV access is not possible, intraosseous (IO) is preferred over endotracheal (ET). IO can be used in both children and adults.
   - Absorption of drugs given via the ET route is considered to be less reliable and predictable. In addition, the optimal dose of most drugs given via the ET route is unknown; the typical dose of drugs administered via the ET route is reported to be 2 to 2.5 times the IV route. Drugs delivered via the ET route should be diluted in 5 to 10 ml of water or normal saline. Advanced cardiac life support (ACLS) drugs that can be given via the ET route are epinephrine, vasopressin, atropine, lidocaine, and naloxone.

5. **In a patient with VF or pulseless VT (Figure 43-1), after the first unsuccessful shock, which two drugs should be considered?**
   - Epinephrine 1 mg IV/IO is the traditional medication to be considered. Additional similar doses of epinephrine can be administered every 3 to 5 minutes. If ET administration is necessary, the suggested dose is epinephrine 1:1000, 2 to 2.5 mg diluted in 5 to 10 ml or water or normal saline, injected directly into the ET tube. Although a mainstay of the American Heart Association's ACLS VT/VF algorithm, it is acknowledged that there is actually very little data to support the use of epinephrine in this situation.
   - One dose of vasopressin 40 mg IV/IO can be considered instead of the first or second dose of epinephrine. Vasopressin is a nonadrenergic peripheral vasoconstrictor that causes coronary and renal vasoconstriction.

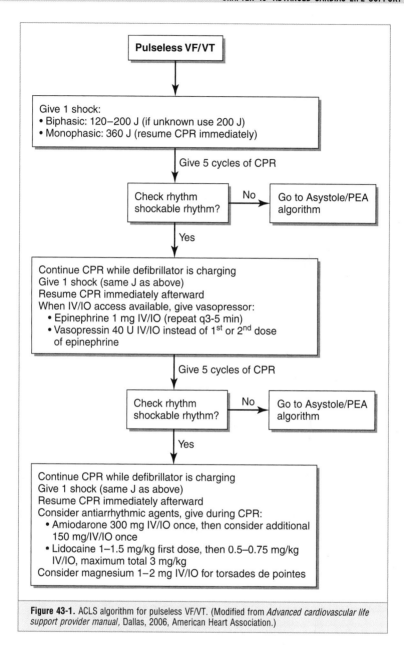

Figure 43-1. ACLS algorithm for pulseless VF/VT. (Modified from *Advanced cardiovascular life support provider manual*, Dallas, 2006, American Heart Association.)

6. **After several unsuccessful shocks, and treatment with epinephrine or vasopressin, what other drugs (and their doses) should be considered?**
Amiodarone or lidocaine should be considered. Soberingly, no antiarrhythmic has ever actually been shown to improve survival to hospital discharge, although amiodarone has been shown to increase rates of survival to hospital admission.

- The dose of amiodarone is 300 mg IV/IO once, with consideration of a subsequent 150 mg IV/IO if indicated 3 to 5 minutes after the first 300-mg dose.
- The dose of lidocaine is 1 to 1.5 mg/kg IV/IO, with subsequent doses of 0.5 to 0.75 mg/kg IV/IO given over 5- to 10-minute intervals, to a maximum total lidocaine dose of 3 mg/kg. The suggested ET dose of lidocaine is 2 to 4 mg/kg.

7. **If the patient is in torsades de pointes, in addition to defibrillation, what medication can be considered?**
   Magnesium, administered as a dose of 1 to 2 g IV/IO, can be given. It is recommended that it be diluted in 10 ml of 5% dextrose in water (D_5W) and administered over 5 to 20 minutes.

8. **After administering a drug via a peripheral IV, what steps should be taken to promote delivery of the drug to the central circulation?**
   After administering a drug via a peripheral IV, a 20-ml bolus of IV fluid should be administered and the extremity should be elevated for 10 to 20 seconds.

9. **Can one shock a hypothermic patient who is in VF/VT?**
   Yes, with caveats. For the hypothermic patient (temperature less than 30° C [86° F]) in VF/VT, a single defibrillation is deemed appropriate. If this is unsuccessful, subsequent defibrillations and drug therapy administration should be deferred until the body core temperature rises above 30° C (86° F). According to the ACLS guidelines, the patient with a hypothermic heart may be unresponsive to drug therapy, defibrillation, and pacemaker therapy.

10. **If a person who was in VF/VT is successfully defibrillated, assuming he or she has not already received any amiodarone, what is the dosing of amiodarone if this is to be started to prevent further VF/VT?**
    The following regimen is what is given in the ACLS booklet and is the "classical" loading of amiodarone. An initial "bolus" of 150 mg IV is given over 10 minutes. This is followed by an infusion of 1 mg/min for 6 hours (total 360 mg), then an infusion of 0.5 mg/min over the next 18 hours (540 mg).

11. **What are the treatable causes of pulseless electrical activity?**
    Because pulseless electrical activity (PEA) has such a poor prognosis unless a reversible cause of the rhythm is quickly identified and addressed, it is important to commit to memory the treatable causes of PEA. The *H*'s and *T*'s of PEA are given in Table 43-1.

TABLE 43-1. POTENTIALLY TREATABLE CAUSES OF PULSELESS ELECTRICAL ACTIVITY	
H's	*T*'s
Hypovolemia	Toxins
Hypoxia	Tamponade (cardiac)
Hydrogen ion (acidosis)	Tension pneumothorax
Hyperkalemia/hypokalemia	Thrombosis (coronary and pulmonary)
Hypoglycemia	Trauma
Hypothermia	

Modified from *Advanced cardiovascular life support provider manual*, Dallas, 2004-2005, American Heart Association.

12. **What drugs can be considered in a patient with PEA?**
Epinephrine and vasopressin can be used, as described earlier for the treatment of VF/VT. Atropine can be considered for asystole or PEA with a slow ventricular rate. The dose of atropine is 1 mg IV/IO, which can be repeated every 3 to 5 minutes, up to a total dose of 3 mg.

13. **In bradycardic patients, such as those with heart block, what are the primary treatments if they are symptomatic and suffering from poor perfusion?**
The immediate use of transcutaneous pacing is now emphasized for patients with symptomatic bradycardia. Although preparations are being made for transcutaneous pacing, the following pharmaceutical interventions should be considered:
   - Atropine 0.5 mg IV: This may be repeated every 3 to 5 minutes to a total dose of 3 mg. The use of atropine should not be relied on in patients with Mobitz II second-degree atrioventricular (AV) block or three-degree (complete) AV block. Some have considered the use of atropine in Mobitz II or three-degree heart block ("infrahisian" heart block) contraindicated, although this is not explicitly stated in the latest ACLS guidelines.
   - Epinephrine 2 to 10 µg/min
   - Dopamine 2 to 10 µg/kg/min

14. **Is transcutaneous pacing recommended for the treatment of a patient in asystole?**
As noted in the ACLS algorithm, several randomized controlled trials have failed to show benefit from attempted transcutaneous pacing in patients in asystole. Thus, it is not currently recommended in this situation.

15. **In a *symptomatic yet stable* patient with a regular narrow complex tachyarrhythmia, what drug is recommended as a first-line agent?**
Adenosine has become the drug of choice for a *symptomatic yet stable* patient with a narrow complex tachyarrhythmia. The distinction between *stable* and *unstable* is subjective, but the symptomatic yet stable patient might be described as one who is slightly lightheaded (systolic blood pressure [SBP] of approximately 80 mm Hg) or having mild shortness of breath or chest discomfort. Patients experiencing more severe symptoms would be those with altered mentation because of low blood pressure or moderate to severe shortness or breath or chest discomfort. Note that although adenosine, which blocks AV conduction, may terminate some narrow complex tachycardias, such as AV nodal reentrant tachycardia (AVNRT) or AV reentrant tachycardia (AVRT), it will not terminate rhythms such as atrial flutter or atrial tachycardia (although it may lead to a transient decrease in conduction through the AV node and slower ventricular response rate, allowing identification of the rhythm). Adenosine would not be expected to terminate an irregular narrow complex tachycardia, because the genesis of these rhythms does not involve the AV node.

16. **What is the dosing regimen for adenosine, and what are its primary side effects?**
The adenosine dosing regimen is 6 mg rapid IV push, followed if no rhythm conversion by 12 mg rapid IV push, with the 12 mg rapid IV push repeated once if necessary. The half-life of adenosine is only several seconds, so every effort must be made to administer this quickly and ensure its quick delivery to the central circulation (see Question 8). The effects of adenosine may be potentiated by dipyrimadole or carbamezepine (consider starting dose of 3 mg) and blocked by theophylline and caffeine. Adenosine may cause the patient to experience flushing, shortness of breath, or chest discomfort. Because it can cause bronchospasm, it should be avoided in patients with significant reactive airway disease. The practitioner should also be aware that because of its profound effects on AV nodal conduction, it may result in asystole for several seconds or more, an often disconcerting occurrence to the practitioner watching the telemetry monitor. Prolonged asystole has been reported in patients with transplanted hearts and following central venous administration; a lower dose of 3 mg should be considered in such situations.

BIBLIOGRAPHY, SUGGESTED READINGS, AND WEBSITES

1. American Heart Association 2005 Guidelines for CPR and ECC: http://www.americanheart.org
2. *Advanced cardiovascular life support provider manual*, Dallas, 2006, American Heart Association.
3. Danger WE, Sanoski CA, Wiggins BS, et al: Pharmacotherapy considerations in advanced cardiac life support, *Pharmacotherapy*, 26(12):1703-1729, 2006.

VII. PRIMARY AND SECONDARY PREVENTION

HYPERTENSION

Gabriel B. Habib, Sr., MD, MS, FACC, FAHA, FCCP

CHAPTER 44

1. **Define *hypertension*. How widespread is it in the United States?**
   The Joint National Committee on Detection, Evaluation, and Treatment of High Blood Pressure, in its seventh report (JNC-7), defined *hypertension* as an average of two or more diastolic readings more than 90 mm Hg on at least two consecutive visits or an average of multiple systolic readings more than 140 mm Hg. Isolated systolic hypertension is diagnosed if systolic blood pressure (BP) is more than 140 mm Hg with a diastolic BP less than 90 mm Hg. A new category called *prehypertension* is now defined as a blood pressure less than the arbitrary cutoff of 140/90 mm Hg for *hypertension* but greater than an *optimal* blood pressure of 120/80 mm Hg. Patients with prehypertension, unlike hypertensive patients, do not require antihypertensive drug therapy but should be counseled to start health-promoting lifestyle modifications aimed at preventing the development of hypertension. Mild, moderate, and severe hypertension subgroups have been defined as well. Based on these definitions, up to 24% of the adult population in the United States suffers from hypertension.

2. **What are the goals of hypertension treatment?**
   Although optimal blood pressure is less than 120/80 mm Hg, the goal of blood pressure treatment is to achieve blood pressure levels less than 140/90 mm Hg in most patients with uncomplicated hypertension and less than 130/80 mm Hg in higher risk hypertensive patients with chronic kidney disease or diabetes mellitus. Ultimately, reducing elevated blood pressure levels is needed primarily to prevent various complications of systemic hypertension such as stroke, heart attacks, heart failure, and renal disease. The best predictor of the efficacy in preventing various cardiorenal complications is the degree of reduction of blood pressure. The risk of cardiovascular disease is lowest at a blood pressure of approximately 115/75 mm Hg and doubles beginning at 115/75 mm Hg with each 20/10 mm Hg increment in blood pressure. Thus, even modest levels of blood pressure reduction can result in signficant reductions in cardiovascular risk.

3. **Is systolic or diastolic blood pressure more powerful as a predictor of cardiovascular complications of hypertension?**
   Systolic and diastolic blood pressure levels are independently predictive of the risk of cardiovascular complications in hypertensive patients. However, systolic blood pressure is more powerful in predicting cardiovascular complications particularly in patients over the age of 50 years. Pulse pressure—the difference between systolic and diastlic blood pressure—is also an independent predictor of cardiovascular complications and is increasingly larger in older patients. A wide pulse pressure is usually indicative of a noncompliant *stiff* aorta with a reduced ability to *distend* and recoil back. Thus, during systolic ejection of blood from the left ventricle into the aorta and systemic circulation, the aorta does *not* distend and the force of ejection is transmitted more forcefully into the peripheral vessels, thus causing an exaggerated systolic blood pressure level recording. During diastole, the elastic recoil of the aorta is more limited, contributing to a lower diastolic blood pressure. Thus, a noncompliant aorta would increase systolic blood pressure and reduce diastolic blood pressure, resulting in a widened pulse pressure.

4. **You have diagnosed a new case of hypertension. What is your next step?**
Arterioles are the vessels that sustain the most damage from persistent elevation of BP. Therefore, the first step is to do a *damage assessment* by evaluating the target organs of hypertension, keeping in mind that their involvement is an expression of arteriolar damage with subsequent ischemia and ischemia-induced changes.

   - **Kidney:** Signs of involvement range from minimal proteinuria or slight increase of serum creatinine to end-stage renal disease. Kidney size is evaluated by a variety of imaging methods and has prognostic significance. Hypertension is the second leading cause of renal failure in the United States, particularly in African Americans.

   - **Brain:** The eye fundus appearance is the *mirror* of the brain circulation. Findings range from minor atherosclerotic changes to papilledema and hemorrhages, which are consistent with malignant hypertension. A careful neurologic examination may reveal signs of previously undiagnosed strokes, and history may reveal previous transient ischemic attacks.

   - **Heart:** The direct consequence is left ventricle hypertrophy (LVH) with increased left ventricular (LV) mass; this is easily documented by electrocardiogram, two-dimensional, and M-mode echocardiogram or cardiac magnetic resonance imaging (MRI). LVH is strongly associated with an increased risk of sudden death and myocardial infarction (MI) and constitutes the basis for decreased LV compliance and subsequent diastolic dysfunction. A thorough evaluation for the presence of coronary artery disease, guided by a skillful interview, is required. Holter monitoring may be necessary for evaluating LVH-associated arrhythmias. The last step in the natural history of the disease is LV dilation and pump failure, with the classical signs of congestive heart failure (CHF).

5. **What is resistant hypertension and how prevalent is it?**
Resistant hypertension is defined as blood pressure that remains above goal in spite of the concurrent use of three antihypertensive agents of different classes. Ideally, one of the three agents should be a diuretic and all agents should be prescribed at optimal dose amounts. Resistant hypertension identifies patients who are at risk of having reversible causes of hypertension or patients who by virtue of persistently elevated blood pressure levels may benefit from special diagnostic and therapeutic considerations. In a recent analysis of the National Health and Nutrition Health and Nutrition Examination Survey (NHANES), only 53% of hypertensive patients were controlled to less than 140/90; the majority of the remaining 47% of these patients probably have resistant hypertension.

6. **What is secondary hypertension?**
Up to 5% of all hypertension cases are *secondary,* meaning that a specific cause can be identified. Some of these cases are curable if the source of hypertension can be treated, such as surgery for an adrenal tumor, stenting of a renal artery stenosis, and correction of an aortic coarctation. Given the low prevalence of secondary hypertension, routine screening for secondary hypertension is not routinely recommended. A targeted approach is much more cost effective, and clinical and laboratory clues are critically important in evaluating patients for specific causes of secondary hypertension. Signs, symptoms, and findings suggestive of secondary hyperension are discussed later and in Table 44-1.

7. **When should one suspect secondary hypertension?**
The following scenarios should trigger a search for possible causes of secondary hypertension (Table 44-2):

   - Onset at a young age (younger than 35 years) in female patients raises the suspicion of renal artery medial fibromuscular dysplasia.

   - Onset at a late age (older than 55 years) suggests atherosclerotic renal vascular disease (renal artery stenosis).

TABLE 44-1. JNC 7 CATEGORIES OF HYPERTENSION

Category	Blood Pressure
Normal	<120/80 mm Hg
Prehypertension	120–130/80–89 mm Hg
Hypertension: Stage 1	140–159/90–99 mm Hg
Hypertension: Stage 2	≥160/100 mm Hg

Modified from the Seventh report of the Joint National Committee on Prevention, Detection, Evaluation, and Treatment of High Blood Pressure (JNC-7), Bethesda, MD, 2003, National Institutes of Health, pp 54-55.

TABLE 44-2. CLINICAL SIGNS, SYMPTOMS, AND FINDINGS SUGGESTIVE OF SECONDARY CAUSES OF HYPERTENSION

Signs, Symptoms, and Findings	Suggested Secondary Cause
Onset at young age (<35 years) in female patient	Renal artery medial fibromuscular dyplasia
Onset at a late age (>55 years), especially in a patient with atherosclerosis	Renal artery stenosis
Exaggerated drop in blood pressure or kidney function with initiation of ACE inhibitor	
Abdominal bruit	
Unexplained hypokalemia	Primary hyperaldosteronism
Paroxysmal episodes of palpitations, sweating, and headaches	Pheochromocytoma
Use of birth control pills, laxatives, or licorice	Drug-induced as a result of mineralocorticoid effects
Renal calculi, elevated calcium level	Hyperparathyroidism
Reduced femoral pulses with high blood pressure values only in the upper extremities	Aortic coarctation
Abdominal striae, truncal obesity	Cushing's disease
Loud snoring, witnessed apnea	Obstructive sleep apnea
Worsening renal function, polycystic kidneys or small kidneys or ultrasound	Renal parenchymal disease

- Unexplained hypokalemia—sometimes manifested by generalized weakness—either in the absence of diuretic use or an exaggerated hypokalemia following low doses of diuretics suggests primary hyperaldosteronism.
- Paroxysmal episodes of palpitations, sweating, and headaches suggest a pheochromocytoma.

- Abdominal/lumbar trauma may result in a perirenal hematoma with subsequent small unilateral kidney.
- A transient episode of periorbital swelling and dark-colored urine that went untreated may point to a chronic glomerulonephritis.
- Multiple episodes of cystitis or urinary infection left untreated or with incomplete treatment will lead to and suggest chronic pyelonephritis.
- Use of birth control pills by young women and laxative use by elderly people or licorice use, which has a mineralocorticoid effect, suggest mineralocorticoid-induced hypertension.
- A history of chronic pain may be the clue for analgesic nephropathy.
- Renal calculi may be the sign of hyperparathyroidism or the cause of obstructive nephropathy.
- Reduced femoral pulses with high BP values only in the upper extremities suggests aortic coarctation.
- Abdominal bruits suggest renal artery stenosis. The cause may be either atherosclerosis in an elderly patient or fibromuscular dysplasia in a young woman. Renal artery stenosis is also suggested by an exaggerated drop in BP following initiation of treatment with angiotensin-converting enzyme (ACE) inhibitors or angiotensin-receptor blockers.
- Bilateral abdominal palpable masses commonly are due to policystic kidney disesase. Typically the history reveals the presence of hypertension with renal failure in other family members.
- Abdominal striae are the sign of Cushing's disease, along with the typical truncal obesity.
- Resistance to a multiple drug regimen can point to a secondary cause of hypertension. In fact, in clinical practice, resistant hypertension with failure to control blood pressure to recommended goals despite at least three antihypertensive agents in optimal diseases is the most important clue that should lead to a thorough evaluation for secnary causes of hypertension.

8. **What is the recommended initial diagnostic workup for a hypertensive patient?**
Any newly diagnosed patient with hypertension should have measurements of serum creatinine, sodium, potassium, calcium and hematocrit, full fasting lipid profile, 12-lead electrocardiogram (ECG), and chest radiograph. Because essential hypertension accounts for the large majority—more than 95%—of all hypertension, a thorough and costly diagnotic workup for secondary causes of hypertension is not routinely recommended unless there are clnical or laboratory clues suggesting secondary hypertension.

9. **What are the most common causes of secondary hypertension among patients with treatment resistant or uncontrolled hypertension, when do you suspect them, and how do you confirm them?**
Secondary hypertension is common among patients with resistant hypertension. The most common causes of secondary hypertension among patients with resistant hypertension are obstructive sleep apnea, renal parenchymal and vascular disease, and, possibly, primary aldosteronism. Rare causes of secondary hypertension include pheochromocytoma, Cushing's syndrome, hyperparathyroidism, aortic coarctation, and intracranial tumors. Following are important clinical or laboratory clues to these secondary hypertension causes:

- **Obstructive sleep apnea:** Untreated obstructive sleep apnea is an increasingly recognized cause of secondary hypertension. Clues include loud snoring, witnessed apnea, and excessive daytime somnolence. Diagnosis is confirmed with a sleep study.
- **Renal artery stenosis:** This is suspected in patients with atherosclerotic peripheral or coronary vascular disease, early age (younger than 35 years) or late age (older than 55 years) at onset of hypertension, abnormal renal function or worsening renal function with the use of an ACE inhibitor or in patients with a unilateral small kidney. Renal ultrasonography is not recommended and magnetic resistance angiography is the most

specific and reliable noninvasive diagnostic imaging modality. Contrast angiography is also useful for the diagnosis and for possible renal angioplasty. It is important to recognize that the anatomic diagnosis of a renal artery stenosis, independent of its cause, does not imply that the stenosis is the cause of hypertension. Causation can be confirmed by documenting the *functionality* of the lesion by measuring renal vein renin activity and documenting a renin activity ratio greater than 1.5 between the two sides.

- **Primary hyperaldosteronism:** This is suspected in hypertensive patients with unexplained hypokalemia. Diagnosis is suspected by a suppressed renin activity and a high 24-hour urinary aldosterone excretion in the course of a high dietary sodium intake and is confirmed radiographically with a localizing imaging procedure such as computed tomography (CT) or MRI with specific adrenal protocol.
- **Renal parenchymal disease:** This is suspected by impaired renal function, but causation is difficult to confirm because longstanding untreated hypertension may also cause renal parenchymal disease. Imaging techniques that evaluate kidney size, presence of hydronephrosis and obstructive nephropathy, calculi, polycystic kidney disease, or congenital malformations are useful to detect specific causes of renal parenchymal disease.
- **Pheocromocytoma:** A rare secondary cause of hypertension that often presents with paroxysmal and postural hypotension, usually in a younger adult, with intermittent episodes of headache, palpitation, and sweating. The best screening test is plasma free metanephrines (normetanephrine and metanephrine).

10. **A 32-year-old man complains of intermittent episodes of headaches, palpitations, and profuse sweating. Over the last year, he has been treated three times in the emergency department for hypertensive crisis. He does not remember what his BP was, but he felt lightheaded when trying to stand, even before reaching the emergency department (ED). In your office, he always has a BP below 120/70 mm Hg. He has noticed low-grade fever at times and has lost a few pounds. After you examine him, he feels funny, so you measure his BP again. This time it is 165/110 mm Hg, with a heart rate of 115 beats/min. Laboratory studies only show a slightly elevated serum glucose and white blood cell count (WBC) of 18,000/ml with a normal differential. What is your diagnosis?**
This is a typical presentation for a pheochromocytoma. The clues given by the patient's history are invaluable for diagnosis: Many patients with pheochromocytoma have a normal baseline BP, with high BP values only on occasion. *Postural hypotension* is a classical feature. High serum catecholamine levels explain the sweating and palpitations and the low fever, elevation of serum glucose, and leukocytosis. Gentle palpation of the abdomen during physical examination may sometimes trigger a crisis. Because of the general and metabolic manifestations of the disease, it may mimic a large variety of conditions (e.g., vasculitis, diabetes), and a high level of suspicion is always necessary.

Some patients present with a high BP that is constant rather than paroxysmal. A *rule of 10* may be applied: 10% of all cases are familial, 10% are bilateral, 10% are due to a malignant adrenal tumor, 10% recur, 10% are extra-adrenal, 10% occur in children, 10% are associated with a multiple endocrine neoplasia (MEN) syndrome, and 10% present with a stroke as the inaugural symptom.

Diagnosis of a pheochromocytoma is rewarding because this very sick patient who is prone to life-threatening complications can be virtually cured. The current recommendation for biochemical diagnosis of pheochromocytoma is urine testing for metanephrines and fractionated catecholamines. These tests only certify the presence of a cathecolamine-secreting tumor; therefore, the next step is to localize it (90% are in the adrenal medulla; the other 10% are scattered where chromaphin tissue is found). The preferred treatment is laparoscopic adrenalectomy.

11. **How important are nonpharmacologic strategies in hypertension treatment?**
Hypertension treatment is a lifelong commitment regardless of the recommended treatment modality. Thus, compliance to treatment is critically important in achieving the expected clinical

benefits of treatments. Hypertensive patients should be appropriately educated about the natural history and complications of hypertension and the critical importance of compliance with any treatment recommendation. Goal blood pressure attainment is much more likely achieved with earlier initiation of combination antihypertensive drug therapies—particularly in stage 2 hypertension, characterized by blood pressure levels greater than 160/100 mm Hg—and by frequent monitoring of blood pressure at home and in the doctor's office and appropriate uptitration of antihypentive medications to reach accepted goals of blood pressure treatments.

Patients and some physicians tend to be skeptical about the importance of lifestyle changes. Often the skepticism of the physician may be communicated to the patient even without the physician's concsious effort. It is critically important that patients and their physicians believe in the benefit of lifestyle changes. Current hypertension guidelines describe lifestyle changes as *therapeutic* to emphasize their proven benefit. Therapeutic lifestyle changes—weight loss; reduced intake of saturated fat and salt; reduced dietary calorie intake; regular exercise and moderation of alcohol intake; consumption of adequate amounts of calcium, potassium, magnesium, and fiber; and smoking cessation—are at the top of the JNC-7 treatment algorithm recommended for all patients. Therapeutic lifestyle changes have been proven to be effective in reducing blood pressure levels by 10 to 20 mm Hg, changes that are at times similar to the efficacy of one additional antihypertensive drug. In patients with prehypertension—with blood pressure levels between 120/80 and 140/90 mm Hg—therapeutic lifestyle changes, but not pharmacologic treatment, are recommended to prevent hypertension development. Pharmacologic treatment is recommended not solely but in addition to and as an adjunct to therapeutic lifestyle changes in *hypertensive* patients—that is, patients with blood pressure levels greater than 140/90 mm Hg. Antihypertensive drug therapy is recommended at lower levels of blood pressure (more than 130/80 mm Hg) in higher risk patients with diabetes mellitus and chronic kidney disease, and goal of blood pressure treatment is also lower, namely less than 130/80 mm Hg. In patients with uncomplicated hypertension, goal BP levels are less than 140/90 mm Hg.

12. **Is an angiotensin-receptor blocker equally effective to an ACE inhibitor in preventing cardiovascular complications of hypertension?**
Until recently, the evidence supporting the importance of angiotensin-receptor blockers as an effective and safe blood pressure–lowering drug class was quite limited. Recently, large prospective, randomized clinical trials have proven angiotensin-receptor blockers to be at least as effective as a beta-blocker and as effective as an ACE inhibitor in preventing major cardiovascular complications. The largest clinical trials that support these conclusions are the Losartan Intervention for Endpoint reduction in hypertension (LIFE) trial and Ongoing Telmisartan Alone and in Combination with Ramipril Global Endpoint (ONTARGET) clinical trials. A recently completed and soon to be reported trial, the largest placebo-controlled clinical trial of an angiotensin-receptor blocker, will provide further insight into the efficacy of angiotensin-receptor blockers in preventing cardiovascular complications among hypertensive patients. In addition to the proven efficacy of angiotensin-receptor blockers in preventing major cardiovascular complications, they have also been proven effective in preventing renal disease progression to end-stage renal disease among diabetics with established diabetic nephropathy, thus supporting their important role as recommended antihypertensive drugs—akin to ACE inhibitors—in patients with diabetic nephropathy.

13. **True or false: Beta-blockers are preferred initial antihypertensive agents in hypertensive patients with no known hypertensive complications**
False. In large placebo-controlled prospective clinical trials, diuretics and beta-blockers as a group have been shown to reduce cardiovascular complications of hypertension. However, the evidence of these cardioprotective effects of thiazide diuretics in hypertensive patients is more compelling, and in clinical trials comparing diuretic and beta-blockers, such as the Medical Research Council (MRC) trial, diuretics were more effective than beta-blockers. Thus, the JNC-7 report recommends thiazide diuretics, not beta-blockers, as preferred initial treatments in patients with uncomplicated hypertension—that is, patients with no compelling comorbid conditions that may favor specific antihypertensive agents.

Compelling indications in hypertensive patients for the use of a beta-blocker as an antihypertensive agent include a history of MI, compensated heart failure, and coronary artery disease (CAD). Contraindications to beta-blockers must be carefully weighed against their potential therapeutic benefits. For example, a beta-blocker should be avoided in a patient admitted to the hospital with acutely decompensated heart failure but may be started at lower doses then gradualy uptitrated in patients with well-compensated and stable heart failure. Withdrawal of beta-blockers, paticularly in patients with CAD, should be performed gradually to avoid rebound increase in anginal symptoms upon their discontinuation.

14. **Are alpha-blockers effective in preventing cardiovascular complications of hypertension, and when is it appropriate to use them in hypertensive patients?**
Alpha-blockers are effective antihypertensive agents but have not been shown in either placebo-controlled or active-controlled clinical prospective trials to be effective in preventing cardiovascular complications of hypertension. In the Antihypertensive and Lipid-Lowering Treatment to Prevent Heart Attack trial (ALLHAT), the largest hypertensive clinical trial that randomized hypertensive patients to an ACE inhibitor, a calcium channel blocker, or an alpha-blocker versus a thiazide diuretic, the alpha-blocker arm of the trial was prematurely terminated because of an almost doubling of the risk of heart failure and a 25% excess cardiovascular death among patients treated with an alpha-blocker compared with a thiazide diuretic. Thus, alpha-blockers are *not* recommended as initial antihypertensive agents.

However, alpha-blockers may be used as a second- or third-line antihypertensive agent to treat hypertension and may be used because of a compelling and specific reason for the use of an alpha-blocker to minimize obstructive urinary symptoms in older men with benign prostatic hyperplasia.

15. **When are ACE inhibitors specifically recommended in hypertensive patients?**
The JNC-7 report recommends a thiazide as an initial antihypertensive agent in patients with uncomplicated hypertension. Compelling indications for the selection of an ACE inhibitor include heart failure, previous MI, diabetes mellitus, chronic kidney disease, and high CAD risk and for recurrent stroke prevention. These recommendations are based on several randomized, prospective, controlled clinical trials confirming the benefits of ACE inhibitors in preventing cardiovascular or renal complications in these patients. ACE inhibitors prevent myocardial remodeling, heart failure progression, progressive ventricular enlargement after a recent MI, MIs, and stroke in patients with cardiovascular disease and have also been proven to prevent progression of renal disease among diabetics with established diabetic renal disease.

BIBLIOGRAPHY, SUGGESTED READINGS, AND WEBSITES

1. The Seventh Report of the Joint National Committee on Prevention, Detection, Evaluation, and Treatment of High Blood Pressure, http://www.nhlbi.nih.gov/guidelines/hypertension/express.pdf
2. ALLHAT Officers and Coordinators for the ALLHAT Collaborative Research Group: Antihypertensive and Lipid Lowering to Prevent Heart Attack Trial (ALLTHAT), *JAMA* 288:2981-2997, 2002.
3. Calhoun D, Jones D, Textor D, et al: Resistant hypertension: diagnosis, evaluation, and treatment: a scientific statement from the American Heart Association Professional Education Committee of the Council for High Blood Pressure Research, *Hypertension* 51(6):1403-1419, 2008.
4. Cusham WC, Ford CE, Cutler JA, et al: For the ALLHAT Collaborative Research Group. Success and predictors of blood pressure control in diverse North American settings: the Antihypertensive and Lipid Lowering to Prevent Heart Attack Trial (ALLHAT), *J Clin Hypertens* 4:393-404, 2002.
5. Cutler JA, Davis BR: Thiazide-type diuretics and ^{2}-adrenergic blockers as first-line drug treatments for hypertension, *Circulation* 117:2691-2705, 2008.
6. Hajjar I, Kotchen TA: Trends in prevalence, awareness, treatment, and control of hypertension in the United States, 1998-2000, *JAMA* 290:199-206, 2003.
7. Lloyd-Jones DM, Evans JC, et al: Differential control of systolic and diastolic blood pressure: factors associated with lack of blood pressure control in the community, *Hypetension* 36:594-599, 2000.

8. The ALLHAT Officers and Coordinators for the ALLHAT Collaborative Research Group: Major cardiovascular events in hypertensive patients randomized to doxazosin vs. chlorthalidone: the Antihypertensive and Lipid-Lowering Treatment to Prevent Heart Attack Trial (ALLHAT), *JAMA* 283:1967-1975, 2000.

9. The ALLHAT Officers and Coordinators for the ALLHAT Collaborative Research Group: Major outcomes in high-risk hypertensive patients randomized to angiotensin-converting enzyme inhibitor or calcium channel blocker vs diuretic: the Antihypertensive and Lipid-Lowering Treatment to Prevent Heart Attack Trial (ALLHAT), *JAMA* 288:2981-2997, 2002.

10. The ONTARGET Investigators: Telmisartan, ramipril or both in patients at high risk for vascular events, *N Engl J Med* 358:1547-1559, 2008.

11. The seventh report of the Joint National Committee on Prevention, Detection, Evaluation, and Treatment of High Blood Pressure: the JNC-7 report, *JAMA* 289(19):2560-2572, 2003. Erratum in: *JAMA* 290(2):197, 2003.

CHAPTER 45

HYPERCHOLESTEROLEMIA

Glenn N. Levine, MD, FACC, FAHA

1. **Who should be screened for hypercholesterolemia?**
   The National Cholesterol Education Program (NCEP) Adult Treatment Panel III (ATP III) recommends that all adults age 20 years or older should undergo fasting lipoprotein profile every 5 years. Testing should include total cholesterol, low-density lipoprotein (LDL) cholesterol, high-density lipoprotein (HDL) cholesterol, and triglycerides.

2. **True or false: Coronary atherosclerosis is common in persons in their 20s and 30s.**
   True. Autopsy and intravascular ultrasound (IVUS) studies have demonstrated detectable atheromas/atherosclerosis in 50% to 69% of asymptomatic young persons.

3. **What are the ATP III classifications of LDL cholesterol, total cholesterol, HDL cholesterol, and triglyceride levels based on measured values?**
   The values, as denoted in ATP III, are given in Table 45-1. Note that since publication of this classification in 2001, a goal of LDL less than 70 mg/dl has emerged as desirable in some very high risk populations and thus an LDL of significantly less than 100 mg/dl would now be considered optimal in such patients. To convert the values in the table to mmol/L, divide by 88.6.

4. **What are important *secondary* causes of hypercholesterolemia?**
   - Diabetes
   - Hypothyroidism
   - Obstructive liver disease
   - Chronic renal failure/nephrotic syndrome
   - Drugs (progestins, anabolic steroids, corticosteroids)

5. **What is a lipoprotein?**
   A lipoprotein is the particle that transports cholesterol and triglycerides. Lipoproteins are composed of proteins (called apolipoproteins), phospholipids, triglycerides, and cholesterol (Fig. 45-1).

6. **What is lipoprotein(a)?**
   Lipoprotein(a), often represented as Lp(a), is an apoB-containing LDL-like particle. It has independently been correlated with an increased risk of adverse cardiovascular event in certain patient populations. According to a 2008 consensus report from the American Diabetes Association and American College of Cardiology Foundation, "the clinical utility of routine measurement of Lp(a) is unclear, although more aggressive control of other lipoprotein parameters may be warranted in those with high concentrations of Lp(a)."

7. **What is the minimal LDL goal for secondary prevention?**
   The minimal LDL goal for secondary prevention in patients with established coronary artery disease (CAD) is an LDL less than 100 mg/dl. This is also now the goal in patients with coronary heart disease risk equivalents (see Question 9). In an update to ATP III, it was

TABLE 45-1. NCEP-ATP III CLASSIFICATION OF LDL, TOTAL CHOLESTEROL, HDL CHOLESTEROL, AND TRIGLYCERIDE LEVELS (IN MG/DL)*

Value (mg/dl)	Classification
LDL Cholesterol	
<100	Optimal
100–129	Near or above optimal
130–159	Borderline high
160–189	High
≥190	Very high
Total Cholesterol	
<200	Desirable
200–239	Borderline high
≥240	High
HDL Cholesterol	
<40	Low
≥60	High
Triglycerides	
<150	Normal
150–199	Borderline high
200–499	High
≥500	Very high

*Note that since publication of this classification, a goal of LDL less than 70 mg/dl has emerged as desirable in some very-high risk populations. To convert to mmol/L, divide by 88.6.

Modified from the Expert Panel on Detection, Evaluation, and Treatment of High Blood Cholesterol in Adults. Executive Summary of The Third Report of The National Cholesterol Education Program (NCEP) Expert Panel on Detection, Evaluation, and Treatment of High Blood Cholesterol in Adults (Adult Treatment Panel III), *JAMA* 285(19):2486-2497, 2001.

emphasized that an LDL less than 100 mg/dl is a *minimal* goal of therapy. In light of more recent studies (Pravastatin or Atorvastatin Evaluation and Infection Therapy [PROVE-IT], Heart Protection Study [HPS], and Treating to New Targets [TNT]), a goal of LDL less than 70 mg/dl should be considered in patients with coronary heart disease at *very high* risk. Patients with coronary heart disease classified as *very high* risk include those with the following:
- Multiple major coronary risk factors (especially diabetes)
- Severe and poorly controlled risk factors (especially continued cigarette smoking)
- Multiple risk factors of the metabolic syndrome (see question 9)
- Acute coronary syndrome

8. **What is a *coronary heart disease risk equivalent*?**
   Patients with established coronary heart disease (those being treated for secondary prevention) have been recommended for the most aggressive treatment for elevated LDL levels. ATP III established *coronary heart disease risk equivalents* to denote those at high risk for cardiovascular disease and events who would warrant equivalently aggressive lipid therapy as

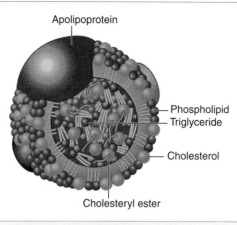

Figure 45-1. A lipoprotein particle. The polar surface coat is composed of apoproteins, phospholipids, and free cholesterol. The nonpolar lipid core is composed of cholesterol esters and triglycerides. (From Genest J, Libby P: Lipoprotein disorders and cardiovascular disease. In Libby P, Bonow RO, Mann DL, Zipes DP: *Braunwald's heart disease: a textbook of cardiovascular medicine*, ed 8, Philadelphia, 2007, Saunders.)

those with established coronary artery disease. ATP III recommends that patients with these risk equivalents should have LDL levels lowered to below 100 mg/dl *at a minimum.* These coronary heart disease risk equivalents include the following:

- Diabetes
- Other clinical forms of atherosclerosis (peripheral arterial disease, abdominal aortic aneurysm, and symptomatic carotid artery disease)
- Multiple cardiac risk factors that confer a 10-year risk for CAD greater than 20% (based on the Framingham risk table)

9. **What factors make up *metabolic syndrome*?**
   - Abdominal obesity (waist circumference in men more than 40 inches/102 cm or in women more than 35 inches/88 cm)
   - Triglycerides 150 mg/dl or more
   - Low HDL cholesterol (less than 40 mg/dl in men or less than 50 mg/dl in women)
   - Blood pressure 135/85 mm Hg or higher
   - Fasting glucose 110 mg/dl or more

10. **What medications should be used to lower LDL levels?**
    Statins are the first-line agents to lower LDL levels. If inadequate LDL lowering is not achieved, a more potent statin can be considered. If adequate LDL is still not achieved, either a bile acid sequestrant, fibrate, or nicotinic acid should be added. Note that patients may need to be followed more carefully for side effects such as liver function test (LFT) elevation and myopathy with certain combination therapies. At the time of this writing, and likely until the results of the Improved Reduction of Outcomes: Vytorin Efficacy International Trial (IMPROVE-IT) are presented, ezetimibe should only be used as a secondary agent if the agents listed here are not tolerated or do not lead to adequate LDL reduction. Table 45-2 summarizes the drugs used to treat hypercholesterolemia, their effects, and their side effects.

TABLE 45-2. DRUGS USED IN THE TREATMENT OF HYPERCHOLESTEROLEMIA

Drug Class	Lipid/Lipoprotein Effects	Side Effects	Contraindications
Statins	LDL ↓ 18%–55% HDL ↑ 5%–15% TG ↓7%–30%	Myopathy Increased LFTs	Absolute: active or chronic liver disease Relative: concomitant use of certain drugs
Bile acid sequestrants	LDL ↓ 15%–30% HDL ↑ 3%–5% TG—no change or increase	Gastrointestinal distress Constipation Decreased absorption of other drugs	Absolute: dysbetalipoproteinemia or TG > 400 mg/dl Relative: TG > 200 mg/dl
Nicotinic acid	LDL ↓ 5%–25% HDL ↑ 15%–35% TG ↓ 20%–50%	Flushing Hyperglycemia Hyperuricemia (or gout) Upper GI distress Hepatotoxicity	Absolute: chronic liver disease or severe gout Relative: diabetes, hyperuricemia, or peptic ulcer disease
Fibric acids	LDL ↓ 5%–20% HDL ↑ 10%–20% TG ↓ 20%–50%	Dyspepsia Gallstones Myopathy	Absolute: severe renal disease or severe hepatic disease
Ezetimibe	LDL ↓ 18%–20% HDL ↑ 1% TG ↓ 5%–11%	Approximately 1% higher rate of LFT elevations when used with statin vs. statin alone	Absolute: active liver disease when used with a statin

GI, Gastrointestinal; *TG*, triglycerides.

Modified from the Expert Panel on Detection, Evaluation, and Treatment of High Blood Cholesterol in Adults. Executive summary of the third report of the National Cholesterol Education Program (NCEP) Expert Panel on Detection, Evaluation, and Treatment of High Blood Cholesterol in Adults (Adult Treatment Panel III), *JAMA* 285(19):2486-2497, 2001.

11. **Is there an age cutoff for secondary prevention therapy with statins?**
No. Older secondary prevention trials with statins included many patients in their 60s and 70s and demonstrated benefit in older and younger patients. Thus, for secondary prevention, according to ATP III, "no hard-and-fast age restrictions appear necessary when selecting persons with established coronary heart disease for LDL-lowering therapy." Since publication of ATP III, the Prospective Study of Pravastatin in the Elderly at Risk (PROSPER), and several other trials were published. In PROSPER, subjects age 70 to 82 with a history of vascular disease or risk factors were randomized to treatment with pravastatin or placebo. After an average of 3.2 years of follow-up, the composite ischemic endpoint was reduced by 15%. The results of PROSPER, HPS, and Anglo-Scandinavian Cardiac Outcomes Trial (ASCOT) reinforce that statin therapy should be used in elderly patients for secondary prevention and should be seriously considered in elderly patients for primary prevention.

12. **What is non-HDL cholesterol?**

The non-HDL cholesterol level is the total cholesterol level minus HDL cholesterol level. It is an approximation of very low density lipoprotein (VLDL) plus LDL levels. VLDL cholesterol is felt in clinical practice to be the most readily available measure of atherogenic remnant lipoproteins. Reduction of non-HDL cholesterol is considered a secondary target of therapy in persons with high triglycerides (200 mg/dl or more). The goals for non-HDL cholesterol are generally 30 mg/dl higher than those for LDL cholesterol. For example, in patients with coronary heart disease and coronary heart disease risk equivalents, the LDL goal is less than 100 mg/dl and the non-HDL goal is less than 130 mg/dl.

13. **What factors and conditions are believed to be associated with or cause low HDL cholesterol?**

   - Elevated triglycerides
   - Overweight and obesity
   - Physical inactivity
   - Type 2 diabetes
   - Cigarette smoking
   - Very high carbohydrate intakes (more than 60% energy)
   - Certain drugs (beta-blockers, anabolic steroids, progestational agents)

14. **What is the difference between myopathy, myalgia, myositis, and rhabdomyolysis?**

   - **Myopathy:** general term referring to any disease of muscles
   - **Myalgia:** muscle ache or weakness without creatine kinase (CK) elevation
   - **Myositis:** muscle symptoms with increased CK levels
   - **Rhabdomyolysis:** muscle symptoms with marked CK elevation (more than 10 times ULN)

15. **What is the incidence of nonspecific muscle aches or joint pains in patients treated with statins?**

In placebo-controlled trials, the incidence of nonspecific muscle aches (myalgia) or joint pains in patients treated with statins is approximately 5%. Interestingly, the rates of these complaints are similar in these trials between active treatment and placebo groups. Nevertheless, it is generally accepted that some patients will have a temporal development of such symptoms after initiation of statin therapy that is likely due to such therapy. The incidence of severe myopathy or overt rhabdomyolysis (creatine kinase [CK] elevation greater than 10 times upper limits of normal) is approximately 1 in 1000 with currently available statins.

BIBLIOGRAPHY, SUGGESTED READINGS, AND WEBSITES

1. Rosenson RS: Overview of Treatment of Hypercholesterolemia: http://www.utdol.com
2. Rosenson RS: Screening Guidelines for Dyslipidemia: http://www.utdol.com
3. Lipids Online: http://www.lipidsonline.com
4. Brunzell JD, Davidson M, Furberg CD, et al: Lipoprotein management in patients with cardiometabolic risk, *J Am Coll Cardiol* 51:1512-1524, 2008.
5. Genest J, Libby P: Lipoprotein disorders and cardiovascular disease. In Libby P, Bonow RO, Mann DL, Zipes DP, editors: *Braunwald's heart disease: a textbook of cardiovascular medicine*, ed 8, Philadelphia, 2007, Saunders.

6. Grundy SM, Cleeman JI, Merz CN, et al: Implications of recent clinical trials for the National Cholesterol Education Program Adult Treatment Panel III guidelines, *J Am Coll Cardiol* 44(3):720-732, 2004.

7. Pasternak RC, Smith SC Jr, Bairey-Merz CN, et al: ACC/AHA/NHLBI clinical advisory on the use and safety of statins, *Circulation* 106(8):1024-1028, 2002.

8. Smith SC Jr, Allen J, Blair SN, et al: AHA/ACC guidelines for secondary prevention for patients with coronary and other atherosclerotic vascular disease: 2006 update: endorsed by the National Heart, Lung, and Blood Institute, *Circulation* 16:113(19):2363-2372, 2006.

DIABETES AND CARDIOVASCULAR DISEASE

Ashish Aneja, MD and Michael E. Farkouh, MD, MSc, FACC

1. **What is the current global burden of diabetes, and what is its impact on the epidemiology of cardiovascular disease?**

   The global burden of diabetes mellitus (DM) in 1985 was an estimated 30 million people. By 2003 it was estimated that there were around 194 million people with diabetes, and this figure is expected to rise to almost 350 million by 2025. At present, the prevalence of DM is much higher in developed countries, but because of adoption of western diets and lifestyles, developing countries are rapidly catching up with their developed counterparts. The disease affects a disproportionately higher number of young people in the developing world. The lifetime risk of diabetes is estimated at 32.8% for U.S. males and 38.5% for U.S. females.

   Knowledge of the epidemiology of DM is important to place the expected contribution of DM to the global CV disease burden into perspective. The relationship between DM type 1 and type 2 and cardiovascular (CV) disease is well established. In particular, DM is a very strong risk factor for the development of coronary artery disease (CAD) and stroke. The hazard ratio for CAD death in diabetic patients is considered as high as 2.03 (95% confidence interval [CI], 1.60 to 2.59) for men and 2.54 (1.84 to 3.49) for women. Atherosclerosis accounts for 80% of all deaths in diabetic persons, compared with about 30% among nondiabetic persons. Atherosclerotic disease also accounts for greater than 75% of hospitalizations for diabetes-related complications. Patients with diabetes but without previous myocardial infarction (MI) carry the same level of risk for subsequent acute coronary events as nondiabetic patients with previous MI. These results have prompted the Adult Treatment Panel III of the National Cholesterol Education Program to establish diabetes as a CAD risk equivalent, mandating aggressive antiatherosclerotic therapy.

2. **What is the impact of diabetes on cardiovascular disease outcomes?**

   In addition to its salutary effects on stable atherosclerotic disease, diabetic patients experience an increased rate of worse early and late complications following acute coronary syndrome. Diabetic patients with non–ST-elevation acute coronary syndromes also experience more in-hospital MIs and associated complications and higher death rates. Diabetic patients also respond less optimally to fibrinolytic therapy, an effect that is sex-dependent—diabetic women fare worse than men. In patients with acute coronary syndromes complicated by hypotension and cardiogenic shock, diabetes is an independent risk variable for adverse outcomes, including death. In the long term, diabetic patients with acute coronary syndromes experience higher rates of heart failure, death, and repeat infarction and require more frequent coronary revascularization.

3. **What effect, if any, does diabetes have on the clinical manifestations and prognosis of peripheral arterial disease and cerebrovascular disease?**

   Diabetes increases the risk of peripheral arterial disease (PAD) about twofold to fourfold. It is more commonly associated with femoral bruits and absent pedal pulses and with a high rate of abnormal ankle-brachial indices, ranging from 11% to 16% in different studies. The duration and severity of diabetes correlate with incidence and extent of PAD. The pattern of PAD in diabetic patients is characterized by a preponderance of infrapopliteal occlusive disease and vascular calcification. Clinically, PAD in diabetic patients manifests more commonly with claudication and also a higher rate of amputation—the most common cause of nontraumatic amputations.

Diabetic patients also have a higher rate of intracranial and extracranial cerebrovascular atherosclerosis and calcifications. Patients with a history of stroke have a threefold higher likelihood of being diabetic than controls, with a risk of stroke that may be up to threefold to fourfold higher than nondiabetic patients. Compared with nondiabetic subjects, the mortality from stroke in diabetic patients is almost threefold higher. Diabetes also results in a disproportionately higher stroke rate in younger patients and increases the risk of severe carotid disease. In patients younger than 55 years, diabetes increases the risk of stroke about 10 times according to one study. Diabetic patients also suffer worse poststroke outcomes, including a higher mortality rate and recurrence risk and a greater probability of vascular dementia.

4. **What is the overall impact of diabetes on the vascular tree?**
Cardiovascular complications in diabetic patients can be the result of macrovascular disease, including CAD, peripheral arterial disease, and cerebrovascular disease, or can be due to microvascular disease that can result in nephropathy, retinopathy, and neuropathy. Many regard diabetic cardiomyopathy as a distinct entity that is thought to result primarily from hyperglycemia-induced myocardial adverse effects.

5. **What is the burden of additional cardiovascular risk factors in diabetic patients, and what is their cumulative impact on the atherosclerosis morphology and burden?**
Diabetic patients are known to bear a higher burden of CV risk factors, including twice the prevalence of hypertension, and a higher prevalence of dyslipidemia, including lower high-density lipoprotein (HDL) cholesterol and higher triglycerides levels. The clustering of CV risk factors appears to have a multiplicative effect in diabetic patients, who experience a threefold higher CV mortality than nondiabetic persons for each risk factor present. In addition, CAD in diabetic patients involves a greater number of coronary vessels and more diffuse atherosclerotic lesions, including significantly more severe proximal and distal CAD.

Atherosclerotic plaque ulceration and thrombosis also occur more often in diabetic patients. Atherosclerotic plaques in diabetic patients are also considered high-risk plaques because of a greater propensity for erosion or rupture, which account for a higher incidence of acute coronary syndromes in this population. Diabetic plaques are also characterized by high levels of inflammatory cell infiltration, large lipid cores, thin fibrous caps, and the presence of new vessel formation (neovascularization) and hemorrhage within the plaque.

6. **What characteristics of the atherosclerotic plaque in diabetic patients make it unstable compared with plaque in nondiabetic patients?**
In addition to its adverse effects on the endothelium, diabetes promotes processes that lead to monocyte transmigration across the endothelium into the vessel wall and uptake of oxidized low-density lipoproteins (LDLs) into these cells, resulting in foam cell and fatty streak formation. In addition to plaque initiation, diabetes renders the atherosclerotic plaque unstable. Endothelial cells in diabetic patients release cytokines and enzymes (matrix metalloproteinases) that not only reduce collagen synthesis by vascular smooth muscle cells but also accelerate its breakdown. Because collagen is an essential component of the plaque fibrous cap, weakening it renders the plaque unstable. Plaque rupture or erosion triggers an intense local prothrombotic milieu, resulting in thrombus formation. Diabetes also results in elevated factor VII levels (procoagulant) and reduced protein C and antithrombin III levels (naturally occurring anticoagulants). Finally, diabetic endothelial cells produce more tissue factor, the major procoagulant found in atherosclerotic plaques.

7. **What broad management strategy is advocated for diabetic patients with cardiovascular disease?**

A multidisciplinary approach is the cornerstone in the successful management of diabetes and cardiovascular disease. Because the presence of diabetes is considered equivalent to having CAD, aggressive management of all potential risk factors, including hypertension, dyslipidemia, and the hypercoagulable state, are recommended. In addition to measures to promote weight loss by dietary modification and exercise, diabetic patients benefit tremendously from aggressively managing conventional risk factors. The strongest evidence supporting a multifaceted and comprehensive approach in the management of diabetic patients comes from the Steno-2 trial. It demonstrated that a strategy including lifestyle and pharmacologic interventions intended to reduce cardiovascular risk in type 2 diabetic patients with microalbuminuria was significantly more effective in reducing cardiovascular events and mortality than usual care in the long term.

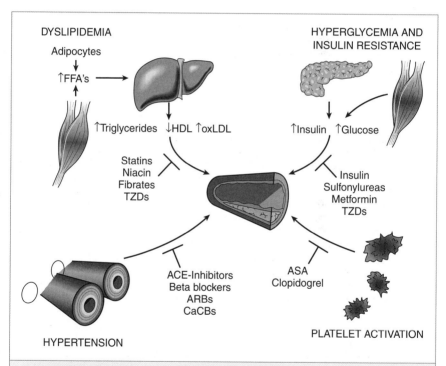

Figure 46-1. Diabetes requires therapy for each metabolic abnormality to stem the onset and progression of atherosclerosis. Statins improve the lipid profile and decrease the risk of MI and death. Treatment of hypertension decreases the rate of MI and stroke in patients with diabetes. Therapy should include ACE inhibitors or ARBs for their microvascular and possible atherosclerosis benefits. The heightened thrombotic potential of the diabetic state supports the use of platelet antagonists, such as aspirin or clopidogrel. Although strict treatment of hyperglycemia does not significantly reduce the incidence of myocardial infarction or death, the improvement in microvascular outcomes itself warrants vigorous pursuit of rigorous glycemic control in diabetes. *FFAs,* Free fatty acids; *HDL,* high-density lipoprotein; *oxLDL,* oxidated low-density lipoprotein; *CaCBs,* calcium channel blockers; *ASA,* aspirin. (Modified from Libby P, Plutzky J: Diabetic macrovascular disease: the glucose paradox? *Circulation* 106:2760, 2002.)

8. **How does the treatment of hyperglycemia and insulin resistance impact outcomes in diabetic patients with cardiovascular disease?**

    Tight glycemic control has been shown to improve microvascular complications, including diabetic nephropathy. The current American Diabetes Association target for HbA_{1C} is less than 7% and for the American College of Clinical Endocrinology less than 6.5%. Diabetic nephropathy occurs in 40% of patients with type 1 and type 2 diabetes, and the main risk factors for its development include poor glycemic control, hypertension, and ethnicity. The Diabetes Control and Complications Trial (DCCT) and the United Kingdom Prospective Diabetes Study group trial (UKPDS) demonstrated that the development and progression of microalbuminuria can be prevented through strict glycemic control. This was also demonstrated for type 2 patients in the ADVANCE trial.

    Despite epidemiologic evidence linking poor glycemic control with cardiovascular disease, the role of aggressive glucose control in reduction of CV risk is controversial and potentially harmful in susceptible populations. This has recently been an area of considerable debate because of the results of two recent large randomized controlled trials: ACCORD and ADVANCE. The means used to attain glycemic control have recently received much scrutiny because of reports suggesting increased risk of cardiovascular disease, including mortality, MI, and fluid retention/heart failure with thiazolidinediones, in particular rosiglitazone. These adverse findings have been reported in several meta-analyses, but evidence from randomized controlled trials to suggest an adverse cardiovascular profile remains equivocal. A scientific statement (reference 17) from the American Diabetes Association, the American Heart Association, and the American College of Cardiology has now been published that addressed the results of these recent studies.

    Metformin remains the first-line treatment option in most type 2 diabetes patients and seems to have a beneficial effect on insulin resistance without an adverse effect on cardiovascular disease. The ongoing Bypass Angioplasty Revascularization Investigation 2 Diabetes (BARI 2D) trial will provide comparative efficacy information for insulin sensitizers and insulin replacement and is expected to provide important information in deciding the ideal means for glycemic control in diabetic patients with CHD.

9. **What are the currently recommended strategies for the management of diabetic dyslipidemia?**

    The lipid abnormalities in diabetes improve with lifestyle modifications, including weight loss, exercise, smoking cessation, and dietary changes, which are the first line of treatment. The most effective intervention in the management of diabetic patients with CAD is the use of statin medications, which have proven especially useful in this population. In the Scandinavian Simvastatin Survival Study (4S) and Cholesterol and Recurrent Events (CARE) trials and the Heart Protection Study, simvastatin demonstrated a significantly greater benefit in mortality and MI compared with nondiabetic subjects. The goal for LDL cholesterol is less than 100 mg/dl for patients without CAD and less than 70 mg/dl for those with CAD.

    In addition to statins, the fibric acid derivatives may be especially beneficial in diabetic patients because of their effects in lowering triglycerides and raising HDL levels. Treatment with gemfibrozil significantly reduced the risk of MI, in the Veterans Affairs High-Density Lipoprotein Cholesterol Intervention (VA-HIT) trial. In addition to the lipid-lowering effect, fibric acid derivates may have antiatherogenic, antithrombogenic, and antiinflammatory effects, which can prove especially useful in diabetic patients. Nicotinic acid also produces a similar favorable effect on the lipid profile in diabetic patients; diabetic patients on niacin require close monitoring of their glucose levels.

10. **What do the current guidelines recommend for management of hypertension in diabetic patients?**

    The goal blood pressure (BP) in diabetic patients is less than 130/80 mm Hg and those with a BP 140/90 mm Hg or more should be given drug therapy in addition to lifestyle and behavioral therapy. It is not uncommon for diabetic patients to require multiple agents for optimal BP control. Unless contraindicated or not tolerated, either an angiotensin-converting enzyme (ACE) inhibitor or an angiotensin-receptor blocker (ARB) should be included in all BP regimens for diabetic patients. Diuretics, beta-blockers, ACE inhibitors, ARBs, and calcium channel antagonists all effectively decrease blood pressure in diabetic patients.

Regardless of the agent chosen, evidence from prior randomized clinical trials overwhelmingly favors strict blood pressure control. The recommendations given here are based on the results of trials of hypertension or cardiovascular prevention. In the Heart Outcomes and Prevention Evaluation (HOPE) study, ramipril significantly decreased the rates of MI, stroke, and death in patients with diabetes and one additional cardiovascular risk factor. The Losartan Intervention for Endpoint Reduction in Hypertension (LIFE) study demonstrated that losartan was more effective than atenolol for reducing cardiovascular mortality in diabetic patients with hypertension and left ventricular hypertrophy (LVH).

11. **What are the principles of management of chronic CAD in diabetic patients?**
Diabetic patients are more likely to experience painless cardiac ischemia and suffer more silent MIs and sudden cardiac death. Evidence from observational studies and randomized trials has shown significant mortality benefit with beta-blockers in diabetic patients. Beta-blockers are well tolerated in diabetic patients; masking or prolongation of hypoglycemic symptoms is infrequent, particularly with cardioselective agents. Recommendations include continuing antiplatelet therapy; ACE inhibitors and ARBs should be used as appropriate for blood pressure control and beta-blockers are recommended in diabetic patients after an MI. The role of aggressive antiplatelet therapy versus conventional treatments is currently being explored in diabetic patients with stable CAD. The multifaceted approach to the diabetic patient is illustrated in Figure 46-1.

12. **What strategies for coronary revascularization are currently recommended for the management of multivessel CAD in diabetic patients?**
The optimal revascularization strategy in stable diabetic patients with multivessel coronary disease has been debated extensively in recent years. The Bypass Angioplasty Revascularization Investigation (BARI) trial substudy of diabetic patients indicated that coronary artery bypass grafting (CABG) offered a clinically meaningful and statistically significant survival advantage in diabetic patients when compared to balloon angioplasty. Even in nondiabetic patients, the need for future revascularization has been traditionally higher in the angioplasty group compared with CABG, and these differences are even more pronounced in diabetic patients. However, BARI was conducted in an era when stents were not available. The BARI 2D trial compares a revascularization strategy with optimal medical management alone in diabetic patients with stable CAD. This trial will report in 2009. Currently the favored stent strategy in diabetic patients is the use of drug-eluting stents, which have reduced restenosis rates significantly, especially among diabetic patients. The ongoing Frequent Optimization Study Using the QuickOpt Method (FREEDOM) compares revascularization with drug-eluting stents versus CABG in diabetic patients with multivessel disease and should be able to address this important question.

BIBLIOGRAPHY, SUGGESTED READINGS, AND WEBSITES

1. Ligaray KPL, Isley WL: Diabetes Mellitus, Type 2: http://www.emedicine.com
2. McCullock DK: Overview of Medical Care in Adults with Diabetes Mellitus: http://www.utdol.com
3. Nesto RW: Coronary Artery Revascularization for Angina in Patients with Diabetes Mellitus: http://www.utdol.com
4. ADVANCE Collaborative Group: Intensive blood glucose control and vascular outcomes in patients with type 2 diabetes, *N Engl J Med* 358(24):2560-2572, 2008.

5. American Diabetes Association: Standards of medical care in diabetes—2006, *Diabetes Care* 29(Suppl 1):S4-S42, 2006.

6. Beckman JA, Creager MA, Libby P: Diabetes and atherosclerosis: epidemiology, pathophysiology, and management, *JAMA* 287(19):2570-2581, 2002.

7. Berry C, Tardif JC, Bourassa MG: Coronary heart disease in patients with diabetes. Part I: Recent advances in prevention and noninvasive management, *J Am Coll Cardiol* 49(6):631-642, 2007.

8. Effects of ramipril on cardiovascular and microvascular outcomes in people with diabetes mellitus: results of the HOPE study and MICRO-HOPE substudy, *Lancet* 355:253-259, 2000.

9. Gaede P, Lund-Andersen H, Parving HH, et al: Effect of a multifactorial intervention on mortality in type 2 diabetes, *N Engl J Med* 358(6):580-591, 2008.

10. Gerstein HC, Miller ME, Byington RP, et al: Effects of intensive glucose lowering in type 2 diabetes, *N Engl J Med* 358(24):2545-2559, 2008.

11. Goldberg RB, Mellies MJ, Sacks FM, et al: Cardiovascular events and their reduction with pravastatin in diabetic and glucose-intolerant myocardial infarction survivors with average cholesterol levels: subgroup analyses in the cholesterol and recurrent events (CARE) trial: the CARE investigators, *Circulation* 98:2513-2519, 1998.

12. Grundy SM, Cleeman JI, Merz CN, et al: Implications of recent clinical trials for the National Cholesterol Education Program Adult Treatment Panel III Guidelines, *J Am Coll Cardiol* 44(3):720-732, 2004.

13. Gu K, Cowie CC, Harris MI: Diabetes and decline in heart disease mortality in US adults, *JAMA* 281:1291-1297, 1999.

14. Malmberg K, Yusuf S, Gerstein HC, et al: Impact of diabetes on long-term prognosis in patients with unstable angina and non-Q-wave myocardial infarction: results of the OASIS (Organization to Assess Strategies for Ischemic Syndromes) registry, *Circulation* 102:1014-1019, 2000.

15. Pyorala K, Pedersen TR, Kjekshus J, et al: Cholesterol lowering with simvastatin improves prognosis of diabetic patients with coronary heart disease, *Diabetes Care* 20:614-620, 1997.

16. Smith SC Jr, Allen J, Blair SN, et al: ACC/AHA guidelines for secondary prevention for patients with coronary and other atherosclerotic vascular disease: 2006 update: endorsed by the National Heart, Lung, and Blood Institute, *Circulation* 113(19):2363-2372, 2006.

17. Skyler JS, Bergenstal R, Bonow RO, et al. Intensive glycemic control and the prevention of cardiovascular events: implications of the ACCORD, ADVANCE, and VA Diabetes Trials: a position statement of the American Diabetes Association and a Scientific Statement of the American College of Cardiology Foundation and the American Heart Association. *J Am Coll Cardiol* 20;53(3):298-304, 2009.

CHAPTER 47

TREATMENT OF TOBACCO USE AND DEPENDENCE

J. Taylor Hays, MD

1. **What is the current prevalence of smoking in the United States, how has it changed over the past 40 years, and what are the demographic characteristics that are more common among smokers?**
   In 2006 an estimated 20.8% (45.3 million) of U.S. adults were current cigarette smokers; of these, 80.1% (36.3 million) smoked every day, and 19.9% (9.0 million) smoked some days. Prevalence is higher among men (23.9%) than women (18.0%). In addition, smoking prevalence is inversely related to highest educational level achieved, with the highest prevalence in adults who have earned a high school diploma equivalent (46.0%) or less (35.4%). Smoking prevalence is highest among adults living below the federal poverty level (30.6%).

2. **What are the most common smoking-attributable conditions and their magnitude?**
   The leading causes of death in the United States are heart disease, cancer, stroke, and chronic lung disease, accounting for 78.5% of all mortality. A significant portion of the mortality from these diseases is attributable to tobacco use (Table 47-1).

TABLE 47-1. DISEASES AND HEALTH CONDITIONS FOR WHICH EVIDENCE HAS ESTABLISHED A DIRECT CAUSAL RELATIONSHIP WITH CIGARETTE SMOKING

Cancer	Cardiovascular	Respiratory	Other
Bladder	Abdominal aortic aneurysm	COPD[a]	SIDS[d]
Cervix	Atherosclerosis	Pneumonia	Low birth weight
Esophagus	Cerebrovascular disease	Respiratory symptoms[b]	Reduced fertility
Kidney	Coronary heart disease		Preterm delivery
Larynx		Reduced lung function[c]	Cataracts
Leukemia			Poor wound healing
Lung			Osteoporosis
Oral			Hip fractures
Pancreas			Peptic ulcer
Stomach			

[a]Chronic obstructive pulmonary disease.
[b]Coughing, phlegm, wheezing, and dyspnea in children, adolescents, and adults.
[c]Includes reduced lung function in infants born to smoking mothers; active smoking and impaired lung growth in childhood and adolescence; early onset of lung function decline in late adolescence; and premature acceleration of age-related decline in adults.
[d]Sudden infant death syndrome.

From Fiore MC, Jaén CR, Baker TB, et al: *Treating tobacco use and dependence: 2008 update. Clinical practice guideline,* Rockville, MD, 2008, U.S. Department of Health and Human Services, Public Health Service.

Cardiovascular Disease

Cardiovascular disease is the most common cause of death in United States (myocardial infarction [MI], sudden death, heart failure, stroke, abdominal aortic aneurysm), and smoking is a major cause for each of these conditions. Particularly striking is the association of smoking and premature coronary heart disease mortality among men and women. There is a strong dose-response for smoking and MI, with risk levels for MI five times higher among heavier smokers compared with former smokers. Unlike the decline in risk for lung cancer after smoking cessation, the risk reduction for mortality with MI occurs rapidly after smoking cessation, usually reaching its nadir within 3 years.

Not surprisingly, cigarette smoking is also strongly associated with stroke (ischemic and subarachnoid hemorrhage) in a dose-response fashion. Consistent with other smoking-related conditions, the risk of stroke declines significantly after smoking cessation. Similar associations exist between smoking and abdominal aortic aneurysm and other peripheral vascular diseases. One exception is the unique and consistent causal association between smoking and thromboangiitis obliterans (Buerger's disease). The only known effective treatment for this condition is smoking cessation.

Cancer

Lung cancer is the leading cause of cancer death in both men and women, accounting for 28% of all cancer mortality. The age-adjusted annual incidence rate for lung cancer is declining steadily in men from a high of 102 per 100,000 in 1984 to approximately 81 per 100,000 in 2000. However, the rate of increase in annual incidence continues to rise for women and is now at approximately 50 per 100,000. A dose-response relationship between tobacco use and lung cancer risk exists, but there is no risk-free level of smoking. The risk of lung cancer declines significantly with prolonged smoking abstinence. For the typical one package per day smoker it will take 15 to 20 years to see lung cancer mortality risk reach its nadir.

Many other cancers are also caused by cigarette smoking. Aside from lung cancer the most common ones associated with tobacco use are aerodigestive tract cancers. This includes cancers of the oral cavity and throat, larynx, esophagus, and stomach. There is a synergistic effect of tobacco use and alcohol consumption, increasing the relative risk of oropharyngeal cancer by 40 to 100 times in people who smoke and drink heavily compared with the nonsmoker, nondrinker. Many other cancers have also been causally related to tobacco use, have a dose-dependent relationship to tobacco use, and have a declining risk after tobacco use is stopped (see Table 47-1).

Chronic Lung Disease

Chronic obstructive pulmonary disease (COPD) is the fourth leading cause of death in the United States. Although other lung conditions may result in COPD, cigarette smoking is by far the major causative agent in the development of COPD. The Surgeon General noted that COPD "could be almost completely prevented with the elimination of smoking." In a recent cohort study, the hazard ratio for COPD death among women in the Nurses' Health Study smoking 35 or more cigarettes per day was 155 compared with women who never smoked. The risk of COPD mortality declines significantly with smoking cessation. Symptoms from COPD also improve after smoking cessation, and lung function is preserved compared with those who continue to smoke.

3. **Why do smokers become addicted to tobacco?**
   Nicotine is the addictive substance in tobacco and is the primary factor in continued and compulsive tobacco use. Nicotine primarily stimulates $\alpha 4 \beta 2$ nicotinic acetylcholine receptors (nAChR) in the central nervous system. Activation of these receptors stimulates release of dopamine in the mesolimbic dopaminergic system (reward center) of the brain, which leads to the pleasurable effects (positive reinforcement) of nicotine such as arousal and relief of anxiety. Decreased levels of dopamine that occur during tobacco abstinence causes withdrawal symptoms (negative reinforcement) resulting in strong craving to smoke.

Because the reinforcement from drugs of abuse is inversely related to the rate of onset of action, the pharmacokinetic profile of nicotine delivered via tobacco smoke significantly contributes to nicotine addiction. Following inhalation, cigarette smoking results in rapidly rising nicotine levels because of the large surface area for absorption in the pulmonary circulation. Nicotine-containing blood enters the left side of the heart and rapidly reaches the cerebral circulation and receptor targets undiluted by the systemic circulation. Human studies confirm an immediate, rapid rise in nicotine levels from cigarette smoking, resulting in an intense subjective response. The positive reinforcing effects occurring in close temporal proximity to environmental triggers results in strong behavioral reinforcement. The subjective response to nicotine becomes so intimately associated with the environmental triggers (e.g., after meals, morning coffee, stress) that exposure to the trigger causes anticipation of nicotine's effects and desire to smoke. On the other hand, the presence of uncomfortable withdrawal symptoms with tobacco abstinence are negatively reinforcing in that relief of these symptoms occurs in seconds after puffing on a cigarette. These factors that both positively and negatively reinforce continued smoking prevent smokers from achieving sustained tobacco abstinence.

4. **What are the most effective pharmacologic treatments for tobacco use and dependence?**
First-line pharmacotherapies recommended in current clinical practice guidelines include nicotine replacement therapy, bupropion sustained-release therapy, and varenicline (Table 47-2).

TABLE 47-2. FIRST-LINE MEDICATIONS FOR THE TREATMENT OF TOBACCO USE AND DEPENDENCE AND ESTIMATED 6-MONTH ABSTINENCE RATES

Medication	Estimated 6-month Abstinence Rate (%)[a]
Varenicline	33.2
Nicotine nasal spray	26.7
High-dose nicotine patch[b]	26.5
Nicotine inhaler	24.8
Nicotine lozenge[c]	24.2
Bupropion SR	24.2
Standard-dose nicotine patch	23.4
Nicotine gum	19

[a]All rates are for each medication provided as monotherapy.
[b]Nicotine patch dose >25 mg per day.
[c]Nicotine lozenge dose of 2 mg per lozenge; results based on a single randomized trial.

From *Clinical practice guideline 2008 update*, 2008, U.S. Department of Health and Human Services, Public Health Services.

Nicotine Replacement Therapies

Nicotine replacement therapy (NRT) works primarily by reducing the severity of nicotine withdrawal symptoms by partially replacing nicotine previously obtained from tobacco. In the United States, NRT is available without a prescription in three different formulations (chewing gum, transdermal patch, and oral lozenge) and with a prescription in two different formulations (intranasal spray and oral inhaler). Meta-analysis has shown the odds ratio (OR) for achieving abstinence with NRT at 6 to 12 months is 1.77 (95% confidence interval [CI], 1.66 to 1.88) compared with placebo, with the highest OR for nasal spray (2.35; 95% CI, 1.63 to 3.38) and the lowest for gum (1.66; 95% CI, 1.52 to 1.81). This meta-analysis concluded that all formulations demonstrated similar efficacy. Excluding trials with shorter follow-up, the percentage of smokers who remained abstinent for more than 12 months ranged from 13.7% with transdermal patches to 24% with intranasal spray. Because all formulations have been shown to have similar efficacy, the choice of formulation should be based on individual patient preference and previous experience with NRT products.

Adverse effects differ among the various NRT formulations. Patch site skin reactions, nausea, vomiting, sweating, alteration in mood, and sleep disturbances are among the more common adverse effects seen with nicotine patch. Common adverse effects associated with nicotine gum include jaw fatigue and soreness, hiccupping, burping, and nausea. Those associated with nicotine inhaler and nasal spray are attributed to local irritation at the site of administration (i.e., mouth or nose). Although concern has been expressed about the safety of NRT in smokers with cardiac disease, a meta-analysis of safety data from clinical studies with the transdermal patch in patients with cardiovascular disease found no evidence of an increased risk of cardiac events associated with NRT treatment. Although NRT can be associated with development of tolerance and physical dependence, the risk that dependence will develop in patients who are using these products as smoking cessation aids is low.

Bupropion SR

The antidepressant agent bupropion sustained release (SR) was the first nonnicotinic agent to be FDA approved for the treatment of tobacco dependence. Bupropion appears to reduce nicotine withdrawal symptoms by simulating the nicotine-mediated activation of brain dopaminergic and noradrenergic reward systems by blocking neuronal dopamine and norepinephrine reuptake, thereby elevating central nervous system (CNS) levels of these transmitters.

Similar to NRT, a recent meta-analysis including studies of more than 6 months' duration demonstrated that bupropion SR 150 to 300 mg/day approximately doubles the odds of smoking cessation compared with placebo when used as sole pharmacotherapy (OR 2.06; 95% CI, 1.77 to 2.40). In addition to reducing withdrawal symptoms, evidence suggests that bupropion SR treatment reduces the weight gain often seen after smoking cessation.

Dry mouth and insomnia were the only adverse events that occurred more commonly with bupropion SR compared with placebo in early smoking cessation trials. Both these adverse events appear to be dose related, and neither is a common cause for drug discontinuation. Bupropion SR has been associated with a small increased incidence of seizures (a rate of 1 in 1000), particularly among those at increased risk because of medical problems that may predispose to seizures.

Varenicline

Varenicline is a partial agonist of the $\alpha4\beta2$ neuronal nAChR, creating a sustained low level of dopamine release in the reward center and reducing nicotine withdrawal symptoms. The drug also acts as an antagonist at the $\alpha4\beta2$ neuronal nAChR, inhibiting the rewarding effects of nicotine and reducing smoking satisfaction.

Two identically designed, randomized, multicenter, phase 3 trials compared varenicline with placebo and bupropion SR in 2052 total subjects. Participants in these studies were randomized to one of three treatments for 12 weeks, with 40 weeks of nontreatment follow-up: varenicline 1 mg twice daily, bupropion SR 150 mg twice daily, or placebo. Continuous abstinence during weeks 9 to 12 was approximately 44% for varenicline compared with approximately 30% for bupropion SR and 18% for placebo. Similarly, during weeks 9 to 52, the continuous abstinence rate was 22% to 23% with varenicline compared with 15% to 16% with bupropion and 8% to 10% with placebo. A third phase 3 trial evaluated the effect of extended therapy with varenicline 1 mg twice daily compared with placebo to delay or prevent relapse following successful abstinence after 12 weeks of open-label varenicline treatment. The continuous abstinence rate and odds of achieving abstinence were significantly greater in subjects receiving active varenicline for 24 weeks compared with placebo-treated subjects at both week 24 (70.5% versus 49.6%; OR 2.48) and week 52 (43.6% versus 36.9%; OR 1.34).

The most common adverse event attributed to varenicline 1 mg twice daily is mild nausea, occurring in approximately one third of treated subjects. Other common adverse events reported with varenicline are headache, insomnia, and abnormal dreams. Insomnia also tends to be mild, and is less common compared with bupropion treatment. Recent labeling changes (addition of a new warning) for varenicline were instituted because of postmarketing surveillance reports noting a possible increased risk of neuropsychiatric symptoms (new onset of depressed mood, suicidal ideation and behavior, and changes in emotion and behavior within days to weeks of initiating treatment). These adverse effects were not noted in any of the clinical trials with varenicline and will require additional study to determine if they are causally related to the use of varenicline. Patients and their families should be apprised of the potential for these adverse effects and to report them if they do occur. If these symptoms occur, the drug should be stopped and the patient assessed immediately.

Combination Treatment

Combination treatment using a short-acting NRT formulation, such as nicotine gum/lozenge plus nicotine patch or combined NRT and bupropion, are generally recommended for patients unable to quit smoking using monotherapy. A meta-analysis of trials combining the nicotine patch with either the gum or spray formulation demonstrated nearly doubled odds of quitting compared with NRT monotherapy. The combined use of bupropion and nicotine patch is superior to monotherapy with nicotine patch but not bupropion alone. Clinical safety and efficacy of varenicline in combination with other smoking cessation therapies have not been evaluated. Varenicline combined with the nicotine patch is associated with an increased incidence of nausea.

BIBLIOGRAPHY, SUGGESTED READINGS, AND WEBSITES

1. U.S. Department of Health and Human Services: The Health Consequences of Smoking. A Report of the Surgeon General: http://www.cdc.gov/tobacco/data_statistics/sgr/sgr_2004/index.htm

2. U.S. Preventive Services Task Force: Counseling to Prevent Tobacco Use and Tobacco-Caused Disease: Recommendation Statement: http://www.ahrq.gov/clinic/3rduspstf/tobacccoun/tobcounrs.pdf

3. Benowitz NL: Clinical pharmacology of nicotine: implications for understanding, preventing and treating tobacco addiction, *Clin Pharmacol Ther* 83:531-541, 2008.

4. Cigarette smoking among adults—United States, 2006, *MMWR Morb Mortal Wkly Rep* 56(44):1157-1161, 2007.

5. Fiore MC, Jaén CR, Baker TB, et al: *Treating tobacco use and dependence: 2008 update. Clinical practice guideline*, Rockville, MD, 2008, U.S. Department of Health and Human Services, Public Health Service.

6. Hughes JR, Stead LF, Lancaster T: Antidepressants for smoking cessation, *Cochrane Database Syst Rev* 4: CD000031, 2004.

7. Jorenby DE, Hays JT, Rigotti NA, et al: Efficacy of varenicline, an alpha4-beta2 nicotinic acetylcholine receptor partial agonist, vs placebo or sustained-release bupropion for smoking cessation: a randomized controlled trial, *JAMA* 296:56-63, 2006.

8. Kenfield SA, Stampfer MJ, Rosner BA, et al: Smoking and smoking cessation in relation to mortality in women, *JAMA* 299:2037-2047, 2008.

9. Mokdad AH, Marks JS, Stroup DF, et al: Actual causes of death in the United States, 2000, *JAMA* 291: 1238-1245, 2004.

10. Peto R, Lopey AD, Boreham J, et al: Mortality from smoking in developed countries 1950-2000. In *Indirect estimates from national vital statistics*, New York, 1994, Oxford University Press.

11. Silagy C, Lancaster T, Stead L, et al: Nicotine replacement therapy for smoking cessation, *Cochrane Database Syst Rev* 3:CD000146, 2004.

12. Steinberg MB, Schmelzer AC, Richardson DL, et al: The case for treating tobacco dependence as a chronic disease, *Ann Intern Med* 148:554-556, 2008.

CHAPTER 48

EXERCISE AND THE HEART

Eric H. Awtry, MD and Gary J. Balady, MD

1. **What is the difference between physical activity and exercise?**
   Physical activity refers to the contraction of skeletal muscle that produces bodily movement and requires energy. *Exercise* is physical activity that is planned and is performed with the goal of attaining or maintaining physical fitness. *Physical fitness* is a set of traits that allows an individual to perform physical activity.

2. **What is the difference between isometric and isotonic exercise?**
   Isotonic muscle contraction produces limb movement without a change in muscle tension, whereas isometric muscle contraction produces muscle tension without a change in limb movement. Most physical activities involve a combination of both forms of muscle contraction, although one form usually predominates. Isotonic exercise (also referred to as aerobic, dynamic, or endurance exercise) involves high-repetition movements against low resistance and includes such activities as walking, running, swimming, and cycling. Isometric exercise (also referred to as resistance exercise or strength training) consists of low-repetition movements against high resistance and includes such activities as weight lifting and body building.

3. **What is the *training effect*?**
   Regular isotonic exercise results in improved exercise capacity, whereas regular resistance exercise results in increased strength. These changes allow an individual to exercise at a higher intensity and for a longer duration while attaining a lower heart rate for a given submaximal level of exercise. This is referred to as the training effect.

4. **What are the acute cardiovascular changes that occur with exercise?**
   Isotonic exercise results in an increase in heart rate and stroke volume that produces a fourfold to sixfold increase in cardiac output in healthy individuals. The increase in heart rate relates both to a withdrawal of vagal tone and an increase in sympathetic tone. Heart rate gradually rises during exercise to a maximal level that can be predicted by the following formula:

   $$\text{Maximum predicted heart rate} = 220 - \text{Age in years}$$

   Stroke volume increases by 20% to 50% as a result of both increased venous return from exercising muscles and more complete left ventricular emptying owing to enhanced myocardial contractility and to decreased peripheral vascular resistance owing to vasodilation in exercising muscle. Vascular beds other than in the heart, brain, and exercising muscle vasoconstrict during exercise. This, in conjunction with the increase in cardiac output, results in a rise in systolic blood pressure. The diastolic blood pressure remains unchanged or falls slightly. Isometric exercise results in a moderate increase in cardiac output, predominantly as a result of an increase in heart rate. Contracting muscle produces a rise in peripheral vascular resistance and may result in an increase in both systolic and diastolic blood pressure.

5. **What are the chronic cardiovascular changes that occur with exercise?**
   The increase in cardiac output associated with isotonic exercise creates a volume load that results in left ventricular dilation with minimal increase in wall thickness. The vasoconstriction and increased afterload associated with isometric exercise produces a pressure load that results in ventricular hypertrophy without dilation.

6. How is exercise intensity defined?

Exercise intensity is defined by the amount of energy required for the performance of the physical activity per unit of time. This can be measured directly using respiratory gas analysis to quantify oxygen uptake during exercise or can be estimated using standard regression models to estimate energy expenditure per a given workrate of exercise. Exercise intensity can also be expressed in terms of resting oxygen requirement (metabolic equivalents [METs]), where one MET equals the amount of oxygen consumed by a resting, awake individual and is equivalent to 3.5 ml O_2/kg of body weight/minute. Light exercise denotes those activities requiring less than 3 METs, moderate activity denotes activities requiring 3 to 6 METs, and vigorous activity denotes activities requiring more than 6 METs.

7. How much exercise is necessary to maintain cardiovascular fitness?

Current guidelines from the American Heart Association (AHA) and the American College of Sports Medicine (ACSM) recommend that all healthy adults perform moderate-intensity aerobic exercise (e.g., brisk walking) for at least 30 minutes on at least 5 days of the week or perform vigorous-intensity aerobic exercise (e.g., jogging) for at least 20 minutes on at least 3 days of the week. In addition, resistance exercise should be performed on at least 2 days of the week. Individuals who wish to improve their level of fitness or achieve substantial weight loss may need to perform significantly greater amounts of exercise. Importantly, exercise need not be performed all at one sitting; 10- or 15-minute periods of exercise can be accumulated throughout the day and applied to the daily exercising goal.

8. What is the effect of exercise on cardiac risk factors?

Exercise has beneficial effects on hypertension, diabetes, hyperlipidemia, and obesity. In addition, exercise has favorable effects on endothelial function, thrombosis, inflammation, and autonomic tone (Table 48-1).

TABLE 48-1. BENEFICIAL EFFECTS OF ENDURANCE EXERCISE ON ATHEROSCLEROTIC RISK FACTORS

Factor	Effect of Exercise
Hypertension	Modest ↓ in both SBP (approximately 4 mm Hg) and DBP (approximately 3 mm Hg)
Diabetes	↑ Insulin sensitivity, ↓ hepatic glucose production, preferential use of glucose over fatty acids by exercising muscle
Hyperlipidemia	Significant ↓ in TG, modest ↑ in HDL, minimal change in LDL
Obesity	Modest weight loss (2–3 kg), ↓ in body fat necessary to maintain weight loss
Thrombosis	↓ Fibrinogen, ↓ platelet activation
Endothelial function	Improved vasodilation, possibly through ↑ NO synthesis
Autonomic tone	↑ Vagal tone, ↓ sympathetic tone
Inflammation	↓ Inflammatory markers (CRP, TNF-α, IL-6)

CRP, C-reactive protein; *DBP*, diastolic blood pressure; *HDL*, high-density lipoprotein; *IL*, interleukin; *LDL*, low-density lipoprotein; *NO*, nitric oxide; *SBP*, systolic blood pressure; *TG*, triglycerides; *TNF*, tumor necrosis factor.

9. **Do endurance training and resistance training have similar benefits?**
   Endurance and resistance training have some similar effects and some complementary effects. Both improve insulin resistance, bone mineral density, and body composition. Endurance training improves peak measured exercise capacity, whereas resistance training improves muscle strength. Endurance training expends a greater amount of calories during exercise, whereas resistance training increases resting energy expenditure because of increased muscle mass.

10. **What is the effect of exercise on mortality?**
    Observational studies demonstrate an inverse linear relationship between the amount of physical activity performed and all-cause mortality. This is true for healthy individuals and for those with chronic diseases including diabetes and cardiovascular disease. A person who adheres to current exercise recommendations may benefit from a 30% to 50% reduction in all-cause mortality, when compared with inactive individuals; however, this benefit has not yet been demonstrated in adequately powered randomized controlled trials. In addition, exercise capacity (as measured in METs) is a strong predictor of the risk of death in patients with and without cardiovascular disease. Greater exercise capacity is associated with longer survival.

11. **Is it ever too late to obtain the benefits of exercise?**
    There does not appear to be an age limit after which exercise confers no benefit, and available data suggest that exercise is associated with a reduction in mortality even in the elderly. Additionally, individuals who are inactive but subsequently become physically active have a decreased risk of cardiovascular events and a lower mortality than those persons who remain inactive. Exercise attenuates, but does not prevent, the gradual decline in exercise capacity that occurs with aging; however, it does increase a person's maximal exercise capacity at any given age. Importantly, exercise that is performed at a young age but is not continued throughout adulthood does not appear to improve long-term survival.

12. **Is it safe for patients with known coronary artery disease to exercise?**
    Yes. Exercise is not only safe in patients with known coronary artery disease (CAD), but it confers multiple benefits. Meta-analyses demonstrate that patients with CAD who are enrolled in cardiac rehabilitation programs have a 20% lower risk of death and a 25% lower risk of cardiac death compared with patients who are not enrolled in an exercise program. Furthermore, patients who undergo exercise training have improvement in various cardiac risk factors, have less angina and less ischemia at a given level of exertion, have increased exercise capacity, and may have a lower risk of recurrent myocardial infarction.

13. **How long after myocardial infarction can a patient begin an exercise program?**
    Patients who are clinically stable after myocardial infarction can begin an exercise program as part of inpatient cardiac rehabilitation within 1 to 2 days of their infarction. Initially activity may be limited to range-of-motion exercises but is rapidly increased to assisted walking. Activity is then gradually increased so that most patients can independently perform activities of daily living at the time of hospital discharge. Current AHA/American College of Cardiology (ACC) guidelines suggest that after myocardial infarction all stable patients should be referred to formal outpatient cardiac rehabilitation programs. This is especially true for patients with multiple cardiac risk factors and for moderate- or high-risk patients (e.g., patients with residual CAD, patients with depressed left ventricle [LV] systolic function) for whom a supervised exercise program is appropriate. Stable patients can usually enroll in these programs 2 to 3 weeks after myocardial infarction.

14. **Is exercise safe for patients with heart failure?**
    Yes, providing that the patient is compensated and not congested. The hemodynamic effects associated with isotonic exercise (increased stroke volume, decreased systolic vascular resistance [SVR]) are beneficial in patients with depressed LV systolic function, and recent data suggest

that exercise training is safe. Although isometric exercise was previously avoided in patients with heart failure, recent data suggest that light to moderate levels of resistance training are well tolerated by patients with heart failure and may yield similar benefits as in healthy individuals.

15. **What is an exercise prescription?**
An exercise prescription is a recommended exercise regimen that is individualized for a particular patient and takes into account the patient's physical abilities, cardiac status, and medical comorbidities. The exercise prescription has four components: *intensity, duration, frequency,* and *modality.*

16. **How is an exercise prescription developed after myocardial infarction?**
Upon entry into a cardiac rehabilitation program, patients undergo formal exercise testing to quantify their exercise capacity, assess for inducible ischemia, and derive an exercise intensity that is both safe and effective. Exercise *intensity* is generally prescribed using a range of heart rates derived from the exercise test that represents 50% to 85% of heart rate reserve, where heart rate reserve is the difference between resting heart rate and peak exercise heart rate. For patients who develop ischemia during the exercise test (manifested by symptoms or electrocardiogram [ECG] changes), the peak training heart rate should be set at 10 beats/min below the rate at which the ischemia occurred. Exercise should then be performed for a minimum *duration* of 20 to 30 minutes and a *frequency* of 3 to 5 days per week. *Modalities* for endurance training commonly include walking/jogging (treadmill), rowing, cycling, and stair climbing.
    Resistance training should be included as part of a comprehensive exercise regimen and appears to be particularly beneficial in the elderly, patients with stable heart failure, and those with diabetes. Resistance training is prescribed at an *intensity* of 10 to 15 repetitions per set to moderate fatigue; *duration* of 1 to 3 sets of 8 to 10 different upper and lower body exercises; performed at a *frequency* of 2 to 3 times/week. Common *modalities* for resistance training include free weights, weight machines, wall pulleys, elastic bands, and calisthenics.

17. **What are the cardiovascular risks of exercise?**
Overall, the risk of adverse cardiovascular events related to exercise in healthy individuals is extremely low and varies depending on an individual's age, gender, level of physical fitness, and medical condition. Most events relate to structural or congenital heart disease in young athletes (e.g., hypertrophic cardiomyopathy, coronary anomalies, right ventricular dysplasia) or CAD in older individuals. The performance of vigorous exercise is associated with a transient increase in myocardial infarction and sudden cardiac death, especially in sedentary individuals with underlying CAD.

18. **Should patients be screened before enrolling in an exercise program?**
The AHA recommends screening of high school and college athletes by obtaining personal and family history and performing a cardiovascular physical examination before competing in sports and every 2 to 4 years thereafter. Further testing is not suggested in the absence of abnormal findings. In general, healthy individuals without symptoms of cardiovascular disease can embark on low- to moderate-intensity exercise programs without preexercise screening. However, preexercise stress testing should be considered in asymptomatic men older than age 45 years and women older than age 55 years (particularly those with multiple cardiovascular risk factors or diabetes) who plan to participate in vigorous exercise, in patients with established CAD, and in those who have exercise-related symptoms that suggest the possibility of CAD.

19. **What are the contraindications to participation in an exercise program?**
Absolute contraindications to exercise include unstable coronary heart disease, decompensated heart failure, symptomatic valvular stenosis, severe systemic hypertension (blood pressure more than 180/110 mm Hg), and uncontrolled arrhythmias. Detailed recommendations regarding athletic competition are provided in the 36th Bethesda Conference on Eligibility Recommendations for Competitive Athletes with Cardiovascular Abnormalities.

BIBLIOGRAPHY, SUGGESTED READINGS, AND WEBSITES

1. American Association of Cardiovascular and Pulmonary Rehabilitation: http://www.aacvpr.org
2. American College of Sports Medicine: http://www.acsm.org
3. American Heart Association (search *Exercise*): http://www.americanheart.org
4. 36th Bethesda Conference: Eligibility Recommendations for Competitive Athletes with Cardiovascular Abnormalities: http://www.csmfoundation.org/36th_Bethesda_Conference_-_Eligibility_Recommendations_for_Athletes_with_Cardiac_Abnormalities.pdf
5. American Diabetes Association: Physical activity/exercise and diabetes, *Diabetes Care* 29:1433-1438, 2006.
6. Awtry EA, Balady GJ: Exercise and physical activity. In Topol EJ, editor: *Textbook of cardiovascular medicine*, ed 3, Philadelphia, 2007, Lippincott Williams and Wilkins.
7. Balady GJ, Ades PA: Exercise and sports cardiology. In Libby P, Bonow R, Mann D, et al, editors: *Braunwald's heart disease: a textbook of cardiology*, ed 8, Philadelphia, 2008, Saunders.
8. Balady GJ, Williams MA, Ades PA, et al: Core components of cardiac rehabilitation/secondary prevention programs: 2007 update. A statement from the American Heart Association, *Circulation*, 115:2675-2682, 2007.
9. Haskell WL, Lee I-M, Pate RP, et al: Physical activity and public health: updated recommendation for adults from the American College of Sports Medicine and the American Heart Association, *Circulation* 116:1081-1093, 2007.
10. Maron BJ, Thompson PD, Ackerman MJ, et al: Recommendations and considerations related to preparticipation screening for cardiovascular abnormalities in competitive athletes: 2007 update. A scientific statement from the American Heart Association Council on Nutrition, Physical Activity, and Metabolism, *Circulation* 115:1643-1655, 2007.
11. Thompson PD, Franklin BA, Balady GJ, et al: Exercise and acute cardiovascular events: placing the risks into perspective: a scientific statement from the American Heart Association Council on Nutrition, Physical Activity, and Metabolism and the Council on Clinical Cardiology, *Circulation* 115:2358-2368, 2007.
12. Thompson PD: Exercise prescription and proscription for patients with coronary artery disease, *Circulation* 112:2354-2363, 2005.
13. Whaley MH, Brubaker PH, Otto RM, eds. *American College of Sports Medicine guidelines for exercise testing and prescription*, ed 7, New York, 2006, Lippincott Williams and Wilkins.
14. Williams MA, Haskell WL, Ades PA, et al: Resistance exercise in individuals with and without cardiovascular disease: 2007 update. A scientific statement from the American Heart Association Council on Clinical Cardiology and Council on Nutrition, Physical Activity, and Metabolism, *Circulation* 116:572-584, 2007.
15. 36th Bethesda Conference: Eligibility recommendations for competitive athletes with cardiovascular abnormalities, *J Am Coll Cardiol* 45:1312-1375, 2005.

CHAPTER 49

METABOLIC SYNDROME

Allison M. Pritchett, MD

1. **What is the metabolic syndrome?**

   The metabolic syndrome is a constellation of metabolic derangements that are commonly found in the same patient. The components of the metabolic syndrome are abdominal obesity, dyslipidemias, hypertension, insulin resistance with or without glucose intolerance, and prothrombotic and proinflammatory states. This clustering of cardiovascular risk factors has also been called *Syndrome X* or the *insulin resistance syndrome*.

   The underlying pathogenesis of the metabolic syndrome remains incompletely understood. Obesity and insulin resistance are two of the most commonly proposed conditions that lead to the other metabolic derangements. Abdominal obesity is a measure of visceral adiposity. Visceral adipose tissue is particularly active as an endocrine organ and produces fatty acids, tumor necrosis factor (TNFα), components of the renin-angiotensin-aldosterone cascade, plasminogen activator inhibitor (PAI-1), and adiponectin. These adipose tissue products can contribute to insulin resistance, hypertension, and proinflammatory and procoagulable states. Insulin resistance is also felt to play a central role, yet its contribution to the other criteria remains poorly defined.

2. **How is it defined?**

   The two most commonly used definitions of the metabolic syndrome are those from the National Cholesterol Education Program's Adult Treatment Panel (ATP III) and the World Health Organization (WHO) and are given in Table 49-1.

   The ATP III definition originally used a fasting glucose of 110 mg/dl or higher. The American Diabetes Association reduced this cut-point down to the current 100 mg/dl or higher to identify those with impaired fasting glucose or diabetes. The definition of the metabolic syndrome has been modified to include this cut-point.

TABLE 49-1. DEFINITIONS OF THE METABOLIC SYNDROME FROM ATP III AND WHO	
ATP III Definition	**WHO Definition**
Three or more of the following criteria:	The presence of diabetes, impaired fasting glucose, or insulin resistance and at least two of the following criteria:
1. Waist circumference >102 cm (40 inches) in men and >88 cm (35 inches) in women	1. Waist-to-hip ratio >0.90 in men or >0.85 in women
2. Triglycerides ≥150 mg/dl	2. Triglycerides ≥150 mg/dl or HDL cholesterol <35 mg/dl in men and <39 mg/dl in women
3. High density lipoprotein (HDL) cholesterol <40 mg/dl in men and <50 mg/dl in women	3. Blood pressure ≥140/90 mm Hg
4. Blood pressure ≥130/85 mm Hg or antihypertensive treatment	4. Urinary albumin excretion rate >20 μg/min or albumin-to-creatinine ratio ≥30 mg/g
5. Fasting glucose ≥110 mg/dl or hypoglycemic therapy	

3. **How is central obesity defined?**
   The definition of central obesity using waist circumference is gender and ethnic-group specific. Table 49-2 lists the International Diabetes Federation's (IDF's) recommended cut-points by ethnic group.

TABLE 49-2. WAIST CIRCUMFERENCE VALUES BY ETHNIC GROUP		
Country/Ethnic Group	Sex	Waist Circumference
USA	Male	≥102 cm or 40 inches
	Female	≥88 cm or 35 inches
European	Male	≥94 cm or 37 inches
	Female	≥80 cm or 32 inches
South Asian/Chinese/	Male	≥90 cm or 35 inches
Japanese	Female	≥80 cm or 32 inches
South/Central American	Use South Asian recommendations until more data available	
African/Eastern Mediterranean/Middle East	Use European recommendations until more data available	

Data from the International Diabetes Federation's *Consensus worldwide definition of the metabolic syndrome*, www.idf.org/webdata/docs/MetSyndrome_FINAL.pdf

4. **Which definition should be used?**
   Published literature has mainly compared the ATP III and WHO definitions. The prevalence of the metabolic syndrome in the adult population of the United States is similar for both definitions (23.9% for ATP III and 25.1% for WHO). The concordance between the two definitions is more than 80%. As detailed under question 6, the metabolic syndrome, as defined by either definition, is associated with increased risk for cardiovascular and overall mortality. The two definitions have similar positive predictive values (31.3% for ATP III and 32.4% for WHO) for cardiovascular disease. The metabolic syndrome, defined by either definition, is a stronger predictor of cardiovascular mortality in women than in men.

5. **What is the prevalence of metabolic syndrome in the United States?**
   - General population:
     The National Health and Nutrition Examination Survey (NHANES) demonstrated an unadjusted prevalence of 26.7% in 1999 to 2000. This was increased from 23.1% in the previous survey in 1988 to 1994. According to NHANES 1999 to 2000, the frequency of each of the individual criteria is abdominal obesity (44%), low high-density lipoprotein (HDL) cholesterol (39.9%), high blood pressure (39.2%), elevated triglycerides (32.6%), hyperglycemia (30.7%).
   - Distribution by age:
     The prevalence of the metabolic syndrome increases with age. NHANES data (1988–1994) reported a prevalence of 6.7% in those age 20 to 29 years, increasing to 43.5% in those 60 to 69 years of age.
   - Distribution by sex:
     Previously the prevalence of metabolic syndrome has been roughly equivalent between the two genders. However, women experienced a 26% relative increase in the prevalence of the metabolic syndrome between the two NHANES surveys compared with a

nonsignificant increase in men. Currently there is a trend toward an increased prevalence in women compared with men.

- Distribution by race/ethnicity:

  In the United States, Mexican Americans have the highest prevalence of metabolic syndrome (31.9%), followed by whites (23.8%), then African Americans (21.6%) and other races (20.3%). The Strong Heart Study has reported a prevalence of 35% in the Native American population.

- Patients with coronary artery disease (CAD)

  In the post–myocardial infarction population, the prevalence of the metabolic syndrome ranges from 29% to 46%.

- Patients with heart failure:

  The prevalence of the metabolic syndrome in the heart failure population ranges from 68% to 78%.

6. **Is the metabolic syndrome linked to worse outcomes?**

   Yes.

   - Overall mortality and cardiovascular mortality

     Both overall and cardiovascular mortality are increased in those with the metabolic syndrome compared with those without the metabolic syndrome. The metabolic syndrome is associated with a hazard ratio for overall mortality of approximately 1:5 and cardiovascular mortality of approximately 2:4.

   - Coronary artery disease

     The risk for developing CAD is approximately two times greater in those with the metabolic syndrome compared with those without. Of the individual components, hyperglycemia, elevated blood pressure, and low HDL are most strongly linked to CAD risk. The risk for CAD increases with an increasing number of metabolic syndrome components.

   - Heart failure

     The metabolic syndrome increases the risk of developing heart failure. Paradoxically, in patients with established heart failure, the metabolic syndrome is associated with improved overall survival. The reason for this phenomenon is not clear, but perhaps patients with more severe heart failure *lose* some of their metabolic parameters (i.e., they have lower blood pressure, cholesterol, and spontaneous weight loss).

   - Diabetes

     Given the inclusion of measures of glucose intolerance or insulin resistance in the definition of the metabolic syndrome, it is not surprising that the presence of the metabolic syndrome predicts the future development of diabetes.

7. **How is the metabolic syndrome treated?**

   Lifestyle modification is considered first line therapy. Gradual weight loss using a modest reduced-energy diet (500–1000 calorie/day reduction) to achieve a realistic goal of approximately 7% to 10% reduction in total body weight is recommended. Dietary composition should consist of increased amounts of fruits, vegetables, and whole grains, with minimal intake of saturated fat, trans fat, cholesterol, and simple sugars. In general, 30 minutes of daily moderate-intensity physical activity is recommended. Implementation of lifestyle modification can reduce total cholesterol, triglycerides, blood pressure, glucose, C-reactive protein (CRP), and plasminogen activator inhibitor 1 (PAI-1); raise HDL; and improve insulin resistance.

   Despite implementation of lifestyle modification, many patients require drug therapy targeted at the individual components of the metabolic syndrome to achieve recommended treatment goals.

   - **Dyslipidemia:** The ATP III recommendations are to first treat the LDL cholesterol to achieve goal levels. The treatment goal for LDL cholesterol is defined by the presence of CAD or the 10-year risk for developing CAD as estimated by the Framingham Risk Score. Statins have been shown to reduce the risk of cardiovascular events in patients with the metabolic syndrome.

   Elevated triglycerides and low HDL cholesterol are secondary targets for therapy. The exception is the case of very high triglycerides (500 mg/dl or more), which requires triglyceride lowering before addressing other lipid abnormalities in order to prevent acute pancreatitis. Otherwise, weight reduction and increased physical activity are recommended as initial interventions. However, pharmacologic therapy with niacin or a fibrate may be added in patients at high risk for CAD and high triglycerides (200–499 mg/dl). Although niacin lowers triglycerides and raises HDL, it can also increase glucose levels and require adjustment in diabetic medications.

Fibrates also lower triglycerides and increase HDL cholesterol. This class of agents has been shown to reduce cardiovascular events when used for secondary prevention in patients with known CAD. Fibrate use in those with the metabolic syndrome has not been studied prospectively, but post hoc analyses of several randomized clinical trials have demonstrated that patients with the metabolic syndrome who were treated with a fibrate had a greater reduction (an overall relative risk reduction of 35%–78%) in cardiovascular endpoints than those without these metabolic abnormalities. The effects of the combination of a statin and fibrate are being evaluated in the ongoing Action to Control Cardiovascular Risk in Diabetes Study (ACCORD trial). This study will provide more information of the safety and efficacy of combination therapy.

- **Elevated blood pressure:** According to the Seventh Report of the Joint National Committee (JNC-7) recommendations, pharmacologic therapy should be initiated when blood pressure is 140/90 mm Hg or more. Diabetics require therapy at lower levels of blood pressure (130/80 mm Hg or more). Individual patients may have specific indications for different pharmacologic antihypertensive agents. Currently no specific agents are recommended for patients with the metabolic syndrome, and the main focus is on reducing the overall blood pressure.
- **Insulin resistance and hyperglycemia:** Two drug classes, metformin and the thiazolidinediones (TZDs), reduce insulin resistance and delay or prevent progression to diabetes. However, no data show that therapy with these agents will reduce the risk of future CAD. Currently these medications are recommended strictly for treating hyperglycemia. Once diabetes is established, glycemic control to achieve a hemoglobin A1c (HbA1c) of less than 7% is recommended to reduce future vascular events.
- **Prothrombotic state:** Fibrinogen, PAI-1, and other coagulation factors are not routinely measured in clinical practice. No specific therapies directly target the levels of these factors. Antiplatelet therapy may be considered. Currently aspirin is recommended for primary prevention of thrombotic events in patients at high risk for CAD.
- **Proimflammatory state:** The proinflammatory state is most commonly defined by an elevated CRP. Several of the lipid-lowering medications will also reduce CRP.

8. **What is the utility of defining the metabolic syndrome as a clinical entity?**
   There are critics of the clinical utility of diagnosing a patient with the *metabolic syndrome*. Some of the arguments against labeling this clustering of cardiovascular risk factors as a syndrome are as follows:
   - Each of the individual variables should not be considered as present or absent, but rather treated as continuous variables that contribute to a spectrum of CAD risk. The rationale for specific cut-points is not well defined.
   - The underlying, unifying pathophysiology of the syndrome is poorly understood.
   - Is the metabolic syndrome useful in predicting CAD risk? As noted earlier, the metabolic syndrome increases risk for CAD. However, the presence of diabetes alone is associated with an even greater risk of CAD than the metabolic syndrome. So should diabetics be included in the definition of the metabolic syndrome? Several studies have excluded diabetics and shown that the metabolic syndrome still predicts an increased risk for CAD. However, the Framingham risk score has a higher sensitivity for predicting events than the presence of the metabolic syndrome. Also, because only three of five metabolic components are required for the diagnosis, different combinations of the risk factors may translate into different risk for CAD. Lastly, other known CAD risk factors are not incorporated into the definition of the metabolic syndrome.

- The treatment of the syndrome is essentially the treatment of each individual component. Currently no treatments, other than lifestyle modification, uniformly treat all the components of the syndrome.

In the end, further research is needed to better understand the underlying etiology of the metabolic syndrome, to reach a consensus on the definition of the metabolic syndrome and its role in predicting risk of CAD, and to improve strategies for treating the various components of the syndrome.

BIBLIOGRAPHY, SUGGESTED READINGS, AND WEBSITES

1. The International Diabetes Federation's Consensus Worldwide Definition of the Metabolic Syndrome: http://www.idf.org

2. World Health Organization: Definition, Diagnosis and Classification of Diabetes Mellitus and its Complications: Report of a WHO Consultation. Part 1: Diagnosis and Classification of Diabetes Mellitus: whqlibdoc.who.int/hq/1999/WHO_NCD_NCS_99.2.pdf

3. Ballantyne CM, Olsson AG, Cook TJ, et al: Influence of low high-density lipoprotein cholesterol and elevated triglyceride on coronary heart disease events and response to simvastatin therapy in 4S, *Circulation* 104: 3046-3051, 2001.

4. Executive summary of the third report of the National Cholesterol Education Program (NCEP) Expert Panel on Detection, Evaluation, and Treatment of High Blood Cholesterol in Adults (Adult Treatment Panel III), *JAMA* 285:2486-2497, 2001.

5. Ford ES, Giles WH, Dietz WH: Prevalence of the metabolic syndrome among U.S. adults—finding from the Third National Health and Nutrition Examination Survey, *JAMA* 287:356-359, 2002.

6. Ford ES, Giles WH, Mokdad AH: Increasing prevalence of the metabolic syndrome among U.S. adults, *Diabetes Care* 27:2444-2449, 2004.

7. Genuth S, Alberti KG, Bennett P, et al: Follow-up report on the diagnosis of diabetes mellitus. The Expert Committee on the Diagnosis and Classification of Diabetes Mellitus, *Diabetes Care* 26:3160-3167, 2003.

8. Ginsberg HN: Treatment for patients with the metabolic syndrome, *Am J Cardiol* 91(Suppl):29E-39E, 2003.

9. Grundy SM, Hansen B, Smith SC, et al: Clinical management of metabolic syndrome—report of the American Heart Association/National Heart, Lung, and Blood Institute/American Diabetes Association Conference on Scientific Issues Related to Management, *Circulation* 109:551-556, 2004.

10. Grundy SM, Brewer B Jr, Cleeman JI, et al: Definition of metabolic syndrome—report of the National Heart, Lung, and Blood Institute/American Heart Association Conference on Scientific Issues Related to Definition, *Circulation* 109:433-438, 2004.

11. Kahn R, Buse J, Ferrannini E, et al: The metabolic syndrome: time for a critical appraisal, *Diabetes Care* 28:2289-2304, 2005.

12. Malik S, Wong ND, Franklin SS, et al: Impact of the metabolic syndrome on mortality from coronary heart disease, cardiovascular disease, and all causes in united states adults, *Circulation* 110:1245-1250, 2004.

13. McNeill AM, Rosamond WD, Girman CJ, et al: The metabolic syndrome and 11-year risk of incident cardiovascular disease in the Atherosclerosis Risk in Communities Study, *Diabetes Care* 28:385-390, 2005.

14. Rubins HB, Robins SJ: Conclusions from the VA-HIT study, *Am J Cardiol* 86:543-544, 2000.

CHAPTER 50

PREVENTIVE CARDIOLOGY

L. Veronica Lee, MD, FACC and
Joanne M. Foody, MD, FACC, FAHA

1. What is preventive cardiology?

Mounting evidence demonstrates that controlling hypertension (HTN) and diabetes mellitus (DM), improving lipid profiles, smoking cessation, and lifestyle modifications reduce the risk of a first or subsequent heart attack. The field of preventive cardiology has evolved to treat the spectrum of coronary disease risk factors and coronary artery disease through the assessment of individual risk and early initiation of interventions to prevent, delay, or modify the development of clinical atherosclerosis (primary prevention), as well as treat individuals after the manifestation of symptomatic coronary artery disease (secondary prevention). Current recommendations based on guidelines by the American College of Cardiology/American Heart Association (ACC/AHA) are summarized in Table 50-1.

2. How is dyslipidemia related to cardiovascular disease (CVD)?

A continuous, independent, and strong relationship between cardiovascular disease and low-density lipoprotein (LDL) cholesterol or total cholesterol (TC) levels is well established. HMG CoA reductase inhibitors (statins) in numerous randomized secondary (i.e., 4S, CARE, LIPID) and primary prevention trials (i.e., WOSCOPS, AFCAPS/TEXCAPS) have demonstrated an overall significant 13% reduction of cardiovascular mortality (10% total mortality) for every 10% fall in TC level. Despite these proven beneficial effects, less than 33% of 5.5 million Americans at risk are treated, and only 33% of those treated and 20% of CVD patients achieve target goals of the National Cholesterol Education Program.

3. What is the relationship between HDL cholesterol and CVD?

Epidemiology has shown that high-density lipoprotein (HDL) cholesterol complex is an independent risk factor (cardiac risk factor) for CVD. There is an inverse relationship between HDL level and cardiovascular risk.

4. Are triglycerides an independent risk factor (cardiac risk factor) for CVD?

A potent independent relationship exists between CVD and triglyceride (TG) level, which is present in insulin resistance and metabolic syndrome and particularly in women and elderly patients. CVD event rates are twice as high in patients with TG more than 200 mg/dl compared with those with normal TG levels. Controversy continues over whether elevated TG levels directly influence plaque formation and stability or whether TG levels are more a marker of other comorbid conditions that contribute to the development of atherosclerotic disease.

5. Describe the current recommendations for the modification of lipids?

- Screening every 5 years is an important first step in adults (older than 20 years) without known CVD.
- Optimal levels of lipids in adults without known CVD are TC less than 150 mg/dl, TG less than 150 mg/dl, and HDL more than 45 mg/dl in men and more than 50 mg/dl in women. Optimal risk is defined as LDL less than 100 mg/dl.

TABLE 50-1. THE ABCDEs FOR CVD PREVENTION IN MEN AND WOMEN

A	ACEI	Post-MI, CHF, LVEF (<40%), LVH, nephropathy, CVD and/or DM, or hypertension. Avoid in pregnancy.
	ARB	DM, nephropathy, hypertension, or LVH. If ACEI intolerant after MI, CHF, LVEF(<40%). Avoid in pregnancy.
	Antiplatelet: ASA, clopidogrel	At risk of CVA, or >65 years without contraindications, known or at high risk of CVD. Clopidogrel if aspirin intolerant or after stent for CVD. Risk of bleeding or other adverse reaction to be considered when prescribing.
	Sleep apnea	Screen all patients with known or at risk of CVD, arrhythmia, hypertension, CHF. Treat if sleep apnea present.
B	β-Blockers	Post-MI, at high risk of CVD, inducible ischemia, symptomatic tachycardias, CHF, LVEF (<40%), and hypertension.
	Blood pressure control	Optimal BP from lifestyle modification (low-sodium, high-potassium [unless kidney disease] diet, folic acid, exercise, stress reduction, smoking cessation) to achieve BP < 120/80 mm Hg. Initiate medical therapy with low CVD risk but BP > 140/90 mm Hg or if at high risk for CVD, DM, nephropathy with BP > 130/80 mm Hg. Therapy should be risk directed.
C	Cholesterol	Lifestyle modification (increases in exercise, weight loss, fish or flaxseed oil; avoid trans fatty acids [hydrogenated or partially hydrogenated oils]; reduce saturated fat <7% of dietary fat per day; and improve glycemic control) to achieve HDL-C <45 mg/dl in men and <50 mg/dl in women, LDL-C <100 mg/dl, and triglycerides <150 mg/dl. For high-risk patients: add medication to lower LDL-C <100 mg/dl or if very high risk to <70 mg/dl. If not at optimal risk, give medical therapy if >130 mg/dl and multiple risk factors, >160 mg/dl and multiple risk factors but a 10-year absolute risk of <10%, or >190 mg/dl regardless of other risk factors.
	Cigarette smoking	Avoid all smoking and secondhand smoke exposure. Institute behavioral modification and counseling. Consider medical therapy (e.g., bupropion, nicotine patch, varenicline).
D	Depression and anxiety	People should be screened and treated for depression and anxiety because both can increase the risk of CVD and make risk factors harder to treat.
	Diabetes	Impaired fasting glucose (glucose of 110–124 mg/dl): implement lifestyle change, weight loss, exercise. Diabetes: improve glycemic control with lifestyle change and medications. Hemoglobin A1c should be <7.0%.
	Diet, weight management	Lifestyle change; portion control and a diet high in fiber, fruits and vegetables, whole grains, low in sodium (<2.3 g/day or 1 tsp), low in saturated fat (<7%) and cholesterol (<300 mg/day), and high in natural foods; BMI of 18.5–24.9 kg/m^2, waist circumference <35 inches, and body fat of <25%. Screen for sleep apnea.

(Continued)

TABLE 50-1. THE ABCDEs FOR CVD PREVENTION IN MEN AND WOMEN (CONTINUED)

E	Exercise	Moderate intensity >30 min/day on most days. Initiate walking regimen with goals using a pedometer if not exercising. For weight loss, increase to 60–90 min/day most days. Resistance training and stretching should be included. Address exercise limitations with physical therapy. Cardiac rehabilitation for patients post-MI, post-revascularization, and with CHF, chronic angina, stroke, and peripheral artery disease.

ACEI, Angiotensin-converting enzyme inhibitor; *ARB*, angiotensin-receptor blocker; *ASA*, acetylsalicylic acid, *BP*, blood pressure; *BMI*, body mass index; *CHF*, congestive heart failure; *CVD*, cardiovascular disease; *HDL-C*, high-density lipoprotein cholesterol; *LDL-C*, low-density lipoprotein cholesterol; *LV*, left ventricular; *LVEF*, left ventricular ejection fraction; *LVH*, left ventricular hypertrophy; *MI*, myocardial infarction.

- Lifestyle modification includes increased exercise, weight loss, dietary changes, avoiding trans fatty acids, reducing saturated fat to less than 7% of daily fat, and use of omega-3–rich oils.
- For most cases of primary prevention, medical therapy should be initiated if, after 3 to 6 months of lifestyle modification, LDL levels remain elevated (130–190 mg/dl, depending on risk factors and 10-year risk of development of CVD).
- Patients with cardiovascular disease should have an LDL level less than 100 mg/dl or, if at very high risk, LDL less than 70 mg/dl.

These issues are discussed further in Chapter 45 on Hyperlipidemia.

6. **What is the significance of hypertension and CVD?**
   A continuous graded relationship exists between increasing systolic and diastolic blood pressure and cardiovascular complications (myocardial infarction [MI], stroke, death). Thirty percent of adult Americans have hypertension. The lifetime risk of developing hypertension is 90%. Hypertension is a primary cause of death in almost 280,000 adults annually, with a cost of $63.5 billion in 2006.

7. **What are the definitions of prehypertension and hypertension?**
   Optimal blood pressure (BP) is defined as less than 120/80 mm Hg. *Prehypertension* is a BP between 120 to 139/80 to 89 mm Hg; and stage I hypertension starts at 140/90 mm Hg.

8. **Should lifestyle modification be recommended in patients with prehypertension or hypertension?**
   Yes. Lifestyle modification in prehypertension or hypertension includes low-sodium, high-potassium (without end-stage renal disease [ESRD]) and high-fiber diet; reducing sodium intake to less than 2.3 g/day; three daily servings of low or nonfat dairy; daily exercise; weight management; smoking cessation; stress and ethanol reduction; and, for women, consideration of folate supplementation. Issues regarding hypertension are discussed further in Chapter 44.

9. **What is the burden of diabetes in America, and what are the diagnostic criteria?**
   Seven percent of Americans have diabetes, and it is the sixth leading cause of death. Adults with DM have twice the mortality of nondiabetic adults of the same age, and 65% will die from MI or cerebrovascular accident (CVA), with an estimated cost of $132 billion in 2002.

10. **What interventions are used to prevent the complications of diabetes?**
    Glycemic control through diet, weight loss, exercise, and medications are the mainstays of complication prevention in patients with DM. Current American Diabetes Association (ADA) guidelines support the use of a target of a hemoglobin A1c below 7.0%, although this should be clinically coordinated with age, comorbidities, and life expectancy.

11. **What is the burden of tobacco abuse in the United States and its impact on CVD?**
    The most preventable cause of CVD is cigarette use, responsible for more than 400,000 deaths and $100 billion a year in the United States. Currently 26% of Americans smoke, the lowest level in decades, but still greater than the national goal set by Healthy People 2000 of 15%. Smoking rates remains higher in women, the young, African Americans, and those with lower education levels.
    Smoking causes increased CVD mortality and a 10-fold increase of sudden cardiac death in men (4.5-fold in women) compared with nonsmokers. CVD risk is related to dose, age of onset, amount of inhalant, and duration and quantity of cigarettes smoked. CVD risk doubles with smoking as few as one to four cigarettes daily. Compared with patients with cardiovascular disease who do not smoke or stop smoking, patients with cardiovascular disease who continue to smoke have a lower quality of life and activity, more angina, more unemployment, more hospital admissions, greater post–acute coronary syndrome (ACS) mortality (at 7 years, 82% versus 37% in quitters), and greater post–coronary artery bypass grafting (CABG) mortality (at 5 years, 31% versus 20% in nonsmokers). Environmental tobacco smoke increases CVD risk in nonsmokers and is believed to lead to 37,000 CVD deaths yearly. These issues are also discussed in Chapter 47 on smoking cessation.

12. **Is sedentary lifestyle a cardiac risk factor for CVD?**
    Sedentary lifestyle is a primary, modifiable cardiac risk factor of CVD, and exercise prevents the development and progression of CVD. Regular exercise improves weight, glycemic control, dyslipidemia, and hypertension and reduces CVD mortality. An inverse and dose-dependent relationship with CVD and CVD mortality exists between increased daily activity and fitness level. Lack of regular exercise is as much of a CVD cardiac risk factor as smoking. Unfortunately, improved functional status decreases all-cause and cardiac mortality 20% to 25% and a 1 metabolic equivalent task (MET) rise in functional capacity reduces cardiovascular risk 8% to 14%. Only 11% to 38% of patients with cardiovascular disease receive cardiac rehabilitation. These issues are also discussed in Chapter 48 on exercise and the heart.

13. **What are the current recommendations regarding exercise and CVD?**
    At present, moderate-intensity aerobic exercise more than 30 min/day most days is recommended. The use of patient activity diaries, goal setting, and use of a pedometer can often improve exercise compliance and results. For weight loss, exercise should be for 60 to 90 minutes a day on most days. Cardiac rehabilitation is suggested after MI, revascularization, congestive heart failure (CHF), CVA, chronic angina, and peripheral artery disease.

14. **What is the obesity epidemic?**
    The current global obesity epidemic has resulted in more than 33% of Americans being obese (body mass index (BMI) greater than 27.8 kg/m^2 in men and 27.3 kg/m^2 in women or 120% ideal weight). Obesity worsens dyslipidemia (elevated TC, TG, small particle LDL, and reduced HDL levels), insulin resistance, and glucose intolerance, and hypertension. It also is associated with procoagulability effects, increased atherosclerosis, and risk for cancer. Visceral adiposity (increased weight hip ratio) is particularly concerning.

15. What kinds of programs improve the chances of weight loss?

Appropriate weight goals with longitudinal reinforcement by the physician, as well as outside programs (e.g., Weight Watchers), improve the chances for lifestyle change and weight loss. Patients need realistic short-term achievable goals, such as a starting goal of 10% weight loss. Further goals of additional 10% increments of weight loss at 6-month intervals can later be set. Weight loss is enhanced by regular aerobic exercise.

BIBLIOGRAPHY, SUGGESTED READINGS, AND WEBSITES

 1. American College of Cardiology Clinical Statements/Guidelines http://www.acc.org/qualityandscience/clinical/statements.htm

 2. American Heart Association Scientific Statements and Practice Guidelines http://www.americanheart.org/presenter.jhtml?identifier=9181

 3. Bonow RO, Bennett S, Casey DE Jr, et al: American College of Cardiology; American Heart Association Task Force on Performance Measures (Writing Committee to Develop Heart Failure Clinical Performance Measures); Heart Failure Society of America. ACC/AHA clinical performance measures for adults with chronic heart failure: a report of the American College of Cardiology/American Heart Association Task Force on Performance Measures (Writing Committee to Develop Heart Failure Clinical Performance Measures) endorsed by the Heart Failure Society of America, *J Am Coll Cardiol* 46(6):1144-1178, 2005.

 4. Ford ES, Ajani UA, Croft JB, et al: Explaining the decrease in U.S. deaths from coronary disease, 1980–2000, *N Engl J Med* 356:2388-2398, 2007.

 5. Grundy SM, Cleeman JI, Daniels SR, et al: Diagnosis and management of the metabolic syndrome: an American Heart Association/National Heart, Lung, and Blood Institute Scientific Statement, *Circulation* 112(17): 2735-2752.

 6. Krumholz HM, Anderson JL, Brooks NH, et al: American College of Cardiology/American Heart Association Task Force on Performance Measures; Writing Committee to Develop Performance Measures on ST-Elevation and Non–ST-Elevation Myocardial Infarction. ACC/AHA clinical performance measures for adults with ST-elevation and non–ST-elevation myocardial infarction: a report of the American College of Cardiology/American Heart Association Task Force on Performance Measures (Writing Committee to Develop Performance Measures on ST-Elevation and Non–ST-Elevation Myocardial Infarction), *Circulation* 113(5):732-761, 2006.

 7. National Center for Health Statistics, Center for Disease Control and Prevention: Compressed mortality file: underlying cause of death 1979–2004. Available at http://wonder.cdc.gov/mortSQL.html, accessed January 15, 2008.

 8. Rosamond W, Flegal K, Furie K, et al: Heart disease and stroke statistics—2008 update: a report from the American Heart Association Statistics Committee and Stroke Statistics Subcommittee, *Circulation* 117:e1-e121, 2008.

 9. Smith SC Jr, Allen J, Blair SN, et al: AHA/ACC guidelines for secondary prevention for patients with coronary and other atherosclerotic vascular disease: 2006 update: endorsed by the National Heart, Lung, and Blood Institute, *Circulation* 113(19):2363-2372. Erratum in *Circulation* 113(22):e847, 2006.

10. Smith SC Jr: Can preventive therapy alter the initial presentation of coronary heart disease? *Ann Intern Med* 144(4):296-297.

11. Smith SC Jr: Current and future directions of cardiovascular risk prediction, *Am J Cardiol* 97(2A):28A-32A, 2006.

12. Smith SC Jr, Clark LT, Cooper RS, et al: Discovering the full spectrum of cardiovascular disease: Minority Health Summit 2003: report of the Obesity, Metabolic Syndrome, and Hypertension Writing Group, *Circulation* 111(10):e134-139.

13. Third report of the National Cholesterol Education Program (NCEP) Expert Panel on detection, evaluation, and treatment of high blood cholesterol in adults (Adult Treatment Panel III), *Circulation* 106:3143, 2002.

HYPERTENSIVE CRISIS

Christopher J. Rees, MD and Charles V. Pollack, Jr., MA, MD, FACEP, FAAEM, FAHA

CHAPTER 51

1. **What is a hypertensive crisis?**

   The term *hypertensive crisis* generally is inclusive of two different diagnoses, *hypertensive emergency* and *hypertensive urgency*. Distinguishing between the two is important because they require different intensities of therapy. It should be noted that older and less specific terminology, such as "malignant hypertension" and "accelerated hypertension", should no longer be used. The Seventh Report of the Joint National Committee on Prevention, Detection, Evaluation, and Treatment of High Blood Pressure (JNC-7) defines hypertensive emergency as being "characterized by severe elevations in blood pressure (more than 180/120 mm Hg), complicated by evidence of impending or progressive target organ dysfunction". JNC-7 defines hypertensive urgency as "those situations associated with severe elevations in blood pressure without progressive target organ dysfunction". There is no absolute value of blood pressure that defines a hypertensive urgency or emergency or separates the two syndromes. Instead, the most important distinction is whether there is evidence of impending or progressive end-organ damage, which defines an emergency or other symptoms that are felt referable to the blood pressure.

2. **How commonly do these situations occur?**

   It is estimated that 50 to 75 million people have hypertension and that 1% of those will have a hypertensive emergency. Hypertension accounts for 110 million emergency department (ED) visits per year, with severe hypertension accompanying as many as 25% of all admissions from the ED.

3. **What are the causes of hypertensive crisis?**

   The most common cause of hypertensive emergency is an abrupt increase in blood pressure in patients with chronic hypertension. Medication noncompliance is a frequent cause of such changes. Blood pressure control rates for patients diagnosed with hypertension are less than 50%. The elderly and African Americans are at increased risk of developing a hypertensive emergency. Other causes of hypertensive emergencies include stimulant intoxication (cocaine, methamphetamine, and phencyclidine), withdrawal syndromes (clonidine, β-adrenergic blockers), pheochromocytoma, and adverse drug interactions with monoamine oxidase (MAO) inhibitors.

4. **What are the common clinical presentations of hypertensive crisis?**

   Typical presentations of hypertensive urgency include severe headache, shortness of breath, epistaxis, or severe anxiety. Clinical syndromes typically associated with hypertensive emergency include hypertensive encephalopathy, intracerebral hemorrhage, acute myocardial infarction, pulmonary edema, unstable angina, dissecting aortic aneurysm, or eclampsia. Note that in hypertensive emergency presentations, there is evidence of impending or progressive target organ dysfunction and that the absolute value of the blood pressure is not pathognomonic.

5. **What historical information should be obtained?**

   A thorough history, especially as it relates to prior hypertension, is important to obtain and document, as most patients with a hypertensive emergency carry a diagnosis of hypertension and are either inadequately treated or are noncompliant with treatment.

   A thorough medication history is also essential. The patient's current medications need to be reviewed and updated to include timing, dosages, recent changes in therapy, last doses taken, and compliance. Patients should also be questioned about over-the-counter medication usage and recreational drug use because these agents may also affect blood pressure.

6. **How should the physical examination be focused?**

   Physical examination should start with recording the blood pressure in both arms with an appropriately sized blood pressure cuff. Direct ophthalmoscopy should be performed with attention to evaluating for papilledema and hypertensive exudates. A brief, focused neurologic examination to assess mental status and the presence or absence of focal neurologic deficits should be performed. The cardiopulmonary examination should focus on signs of pulmonary edema and aortic dissection, such as rales, elevated jugular venous pressure, or cardiac gallops. Peripheral pulses should be palpated and assessed. Abdominal examination should include palpation for abdominal masses and tenderness and auscultation for abdominal bruits.

7. **What laboratory and ancillary data should be obtained?**

   All patients should have an electrocardiogram performed to assess for left ventricular hypertrophy, acute ischemia or infarction, and arrhythmias. Urinalysis should be performed to evaluate for hematuria and proteinuria as signs of acute renal failure. Women of child-bearing age should have a urine pregnancy test performed. Laboratory studies should include a basic metabolic profile with blood urea nitrogen (BUN) and creatinine and a complete blood cell count (CBC) with a peripheral smear to evaluate for signs of microangiopathic hemolytic anemia. If acute coronary syndrome is suspected, cardiac biomarkers should be assessed. Choice of radiographic studies, if any, should be based on the presentation and diagnostic considerations. A chest radiograph is often ordered to evaluate for pulmonary edema, cardiomegaly, and mediastinal widening. If there are any focal neurologic findings, a computed tomography (CT) scan of the brain should be performed to evaluate for hemorrhage.

8. **What are the cardiac manifestations of hypertensive emergencies?**

   Cardiac manifestations of hypertensive emergency include acute coronary syndromes, acute cardiogenic pulmonary edema, and aortic dissection. The latter deserves special attention because it has much higher short-term morbidity and mortality, requires more urgent and rapid reduction in blood pressure, and also requires specific inhibition of the reflex tachycardia often associated with blood pressure–lowering agents. It is recommended that patients with aortic dissection have their systolic blood pressure reduced to at least 120 mm Hg within 20 minutes, a much more rapid decrease than is recommended for other syndromes associated with hypertensive emergency.

9. **What are the central nervous system manifestations of hypertensive emergency?**

   Neurologic emergencies associated with hypertensive emergency include subarachnoid hemorrhage, cerebral infarction, intraparenchymal hemorrhage, and hypertensive encephalopathy. Patients with hemorrhage and infarction usually have focal neurologic findings and may have corresponding findings on head CT or magnetic resonance imaging (MRI) of the brain. Hypertensive encephalopathy is more difficult to diagnose with patients with severe headache, vomiting, drowsiness, confusion, visual disturbances, and seizures; coma may ensue. Papilledema is often present on physical examination.

10. **What are the renal manifestations of hypertensive emergencies?**
    Renal failure can both cause and be caused by hypertensive emergency. Typically, hypertensive renal failure presents as nonoliguric renal failure, often with hematuria.

11. **What are the pregnancy-related issues with hypertensive emergency?**
    Preeclampsia is a syndrome that includes hypertension, peripheral edema, and proteinuria in women after the twentieth week of gestation. Eclampsia is the more severe form of the syndrome, with severe hypertension, edema, proteinuria, and seizures.

12. **What are general issues in the treatment of hypertensive urgency?**
    Patients with hypertensive urgencies often have elevated blood pressure and nonspecific symptoms but no evidence of progressive end-organ damage. These patients do not often require urgent treatment with parenteral antihypertensives. There is no evidence to suggest that urgent treatment of patients with hypertensive urgencies in an emergency department setting reduces morbidity or mortality. In fact, there is evidence that too-rapid treatment of asymptomatic hypertension has adverse effects. Rapidly lowering blood pressure below the autoregulatory range of an organ system (most importantly the cerebral, renal, or coronary beds) can result in reduced perfusion, leading to ischemia and infarction. It is usually appropriate in these situations instead to gradually reduce blood pressure over 24 to 48 hours. Most patients with hypertensive urgency can be treated as outpatients, but some may need to be admitted as dictated by symptoms and situation and to ensure close follow-up and compliance. The most important intervention for hypertensive urgency is to ensure good follow-up, which helps to promote ongoing, long-term control of blood pressure. No guidelines and no evidence support a specific blood pressure *target* number that must be achieved in order to safely discharge a patient with hypertensive urgency.

13. **What are general issues in treating hypertensive emergencies?**
    JNC-7 recommends that patients with hypertensive emergencies be treated as inpatients in an intensive care setting with an initial goal of reducing mean arterial blood pressure by 10% to 15%, but no more than 25%, in the first hour and then, if stable, to a goal of 160/100-110 mm Hg within the next 2 to 6 hours. This requires parenteral agents. Aortic dissection is a special situation that requires reduction of the systolic blood pressure to at least 120 mm Hg within 20 minutes. Treatment is also required to help blunt the reflex tachycardia associated with most antihypertensive agents. Ischemic stroke and intracranial hemorrhage are also special situations, and guidelines exist for the treatment of hypertension in these settings from multiple experts, including guidelines from the American Stroke Association/American Heart Association (ASA/AHA). These guidelines state that "there is little scientific evidence and no clinically established benefit for rapid lowering of blood pressure among persons with acute ischemic stroke." Too rapid a decline in blood pressure during the first 24 hours after presentation of an intracranial hemorrhage has been independently associated with increased mortality. The overall weight of evidence currently supports only judicious use of antihypertensive agents in the treatment of acute ischemic or hemorrhagic stroke. Expert guidance is recommended, especially if fibrinolytic therapy is being considered for acute ischemic stroke.

14. **What specific agents are used for treating patients with hypertensive emergencies?**
    Table 51-1 reviews specific agents available for use.

15. **Are different agents more helpful for different clinical situations?**
    Table 51-2 reviews specific agents recommended for specific situations.

TABLE 51-1. PARENTERAL AGENTS FOR USE IN HYPERTENSIVE EMERGENCIES

Drug	Class/ Mechanism	Usual Dose	Onset	Effect Duration After D/C	Advantages	Disadvantages/ Adverse Effects	Common Uses
Sodium nitroprusside	Direct arterial and venous vasodilator via cGMP	0.25–10 μg/kg/min Average effective dose 3 μg/kg/min	1–2 min	3–4 min after infusion stopped	Large amount of experience with use	Nausea, vomiting, muscle twitching, diaphoresis Cyanide toxicity, especially with renal insufficiency and prolonged infusions (>48 hours) Inactivated by light; needs to be given in light-protected delivery system Usually requires invasive intraarterial blood pressure monitoring Use cautiously with ↑ ICP; can worsen Use cautiously in ACS; can cause coronary steal	Has been used in all syndromes of HE
Clevidipine	Ultra short acting dihydropyridine Calcium channel blocker Vasodilator	2–16 μg/kg/min	1–5 min	T ½ 1 min; effect lasts 5–10 min after stopping	Ultra short acting with rapid onset, offset of effect Little to no reflex tachycardia Metabolism independent of renal and hepatic function Arterial line not required No special delivery system needed; used with peripheral IV access		Studied in postoperative hypertension, post-cardiac surgery, and ED treatment of HE Potentially useful for all types of HE syndromes

Drug	Class/Mechanism	Dose	Onset	Duration	Uses	Side effects	Comments
Fenoldopam	Peripheral, dopamine-1 receptor agonist, causes vasodilation especially in renal, cardiac, sphlanchic beds	0.1 µg/kg/min to max 1.6 µg/kg/min Titrate in 0.05–0.1 µg/kg/min increments	10 min Max effect in 30 min	1 hour after stopping	Increases renal blood flow, improving CrCl especially in setting of impaired renal function Used without invasive BP monitoring	Reflex tachycardia HA, dizziness, flushing, nausea Worsening angina A-fibrillation tachyphylaxis after 48 hours Contraindicated in glaucoma; causes dose-related increase in IOP	Especially useful in HE syndromes complicated by renal insufficiency or failure
Nicardipine	Dihydropyridine Calcium channel blocker Vasodilator	5 mg/hr; can ↑ by 2.5 mg/hr to max 15 mg/hr	Within 10 min	2–6 hours after stopping	Dilates coronary vessels; can use with known CAD Used without invasive BP monitoring	HA, flushing, dizziness, hypotension, digital dysesthesias Abrupt withdrawal can cause or worsen angina or hypertension Metabolized in liver; use with caution in cirrhotics	Has been used extensively in postoperative hypertension, especially after CT surgery
Nitroglycerin	Direct venous vasodilator	5 µg/kg/min to max 100 µg/kg/min	2–5 min	5–10 min	Dilates coronary vessels	Ineffective arterial vasodilator HA, hypotension, tachycardia	Not used for most HE; reserved for cardiac ischemia and cardiogenic pulmonary edema

(Continued)

TABLE 51-1. PARENTERAL AGENTS FOR USE IN HYPERTENSIVE EMERGENCIES (CONTINUED)

Drug	Class/Mechanism	Usual Dose	Onset	Effect Duration After D/C	Advantages	Disadvantages/Adverse Effects	Common Uses
Enalaprilat	ACE inhibitor	1.25 mg IVP at 4–6 hr intervals; max 5 mg in 6 hours	15 min–4 hours to peak effect	12–24 hours		BP response variable, unpredictable, and not dose related May not peak for 4 hours Contraindicated in pregnancy	Not generally useful for HE syndromes
Hydralazine	Direct arterial vasodilator	10–20 mg IV	10–20 min	1–4 hours	Increases uterine blood flow	Flushing, HA, nausea Sig reflex tachycardia Has precipitated MI Use cautiously in CKD, CAD, CVD	Used only for eclampsia/preeclampsia
Esmolol	Selective β₁ receptor blocker	Load 250–500 µg/kg over 1–3 min Can infuse at 50–100 µg/kg/min Titrate every 5 min with repeat bolus and ↑ drip by 50 µg/kg/min to max dose 300 µg/kg/min	6–20 min after bolus Max effect 5 min	Effects last for 20 min after stopping	Ultra short acting	Bradycardia Hypotension Bronchospasm Seizure Acute pulmonary edema Abrupt withdrawal can precipitate chest pain Requires central access; extravasation can cause local tissue necrosis and can cause small vein phlebitis Use with caution in CKD	Often used in combination with vasodilators to reduce reflex tachycardia

| Labetolol | Combined α- and β-adrenergic receptor blocker | 20 mg IV over 2 min Additional boluses every 10 min with escalating doses of 40, 80 to max; cumulative dose of 300 mg Can start infusion with 1–2 mg/min | 2–5 min after bolus with peak in 5–15 min | 2–4 hours after stopping infusion or last bolus | Decreases reflex tachycardia from other agents Does not affect cerebral blood flow Doesn't decrease cardiac blood flow or CO Doesn't affect renal function | Profound orthostasis Contraindicated in decompensatred CHF, heart block, asthma, pheochromocytoma Can cause profound hypotension Dizziness, nausea, vomiting, paresthesias, scalp tingling, bronchospasm | Often used in combination with vasodilators to reduce reflex tachycardia associated with those agents. |
| Phentolamine | Pure α-adrenergic antagonist | 5–20 mg IV bolus every 5 min Can infuse at 0.2–0.5 mg/min | 1–2 min | 10–30 min | Used for catecholamine-induced HE | Sig tachycardia CAD, CVD, has caused or precipitated MI and stroke Contraindicated with history of significant arrhythmia Use cautiously in CKD Use cautiously or not at all if recent phosphodiesterase-5 inhibitor (sildenafil, tadalifil, vardenafil) use; can cause vasospasm | Used only for catecholamine-induced HE, such as cocaine-induced HE, pheochromocytoma, and MAOI tyramine-induced HE |

ACE, Angiotensin-converting enzyme; ACS, acute coronary syndrome; BP, Blood pressure; CAD, coronary artery disease; CHF, congestive heart failure; HE, hypertensive emergency; ICP, intracranial pressure; IV, intravenously; MI, myocardial infarction.

TABLE 51-2. SPECIFIC ANTIHYPERTENSIVE AGENTS SUGGESTED FOR SPECIFIC HYPERTENSIVE EMERGENCY (HE) SYNDROMES

Syndrome	Suggested Antihypertensive Agents
Aortic dissection	Nitroprusside, often in combination with (esmolol, labetolol) Nicardipine with beta-blocker Beta-blocker alone
Acute pulmonary edema	Nitroglycerin preferred Fenoldopam Nicardipine Clevidipine
Acute coronary syndrome	Beta-blocker Nitroglycerin Clevidipine
HE with acute or chronic renal failure	Labetolol Nicardipine Fenoldopam Clevidipine
Eclampsia	Labetolol Nicardipine Hydralazine (all in conjunction with magnesium sulfate)
Acute ischemic stroke or ICH (if expert guidance deems blood pressure control necessary)	Nicardipine Labetolol Clevidipine
Hypertensive encephalopathy	Clevidipine Labetolol Esmolol Nicardipine Fenoldopam Nitroprusside
Adrenergic crisis with HE	Phentolamine Nitroprusside Beta-blocker

HE, Hypertensive emergency; *ICH*, intracranial hemorrhage.

BIBLIOGRAPHY, SUGGESTED READINGS, AND WEBSITE

1. Adams HP Jr, DelZoppo G, Alberts MJ, et al: Guidelines for the early management of adults with ischemic stroke: A guideline from the American Heart Association/American Stroke Association Council, Clinical Cardiology Council, Cerebrovascular Radiology and Intervention Council, and the Atherosclerotic Peripheral Vascular Disease and Quality of Care Outcomes in Research Interdisciplinary Working Groups, *Stroke* 38(5):1655-1711, 2007.

2. Amin A: Parenteral medication for hypertension with symptoms, *Ann Em Med* 51(3):S1-S15, 2008.

3. Elliott WJ: Clinical features in the management of selected hypertensive emergencies, *Progress Cardiovasc Dis* 48(5):316-325, 2006.

4. Flanigan JS, Vitberg D: Hypertensive emergencies and severe hypertension: what to treat, who to treat, and how to treat, *Med Clin North Am* 90:439-451, 2006.

5. Gray RO: Hypertension. In Marx: *Rosen's emergency medicine: concepts and clinical practice*, ed 6, Philadelphia, 2006, Mosby.

6. Haas AR, Marik PE: Current diagnosis and management of hypertensive emergency, *Sem Dialysis* 19(6): 502-512, 2006.

7. Marik PE, Varon J: Hypertensive crisis: challenges and management, *Chest* 131(6):1949-1962, 2007.

8. National Heart, Lung, and Blood Institute: *Seventh report of the Joint National Committee on Prevention, Detection, Evaluation, and Treatment of High Blood Pressure (JNC-7)*, Publication no. NIH 03-5233. Bethesda, MD, 2003, pp. 54-55.

9. Qureshi AI, Bliwise DL, Bliwise NG, et al: Rate of 24-hour blood pressure decline and mortality after spontaneous intracerebral hemorrhage: a retrospective analysis with a random effects regression model, *Crit Care Med* 27:480-485, 1999.

10. Stewart DL, Feinstein SE, Colgan R: Hypertensive urgencies and emergencies, *Prim Care Clin Off Practice* 33:613-623, 2006.

11. Strandgaard S, Olesen J, Skinhoj E, et al: Autoregulation of brain circulation in severe arterial hypertension, *Br Med J* 1:507-510, 1973.

12. Zampaglione B, Pascale C, Marchisio M, et al: Hypertensive urgencies and emergencies: prevalence and clinical presentation, *Hypertension* 27(1):144-147, 1996.

CHAPTER 52

THORACIC AORTIC ANEURYSM AND DISSECTION

Jean Bismuth, MD, Christof Karmonik, PhD, and Alan B. Lumsden, MD, FACS

1. **What are the primary thoracic aortic pathologies?**

   Aneurysm and dissection are the principal aortic diseases. Other more rare conditions of the thoracic aorta include aortic coarctation. In a recent Swedish population study, a significant increase in the incidence of aneurysms and dissections of the thoracic aorta from 1987 through 2002 was shown. The increase was from 10.7 per 100,000 per year in 1987 to 16.3 per 100,000 per year in 2002 (52% increase) for men, whereas women showed a more modest increase from 7.1 per 100,000 per year in 1987 to 9.1 per 100,000 per year in 2002 (28% increase). During this same period, the median age at diagnosis decreased from 73 to 71 years.

2. **What is the cause of thoracic aortic aneurysms?**

   Aneurysms of the ascending thoracic aorta most often result from the process of cystic medial degeneration, which is also found in virtually all cases of Marfan syndrome. Aneurysms of the descending aorta are most commonly degenerative—that is, caused by atherosclerosis. Aneurysms of the aortic arch are generally contiguous with either ascending or descending aneurysms and as such are more mixed in their etiology. Other causes include aortic dissection and the more rare infectious causes such as syphilis and infectious aortitis.

3. **What are the survival rates for untreated thoracic aortic aneurysms?**

   Survival rates for thoracic aortic aneurysms not undergoing surgical repair are as follows:
   - 65% at 1 year
   - 36% at 3 years
   - 20% at 5 years

   Aneurysm rupture occurs in 32% to 68% of patients not treated surgically, with rupture accounting for 32% to 47% of all deaths. It is estimated that less than one half of patients with rupture actually arrive to the hospital alive. The mortality rates for aneurysmal rupture are 54% at 6 hours and 76% at 24 hours. Because death is the most likely outcome after unexpected rupture, more patients should be encouraged to undergo elective repair and those managed conservatively should have risk factors aggressively controlled.

4. **List the risk factors for rupture of thoracic aortic aneurysms.**

   Risk factors for rupture can be divided into dimensional and nondimensional factors. The dimensional factors include size and growth rate; nondimensional factors include smoking/chronic obstructive lung disease (COPD), age, hypertension, renal failure, and pain.

5. **How fast does an aortic aneurysm grow?**

   Aneurysms expand exponentially; that is, the larger the aneurysm the more rapid the growth. The aneurismal thoracic aorta grows on average at a rate of 0.10 cm per year. On average, the descending thoracic aorta grows faster than the ascending thoracic aorta (0.19 cm/year versus 0.07 cm/year). The annual growth rates of aneurysms in patients with chronic dissections are significantly higher, ranging from 0.24 cm/year for small (4.0 cm) aneurysms to 0.48 cm/year for large (8.0 cm) aneurysms.

6. **At what size should an aneurysm be repaired electively? What is the management of symptomatic aneurysms?**

Studies have shown that the critical size for the thoracic aorta is 6.0 cm, at which point 31% of patients have suffered from rupture or dissection. For the descending thoracic aorta the critical size is 7.0 cm, at which point 43% of patients have experienced rupture or dissection. These numbers relate to median value and as such repair of an aneurysm should ideally occur earlier; otherwise one would potentially be approaching a complication rate of 50%. The threshold for intervention in patients with connective tissue disorders such as Marfan syndrome should be significantly lower than in other patients because of the higher risk of complications. If the patient has a symptomatic aneurysm, all the statistics are moot and the patient should be managed operatively. Suggested criteria for referral for aneurysm repair are given in Table 52-1.

TABLE 52-1. CRITERIA FOR SURGICAL INTERVENTION IN THE THORACIC AORTA			
	Non-Marfan	Marfan Disease	Dissection
Ascending	5.5 cm	5.0 cm	Any size
Descending	6.5 cm	6.0 cm	6.0 cm

7. **What is the definition of a dissection?**

The essential feature of aortic dissection is a tear in the intima, which consequently allows medial disruption with formation and propagation of a subintimal hematoma, often occupying half of the aortic circumference. This can lead to branch vessel compromise and effects such as mesenteric ischemia, stroke, and renal failure.

8. **What is the criteria for classifying a dissection as either acute or chronic?**

Acute dissections are those that are of less than 14 days duration from onset of symptoms, whereas beyond this time frame dissections are considered chronic. Some authors consider the period between 14 to 60 days as *subacute* dissections. This 14-day period is chosen based on the facts that this is the period during which the highest morbidity and mortality rates are observed and that surviving patients will generally stabilize during these 14 days.

9. **What are the most reliable symptoms/signs/radiographic findings associated with dissection?**

The most reliable symptoms/signs/radiographic findings associated with dissection include chest/back pain (86%), abrupt onset of pain (89%), hypertension (69%), any pulse loss (21%), and migrating pain (24%). Widened mediastinum is found in up to 56% of patients.

10. **How are aortic dissections classified?**

In general terms, most classification systems for location identify the dissection's position relative to the origin of the subclavian artery. That is, the dissections involve either the ascending aorta, descending aorta, or both. Ninety percent of thoracic dissections involve the first 10 cm of the aorta. The accepted classification systems are DeBakey and Stanford. In the DeBakey classification, type I aortic dissections involve the ascending and descending aorta, type II dissections involve the ascending aorta alone, and type III dissections are limited to the descending aorta (thoracic alone [IIIa] or with the abdominal aorta [IIIb]). The Stanford classification condenses DeBakey's classification so that type A refers to ascending dissections while type B to descending dissections. Although the Stanford classification more succinctly emphasizes a patient's need for emergent surgery (type A), it ignores what is happening in the remainder of the aorta, which is important for follow-up. These classifications are illustrated in Figure 52-1.

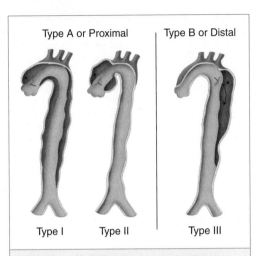

Figure 52-1. Classification systems for aortic dissection based on the DeBakey classification system (type I, II, or III) or the Stanford system (type A or B). (From Isselbacher EM: Diseases of the aorta. In Braunwald E, Zipes DP, Libby P, Bonow RO: *Braunwald's heart disease: a textbook of cardiovascular medicine*, ed 7, Philadelphia, 2004, Saunders.)

11. **Is there a need to distinguish intramural hematoma (IMH) and penetrating atherosclerotic ulcer (PAU) from aortic dissection?**
    The diagnoses of intramural hematoma (IMH) and penetrating atherosclerotic ulcer (PAU) are mostly a consequence of the refined diagnostic modalities available today. There are, though, at least three reasons why intramural hematoma and penetrating atherosclerotic ulcer are of great concern:
    1. The rate of rupture on initial presentation is high (45%).
    2. The rate of radiographic advancement is significant (50%).
    3. Delayed rupture occurs with great frequency and is fatal.

12. **What is the ideal treatment of aortic dissection?**
    Type A dissection is managed surgically. Acute uncomplicated type B dissection has a favorable early outcome, with 85% to 90% of patients able to leave the hospital on medical therapy. On the other hand, *complicated* acute type B dissections have a greater than 50% mortality rate and therefore need intervention (e.g., open repair, stentgraft, fenestration).

13. **What constitutes optimal medical therapy for aortic dissection?**
    The aims of medical therapy are to decrease the force of the left ventricular contractions, to reduce the steepness of the rise of the aortic pulse wave (dP/dt), and to reduce the systemic arterial pressure as low as possible without affecting vital organ perfusion. Beta-blockers are considered the optimal drug in reaching this goal. Esmolol is generally the drug of choice, but labetalol (which also adds alpha antagonist activity) and metoprolol can also be used. If the target blood pressure cannot be achieved with a beta-blocker alone, then a second agent such as nitroprusside or nicardipine can be used.

14. **List the anomalies associated with aortic coarctation.**
Anomalies associated with aortic coarctation include hypoplastic left-sided heart, severe mitral or aortic valve disease (bicuspid aortic valve in more than 70% of patients), ventricular septal defect, transposition of the great arteries, and variations of double-outlet or single ventricle.

15. **Describe the range of clinical presentations in aortic coarctation.**
Presentations can vary drastically from left-sided heart failure in children to otherwise asymptomatic hypertension in adults. The classic finding is a pulse disparity between the upper and lower extremities and palpable pulsatility of the intercostals arteries.

16. **What are the best options for imaging thoracic aortic dissections?**
- **Computed tomography (CT) scan:** Sensitivities of 83% to 94% and specificities of 87% to 100% have been reported with the use of CT scanning for the diagnosis of aortic dissection, and this is increased with the use of modern helical CT scanners (Fig. 52-2, *A*).
- **Magnetic resonance imaging (MRI):** Both the sensitivity and the specificity of MRI are in the range of 95% to 100%. Particularly useful tools are the dynamic images of MRI, which afford the physician further information.
- **Transesophageal echo (TEE):** The sensitivity of transesophageal echocardiography has been reported to be as high as 98%, and the specificity ranges from 63% to 96%.

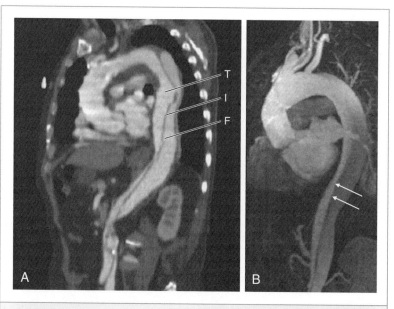

Figure 52-2. CT and MRI images of aortic dissections. **A,** CT demonstrating aortic dissection. Shown is a contrast-enhanced spiral CT scan of the chest at the level of the pulmonary artery showing an intimal flap *(I)* in the descending thoracic aorta separating the two lumina in a type B aortic dissection. *F,* False lumen; *T,* true lumen. **B,** Gadolinium-enhanced magnetic resonance angiography (MRA) of a patient with aortic dissection. The intimal flap *(arrows)* is clearly delineated. (**A** from Libby P, Bonow RO, Mann DL, et al: *Braunwald's heart disease: a textbook of cardiovascular medicine,* ed 8, Philadelphia, 2008, Saunders. **B** from Adam: *Grainger & Allison's diagnostic radiology,* ed 5, Philadelphia, 2008, Churchill and Livingstone. Courtesy Dr Sanjay K. Prasad.)

17. **List the main indications for surgical intervention on the thoracic aorta.**
    Indications for surgical intervention include the following:
    - Fusiform aneurysm of 5.5 cm or twice the diameter of the normal contiguous aorta
    - Saccular width of 2 cm or total aortic size of 5 cm
    - Acute type B dissection with distal ischemia, rupture, or leak for any reason
    - Aortic coarctation
    - Pseudoaneurysm
    - Mycotic aneurysm

18. **Is endovascular exclusion always a good option?**
    Degenerative aneurysms can be treated either by endovascular techniques or open surgical procedures with equivalent midterm results. The only randomized trial for chronic dissections, the INSTEAD Trial, did not appear to support prophylactic stent grafting in asymptomatic, medically controlled patients.

BIBLIOGRAPHY, SUGGESTED READINGS, AND WEBSITES

1. Aortic Dissection: http://www.aorticdissection.com
2. Manning WJ: Clinical Manifestations and Diagnosis of Aortic Dissection: http://www.utdol.com
3. Woo YJ, Mohler ER: Management and Outcome of Thoracic Aortic Aneurysm: http://www.utdol.com
4. Elefteriades JA: Natural history of thoracic aortic aneurysms: indications for surgery, and surgical versus nonsurgical risks, *Ann Thorac Surg* 74(5):S1877-S1880; discussion S1892-1898, 2002.
5. Griepp RB, Ergin MA, Galla JD, et al: Natural history of descending thoracic and thoracoabdominal aneurysms, *Ann Thorac Surg* 67(6):1927-1930; discussion 1953-1958, 1999.
6. Khan IA, Nair CK: Clinical, diagnostic, and management perspectives of aortic dissection, *Chest* 122(1): 311-328, 2002.
7. Olsson C, Thelin S, Ståhle E, et al: Thoracic aortic aneurysm and dissection: increasing prevalence and improved outcomes reported in a nationwide population-based study of more than 14,000 cases from 1987 to 2002, *Circulation* 114(24):2611-2618, 2006.
8. Suzuki T, Mehta RH, Ince H, et al: Clinical profiles and outcomes of acute type B aortic dissection in the current era: lessons from the International Registry of Aortic Dissection (IRAD), *Circulation* 108(Suppl 1):1312-1337, 2003.
9. Svensson LG, Kouchoukos NT, Miller DC, et al: Expert consensus document on the treatment of descending thoracic aortic disease using endovascular stent-grafts, *Ann Thorac Surg* 85(Suppl 1):S1-S41, 2008.

PERICARDITIS, PERICARDIAL CONSTRICTION, AND PERICARDIAL TAMPONADE

Brian D. Hoit, MD

1. **The pericardium is not necessary for life. What does it do? Why is it important?**
The pericardium serves many important but subtle functions. It limits distension and facilitates interaction of the cardiac chambers, influences ventricular filling, prevents excessive torsion and displacement of the heart, minimizes friction with surrounding structures, prevents the spread of infection from contiguous structures, and equalizes gravitational, hydrostatic, and inertial forces over the surface of the heart. The pericardium also has immunologic, vasomotor, fibrinolytic, and metabolic activities. Therapeutically, the pericardial space can be used for drug delivery.

2. **What diseases affect the pericardium?**
The pericardium is affected by virtually every category of disease (Box 53-1), including idiopathic, infectious, neoplastic, immune/inflammatory, metabolic, iatrogenic, traumatic, and congenital.

BOX 53-1. CAUSES OF PERICARDIAL HEART DISEASE

- **Idiopathic**
- **Infectious**
  Bacterial, viral, mycobacterial, fungal, protozoal, HIV-associated
- **Neoplastic**
- **Metastatic** (breast, lung, melanoma, lymphoma, leukemia), primary (mesothelioma, fibrosarcoma)
- **Immune/inflammatory**
  Connective tissue disease, arteritis, acute myocardial infarction, post–pericardial injury syndrome
- **Metabolic**
  Nephrogenic, myxedema, amyloidosis, aortic dissection
- **Iatrogenic**
  Drugs, radiation therapy, device/instrumentation, cardiac ressuscitation
- **Traumatic**
  Blunt, penetrating, surgical
- **Congenital**
  Pericardial cysts, congenital absence of pericardium, mulibrey nanism

---

Modified from Hoit BD: Diseases of the pericardium. In Fuster V, O'Rourke RA, Walsh RA, et al, eds: *Hurst's the heart*, ed 12, New York, McGraw-Hill, 2008.

3. **What is pericarditis? What are the clinical manifestations? What are the causes?**
   Acute pericarditis is a syndrome of pericardial inflammation characterized by typical chest pain
   (sharp, retrosternal pain that radiates to the trapezius ridge, often aggravated by lying down
   and relieved by sitting up), a pathognomonic pericardial friction rub (characterized as superficial,
   scratchy, *crunchy*, and evanescent), and specific electrocardiographic changes (diffuse ST-T
   wave changes [Fig. 53-1] with characteristic evolutionary changes and PR segment depression).
   Causes include infectious (viral, bacterial, fungal, mycobacterial, human immunodeficiency
   virus [HIV] associated), neoplastic (usually metastatic from lung or breast; melanoma,
   lymphoma, or acute leukemia), myocardial infarction, injury (postpericardiotomy, traumatic),
   radiation, myxedema, and connective tissue disease.

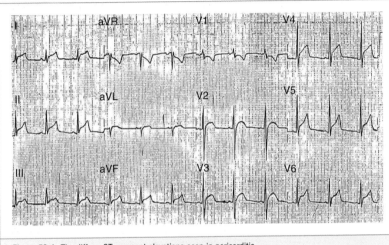

Figure 53-1. The diffuse ST-segment elevations seen in pericarditis.

4. **Should patients presenting with acute pericarditis be hospitalized? Why?**
   Hospitalization is warranted for high-risk patients with an initial episode of acute pericarditis in
   order to determine a cause and to observe for the development of cardiac tamponade;
   close, early follow-up is critically important for the remainder of patients not hospitalized.
   Features indicative of high-risk pericarditis include fever greater than 38° C, subacute onset, an
   immunosuppressed state, trauma, oral anticoagulant therapy, myopericarditis, a moderate or
   large pericardial effusion, cardiac tamponade, and medical failure.

5. **What is the treatment for acute pericarditis?**
   Acute pericarditis usually responds to oral nonsteroidal antiinflammatory agents (NSAIDs),
   such as aspirin (650 mg every 3 to 4 hours) or ibuprofen (300–800 mg every 6 hours).
   Indomethacin reduces coronary blood flow and should be avoided. Colchicine (1 mg/day) may
   be used to supplement the NSAIDs or as monotherapy. Chest pain is usually alleviated in
   1 to 2 days, and the friction rub and ST-segment elevation resolve shortly thereafter. Most mild
   cases of idiopathic and viral pericarditis are adequately treated with 1 to 4 days of treatment,
   but the duration of therapy is variable and patients should be treated until an effusion, if present,
   has resolved. The intensity of therapy is dictated by the distress of the patient, and narcotics
   may be required for severe pain. Corticosteroids should be avoided unless there is a specific
   indication (such as connective tissue disease or uremic pericarditis) because they enhance
   viral multiplication and may result in recurrences when the dosage is tapered. Although the
   European Society of Cardiology (ESC) recently published guidelines for the diagnosis and
   management of pericardial diseases, there are few randomized, placebo-controlled trials from
   which appropriate therapy may be selected.

6. **What is recurrent pericarditis? How is it treated?**
Recurrences of pericarditis (with or without pericardial effusion) occur with highly variable frequency over a course of many years. Although they may be spontaneous, occurring at varying intervals after discontinuation of drug, they are more commonly associated with either discontinuation or tapering of antiinflammatory drugs. Painful recurrences of pericarditis may respond to NSAIDs and colchicine but commonly require corticosteroids. Once steroids are administered, dependency and the development of steroid-induced abnormalities are potential perils. Pericardiectomy should be considered only when repeated attempts at medical treatment have clearly failed.

7. **What is PPIS?**
Postpericardial injury syndrome (PPIS) refers to pericarditis or pericardial effusion that results from injury of the pericardium. The principal conditions considered under these headings include post–myocardial infarction syndrome, postpericardiotomy syndrome, and traumatic (blunt, sharp, or iatrogenic) pericarditis. Clinical features include the following:
- Prior injury of the pericardium, myocardium, or both
- A latent period between the injury and the development of pericarditis or pericardial effusion
- A tendency for recurrence
- Responsiveness to NSAIDs and corticosteroids
- Fever, leukocytosis, and elevated erythrocyte sedimentation rate (and other markers of inflammation)
- Pericardial and sometimes pleural effusion, with or without a pulmonary infiltrate
- Alterations in the populations of lymphocytes in peripheral blood

When the pericardial injury syndrome occurs after an acute myocardial infarction, it is also known as Dressler's syndrome, which is now much less common than in the past.

8. **What are the pericardial compressive syndromes? What are their variants?**
The complications of acute pericarditis include cardiac tamponade, constrictive pericarditis, and effusive-constrictive pericarditis. Cardiac tamponade is characterized by the accumulation of pericardial fluid under pressure and may be acute, subacute, low pressure (occult), or regional. Constrictive pericarditis is the result of thickening, calcification, and loss of elasticity of the pericardial sac. Pericardial constriction is typically chronic but may be subacute, transient, and occult. Effusive-constrictive pericarditis is characterized by constrictive physiology with a coexisting pericardial effusion, usually with tamponade. Elevation of the right atrial and pulmonary wedge pressures persists after drainage of the pericardial fluid.

9. **What are similarities between tamponade and constrictive pericarditis?**
Characteristic of both tamponade and constrictive pericarditis is greatly enhanced ventricular interaction (interdependence), in which the hemodynamics of the left and right heart chambers are directly influenced by each other to a much greater degree than normal. Other similarities include diastolic dysfunction and preserved ventricular ejection fraction; increased respiratory variation of ventricular inflow and outflow; equally elevated central venous, pulmonary venous, and ventricular diastolic pressures; and mild pulmonary hypertension.

10. **What are the differences between tamponade and constrictive pericarditis?**
In tamponade, the pericardial space is open and transmits the respiratory variation in thoracic pressure to the heart, whereas in constrictive pericarditis the cavity is obliterated and the pericardium does not transmit these pressure changes. The dissociation of intrathoracic and intracardiac pressures (along with ventricular interaction) is the basis for the physical, hemodynamic, and echocardiographic findings of constriction.

In tamponade, systemic venous return increases with inspiration, enlarging the right side of the heart and encroaching on the left, whereas in constrictive pericarditis, systemic venous return does not increase with inspiration. The mechanism of diminished left ventricular and increased right ventricular volume in constrictive pericarditis is impaired left ventricular filling because of a lesser pressure gradient from the pulmonary veins.

In tamponade, early ventricular filling is impaired, whereas it is enhanced in constriction.

11. **What are the physical findings of tamponade?**
Cardiac tamponade is a hemodynamic condition characterized by equal elevation of atrial and pericardial pressures, an exaggerated inspiratory decrease in arterial systolic pressure (pulsus paradoxus), and arterial hypotension. The physical findings are dictated by both the severity of cardiac tamponade and the time course of its development. Inspection of the jugular venous pulse waveform reveals elevated venous pressure with a loss of the Y descent (because of the decrease in intrapericardial pressure that occurs during ventricular ejection, the systolic atrial filling wave and the X descent are maintained). Pulsus paradoxus is an inspiratory decline of systolic arterial pressure exceeding 10 mm Hg, which is measured by subtracting the pressure at which Korotkoff's sounds are heard only during expiration from the pressure at which sounds are heard throughout the respiratory cycle. Tachycardia and tachypnea are usually present.

12. **What are the physical findings of constrictive pericarditis?**
Constrictive pericarditis resembles the congestive states caused by myocardial disease and chronic liver disease. Physical findings include ascites, hepatosplenomegaly, edema, and, in long-standing cases, severe wasting. The venous pressure is elevated and displays deep Y and often deep X descents. The venous pressure fails to decrease with inspiration (Kussmaul's sign). A pericardial knock that is similar in timing to the third heart sound is pathognomonic but occurs infrequently. Except in severe cases, the arterial blood pressure is normal.

13. **What is the role of echocardiography in tamponade?**
Although tamponade is a clinical diagnosis, echocardiography plays major roles in the identification of pericardial effusion and in the assessment of its hemodynamic significance (Fig. 53-2). The use of echocardiography for the evaluation of all patients with suspected pericardial disease was given a class I recommendation by a 2003 task force of the American College of Cardiology (ACC), the American Heart Association (AHA), and the American Society of Echocardiography (ASE). Except in hyperacute cases, a moderate to large effusion is usually present and swinging of the heart within the effusion may be seen. Reciprocal changes in left and right ventricular volumes occur with respiration. Echocardiographic findings suggesting hemodynamic compromise (atrial and ventricular diastolic collapses) are the result of transiently reversed right atrial and right ventricular diastolic transmural pressures and typically occur before hemodynamic embarrassment. The respiratory variation of mitral and tricuspid flow velocities is greatly increased and out of phase, reflecting the increased ventricular interaction. Less than a 50% inspiratory reduction in the diameter of a dilated inferior vena cava reflects a marked elevation in central venous pressure, and abnormal right-sided venous flows (systolic predominance and expiratory diastolic reversal) are diagnostic. In patients who do not have tamponade on first assessment, repeat echocardiography during clinical follow-up was given a class IIa recommendation by the 2003 ACC/AHA/ASE task force.

14. **What is the role of echocardiography in constrictive pericarditis?**
Echocardiography is an essential adjunctive procedure in patients with suspected pericardial constriction. The use of echocardiography for the evaluation of all patients with suspected pericardial disease is a class I ACC/AHA/ASE task force recommendation. Echo findings to be

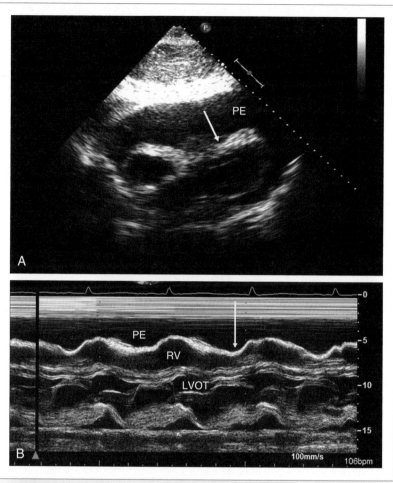

Figure 53-2. Echocardiography in cardiac tamponade. **A,** Subcostal two-dimensional echo. A large effusion (PE) with marked compression of the right ventricle *(arrow)* is seen. **B,** M-mode of the parasternal long axis. Note the right ventricular *(long arrow)* collapse. *LVOT,* left ventricular outflow tract; *PE,* pericardial effusion; outflow tract; *RV,* right ventricular.

sought include increased pericardial thickness (best with transesophageal echo), abrupt inspiratory posterior motion of the ventricular septum in early diastole, plethora of the inferior vena cava and hepatic veins, enlarged atria, and an abnormal contour between the posterior left ventricular the left atrial posterior walls. Although no sign or combination of signs on M-mode is diagnostic of constrictive pericarditis, a normal study virtually rules out the diagnosis. Doppler is particularly useful, showing a high *E* velocity of right and left ventricular inflow and rapid deceleration, a normal or increased tissue Doppler *E'*, and a 25% to 40% fall in transmitral flow and marked increase of tricuspid velocity in the first beat after inspiration. Increased respiratory variation of mitral inflow may be missing in patients with markedly elevated left atrial pressure but may be brought out by preload reduction (e.g., head-up tilt).

Hepatic vein flow reversals increase with expiration, reflecting the ventricular interaction and the dissociation of intracardiac and intrathoracic pressures, and pulmonary venous flow shows marked respiratory variation.

15. **Are other imaging modalities useful in pericardial disease?**
Other imaging techniques, such as computed tomography (CT) and cardiovascular magnetic resonance (CMR) are not necessary if two-dimensional and Doppler echocardiography are available. However, pericardial effusion may be detected, quantified, and characterized by CT and CMR. CT scanning of the heart is extremely useful in the diagnosis of constrictive pericarditis; findings include increased pericardial thickness (greater than 4 mm) and calcification. CMR provides direct visualization of the normal pericardium, which is composed of fibrous tissue and has a low magnetic resonance imaging (MRI) signal intensity. CMR is claimed by some to be the diagnostic procedure of choice for the detection of constrictive pericarditis (Fig. 53-3).

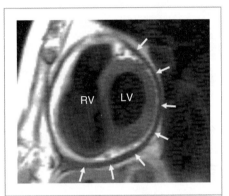

Figure 53-3. MRI demonstrating thickened pericardium encasing the heart *(arrows)*. (Reproduced with permission from Pennell D: Cardiovascular magnetic resonance. In Libby P, Bonow R, Mann D, et al: *Braunwald's heart disease: a textbook of cardiovascular medicine,* ed 8, Philadelphia, 2008, Saunders.)

16. **Constrictive pericarditis is a surgical disease, except when very early constriction or in severe, advanced disease. What is the role for medical therapy in constrictive pericarditis?**
Medical therapy of constrictive pericarditis plays a small but important role. Diuretics and digoxin (in the presence of atrial fibrillation) are useful in patients who are not candidates for pericardiectomy because of their high surgical risk. Preoperative diuretics should be used sparingly with the goal of reducing, not eliminating, elevated jugular pressure, edema, and ascites. Postoperatively, diuretics should be given if spontaneous diuresis does not occur; the central venous pressure may take weeks to months to return to normal after pericardiectomy. In some patients, constrictive pericarditis resolves either spontaneously or in response to various combinations of NSAIDs, steroids, and antibiotics (transitory constriction). Therefore, before pericardiectomy is recommended, conservative management for 2 to 3 months in hemodynamically stable patients with subacute constrictive pericarditis is recommended.

BIBLIOGRAPHY, SUGGESTED READINGS, AND WEBSITES

1. Cheitlin MD, Armstrong WF, Aurigemma GP, et al: ACC/AHA/ASE 2003 Guidelines for the Clinical Application of Echocardiography: http://www.acc.org/qualityandscience/clinical/statements.htm

2. Hoit BD: Diseases of the pericardium. In Fuster V, O'Rourke RA, Walsh RA, et al, editors: *Hurst's the heart*, ed 12, New York, 2008, McGraw-Hill.

3. Hoit BD: Management of effusive and constrictive pericardial heart disease, *Circulation* 105:2939-2942, 2002.

4. Hoit BD: Treatment of pericardial disease. In *Cardiovascular therapeutics*, ed 2, Philadelphia, 2002, Saunders.

5. Little WC, Freeman GL: Pericardial disease, *Circulation* 113:1622, 2006.

6. Maisch B, Seferovic PM, Ristic AD, et al: Guidelines on the diagnosis and management of pericardial diseases executive summary; The Task Force on the Diagnosis and Management of Pericardial Diseases of the European Society of Cardiology, *Eur Heart J* 25:587-610, 2004.

7. Shabetai R: *The pericardium*, Norwell, Mass, 2003, Kluwer Academic Publishers.

CHAPTER 54

SYNCOPE

Glenn N. Levine, MD, FACC, FAHA

1. **What is the word *syncope* derived from?**
   According to text in the European Society of Cardiology (ESC) Guidelines on the Management of Syncope, the word *syncope* is derived from the Greek words *syn,* meaning "with," and the verb *kopto,* meaning "I cut" or "I interrupt."

2. **What is the underlying mechanism causing syncope?**
   Transient global cerebral hypoperfusion. Note that other conditions that do not cause transient global cerebral hypoperfusion can cause a transient loss of consciousness, and some experts believe these conditions should be referred to as *transient loss of consciousness* instead of syncope.

3. **Cessation of cerebral blood flow of what duration causes syncope?**
   Cessation of cerebral blood flow for as short a period as 6 to 8 seconds can precipitate syncope.

4. **What is the most common cause of syncope in the general population?**
   Neurocardiogenic syncope is the most common cause of syncope in the general population. This is also variably referred to in the literature as *vasovagal syncope, neurally mediated syncope,* and *vasodepressor syncope.*

5. **What are the most common causes of syncope in pediatric and young patients?**
   According to the scientific statement on syncope from the 2006 American Heart Association/ American College of Cardiology Foundation (AHA/ACCF), the most common causes of syncope in pediatric and young patients are neurocardiogenic syncope, conversion reactions (psychiatric causes), and primary arrhythmic causes (e.g., long QT syndrome, Wolff-Parkinson-White syndrome). In contrast, elderly patients have a higher frequency of syncope caused by obstructions to cardiac output (e.g., aortic stenosis, pulmonary embolism) and by arrhythmias resulting from underlying heart disease.

6. **What is the most common cause of sudden cardiac death in young athletes?**
   Hypertrophic cardiomyopathy, followed by anomalous origin of a coronary artery. Other causes of sudden cardiac death in younger persons in general include long QT syndrome, Brugada syndrome, and arrhythmogenic right ventricular dysplasia/cardiomyopathy (ARVD/C), as well as pulmonary embolism (Box 54-1).

7. **What are the common causes of syncope?**
   - **Neurocardiogenic:** This is the most common cause of syncope in otherwise healthy persons, particularly younger persons. It is often precipitated by fear, anxiety, or other types of emotional distress. Its course is usually benign.
   - **Orthostatic hypotension:** Orthostatic hypotension results from venous pooling and decreased cardiac output and fall in blood pressure. It may be due to volume depletion, anemia or acute bleeding, peripheral vasodilators (most notoriously the alpha receptor

BOX 54-1. CAUSES OF SYNCOPE AND LOSS OF CONSCIOUSNESS

Nonsyncope "Loss of Consciousness"
- Seizures
- Hypoglycemia
- Hypoxemia
- Psychogenic

Noncardiac
- Neurocardiogenic
- Carotid sinus hypersensitivity
- Situational (e.g., micturation, defecation, cough, swallowing)
- Orthostatic hypotension (volume depletion, anemia/bleeding, drugs, autonomic dysfunction)
- Subclavian steal
- Vertebrobasilar disease (very rarely, severe bilateral carotid disease)

Cardiac

1. Structural/Functional
- Aortic stenosis
- Hypertrophic cardiomyopathy
- Left atrial myxoma
- Pulmonary embolism

2. Arrhythmic

   a. *Bradyarrhythmic*
   - Profound (sinus) bradycardia
   - Sick sinus syndrome/ tachy-brady syndrome
   - Heart block
   - Pacemaker malfunction

   b. *Tachyarrhythmia*
   - SVT
   - VT/torsades de pointes

blockers used to treat benign prostatic hypertrophy), or autonomic dysfunction (e.g., diabetic neuropathy, dysautonomia caused by central nervous system [CNS] disease).

- **Carotid sinus hypersensitivity:** This condition is suggested by syncope precipitated by neck movement, or by tight collars or ties. The diagnosis is made by carotid sinus massage (see Question 10).
- **Cerebrovascular disease:** Carotid artery stenosis usually leads to focal neurologic deficits rather that frank syncope (except perhaps in the very rare case of severe bilateral carotid artery disease, in which global cerebral hypoperfusion can occur). Vertebrobasilar disease is more likely to lead to syncope, although this is a rare cause of syncope in the general population.
- **Tachyarrhythmias:** Ventricular tachycardia (VT) and torsades de pointes are the most ominous cause of syncope. In patients with a history of prior myocardial infarction or those with significantly depressed left ventricular ejection fraction (less than 30% to 35%), the presumptive cause of syncope is VT until proven otherwise. Polymorphic VT and torsades de pointes is the presumptive cause of syncope in those with prolonged QT intervals because of drugs or congenital long QT syndrome and in those with Brugada syndrome (see Question 14). Supraventricular tachycardia (SVT) may produce presyncope but does not usually produce overt syncope.

- **Bradyarrhythmias:** Syncope may be caused by intermittent complete heart block. *Sick sinus syndrome* is a general term covering multiple disorders of the conduction system. *Tachy-brady syndrome* is the more appropriate term used to describe patients with intermittent atrial fibrillation who, when the atrial fibrillation terminates, then have a several or more second period of asystole before normal sinus rhythm and ventricular depolarization resume.
- **Structural/Functional:** Aortic stenosis is the most common structural cause of syncope in older patients. The dynamic obstruction that occurs in hypertrophic cardiomyopathy (see Chapter 29) is the most common cause of structural/functional–mediated syncope in younger patients. Left atrial myxoma, causing functional mitral stenosis, is an extremely rare cause of syncope. Syncope can also occur with massive pulmonary embolism, which obstructs the pulmonary artery to an extent that it compromises blood flow to the left ventricle.

8. **What is the approach to the patient with syncope?**
   The goals of the evaluation of patients with syncope are not only to identify the cause of syncope but also to determine if the cause is cardiac or noncardiac. Noncardiac causes of syncope generally have a relatively benign course (overall 1-year mortality rates of 0% to 12% and an approximately 0% mortality rate with neurally mediated syncope). Unexplained/undiagnosed causes have an intermediate 1-year mortality rate of 5% to 6%. Cardiac causes, in contrast, are associated with 1-year mortality risk of 18.5% to 33%. Thus, there is a premium on excluding a cardiac cause of syncope, even if the exact cause of syncope cannot be determined.

   A detailed history and physical examination, along with electrocardiogram (ECG) examination, can identify the presumptive cause of syncope in 40% to 50% of cases. Premonitory symptoms such as nausea or diaphoresis, especially in a younger person, or symptoms caused by anxiety, pain, or emotional distress, suggest neurocardiogenic syncope. Syncope during or immediately after urination, defecation, or certain other activities suggests situational syncope. Recent initiation of certain blood pressure–lowering medications, particularly alpha receptor blockers (such as used to treat benign prostatic hypertrophy), raise suspicion for orthostatic hypotension, which can be confirmed on examination. A history of prior myocardial infarction or depressed ejection fraction raises the concern for ventricular tachycardia. Cardiac systolic murmurs suggest aortic stenosis or hypertrophic cardiomyopathy. Table 54-1 gives the factors on history, physical examination, and electrocardiogram that may suggest a specific cause for the patient's syncope.

TABLE 54-1. SYMPTOMS AND FINDINGS OBTAINED ON THE HISTORY, PHYSICAL DIAGNOSIS, AND ELECTROCARDIOGRAM, AND CAUSES FOR SYNCOPE THEY SUGGEST

Symptoms/Findings	Cause
History	
Postepisode fatigue or weakness	Suggests neurocardiogenic syncope
Syncope precipitated by anxiety, pain, or emotional distress	Suggests neurocardiogenic syncope
Auras, postictal confusion, focal neurologic signs/symptoms	Favors a neurologic cause
History of MI, depressed EF, or repaired congenital heart disease	Raises concern of a ventricular arrhythmia
Syncope precipitated by neck turning	Suggests carotid sinus hypersensitivity

(Continued)

TABLE 54-1. SYMPTOMS AND FINDINGS OBTAINED ON THE HISTORY, PHYSICAL DIAGNOSIS, AND ELECTROCARDIOGRAM, AND CAUSES FOR SYNCOPE THEY SUGGEST (CONTINUED)

Symptoms/Findings	Cause
Sudden onset shortness of breath or chest pain	Suggests pulmonary embolism or arrhythmia
Syncope related to micturation, coughing, swallowing, or defecation	Suggests "situational syncope"
Arm movement and use precipitate syncope	Suggests subclavian steal
Palpitations	Suggests cardiac tachyarrhythmia
Family history of sudden cardiac death	Suggests hypertrophic cardiomyopathy, long QT syndrome, or Brugada syndrome
Physical Examination	
Orthostatic changes	Suggests orthostatic hypotension caused by dehydration, drugs, or autonomic dysfunction
Carotid sinus hypersensitivity	Suggests carotid sinus hypersensitivity
Carotid bruit	Suggests underlying coronary artery disease, as well as possible carotid stenosis
Systolic ejection murmur	Suggests aortic stenosis or hypertrophic cardiomyopathy
Unequal blood pressures, bruit over subclavian area	Suggests subclavian steal
Electrocardiogram	
Prolonged PR interval +/- bundle branch block	Suggests heart block as cause
Marked sinus bradycardia	Raises the possibility of sick sinus syndrome
Prolonged QT interval	Raises the possibility of ventricular tachycardia/torsades de pointes as a result of congenital long QT syndrome or drugs
Marked left ventricular hypertrophy	Raises possibility of hypertrophic cardiomyopathy
Q waves	Suggests old MI and possibility of ventricular tachycardia
Unusual ST segment elevation in V1-V2	Suggests Brugada syndrome and polymorphic VT

EF, Ejection fraction; *MI,* myocardial infarction.

9. **How does one _properly_ test for orthostatic hypotension?**

Recommendations vary, but according to the ESC Guidelines on the Management of Syncope, one first has the patient lie supine for 5 minutes. Blood pressure is then measured 3 minutes after the patient stands, with subsequent blood pressure measurements each minute thereafter if the blood pressure falls and continue to fall compared with supine values. Orthostatic hypotension is defined as a 20 mm Hg or greater drop in systolic blood pressure or systolic blood pressure falling to less than 90 mm Hg. Some other experts also consider falls of diastolic blood pressure of 10 mm Hg or more or increases in heart rate of 20 beats/min or more as criteria to diagnose orthostatic hypotension.

When the diagnosis is still not clear, echocardiography can be obtained, looking for unsuspected depressed left ventricular ejection fraction or right ventricular dysfunction, hypertrophic cardiomyopathy (which may predispose to ventricular tachycardia), or obstructive heart disease (aortic stenosis, hypertrophic cardiomyopathy, rare left atrial myxoma). Note that although echocardiography has become part of the _shotgun_ evaluation of syncope for many practitioners and is recommended as a diagnostic test to consider by both the AHA/ACCF and the ESC, its yield in patients with unremarkable cardiac histories, physical examination, and electrocardiograms is low. In cases in which neurocardiogenic syncope is suspected and further testing is desired, a tilt table test can be obtained. Exercise stress testing has been suggested by some to assess for cardiac ischemia or exercise-induced arrhythmias in appropriately selected patients. In patients in whom a bradyarrhythmia or tachyarrhythmia is suspected, a Holter monitor, event monitor, or implantable loop recorder can be considered or, under certain circumstances, electrophysiologic testing can be performed.

10. **During carotid sinus massage, what is considered a _diagnostic_ response?**

According to the ESC Guidelines on Management of Syncope, a ventricular pause lasting 3 seconds or longer or a fall in systolic blood pressure of 50 mm Hg or more is considered abnormal and defines carotid sinus hypersensitivity. Note that carotid sinus massage should not be performed in patients with a recent transient ischemic attack (TIA) or stroke or those with carotid bruits.

11. **What is a tilt table test?**

Tilt table testing is most commonly performed on patients with neurally mediated syncope (e.g., neurocardiogenic syncope). The patient first lies supine on a board with a foot support. The table is then rotated to a tilt angle of 60 to 80 degrees, so that the patient is almost in the standing position. This maneuver leads to venous pooling and later loss of plasma volume as a result of movement in to interstitial spaces. Overall, there is an approximate 15% to 20% (700 ml) decrease of plasma volume. The normal neuroregulatory mechanisms of the body will usually compensate for this, maintaining blood pressure. Vasovagal reactions can occur during monitoring, leading to decrease in heart rate and blood pressure. In a typical protocol the patient is tilted for 30 minutes, and if no loss of consciousness has occurred, isoproternol infusion is started and the patient retilted. Other protocols may administer different provocative agents, such as nitroglycerin or adenosine. Criteria have been established to classify the patient responses as cardioihibitor, vasodepressor, or mixed, based on falls in heart rate, blood pressure, and the occurrence of syncope.

12. **How should one decide between ordering a Holter monitor, an event monitor, or an implantable loop monitor?**

A Holter monitor, which is usually worn for 24 to 48 hours, is useful if the patient experiences syncope or presyncope at least once a day. An event monitor, which most commonly is ordered for approximately 4 to 8 weeks, is useful if the patient experiences symptoms at least once a month. An implantable loop monitor is reasonable to consider in a patient with occasional symptoms that occur less than once per month.

13. Should a *shotgun* neurologic evaluation, including computed tomography (CT) scan, carotid ultrasound, and electroencephalogram, be ordered in all patients with syncope?

No. True syncope (or loss of consciousness) is a unusual manifestation of neurologic syncope (excluding causes such as reflex, situational or neurocardiogenic syncope and dysautonomia). In one report, electroencephalogram provided diagnostic information in less than 2% of cases of syncope, and almost all those patients had a history of seizures or symptoms suggesting seizure. Neurologic workup should only be undertaken if a neurologic cause is suggested by the history or physical examination. TIAs usually do not cause syncope. Carotid disease and stroke more likely lead to focal neurologic deficits than *global* neurologic ischemia and syncope (the rare exception being severe bilateral carotid artery disease). Severe bilateral vertebrobasilar disease can cause syncope but is not easily diagnosed by screening studies. Importantly, cerebral hypoperfusion caused by ventricular tachycardia can result in seizurelike activity, and the report by family members or other witnesses of the event of "seizurelike" activity in the patient should not cause one to be misled down a search for neurologic causes based on this alone.

14. What is long QT syndrome?

Long QT syndrome is characterized by a corrected QT interval (QTc) of greater than 450 msec (Fig. 54-1). The QT interval is prolonged because of delayed repolarization as a result of a genetic defect in either potassium or sodium channels. Syncope in patients in long QT syndrome likely is due to torsade des pointes. The onset of symptoms most commonly occurs during the first two decades of life. The risk of developing syncope or sudden cardiac death increases with QTc, with lifetime risks of approximately 5% in those with QTc less than 440 msec but 50% in those with QTc more than 500 msec. Patients with long QT syndrome should be referred to electrophysiologists for further evaluation and treatment, which may include medicines or placement of an implantable cardioverter defibrillator (ICD).

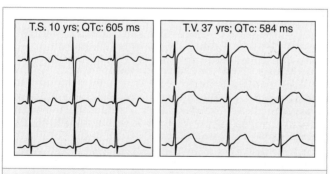

Figure 54-1. Typical electrocardiogram of two long QT syndrome patients showing QT-interval prolongation and T-wave morphologic abnormalities. (From Libby P, Bonow R, Mann D, et al: *Braunwald's heart disease: A textbook of cardiovascular medicine,* ed 8, Philadelphia, 2007, Saunders.)

15. What is Brugada syndrome?

Brugada syndrome is a disorder of sodium channels, resulting in sometimes intermittent unusual ST-segment elevation in leads V1-V3, as well as a right bundle branch block–like pattern (Fig. 54-2). Such patients are susceptible to developing polymorphic VT. Patients with suspected Brugada syndrome should be referred for specialized cardiac evaluation and a probable ICD.

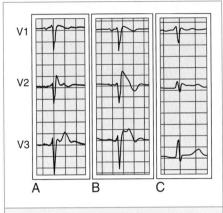

Figure 54-2. Example of the ST-segment elevations in leads V1-V3 seen in patients with Brugada syndrome. (From Libby P, Bonow R, Mann D, et al: *Braunwald's heart disease: A textbook of cardiovascular medicine,* ed 8, Philadelphia, 2007, Saunders.)

BIBLIOGRAPHY, SUGGESTED READINGS, AND WEBSITES

1. Dave J: Syncope: http://www.emedicine.com

2. Syncope: http://www.merck.com/mmpe

3. Brignole M, Alboni P, Benditt DG, et al: Guidelines on management (diagnosis and treatment) of syncope-update. Executive summary, *Eur Heart J* 25:2054-2072, 2004.

4. Calkins H, Zipes DP: Hypotension and syncope. In Libby P, Bonow R, Mann D, et al, editors: *Braunwald's heart disease: a textbook of cardiovascular medicine*, ed 8, Philadelphia, 2007, Saunders.

5. Fogel RI, Varma J: Approach to the patient with syncope. In Levine GN, Mann DL, editors: *Primary care provider's guide to cardiology*, Philadelphia, 2000, Lippincott Williams & Wilkins.

6. Kapoor WN: Syncope, *Eur Heart J* (22):2054-2072, 2004.

7. Priori SG, Napolitano C, Schwartz PJ: Genetics of cardiac arrhythmias. In Libby P, Bonow R, Mann D, et al, editors: *Braunwald's heart disease: a textbook of cardiovascular medicine*, ed 8, Philadelphia, 2007, Saunders.

8. Strickberger SA, Benson DW, Biaggioni I, et al: AHA/ACCF scientific statement on the evaluation of syncope, *J Am Coll Cardiol* 47(2):473-484, 2006.

CHAPTER 55

STROKE AND TIA

Sharyl R. Martini, MD, PhD and Thomas A. Kent, MD

1. **What is stroke? How common is stroke? How common is it in the setting of cardiac disease?**

   Stroke is a focal disturbance of blood flow to the brain. It can be classified as either primarily ischemic (80%) or hemorrhagic (20%). Ischemic strokes can develop a hemorrhagic component, termed hemorrhagic conversion, especially if large. There are approximately 700,000 strokes per year in the United States, and it is the number one cause of morbidity. The biggest risk factor for stroke is prior stroke, and the second biggest risk factor is age. Risk factors common to both stroke and atherosclerotic cardiac disease include hypertension, diabetes, and smoking. In addition, cardiac diseases such as atrial fibrillation and valvular disease are risk factors for stroke. Strokes can occur after cardiac procedures at a rate of 0.7% to 7%, depending on the procedure, and may be due to intrinsic disease or emboli/microemboli from the procedure itself. Stroke is not a single disease but the end result of many different pathophysiologies that lead to cerebrovascular occlusion or rupture.

2. **What is a transient ischemic attack, and why is the clinical recognition of it important?**

   Transient ischemic attack (TIA) is a neurologic deficit that by definition resolves within 24 hours, although most resolve within minutes. It is important to identify TIAs because they represent an opportunity to intervene with appropriate strategies to prevent future strokes and permanent disability. Ninety-day stroke rates for patients with TIA are in excess of 10% in some series, with the greatest risk within the first week after the TIA.

3. **What are the major causes of stroke and TIA?**

   The major categories of ischemic stroke are large vessel atherosclerosis (including embolization from carotid to cerebral arteries), small vessel vasculopathy or lacunar type (Fig. 55-1), and cardioembolic. Hemorrhagic strokes are classified by their location: subcortical (associated with uncontrolled hypertension in 60% of cases) versus cortical (more concerning for underlying mass, arteriovenous malformation, or amyloidosis). Table 55-1 summarizes the major causes of stroke and their relative frequency.

   Among the other potential causes of stroke, dissection of the blood vessels needs to be considered, especially if there is a history of trauma. Illicit drug use is a possible cause of either ischemic stroke (cocaine-induced spasm) or hemorrhagic stroke (as a result of vascular injury or sudden massive increase in blood pressure). Patent foramen ovale (PFO) remains a controversial cause of stroke for which optimal treatment remains unknown. The authors encourage the enrollment of patients with PFO and stroke into ongoing trials comparing intervention with medications. Other rarer causes of stroke include hypercoagulable states (e.g., lupus/antiphospholipid antibody syndrome) and genetic disorders such as homocystinuria and fibromuscular dysplasia.

4. **How are stroke and TIA diagnosed?**

   Stroke and TIA are diagnosed clinically, and no imaging correlation is required. Focal neurologic deficits with sudden onset should be considered vascular until proven otherwise. Focal weakness, numbness, facial asymmetry, or speech difficulties are classic presentations. Altered level of consciousness and cranial nerve deficits are often seen with vertebrobasilar/brainstem

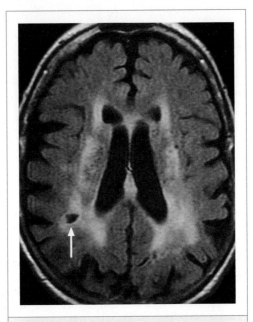

Figure 55-1. MRI demonstrating small vessel ischemic change in deep and periventricular cerebral white matter. There is a mature lacunar infarct in the right parietal lobe *(arrow)*. (From Adam A, Dixon AK: Grainger & Allison's *diagnostic radiology: a textbook of medical imaging*, 5th ed, Philadelphia, Churchill Livingstone, 2008.)

TABLE 55-1. APPROXIMATE DISTRIBUTION OF STROKE BY CLINICAL SUBTYPES	
Large-Vessel Thrombotic Stroke	35%
Embolic Stroke	15%
Lacunar Stroke	20%
Cryptogenic	5%
Subarachnoid Hemorrhage	10%

strokes. Table 55-2 lists the clinical signs and symptoms of the major subtypes of stroke: large vessel atherosclerosis/thrombosis, cardioembolic stroke, and small vessel stroke.

5. **What should be done in cases of suspected stroke or TIA?**
A head computed tomography (CT) must be performed immediately to distinguish ischemic from hemorrhagic strokes because these are managed very differently. The CT itself does not diagnosis stroke; it is primarily used to rule out causes other than ischemic stroke, including hemorrhagic infarction, tumor, subdural hematoma, and other causes. Figure 55-2 demonstrates the CT findings of an acute hemorrhagic stroke.

In cases of suspected stroke, one should page the stroke team (when one exists) or neurology service—every minute counts. Immediately check blood glucose because hypoglycemia or hyperglycemia can cause focal neurologic deficits mimicking stroke. Also obtain an

TABLE 55-2. CLINICAL FEATURES OF THE THREE MOST COMMON TYPES OF STROKE

	Clinical Features	Classic Syndromes
Large-vessel atherosclerosis	Often occur on waking; may have history of TIAs in same vascular distribution, symptoms may fluctuate. Often caused by carotid disease with artery-to-artery embolism. Associated trauma suggests dissection as source of artery-to-artery embolism (may see ipsilateral Horner's syndrome).	*Anterior circulation:* arm and face > leg weakness, plus word-finding difficulty sensory loss, difficulty understanding commands, contralateral neglect, visual field cut *Posterior circulation:* cerebellar or cranial nerve abnormalities predominate, but can begin with confusional state (bilateral hippocampal ischemia caused by basilar artery thrombosis)
Small-vessel subcortical stroke	Strong association with hypertension and microbleeds; occur in subcortical regions such as basal ganglia or brainstem—as such never see cortical findings of language disturbance or neglect; may have TIAs with similar symptoms. These small strokes can also be due to large vessel atherosclerosis or small emboli (see next).	*Pure motor:* contralateral face/arm/leg weakness *Pure sensory:* contralateral face/arm/leg sensory loss *Sensorimotor:* loss of face/arm/leg motor and sensory *Ataxic hemiparesis:* contralateral ataxia out of proportion to mild weakness *Clumsy hand dysarthria:* weak face and clumsy ipsilateral hand, dysarthria and dysphagia
Cardioembolic stroke	Associated history or clinical features of heart disease. Stroke symptoms are maximal at onset because the clot is preformed. TIA symptoms are usually different from one another, representing emboli to different vascular distributions. Often occur during waking hours; can be associated with valsalva maneuvers. Caused by embolism, usually from left atrial appendage (in setting of atrial fibrillation) or left ventricle (in case of akinetic segment). Emboli from infected valves (septic emboli) are likely to bleed and should not be treated with tPA.	Dependent on area of embolization; often middle cerebral artery territory

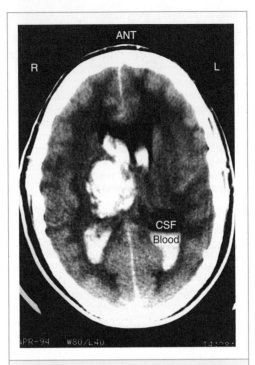

Figure 55-2. Intracerebral hemorrhage. Noncontrasted computed tomography (CT) scan demonstrates a large area of fresh blood in the region of the right thalamus. Blood also is seen in the anterior and posterior horns of the lateral ventricles. Because blood is denser than cerebrospinal fluid (CSF), it is layered dependently. (From Mettler FA: *Essentials of radiology*, 2nd ed, Philadelphia, Saunders, 2005.)

electrocardiogram (ECG) and basic blood analysis (complete blood cell count, coagulation studies, and renal/electrolyte panel). The ECG and cardiac workup initially can reveal atrial fibrillation or the surprisingly common coexistance of various kinds of acute cardiac syndromes and stroke.

6. **How are ischemic acute strokes treated?**
   Three possible treatments are now suggested to improve outcomes after acute ischemic stroke: (1) intravenous tissue plasminogen activator (tPA); (2) aspirin; and, in the case of large strokes, (3) hemicraniectomy performed before clinical herniation.

tPA

The only medication approved by the Food and Drug Administration (FDA) for acute ischemic strokes is intravenous (IV) tPA, administered within 3 hours of symptom onset. **Note, however, that the earlier tPA is given, the better the clinical outcome.** The greatest benefit of tPA occurs at earlier timepoints: It is estimated that 100,000 neurons die each minute during an acute ischemic stroke, so it is critical to give tPA as soon as possible if head CT does not reveal signs of hemorrhage or hypointensities. Note also that only alteplase is approved for this use. Only eight stroke patients need to be treated with IV tPA to give one patient a complete or near-complete recovery, and this number needed to treat (NNT) takes into account the increased risk of hemorrhage after tPA administration. Patients of any age benefit from tPA.

Contraindications to IV tPA include the following:

- Patients who present outside the 3-hour time window
- Those with minor or rapidly resolving deficits (including TIA)
- Uncontrolled hypertension greater than 185/110 mm Hg despite antihypertensive treatment
- Surgery within 2 weeks
- Gastrointestinal (GI) or urinary hemorrhage within 3 weeks
- Stroke, head trauma, or myocardial infarction within 3 months

International normalized ratio (INR) should be 1.5 or lower and platelets 100,000 mm^3 or more. Importantly, patients who have their strokes after cardiac catheterization and meet these criteria may still benefit from tPA, despite the recent administration of heparin and GPIIb/IIIa inhibitors, although this is outside the usual protocols. In this situation, various treatments have been reported, including intraarterial therapy or IV abciximab, but these remain investigational.

After tPA administration, frequent clinical examinations are crucial and blood pressure must be controlled to less than 180/105 mm Hg. Subcutaneous heparin and antiplatelet agents are usually held for 24 hours until follow-up imaging confirms absence of hemorrhagic conversion.

In patients with ischemic stroke who are not candidates for tPA, optimal blood pressure is not known but is often permitted to run high (up to 220/120) as long as there are not signs of hypertensive end-organ damage. This is theoretically designed to increase perfusion of brain tissue at continued risk for ischemia, but it is not known if outcome is improved. Cautious control of blood pressure is recommended to avoid sudden drops or rises. Any hypotension or relative hypotension associated with neurologic worsening should be treated with pressors until clinical examination improves or upper limits prespecified earlier are reached.

Endovascular devices for cerebral clot disruption/retrieval are FDA approved, although their efficacy has yet to be rigorously studied and any procedural delays that delay treatment probably do more harm than good.

Aspirin

In patients not treated with thromboytic therapy, aspirin is given (orally or rectally) as soon as possible and has shown to reduce the chances of recurrent stroke. In patients not treated with thrombolytic therapy, subcutaneous heparin should be started as soon as possible if the patient is not able to ambulate as long as it is not contraindicated.

7. **How are hemorrhagic strokes managed?**
   Hemorrhagic strokes are managed by reversing any coagulopathy and withholding administration of subcutaneous heparin and antiplatelet agents. Controlling blood pressure is a focus of interest because high blood pressure is associated with rebleeding. It is considered safe to decrease blood pressure by up to 25% in the first 2 to 6 hours as long as findings on neurologic examination do not worsen.

8. **What other measures are important in the management of all strokes?**
   In all cases of stroke, ensure adequate deep vein thrombosis (DVT) prophylaxis (anticoagulation or other methods, depending on potential contraindications) and obtain swallow evaluations to prevent aspiration.

9. **Is the presence of atrial fibrillation in patients with stroke or TIA an important consideration for future managment?**
   Yes. Any patient with atrial fibrillation who has had a stroke or TIA is considered high risk for future strokes without anticoagulation (see Question 11). As such, all patients should be monitored with telemetry to optimize identification of intermittent atrial fibrillation because intermittent atrial fibrillation is as much of a risk factor for stroke as persistent atrial fibrillation. A single ECG (unless it reveals atrial fibrillation) is inadequate for detection of this important and modifiable risk factor.

10. **What is the utility of echocardiogram for workup of acute stroke?**
In patients with a suspected cardioembolic cause, echocardiogram is indicated (see also Chapter 6 on echocardiography). Transesophageal echocardiogram is indicated in patients with embolic stroke and a nondiagnostic transthoracic echocardiogram. An echocardiogram is not needed to determine secondary stroke prevention for stroke patients with atrial fibrillation because these patients should be anticoagulated; however, identification of a cardiac thrombus would affect timing of anticoagulation initiation (see later).

11. **Which patients with atrial fibrillation merit anticoagulation therapy for the prevention of stroke?**
All patients with history of stroke *and* atrial fibrillation merit consideration for anticoagulation because the risk of subsequent stroke in these patients is 2% to 5% per year and anticoagulation results in a greater than 60% reduction in ischemic strokes. Other high-risk groups include those over the age of 75 (especially women) and those with the following risk factors: poorly controlled hypertension, diabetes, and poor left ventricular function or recent heart failure. A number of risk stratification schemes can help determine which patients should be anticoagulated to prevent stroke. These include CHADS2, SPAF, AFI, and Framingham, among others. These schemes integrate risk factors to assist in the decision for anticoagulation therapy: The greater the number of risk factors, the higher the risk of stroke. It is important to note that these schemes relate to *primary* prevention in atrial fibrillation; a stroke or TIA automatically places a patient in the high-risk category for each of these schemes. As such, secondary prevention of stroke in patients with atrial fibrillation should involve anticoagulation unless there is a contraindication. The elderly also appear to benefit from anticoagulation for secondary stroke prevention; thus, age alone is not a contraindication, although elderly patients are at higher risk for bleeding.

Contraindications to preventive anticoagulant therapy include history of severe GI bleeding and history of falls or extremely high fall risk. After stroke, many patients are at risk for falls. As they improve, their fall risk status may also improve, so it is important to reconsider anticoagulation at future visits. Goal INR for secondary stroke prevention is 2 to 3; studies have demonstrated that many stroke prevention *failures* are the result of subtherapeutic INRs. The most serious bleeding risk associated with anticoagulation is intracerebral hemorrhage. This risk is probably higher for patients with extensive small vessel disease or microhemorrhages than for those with healthier brain parenchyma. The decision for antocoagulation in particular patients should be a collaborative one, with the risks, benefits, and monitoring schedule clearly explained so that the patient can make an informed decision.

12. **Which patients merit antiplatelet therapy for prevention of stroke? What is the benefit? What are the risks?**
All patients who do not meet criteria for anticoagulation after stroke should receive antiplatelet therapy with either (a) aspirin, (b) clopidogrel, or (c) aspirin plus extended release dipyridamole. These three agents are similarly efficacious for stroke prevention, decreasing risk of second stroke by 14% to 18%. Ensuring optimal compliance with antiplatelet therapy is more important than the individual agent used, so the choice of agent should be guided by comorbidities, tolerability, and cost. Clopidogrel may be preferred in patients with history of significant GI bleeding, peripheral vascular disease, or drug-eluting cardiac stents. Extended-release dipyridamole does not compromise cardiac function and can be used safely in cardiac patients. In fact, meta-analyses have suggested that extended release dipyridamole may protect against nonstroke vascular events. Aspirin plus dipyridamole can cause headaches initially and so may be difficult for patients with chronic headache to tolerate. Also, the capsule does not fit down most feeding tubes and its extended release formulation may not be crushed, so it is not a good choice for patients requiring feeding tubes. Aspirin plus extended release dipyridamole have recently been compared with clopidogrel in the PROFESS trial. At the time of this writing, the results have not been published, but initial reports suggest no superiority to clopidogrel and

a somewhat higher hemorrahge rate. Aspirin alone may be a good choice when not contraindicated, particularly when cost of the alternative agents would hinder compliance.

Aspirin should not be used in combination with clopidogrel *for secondary stroke prevention,* as the combination showed an unacceptably high bleeding risk without additional protection from strokes compared with clopidogrel alone. Patients may require both aspirin and clopidogrel for cardiac conditions such as drug-eluting stents, and such patients may be continued on this combination regimen after stroke. At the time of this writing, investigation comparing aspirin alone versus aspirin plus clopidogrel for small-vessel stroke is ongoing.

13. **How soon after a stroke or TIA should anticoagulation or antiplatelet therapy be initiated?**

In general, antiplatelet therapy can be initiated immediately in patients who are not candidates for tPA and do not have any indication of hemorrhagic component and after 24 hours in patients who received tPA once lack of hemorrhage has been confirmed by CT or magnetic resonance imaging (MRI). Timing of anticoagulation is highly case specific. Larger strokes are more likely to bleed than small strokes, especially early on. The risk of a second stroke in the 2 weeks after initial stroke in patients with atrial fibrillation is only 0.5%. The risk of bleeding from heparinazation has been estimated at 5% based on the TOAST trial. Because of this, it is common practice to wait 1 month after a large stroke before initiating anticoagulation (although such a strategy has not been prospectively studied in a large trial). Patients with very small strokes may be started on anticoagulation within 1 or 2 days of stroke. The decision is much more difficult in patients with large strokes at higher risk for embolization, such as those with mechanical valves or demonstrated cardiac thrombus. In such cases, oral anticoagulation may be started cautiously after 5 to 15 days, depending on the individual situation. Retrospective data suggest bridging with heparin or low-molecular-weight heparin causes higher bleeding risk. In the absence of clinical or laboratory evidence of a hypercoaguable state, it is probably acceptable to start warfarin at low doses to achieve therapeutic anticoagulation slowly.

14. **How should patients with carotid stenosis be managed?**

Patients with symptomatic carotid stensosis greater than 70% should be treated with carotid endarterectomy within 2 weeks of a TIA or nondisabling stroke because their risk of recurrent stroke is 15% over 5 years, and CEA cuts this rate in half. Patients with symptomatic stenosis 50% to 70% benefit less from CEA but have the same up-front surgical risk, so close monitoring with aggressive risk factor management is usually advised for these patients. Asymptomatic patients at all levels of stenosis have a 4% stroke rate, which is also cut in half after CEA, but up-front risk of death or stroke from the procedure is 3% to 6%, so overall benefit is less. The CREST trial comparing stenting with endarterectomy is ongoing. Carotid artery disease is discussed in more detail in Chapter 54.

BIBLIOGRAPHY, SUGGESTED READINGS, AND WEBSITES

1. Caplan LR: Overview of the Evaluation of Stroke: http://www.utdol.com
2. Giraldo EA: Stroke: http://www.merck.com/mmpe
3. Jauch EC, Kissela B: Acute Stroke Management: http://www.emedicine.com
4. Kistler JP, Furie KL, Ay H: Etiology and Clinical Manifestations of Transient Ischemic Attack: http://www.utdol.com
5. Schneck MJ, Xu L, Palacio S: Cardioembolic Stroke: http://www.emedicine.com
6. Adams HP Jr, Bendixen BH, Kappelle LJ, et al: Classification of subtype of acute ischemic stroke. Definitions for use in a multicenter clinical trial. TOAST: Trial of Org 10172 in Acute Stroke Treatment, *Stroke* 24(1):35-41, 1993.
7. Adams HP Jr, del Zoppo G, Alberts MJ, et al: Guidelines for the early management of adults with ischemic stroke, *Circulation* 115(20):e478-534, 2007. Erratum in: *Circulation* 116(18):e515, 2007.

8. Anderson CS, Huang Y, Wang JG, et al: Intensive blood pressure reduction in acute cerebral haemorrhage trial (INTERACT): a randomised pilot trial, *Lancet Neurol* 7(5):391-399, 2008.

9. Broderick J, Connolly S, Feldman E, et al: Guidelines for the management of spontaneous intracerebral hemorrhage in adults, *Circulation* 116(16):e391-e413, 2007.

10. Khatri P, Taylor RA, Palumbo V, et al: The safety and efficacy of thrombolysis for strokes after cardiac catheterization, *J Am Coll Cardiol* 51(9):906-911, 2008.

11. Risk factors for stroke and efficacy of antithrombotic therapy in atrial fibrillation. Analysis of pooled data from five randomized controlled trials, *Arch Intern Med* 154(13):1449-1457, 1994.

12. Sacco RL, Adams R, Albers G, et al: Guidelines for prevention of stroke in patients with ischemic stroke or transient ischemic attack, *Stroke* 37:577-617, 2006.

13. The National Institute of Neurological Disorders and Stroke rt-PA Stroke Study Group: Tissue plasminogen activator for acute ischemic stroke, *N Engl J Med* 333:1581-1587, 1995.

CHAPTER 56

TRAUMATIC HEART DISEASE

Fernando Boccalandro, MD, FACC, FSCAI

1. **What is the most common cause of cardiac injury?**
   Motor vehicle accidents are the most common cause of cardiac injury.

2. **List the physical mechanisms of injury in cardiac trauma.**
   Physical mechanisms of injury include penetrating trauma (e.g., ribs, foreign bodies, sternum); nonpenetrating trauma; massive chest compression or crush injury; deceleration, traction, or torsion of the heart or vascular structures; sudden rise in blood pressure caused by acute abdominal compression; and myocardial contusion.

3. **What is myocardial contusion?**
   Myocardial contusion is a common, reversible injury and is the consequence of a nonpenetrating trauma to the myocardium. It is detected by elevations of specific cardiac enzymes with no evidence of coronary occlusion and by reversible wall motion abnormalities detected by echocardiography. It can manifest in the electrocardiogram (ECG) by ST/T changes or by more complex arrhythmias. Myocardial contusion is pathologically characterized by areas of myocardial necrosis and hemorrhagic infiltrates that can be recognized on autopsy.

4. **Which major cardiovascular structures are most commonly involved in cardiac trauma?**
   Cardiac trauma most commonly involves traumatic contusion or rupture of the right ventricle, aortic valve tear, left ventricle or left atrial rupture, innominate artery avulsion, aortic isthmus rupture, left subclavian artery traumatic occlusion, and tricuspid valve tear.

5. **What bedside findings can be found in patients with suspected major cardiovascular trauma?**
   Obvious clinical signs in patients with nonpenetrating trauma are rare. However, a bedside evaluation by an astute clinician to detect possible life-threatening cardiovascular and thoracic complications can reveal important signs in just a few minutes (Table 56-1).

6. **Can an acute myocardial infarction complicate cardiac trauma?**
   Chest trauma can injure a coronary artery leading to myocardial infarction based on coronary spasm, thrombosis, or dissection of the arterial wall. Patients with established severe coronary artery disease have favorable pathophysiologic conditions to suffer an acute myocardial event during significant trauma as a result of limited coronary flow reserve, excess of circulating catecholamines, hypoxia, blood loss, and hypotension. Always consider the possibility that when a patient has a myocardial infarction and trauma, the acute coronary syndrome could be the primary cause of the traumatic event because of cardiac syncope. Chest trauma can elevate cardiac-specific enzymes without significant coronary stenosis; therefore, careful interpretation of these indicators in a trauma victim is warranted.

TABLE 56-1. IMPORTANT SIGNS OF CARDIOVASCULAR AND THORACIC TRAUMA

Finding	Suggested Lesions
Pale skin color, conjunctiva, palms, and oral mucosa	Suggests important blood loss
Decreased blood pressure in the left arm	Seen in patients with traumatic rupture of the aortic isthmus, pseudocarctation, or traumatic thrombosis of the left subclavian artery
Decreased blood pressure in the right arm	Consider innominate artery avulsion
Subcutaneous emphysema and tracheal deviation	Consider pneumothorax
Elevated jugular venous pulse with inspiratory raise (i.e., Kussmaul's sign)	Suggests cardiac tamponade or tension pneumothorax
Prominent systolic V wave in the venous pulse examination	Suggests tricuspid insufficiency as a result of tricuspid valve tear
Nonpalpable apex or distant heart sounds	Suspect cardiac tamponade
Pericardial rub	Diagnostic for pericarditis
Pulsus paradoxus	Seen in patients with cardiac tamponade, massive pulmonary embolism, or tension pneumothorax
Continuous murmurs or thrills	Consider a traumatic arteriovenous fistula or rupture of the sinus of valsalva
Harsh holosystolic murmurs	Suspect a traumatic ventricular septal defect
Cervical and supraclavicular hematomas	Seen in traumatic carotid rupture

7. **What is the most common type of myocardial infarction suffered in trauma victims?**
According to the most recent definition of myocardial infarction, patients who have myocardial necrosis during trauma usually suffer a type 2 myocardial infarction. This type of myocardial infarction is secondary to ischemia as a result of either increased oxygen demand or decreased supply (e.g., coronary artery spasm, coronary embolism, anemia, arrhythmias, hypertension, or hypotension), rather than coronary occlusion caused by advanced atherosclerosis (type 1 myocardial infarction).

8. **What is the preferred treatment for an ST-elevation acute myocardial infarction in the event of chest trauma?**
The treatment of choice is emergent coronary angiography. Thrombolytics should be limited to minimize bleeding. Also, withholding nitrates, angiotensin-converting enzyme (ACE) inhibitors, and beta-blockers until the patient is hemodynamically stable should be considered. Aspirin may be used in patients with no evidence of severe bleeding. Aortic balloon contrapulsation is contraindicated in patients with acute myocardial infarction and cardiogenic shock with acute traumatic aortic regurgitation or any suspected aortic lesions. If a coronary intervention is needed, percutaneous thrombectomy and balloon angioplasty without stenting are preferred, but if stenting is needed, a bare-metal stent should be considered to limit the risk of in-stent thrombosis in patients who are not candidates for antiplatelet therapy with aspirin and thienopyridines because of an increased risk of bleeding.

9. **List the causes of shock in patients with heart trauma.**
The first cause to address is hypovolemic shock caused by acute blood loss, usually from an abdominal source. If the shock persists despite fluid resuscitation or the degree of hemodynamic compromise is not in proportion to the degree of blood loss, consider cardiogenic causes. Two other important causes are cardiac tamponade and ventricular akinesia or hypokineisa. Rupture of any intrapericardial vessel or cardiac structure (e.g., coronary arteries, proximal aorta, great veins, ventricle) produces a rapid state of shock because of cardiac tamponade, unless there is a concomitant pericardial tear. Cardiac akinesia or severe hypokinesia with temporary myocardial stunning could be a consequence of cardiac trauma and could lead to cardiogenic shock or acute heart failure. Cardiac akinesia or severe hypokinesia requires volume resuscitation to increase the cardiac preload and inotropic support until contractile recovery is achieved.

10. **What workup should be considered in a patient with suspected heart trauma?**
   - **Laboratory testing:** Hemoglobin, hematocrit, chemistries, cardiac enzymes, blood typing, and coagulation panel are routine.
   - **Chest radiograph:** Radiographs are used to evaluate the cardiac silhouette, mediastinum, and lung fields.
   - **Electrocardiogram:** Not a sensitive or specific test, but this may reveal nonspecific ST/T changes, conduction abnormalities, sinus tachycardia, premature atrial contractions, ventricular premature beats, or more complex arrythmias suggestive of myocardial contusion. Low voltage is suggestive of pericardial effusion, whereas electrical alternans is very suspicious for impending cardiac tamponade. If the patient is stable, no further workup may be needed.

If more complex heart lesions are suspected, including any pericardial involvement, an echocardiogram (echo) with Doppler imaging is the test of choice. This test is fast, inexpensive, and readily available to provide a vast amount of information regarding the pericardial space, wall motion, valvular function, myocardium, and proximal aorta. Pay special attention to the right ventricle because of its anterior location close to the sternum, and to the possible presence of ventricular thrombus. Transthoracic echo may have important limitations in patients with complicated trauma (e.g., unstable chest, ventilated patients, chest tube drainages) because of limited windows. Echo-contrast agents and transesophageal echocardiogram could play an important role in this group of patients. Transesophageal echo may not be possible in those with an unstable neck or facial trauma. In suspected aortic involvement, a contrast computed tomography (CT) is the test of choice.

11. **What are the signs of cardiac tamponade?**
Classical signs for cardiac tamponade include three signs, known as Beck's triad: hypotension caused by decreased stroke volume, jugular-venous distension as a result of impaired venous return to the heart, and muffled heart sounds caused by fluid inside the pericardial sac. Other signs of tamponade include pulsus paradoxus and general signs of shock such as tachycardia, tachypnea, and decreasing level of consciousness.

12. **Can a patient suffering from traumatic cardiac tamponade have a normal jugular venous pulse?**
In hypovolemic patients, the jugular-venous distension may be difficult to interpret even in the presence of cardiac tamponade. Thus, attention to the volume status is important while examining the venous pulse in trauma victims.

13. **How can I confirm the diagnosis in a patient with suspected pericardial tamponade?**
A large cardiac silhouette by chest radiograph and low-voltage QRS complexes or electrical alternans in the ECG can suggest the presence of cardiac tamponade. CT can identify the size of

an effusion but cannot confirm the diagnosis. Echocardiography can confirm the diagnosis of tamponade and is the test of choice. It allows to examine not only the amount of pericardial fluid and two-dimensional sings of cardiac tamponade (i.e., right ventricular and atrial collapse, paradoxical septal motion) but, more importantly, to evaluate the degree of hemodynamic compromise caused by the pericardial effusion using Doppler examination during the respiratory cycle.

14. **How can I treat a patient with pericardial tamponade?**
Pericardial tamponade requires immediate treatment with a surgical subxyphoid approach as the preferred option or with a percutaneous approach using bedside echocardiography or under fluoroscopic guidance.

15. **What interventions during resuscitation and management of an unstable trauma patient can precipitate cardiac tamponade in a patient with a pericardial effusion?**
In a patient with a moderate to large effusion, cardiac tamponade can be precipitated by hypovolemia or positive-pressure ventilation during trauma management. Therefore, meticulous attention of the patient's hemodynamics is needed in these circumstances.

16. **What are the mechanisms of injury of the thoracic great vessels?**
Deceleration and traction are the most common mechanisms of injury of the thoracic arteries. Sudden horizontal deceleration creates marked shearing stress at the aortic isthmus (i.e., the junction between the mobile aortic arch and the fixed descending aorta), whereas vertical deceleration displaces the heart caudally and pulls the ascending aorta and the innominate artery. Rapid extension of the neck or traction on the shoulder can also overstretch the arch vessels and produce tears of the intima, disruption of the media, or complete rupture of the vessel wall, leading to bleeding, dissection, thrombosis, or pseudoaneurysm formation. Aortic rupture leads to immediate hypovolemic shock and death in the vast majority of cases.

17. **Describe the management of thoracic arterial lesions.**
Usually, all arterial lesions require surgical repair, except benign ones like wall hematomas and limited dissections. An effort should be made to control the blood pressure with beta-blockers in all arterial lesions if the patient is hemodynamically stable. Venous lesions caused by low pressure usually do not lead to a rapid hemodynamic compromise unless the implicated vessel drains to the pericardium, possibly leading to cardiac tamponade.

18. **What are potential late complications of heart trauma?**
Late complications can include fistulas between different structures, constrictive pericarditis as a late consequence of hemopericardium, embolization from a mural thrombus, ventricular aneurysm formation, valvular insufficiency, and postpericardiotomy syndrome.

19. **What is commotio cordis?**
Sudden death after a blunt chest trauma is a rare phenomenon known as commotio cordis. It is theorized that commotio cordis is caused by ventricular fibrillation secondary to an impact-induced energy transmission via the chest wall to the myocardium during the vulnerable repolarization period. This can cause lethal arrhythmias resulting in sudden death.

20. **Describe the cardiac complications of electrical or lightning injuries.**
Patients in whom an electric current has a vertical pathway are at high risk for cardiac injury. Arrhythmias are frequently seen. Damage to the myocardium is uncommon and occurs mainly because of heat injury or coronary spasm, causing myocardial ischemia. Direct current (DC) and high-tension alternate current (AC) are more likely to cause ventricular asystole, whereas

low-tension AC produces ventricular fibrillation. The most common ECG abnormalities are sinus tachycardia and nonspecific ST-T–wave changes.

The effect of lightning on the heart has been called *cosmic cardioversion* and results in ventricular standstill and, in some reports, ventricular fibrillation. Standstill usually returns to sinus rhythm, but often the patient has a persistent respiratory arrest that causes deterioration of the rhythm. If initial ECG changes are not seen, it is unlikely that significant arrhythmias will occur later.

21. **Can a patient develop a *trauma-related* cardiomyopathy?**
   Takotsubo cardiomyopathy, also known as *transient apical ballooning, stress-induced cardiomyopathy,* and simply *stress cardiomyopathy,* is a nonischemic cardiomyopathy in which there is sudden temporary left ventricular systolic dysfunction. The cause appears to involve high circulating levels of catecholamines and is not specific for mechanical trauma but can be seen in patients after both emotional and physical trauma. Because this finding is associated with emotional stress, the condition is also known as *broken heart syndrome.* The typical presentation of someone with takotsubo cardiomyopathy is a sudden onset of congestive heart failure or chest pain associated with ECG changes suggestive of an anterior wall myocardial infarction after a major trauma. During the course of evaluation, dilation of the left ventricular apex with a hypercontractile base of the left ventricle is often noted by echocardiography. It is this finding that earned the syndrome its name *takotsubo,* or "octopus trap," in Japan, where it was first described. Evaluation of individuals with takotsubo cardiomyopathy may include a coronary angiogram, which generally does not reveal any significant coronary artery disease. Provided that the individual survives the initial presentation, the left ventricular function usually improves within several months with medical therapy.

BIBLIOGRAPHY, SUGGESTED READINGS, AND WEBSITES

1. Bansal MK, Maraj S, Chewaproug D, et al: Myocardial contusion injury: redefining the diagnostic algorithm, *Emerg Med J* 22(7):465-469, 2005.
2. Gianni M, Dentali F, Grandi AM, et al: Apical ballooning syndrome or takotsubo cardiomyopathy: a systematic review, *Eur Heart J* 27(13):1523-1529, 2006.
3. Holanda MS, Domínguez MJ, López-Espadas F, et al: Cardiac contusion following blunt chest trauma, *Eur J Emerg Med* 13(6):373-376, 2006.
4. Karmy-Jones R, Jurkovich GJ: Blunt chest trauma, *Curr Probl Surg* 41(3):211-380, 2004.
5. Khandhar SJ, Johnson SB, Calhoon JH: Overview of thoracic trauma in the United States, *Thorac Surg Clin* 17(1):1-9, 2007.
6. Madias C, Maron BJ, Weinstock J, et al: Commotio cordis—sudden cardiac death with chest wall impact, *J Cardiovasc Electrophysiol* 18(1):115-122, 2007.
7. Mandavia DP, Joseph A: Bedside echocardiography in chest trauma, *Emerg Med Clin North Am* 22(3):601-619, 2004.
8. McGillicuddy D, Rosen P: Diagnostic dilemmas and current controversies in blunt chest trauma, *Emerg Med Clin North Am* 25(3):695-711, viii-ix, 2007.
9. Ritenour AE, Morton MJ, McManus JG, et al: Lightning injury: a review, *Burns* 34(5):585-594, 2008.
10. Thygesen K, Alpert JS, White HD: Joint ESC/ACCF/AHA/WHF Task Force for the Redefinition of Myocardial Infarction. Universal definition of myocardial infarction, *J Am Coll Cardiol* 50(22):2173-2195, 2007.

CHAPTER 57

CARDIAC TUMORS

Glenn N. Levine, MD, FACC, FAHA

1. **Which are more common, primary cardiac tumors or metastatic tumors to the heart?**

   Metastatic tumors to the heart are markedly more common than primary cardiac tumors; with one source reporting metastatic involvement of the heart to be 20 to 40 times more prevalent than primary cardiac tumors. Primary cardiac tumors are extremely rare, occurring in one autopsy series in less than 0.1 % of subjects.

2. **What are the most common tumors that metastasize to the heart?**

   The most common tumors that spread to the heart are lung (bronchogenic) cancer, breast cancer, melanoma, thyroid cancer, esophageal cancer, lymphoma, and leukemia. Malignant melanoma has the greatest propensity to spread to the heart, with 50% to 65% of patients with malignant melanoma having cardiac metastases. Tumors may spread to the heart via direct extension, the circulatory system, or via lymphatics. Renal cell carcinoma may extend up the inferior vena cava all the way into the heart.

3. **What are the most common primary cardiac tumors?**

   Benign tumors are more common than malignant tumors, occurring approximately three times as often as malignant tumors. The most common benign cardiac tumors are myxomas; other common benign cardiac tumors are lipomas and papillary fibroelastomas. Rhabdomyomas are the most common benign tumor occurring in infants and children. Interestingly, they usually regress over time and do not require specific treatment in asymptomatic individuals.

4. **In what chamber do most myxomas occur?**

   Approximately 75% to 80% of myxomas occur in the left atrium (Fig. 57-1), with 15% to 20% occurring in the right atrium. Only 3% to 4% of myxomas arise in the left ventricle and 3% to 4% arise in the right ventricle. Myxomas are usually pedunculated and typically arise from the interatrial septum via a *stalk*. They are described on gross pathological examination as *gelatinous* in consistency. They most commonly occur between the third and sixth decades of life, and more frequently occur in women. They can cause effective obstruction of filling of the left or right ventricles, leading to left or right heart failure symptoms and findings, mimicking the symptoms and findings of mitral or tricuspid valve stenosis. Systemic embolism occurs in 30% to 40% of patients. Constitutional symptoms and findings (see Question 6) are also common.

5. **What are the most common primary malignant tumors?**

   The most common primary malignant tumors are sarcomas (Fig. 57-2). Such sarcomas include angiosarcomas (the most common), rhabdomyocarcomas, fibrosarcomas, and leimyosarcomas. The results of surgery or chemotherapy in the treatment of cardiac sarcomas have been generally poor, with mean survival of only 6 to 12 months.

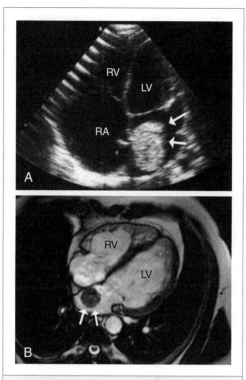

Figure 57-1. A, Left atrial myxoma, as visualized on transthoracic echocardiogram and, **B,** on cardiac MRI. (**A** modified from Erdol C, Ozturk C, Ocal A, et al: Contralateral recurrence of atrial myxoma—case report and review of the literature, *Images Paediatr Cardiol* 8:3-9, 2001.)

6. **What symptoms do cardiac tumors cause?**

    This depends on the location of the tumor, as well as the tumor itself. Left atrial myxomas may cause effective mitral valve stenosis (or regurgitation). Tumors may also cause hemodynamic effects via compression or mass effects. Tumors may lead to atrial or ventricular arrhythmias. Tumors (including myxomas and papillary fibroelastomas) may embolize, leading to transient ischemic attack (TIA) or stroke. Tumors involving the pericardium can cause pericardial effusion and tamponade. Constitutional symptoms (fatigue, weight loss, fever) occur not infrequently, as well as anemia, elevated erythrocyte sedimentation rate, elevated C-reactive protein, and other nonspecific laboratory findings. In patients with known noncardiac cancer, the development of arrhythmias (particularly atrial fibrillation) or development of findings suggesting pericardial effusion/tamponade (distended neck veins, hypotension, pulses paradox, new low voltage on the electrocardiogram [ECG]) should prompt immediate evaluation for cardiac/pericardial metastasis.

7. **What is the workup for suspected cardiac tumors?**

    The initial workup is a transthoracic echocardiogram (echo). Many tumors will also be discovered incidentally or surreptitiously by cardiac echo. Tumors may be further evaluated with transesophageal echo, cardiac magnetic resonance imaging (MRI), or cardiac computed tomography (CT). The role of positron emission tomography (PET) in the evaluation of cardiac tumors is in evolution. Only anecdotal reports exist of the possible role of endomyocardial biopsy for tumor histology.

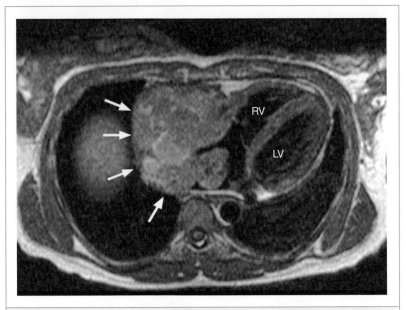

Figure 57-2. Massive angiosarcoma arising from the right atrium, as visualized by MRI. (Modified from Sparrow PJ, Kurian JB, Jones TR, et al: MR imaging of cardiac tumors, *Radiographics* 25(5):1255-1276, 2005.)

8. **What is a *tumor plop*?**
   A tumor plop is a sound heard in early diastole during auscultation produced when a left atrial myxoma prolapses into the left ventricle during diastole. The sound may be due to the tumor striking the left ventricular wall or to tension created on the tumor stalk.

9. **What is lipomatous hypertrophy of the interatrial septum?**
   Lipomatous hypertrophy is an abnormal, exaggerated growth of normal fat cells. It occurs in the interatrial septum, resulting in the appearance of a thickened atrial septum. The finding itself is benign.

10. **What is the Carney complex?**
    Known by various names and acronyms, the Carney complex is an autosomal-dominant syndrome consisting of cardiac myxomas, cutaneous myxomas, spotty pigmentation of the skin, endocrinopathy, and other tumors. Myxomas occurring as part of the Carney complex are reported to account for 7% of all cardiac myxomas.

BIBLIOGRAPHY, SUGGESTED READINGS, AND WEBSITES

1. Goodkind MJ: Cardiac Tumors: http://www.merck.com/mmpe
2. Firstenberg MS: Benign Cardiac Tumors: http://www.emedicine.com
3. Sharma GK: Atrial Myxoma: http://www.emedicine.com

4. Basson CT: Carney Complex: http://www.emedicine.com
5. Kapoor A: *Cancer of the heart*, New York, 1986, Springer Verlag.
6. Reardon MJ, Walkes JC, Benjamin R: Therapy insight: malignant primary cardiac tumors, *Nat Clin Pract Cardiovasc Med* 3(10):548-553, 2006.
7. Reynen K: Cardiac myxomas, *N Engl J Med* 333:1610-1617, 1995.
8. Sparrow PJ, Kurian JB, Jones TR, et al: MR imaging of cardiac tumors, *Radiographics* 25(5):1255-1276, 2005.

4. **List the four**
Different classif
four types:
   - Membran
     small local
     of VSD se
   - Muscular
   - Inlet VSDs
     mitral valv
   - Outlet VSI
     septum th

ADULT

Luc M. Bea

1. **Which pat**
   prophylaxi
   The indicatic
   American He
   congenital h
   is now indic
   - Unrepa
   - Prosthe
   - Residu
   - The fir:
   - Patient
   The new
   or gastroint
   prophylaxis

2. **What are**
   associate
   The three m
   The secund
   usually pres
   septum adj
   defect (end
   sinus venos
   part. In the
   or drainage

3. **When she**
   percutane
   ASDs vary
   sided volun
   leads to pu
   atrial dilatic
   significant
   associated
   hemodyna
   is placed.
   and with tr
   closed per
   require su

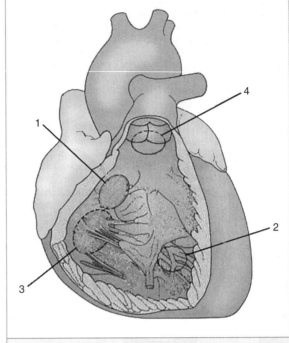

Figure 58-2. Ventricular septal defects: *1*, perimembranous; *2*, muscular; *3*, inlet; *4*, outlet. (Modified from Gatzoulis MA, Webb GD, Daubeney PEF, et al: *Diagnosis and management of adult congenital heart disease*, 2003, Edinburgh, Churchill Livingstone, p. 171.)

5. **What are the long-term complications of a small VSD in the adult patient?**
   In the adult, there are two groups of patients with unrepaired VSD. The smallest group consists of patients with a large VSD that has been complicated by severe pulmonary hypertension (Eisenmenger's syndrome). However, the vast majority of adult patients with VSDs have small defects that are hemodynamically insignificant (i.e., do not cause left ventricular dilation or pulmonary hypertension). As a rule these patients have a benign natural history. Rarely, some patients develop complications such as endocarditis, atrial arrhythmias, tricuspid regurgitation, aortic regurgitation, and double-chamber right ventricle.

6. **What are the complications of a bicuspid aortic valve?**
   A bicuspid aortic valve is present in 0.5% to 2% of the population. The main complications are progressive aortic stenosis, aortic regurgitation, or a combination of both. Other complications include endocarditis and aortopathy. Although infrequent, aortic coarctation is also a well-described association and must be ruled out in these patients. Patients in whom the bicuspid valve demonstrates signs of valve degeneration on echocardiography are at an increased risk of cardiovascular events and need close regular follow-up.

7. **How is hemodynamic severity of coarctation of the aorta assessed in the adult patient?**
   In coarctation of the aorta the narrowing is typically in the proximal portion of the descending aorta just distal to the left subclavian artery. Adult patients can be divided into two groups: those with *native* (i.e., unrepaired) coarctation and those who are post-repair (some of which

have residual stenosis). Some coarctations are mild and not hemodynamically significant. Findings suggestive of a hemodynamically significant coarctation include small diameter (less than 10 mm or less than 50% of reference normal descending aorta at the diaphragm), presence of collaterals, and elevated gradient (more than 20–30 mm Hg clinically, by catheterization or by echocardiogram). The clinical gradient is measured by comparing the highest arm systolic pressure (left or right) to the systolic pressure in the leg (typically measured by palpation of the pedal pulses while inflating a cuff at the calf level). Patients with hemodynamically significant coarctations are at risk of a number of complications, including refractory hypertension, accelerated atherosclerosis, cerebrovascular disease, and aortopathy.

8. **In coarctation of the aorta, when should percutaneous stenting be considered?**
Most clinicians think that patients with significant coarctation of the aorta should be considered for intervention. Although surgery has been available for several decades, percutaneous dilation with stenting has evolved as an alternative. In the adult patient with residual stenosis after repair, stenting has become the first-line therapy at most centers. For adults with native coarctation, stenting has also become first-line therapy at many centers. In patients who undergo percutaneous stenting, the anatomy needs to be suitable (i.e., no significant arch hypoplasia). In adult patients who undergo surgery, the usual procedure is placement of an interposition graft.

9. **Which adult patients with patent ductus arteriosus (PDA) require percutaneous device closure?**
A PDA connects the proximal part of the left pulmonary artery to the proximal descending aorta, just distal to the left subclavian artery. The unrepaired ductus in an adult is usually small in diameter and the resultant left to right shunt is hemodynamically insignificant. However, in some patients the ductus diameter is large and results in severe pulmonary hypertension (Esienmenger's syndrome). Occasionally, some adults have moderate-size ducts resulting in shunting that is not negligible but not significant enough to cause severe pulmonary hypertension. In these patients the left ventricle will be dilated and the pulmonary pressure may be somewhat elevated. Clinically they will have a continuous murmur, a large pulse pressure, and signs of ventricular dilation. This latter group should undergo percutaneous closure in an attempt to prevent long-term complications. Although controversial, many centers advocate routine closure of small PDAs to prevent endarteritis.

10. **How is Marfan syndrome diagnosed?**
The criteria for the diagnosis of Marfan syndrome have evolved over the years. The discovery of the main culprit gene in 1991 (FBN-1) led to the creation of a more selective diagnostic classification; the Ghent criteria. This classification requires presence of specific features involving multiple organ systems. Although molecular testing is available, it is, at the present time, only clinically useful in selected circumstances. In addition to the cardiology workup, patients with suspected Marfan syndrome should be referred to a geneticist.

11. **When should Marfan patients with aortic root dilation be referred for surgery?**
Although any part of the aorta can be involved in Marfan syndrome, the root is usually affected. Surgery (for root dilation) is done to prevent aortic dissection or rupture and is generally recommended when the aortic diameter is greater than 50 mm. For patients with rapid progression (more than 5 mm/year) or a family history of dissection, intervention is recommended by some specialists at 45 mm. In the Bentall procedure for root dilation, the native aortic valve and root are replaced with a composite conduit (a tube graft attached to a prosthetic valve). A more recently introduced surgical technique is a valve-sparing procedure in which the root is replaced by a prosthetic conduit and the native valve is kept in place.

12. **What is tetralogy of Fallot, and what is the main complication seen in the adult?**
Tetralogy of Fallot (TOF) consists of four features: right ventricular outflow tract (RVOT) obstruction, a large VSD, an overriding ascending aorta, and right ventricular hypertrophy. The RVOT obstruction is the clinically important lesion and may be subvalvular, valvular, or supravalvular or may be at multiple levels. Repair involves closing the VSD and relieving the RVOT obstruction. In many patients, to relieve the RVOT obstruction, surgery on the pulmonary annulus and valve leaflets is required and is usually complicated by severe residual pulmonary insufficiency. Over time, chronic severe pulmonary insufficiency often leads to right ventricular dysfunction and exercise intolerance, for which a pulmonary valve replacement (PVR) may be necessary. When PVR is performed, a tissue prosthesis is usually placed (homograft or porcine/bovine prosthesis). The problem with tissue prostheses in young adults is that they require replacement at 10- to 15-year intervals. A percutaneous pulmonary valve prosthesis is now available in certain countries, but experience is limited at the present time. Other complications in TOF include residual RVOT obstruction, residual VSD leak, right ventricular dysfunction, aortic root dilation, and arrhythmias.

13. **What are the three *D*s of Ebstein's anomaly?**
Ebstein's anomaly is characterized by an apically *displaced* tricuspid valve that is *dysplastic* with a right ventricle that may be *dysfunctional*. The displacement affects predominantly the septal and posterior leaflets of the valve. The leaflets are usually diminutive and tethered to the ventricular wall. Characteristically, the anterior leaflet is unusually elongated. The right ventricle is often thin and can have both diastolic and systolic dysfunction. Half of patients have an interatrial communication patent foramen ovale [PFO] or atrial septal defect [ASD]. Fifteen percent of patients have accessory pathways, which will manifest clinically as Wolf-Parkinson-White syndrome. The primary complication of Ebstein's anomaly is tricuspid regurgitation and right-sided heart failure. If significant enough, placement of a tissue prosthesis or valve repair (if the valve anatomy is suitable) is indicated.

14. **What drug therapy should now be considered in all patients with Eisenmenger's syndrome?**
Eisenmenger's syndrome refers to markedly elevated pulmonary pressures caused by a longstanding left to right shunt between the systemic and pulmonary artery circulations because of a congenital defect. Initially, *left to right* shunting leads to increased pulmonary vascular flow, which over time induces changes in the pulmonary vasculature leading to increased pulmonary vascular resistance. When the pulmonary vascular resistance is near, or exceeds, the systemic vascular resistance, the shunt reverses. The resultant *right to left* shunting results in hypoxia and cyanosis. The most common defect causing Eisenmenger's syndrome is a VSD. Other causes include, among others, PDAs, atrioventricular septal defects, and ASDs. Traditionally these patients have been treated with supportive measures. However, recent data support the use of oral pulmonary vasodilators, bosentan (an endothelin blocker), and sildenafil (a nitric oxide promoter). These agents decrease pulmonary artery pressure and improve functional capacity. However, these medications are costly and it remains unclear which patients benefit most. Long-term data, including the effect on mortality, are also lacking. Regardless, all Eisenmenger's patients should be assessed by an appropriate specialist regarding use of pulmonary vasodilator.

15. **When should an Eisenmenger's patient be phlebotomized?**
In Eisenmenger's syndrome, hypoxia resulting from the right to left shunt stimulates marrow production of red blood cells and leads to an elevated hematocrit. Historically, Eisenmenger's patients were phlebotomized routinely because an elevated hematocrit was thought to predispose to a thrombotic event, as with patients with the hematologic condition polycythemia vera. However, in recent years, data suggest that prophylactic phlebotomy in Eisenmenger's patients may be

more harmful than beneficial (i.e., it causes iron deficiency, decreases exercise tolerance, potentially increases the risk of stroke). As such, the use of phlebotomy has become more restrictive and should only be considered in (1) patients with symptoms of hyperviscosity (headaches, dizziness, fatigue, achiness), who have an hematocrit more than 65% with no evidence of iron deficiency; and (2) preoperatively, to improve hemostasis (goal hematocrit less than 65%). In modern practice, only a few Eisenmenger's patients should undergo phlebotomy.

16. **Which types of congenital heart disease lesions have particularly poor outcomes in pregnancy?**
   Very high risk congenital heart disease lesions include the following:
   - Unrepaired cyanotic heart disease
   - Eisenmenger's syndrome
   - Severe aortic stenosis
   - Marfan syndrome with a dilated aortic root (greater than 40 mm)
   - Mechanical valve prosthesis
   - Significant systemic ventricular dysfunction (EF 40% or less).

   These patients should be counseled accordingly about the significant maternal risks and poor fetal outcomes that are associated with pregnancy.

17. **What are the two types of transpositions?**
   Transposition complexes can be divided into two groups. In complete transposition of the great arteries (D-TGA), the anomaly can be simplistically conceptualized as an *inversion of the great vessels* (Fig. 58-3, *A*). The aorta comes out of the right ventricle, and the pulmonary artery comes out of the left ventricle. Desaturated blood is pumped into the systemic circulation, whereas oxygenated blood is pumped into the pulmonary circulation. Without intervention, this condition is associated with very poor outcomes in early infancy.
   Congenitally corrected transposition of the great arteries (L-TGA) can be conceptualized as an *inversion of the ventricles* (Fig. 58-3, *B*). Desaturated blood and oxygenated blood are thus

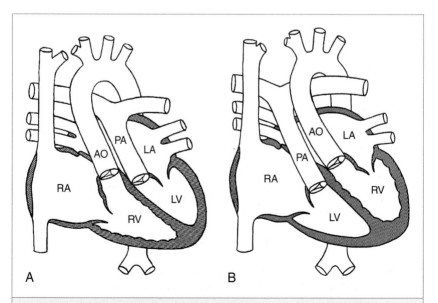

Figure 58-3. A, D-TGA. **B,** L-TGA. (Modified from Mullins CE, Mayer DC: *Congenital heart disease, a diagrammatic atlas*, 1988, New York, Wiley-Liss, pp. 164, 182.)

pumped in the appropriate arterial circulations. In many cases, associated anomalies, such as a VSD, pulmonary stenosis, an abnormal tricuspid valve, and heart block, are present. These patients can survive or present de novo in adulthood without surgical intervention.

18. **What is meant by a *systemic* right ventricle?**

A *systemic right ventricle* refers to a heart anomaly where the *morphologic* right ventricle pumps blood into the aorta. Ventricular morphology is determined by anatomic features typical to each ventricle. For example, the morphologic right ventricle has a tricuspid atrioventricular valve (with attachments to the septum and apical displacement compared with the mitral valve) and coarse apical trabeculations. L-TGA (see Question 17) is a congenital heart defect in which there is a systemic right ventricle. In the first few decades of life, the right ventricle is able to handle pumping into the high-pressure systemic circulation; however, in adulthood, the right ventricular function begins to deteriorate in many patients. This is usually associated with tricuspid regurgitation and manifests clinically as heart failure.

19. **What is the difference between an *atrial* and an *arterial* switch?**

An *atrial* switch is a surgical procedure that was previously done for patients born with D-TGA (Fig. 58-4, *A*). The Mustard and Senning procedures are both examples of an atrial switch and involve rerouting systemic and pulmonary venous flow to the respective pulmonary and systemic ventricles. This procedure was replaced by the *arterial* switch, which consists of "switching" the great arteries and reimplanting the coronary arteries to the *new* aorta (Fig. 58-4, *B*). The arterial switch is performed in the first few weeks after birth and has been the standard of care for patients born with D-TGA for more than two decades.

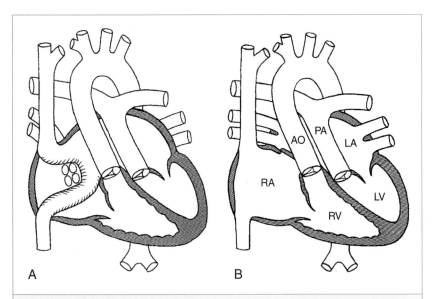

Figure 58-4. A, *Atrial* switch for D-TGA (Mustard or Senning procedure). (Modified from Mullins CE, Mayer DC: *Congenital heart disease, a diagrammatic atlas,* 1988, New York, Wiley-Liss, 1988, p. 296.) **B,** *Arterial* switch for D-TGA. (From Mullins CE, Mayer DC: *Congenital heart disease, a diagrammatic atlas,* 1988, New York, Wiley-Liss, p. 300.)

BIBLIOGRAPHY, SUGGESTED READINGS, AND WEBSITES

1. Nevil Thomas Adult Congenital Heart Library. http://www.achd-library.com
2. Canadian Adult Congenital Heart (CACH) Network. http://www.cachnet.org
3. The National Marfan Foundation. http://www.marfan.org
4. Galié N, Beghetti M, Gatzoulis MA, et al: Bosentan therapy in patients with Eisenmenger Syndrome. A multicenter, double-blind, randomized, placebo-controlled study, *Circulation* 114:48-54, 2006.
5. Gatzoulis MA, Webb GD, Daubeney PEF: *Diagnosis and management of adult congenital heart disease*, Philadelphia, Churchill Livingstone, 2003.
6. Gersony WM, Rosenbaum MS: *Congenital heart disease in the adult*, New York, McGraw-Hill, 2002.
7. Maron BJ, Zipes DP, Ackerman MJ, et al: Bethesda Conference report: 36th Bethesda Conference. Eligibility recommendations for competitive athletes with cardiovascular abnormalities, *J Am Coll Cardiol* 45:1312-1375, 2005.
8. Michelena HI, Desjardins VA, Avierinos JF, et al: Natural history of asymptomatic patients with normally functioning or minimally dysfunctional bicuspid aortic valve in the community, *Circulation* 117:2776-2784, 2008.
9. Siu SC, Colman JM, Sorensen S, et al: Adverse neonatal and cardiac outcomes are more common in pregnant women with cardiac disease, *Circulation* 105:2179-2184, 2002.
10. Spence MS, Balaratnam MS, Gatzoulis MA: Clinical update: cyanotic adult congenital heart disease, *Lancet* 370:1530-1532, 2007.
11. Therrien J, Dore A, Gersony W, et al: Canadian Cardiovascular Society Consensus Conference 2001 update: recommendations for the management of adults with congenital heart disease. Part I: review, *Can J Cardiol* 17(9):940-959, 2001.
12. Therrien J, Gatzoulis M, Graham T, et al: Canadian Cardiovascular Society Consensus Conference 2001 update: Recommendations for the management of adults with congenital heart disease. Part II: review, *Can J Cardiol* 17(10):1029-1050, 2001.
13. Therrien J, Warnes C, Daliento L, et al: Canadian Cardiovascular Society Consensus Conference 2001 update: recommendations for the management of adults with congenital heart disease. Part III: review, *Can J Cardiol* 17(11):1135-1158, 2001.
14. The Task Force on the Management of Grown Up Congenital Heart Disease of the European Society of Cardiology: Management of grown up congenital heart disease, *Eur Heart J* 24(11):1035-1084, 2003.
15. Wilson W, Taubert KA, Gewitz M, et al: AHA guideline: prevention of infective endocarditis. A guideline from the American Heart Association Rheumatic Fever, Endocarditis, and Kawasaki Disease Committee, Council on Cardiovascular Disease in the Young, and the Council on Clinical Cardiology, Council on Cardiovascular Surgery and Anesthesia, and the Quality of Care and Outcomes Research Interdisciplinary Working Group, *Circulation* 116:1736-1754, 2007.

CHAPTER 59

PERIPHERAL ARTERIAL DISEASE

*Thomas J. Kiernan, MD, MRCPI, Bryan P. Yan, MBBS, FRACP,
Glenn N. Levine, MD, FACC, FAHA, and Kenneth A. Rosenfield, MD*

1. **What is the difference between the terms peripheral arterial disease and peripheral vascular disease?**
   According to the American College of Cardiology/American Heart Association (ACC/AHA) 2005 guidelines, the term *peripheral arterial disease* includes a diverse group of disorders that lead to progressive stenosis or occlusion or aneurismal dilation of the aorta and its noncoronary branch arteries, including the carotid, upper extremities, visceral, and lower extremity arterial branches. *Peripheral vascular disease* is a historical term that includes those diseases that affect circulation as a whole and includes all arterial, venous, and lymphatic circulations and all vascular diseases that alter end-organ perfusion. Thus, *peripheral arterial disease (PAD)* is the preferred term to denote stenotic, occlusive, and aneurismal disease of the aorta and its branch arteries and will be used in this chapter.

2. **What are the key components of the vascular physical examination?**
   According to the ACC/AHA guidelines on peripheral arterial disease, the key components of the vascular physical examination include the following:
   - Blood pressure measurements in both arms
   - Carotid pulse palpation for upstroke and amplitude and auscultation for bruits
   - Auscultation of the abdomen and flank for bruits
   - Palpation of the abdomen for aortic pulsation and its maximal diameter
   - Palpation of brachial, radial, ulnar, femoral, popliteal, dorsalis pedis, and posterior tibial pulses; pulse intensity is scored as: 0 = absent, 1 = diminished, 2 = normal, 3 = bounding
   - Performance of Allen's test when knowledge of hand perfusion is needed
   - Auscultation of the femoral arteries for the presence of bruits
   - Inspection of the feet for color, temperature, and integrity of the skin and for ulcers
   - Observation of other findings suggestive of severe PAD, including distal hair loss, trophic skin changes, and hypertrophic nails

3. **Can the location of the patient's lower extremity claudication help to localize the site of occlusive disease?**
   The answer is a qualified yes. Because the pathophysiology of claudication is complex, there is not a perfect correlation between anatomic site of disease and location of symptoms. However, in general, the following statements can be made:
   - Occlusive iliac artery disease may produce hip, buttock, and thigh pain, as well as calf pain.
   - Occlusive femoral and popliteal artery disease usually produces calf pain.
   - Occlusive disease in the tibial arteries may produce calf pain or, more rarely, foot pain and numbness.

4. **What are causes of *pseudoclaudication*?**
   Symptoms that may to some extent mimic claudication caused by PAD can be caused by severe peripheral venous obstructive disease, chronic compartment syndrome, lumbar disease and spinal stenosis, osteoarthritis, and inflammatory muscle diseases. Arterial compromise from conditions other than atherosclerosis can lead to claudication-like symptoms. (See Question 18 on lower limb arterial disease in young patients.)

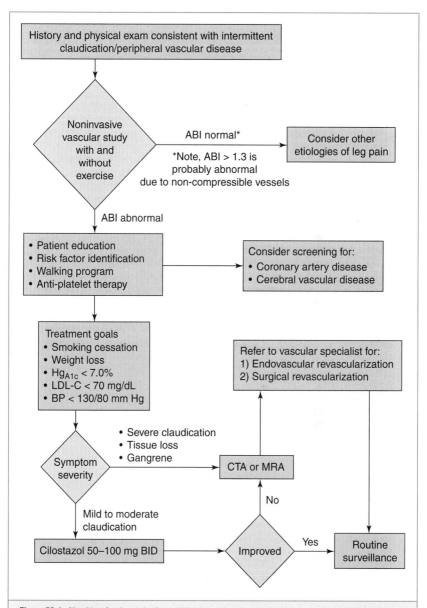

Figure 59-1. Algorithm for the evaluation and management of patients with suspected lower extremity peripheral artery disease. (From Toth PP, Shammas NW, Dippel EJ, et al: Cardiovascular disease. In Rakel: *Textbook of family medicine*, ed 7, Philadelphia, 2007, Saunders.)

5. **What noninvasive tests are used in the assessment of lower limb claudication?**
   - **Ankle-brachial index (ABI):** The ankle-brachial index is the ankle systolic pressure (as determined by Doppler) divided by the brachial systolic pressure. An abnormal index is less than 0.90. The sensitivity is approximately 90% for diagnosis of PAD. (See Question 6 for further details.)

- **Pulse volume recordings (PVRs):** Pulse volume recordings measure changes in volume of toes, fingers, or parts of limbs that occur with each pulse beat as blood flows into or out of the extremity. A toe:brachial index of less than 0.6 is abnormal, and values of less than 0.15 are seen in patients with rest pain (toe pressures of less than 20 mm Hg).
- **Duplex ultrasonography:** Duplex ultrasonography is a noninvasive method of evaluating arterial stenosis and blood flow. This method can localize and quantify the degree of stenosis. Ultrasonography is dependent on operator skill.
- **Transcutaneous oxygen tension measurements:** These measurements are useful in assessing tissue viability for wound healing. Measurements greater than 55 mm Hg are considered normal and less than 20 mm Hg are associated with nonhealing ulcers.
- **Exercise testing:** This testing determines treadmill walking time and preexercise and postexercise ABI. In those without significant PAD, the ABI is unchanged after exercise. In patients with PAD, the ABI falls after exercise. This test is more sensitive for detecting disease than a resting ABI alone.

6. **What is the ankle-brachial index?**
The ABI is the ratio of systolic blood pressure at the level of the ankle to the systolic blood pressure measured at the level of the brachial artery. More specifically, blood pressure is measured in both brachial arteries (with the higher systolic blood pressure being used) and is measured, using a Doppler instrument with a blood pressure cuff on the lower calf, in both posterior tibial and dorsalis pedis arteries. Pulse wave reflections in healthy persons should result in higher blood pressures in the ankle vessel pressure (10–15 mm Hg higher than in the brachial arteries), and thus a normal ankle-brachial index should be greater than 1.00. Using a diagnostic threshold of 0.90 to 0.91, several studies have found the sensitivity of the ABI to be 79% to 95% and the specificity to be 96% to 100% to detect stenosis of 50% or more reduction in lumen diameter.

Experts emphasize that the ABI is a continuous variable below 0.90. Values of 0.41 to 0.90 are considered to be mildly to moderately diminished; values of 0.40 or less are considered to be severely decreased. An ABI of 0.40 or less is associated with an increased risk of rest pain, ischemic ulceration, or gangrene. Patients with long-standing diabetes or end-stage renal disease on dialysis and elderly patients may have noncompressible leg arterial segments caused by medial calcification, precluding assessment of the ABI. A system for interpretation of the ABI is given in Table 59-1.

TABLE 59-1. INTERPRETATION OF THE ABI	
ABI	Interpretation
>1.30	Noncompressible
1.00–1.29	Normal
0.91–0.99	Borderline (equivocal)
0.41–0.90	Mild to moderate PAD
0.00–0.40	Severe PAD

Modified from Hiatt WR: Medical treatment of peripheral arterial disease and claudication, *N Engl J Med* 344:1608-1621, 2001.

7. **What are the recommended medical therapies and lifestyle interventions in patients with lower extremity PAD?**

A supervised exercise regimen is recommended as the initial treatment modality for patients with intermittent claudication. Supervised exercise training is recommended over unsupervised exercise training. Cilostizol treatment can lead to a modest increase in exercise capacity. Because agents with similar biologic effects have been shown to increase mortality in patients with heart failure, this drug should not be used in patients with heart failure. Smoking cessation must be strongly emphasized to the patient. Other measures include general secondary prevention interventions. Recommended medical therapies and lifestyle interventions in patients with lower extremity PAD are summarized in Table 59-2.

TABLE 59-2. RECOMMENDED MEDICAL THERAPIES AND LIFESTYLE INTERVENTIONS IN PATIENTS WITH LOWER EXTREMITY PAD

- Statin Treatment to Lower LD Level to $<70–100$ mg/dl
- Antihypertensive therapy to lower blood pressure to $<140/90$ mm Hg ($<130/80$ mm Hg in patients with diabetes or those with chronic kidney disease)
  - Beta-blockers are not contraindicated in patients with PAD.
  - The use of ACE inhibitors is reasonable in symptomatic lower extremity PAD patients to reduce the risk of adverse cardiovascular events.
- Patients with PAD Should Be Offered Smoking Cessation Interventions
- Antiplatelet therapy is indicated to reduce the risk of MI, stroke, or vascular death
  - Aspirin in doses of 75–325 mg is recommended.
  - Clopidogrel can be used as an alternate therapy to aspirin.
- Supervised exercise training is the recommended initial treatment modality for intermittent claudication.
  - Exercise should be for a minimum of 30–45 minutes at least three times per week.
- Cilostazol (100 mg orally twice a day) is recommended to improve symptoms and increase walking distance in patients with intermittent claudication. (Cilostazol should not be used in patients with heart failure.)

ACE, Angiotensin-converting enzyme.

Modified from Hirsch AT, Haskal ZJ, Hertzer NR, et al: ACC/AHA guidelines for the management of patients with peripheral arterial disease, *J Am Coll Cardiol* 47(6):1239-1312, 2006.

---

8. **What is critical limb ischemia, and how is it graded clinically?**

Whereas claudication is produced by decreased perfusion to the muscles with exercise, *limb-threatening ischemia* refers to inadequate tissue perfusion *at rest*. It is characteristically manifested as rest pain or tissue loss. One widely used scheme for classifying limb ischemia is given in Table 59-3.

9. **What are the causes of renal artery stenosis?**

Approximately 90% of all renal arterial lesions are due to atherosclerosis. Atherosclerotic-related lesions usually affect the ostium and the proximal 1 cm of the main renal artery. Fibromuscular dysplasia (FMD) is the next most common cause. Although it classically occurs in a young woman, it can affect both genders at any age. Less common causes of renovascular hypertension include renal artery aneurysms, Takayasu's arteritis, atheroemboli, thromboemboli, William's syndrome, neurofibromatosis, spontaneous renal artery

TABLE 59-3. CLINICAL CATEGORIES OF CHRONIC LIMB ISCHEMIA		
Grade	Category	Clinical Description
	0	Asymptomatic, not hemodynamically correct
I	1	Mild claudication
	2	Moderate claudication
	3	Severe claudication
II	4	Ischemic rest pain
	5	Minor tissue loss: nonhealing ulcer, focal gangrene with diffuse pedal ulcer
III	6	Major tissue loss extending above transmetatarsal level, functional foot no longer salvageable

(From Rutherford RB, Baker JD, Ernst C, et al: Recommended standards for reports dealing with lower extremity ischemia: revised version, *J Vasc Surg* 26:517, 1997.)

dissection, atriovenous malformations (AVMs) or fistulas, retroperitoneal fibrosis, and prior abdominal radiation therapy.

10. **What are ACC/AHA class I indications for the referral for diagnostic study to identify clinically significant renal artery stenosis?**
    Clinical scenarios that are recognized as class I indications for the performance of a diagnostic study to identify renal artery stenosis include the following:
    - Onset of hypertension before age 30
    - Onset of hypertension after age 55
    - Accelerated hypertension (sudden and persistent worsening of previously controlled hypertension), resistant hypertension (failure to achieve blood pressure goal with full adherences to full doses of an appropriate three-drug regimen that includes a diuretic), and malignant hypertension (hypertension with acute end-organ damage)
    - New azotemia or worsening renal function after angiotensin-converting enzyme (ACE) inhibitor or angiotensin-receptor blocker (ARB) treatment
    - Unexplained atrophic kidney or discrepancy in size between the two kidneys of more than 1.5 cm
    - Sudden, unexplained pulmonary edema (especially in azotemic patients)

11. **What diagnostic tests can be used to identify renal artery stenosis?**
    Duplex ultrasonogrpahy, computed tomographic angiography (if no significant risk of contrast nephropathy), and magnetic resonance angiography (MRA) are all accepted class I noninvasive methods of study. Catheter angiography is recommended if the clinical suspicion for renal artery stenosis (RAS) is high and noninvasive testing is inconclusive (class I recommendation). Captopril renal scintigraphy and selective renal vein rennin measurements are not recommended as useful screening tests (class III recommendation).

12. **What are the main indications for RAS percutaneous revascularization?**
    Most ACC/AHA indications for percutaneous revascularization are class IIa recommendations, meaning the procedure is *reasonable*.

Class I (Indicated):

- Hemodynamically significant RAS and recurrent, unexplained congestive heart failure or sudden, unexplained pulmonary edema

Class IIa (Reasonable):

- Hemodynamically significant RAS and accelerated hypertension, resistant hypertension, malignant hypertension, hypertension with an unexplained unilateral small kidney, and hypertension with intolerance to medication
- Hemodynamically significant RAS and unstable angina
- RAS and progressive chronic kidney disease with bilateral RAS or a RAS to a solitary functioning kidney

Although percutaneous intervention is generally the procedure of choice for lesions and disease involving the proximal and main renal artery, surgical revascularization is generally recommended for those cases with complex disease involving branching/segmental arteries or when aortic surgery is also indicated.

13. **What are the predictors of response to renal artery revascularization in patients with renal artery stenosis?**

It is difficult to predict which patients will benefit from renal artery stenting. A number of clinical characteristics have been shown to be associated with poor outcome or an increased risk of complications with percutaneous renal artery intervention, including decreased baseline renal size (less than 8 cm), advanced baseline renal dysfunction (serum creatinine more than 3.0–4.0 mg/dl), concomitant medical renal disease (e.g., diabetes mellitus, amyloidosis), long-standing hypertension, high baseline renal resistive index identified on duplex ultrasonography, and extensive burden of aortic atherosclerosis. Some studies have suggested that patients with bilateral disease may have a greater improvement in blood pressure and stabilization of renal function but may also have a higher risk of potential complications with percutaneous intervention. A recent report suggested that patients with a higher baseline level of brain natriuretic peptide (BNP) had a more favorable blood pressure response to percutaneous intervention. The most important predictor of a favorable response to revascularization in ischemic nephropathy appears to be the rate of decline (slope of regression lines based on the reciprocal of the serum creatinine measurement) in renal function before the intervention. Patients with a rapid deterioration in renal function experience greater benefit in renal function with stent revascularization than those with stable chronic renal impairment.

14. **What is the *average* rate of expansion of aortic aneurysms?**

Although the rate of expansion can vary significantly from patient to patient, in general, the larger the aneurysm, the greater the average yearly expansion of the aneurysm. For aortic aneurysms less than 4 cm in diameter at the time of their discovery, the average annual rate of expansion is 1 to 4 mm; for aneurysms 4 to 6 cm it is 4 to 5 mm; and for larger aneurysms it is as much as 7 to 8 mm.

15. **In general, when should patients with an infrarenal or juxtarenal abdominal aortic aneurysm undergo repair?**

Current recommendations are that patients with an infrarenal or juxtarenal abdominal aortic aneurysm (AAA) should undergo repair when the aneurysm measures 5.5 cm or greater (although it is also a class IIa recommendation that it *can be beneficial* to repair aneurysms 5.0 to 5.4 cm in diameter). Patients with infrarenal or juxtarenal AAA measuring 4.0 to 5.4 cm in diameter should be monitored by ultrasound or computed tomography (CT) scans every 6 to 12 months. In those with AAA smaller than 4.0 cm, ultrasound examination every 2 to 3 years is felt to be reasonable.

16. **What is the significance of detecting a carotid artery bruit?**
    Approximately 35% of patients with a carotid bruit will have a greater than 50% stenosis of the artery. Those with an audible bruit should be referred for duplex scanning. Unfortunately, auscultation is not a perfect *screening test* for carotid artery disease because only 50% of patients with significant hemodynamic carotid stenosis have an audible bruit that is noted during physical examination.

17. **What are the primary indications for carotid endarterectomy (CEA)?**
    In very general terms, indications for CEA are as follows:
    - Symptomatic stenosis 50% to 99% diameter if the risk of perioperative stroke or death is less than 6%
    - Asymptomatic stenosis greater than 60% to 80% diameter if the expected perioperative stroke rate is less than 3%

    These recommendations are actually more nuanced, and the reader is encouraged to review the AHA/ASA guidelines for prevention of stroke in patients with ischemic stroke or transient ischemic attack (see Bibliography). Formal indications for carotid artery stenting are in evolution. This subject is addressed in an expert consensus document on carotid stenting (see Bibliography).

18. **What causes lower limb arterial disease in young patients?**
    Atherosclerosis tends to primarily affect older persons; however, it can manifest in younger patients who have familial hyperlipidemic syndromes, Buerger's disease (thromboangitis obliterans), or hypercoagulable disorders. Popliteal entrapment syndrome is an anatomic abnormality in which the popliteal artery gets compressed either by an abnormal muscle band or because it has taken an abnormal (medial) course behind the knee and is compressed by a normal gastrocnemius muscle. Popliteal adventitial cystic disease is also in the differential diagnosis of claudication in young patients; it produces a popliteal stenosis that gives a classic "scimitar sign" on angiography. Exercise-induced compartment syndrome may produce similar symptoms of leg pain with exercise that is relieved by rest.

19. **What is fibromuscular dysplasia (FMD)?**
    Fibromuscular dysplasia (FMD), formerly called fibromuscular fibroplasia, is a group of nonatherosclerotic, noninflammatory arterial diseases that can affect almost any artery but most commonly involves the renal arteries. Histologic classification discriminates three main subtypes, intimal, medial and perimedial, which may be found in a single patient. Angiographic classification includes the following:
    - Multifocal type, with multiple stenoses and the "string-of-beads" appearance that is classic for medial fibroplasias
    - Focal type, which is more suggestive of intimal fibroplasia

20. **What is Buerger's disease?**
    Buerger's disease, more appropriately called thromboangiitis obliterans, is a disease of small and medium-sized arteries, as well as veins and nerves. Buerger's disease is a nonatherosclerotic disease instead caused by inflammatory processes and thrombosis. Clinically, it presents most commonly with ischemia of the digits and hand, arm, feet, or calf claudication. Ischemic ulcers may also occur. It occurs almost exclusively in tobacco users, and the only true "treatment" is smoking cessation.

21. **What is Takayasu's arteritis?**
    Takayasu's arteritis is a vasculitis of unknown cause, primarily affecting the aorta and its primary branches. It is more common in Asian populations and predominantly affects women. Over time it can lead to narrowing or occlusion of the aorta and its branches, such as the subclavian artery. Clinically, patients most commonly manifest upper arm claudication but may also develop neurologic symptoms as a result of vertebrobasilar ischemia.

22. **What is May-Thurner syndrome?**

Iliocaval compression, or May-Thurner syndrome (MTS), was initially described as the development of spurs in the left iliac vein as a consequence of compression from the contralateral right common iliac artery against the lumbar vertebra. The pathogenesis of MTS is not completely understood, but it is theorized that it may be a combination of both mechanical compression and arterial pulsations by the right iliac artery that leads to the development of intimal hypertrophy within the wall of the left common iliac vein. This can lead to potential endothelial changes and thrombus formation. Patients with MTS tend to be young women in the second to fourth decade of life who develop the syndrome after periods of prolonged immobilization or pregnancy. Patients may have a history of several days or more of persistent, unexplained pain and swelling of the left thigh and calf. Duplex ultrasound characteristically may reveal left common iliac vein thrombosis. Management of symptomatic MTS in association with deep vein thrombosis may involve catheter-directed thrombolysis, anticoagulation, and potentially iliocaval stenting.

BIBLIOGRAPHY, SUGGESTED READINGS, AND WEBSITES

1. Inter-Society Consensus (TASC) II Guidelines: http://www.tasc-2-pad.org

2. Mohler ER: Clinical Features, Diagnosis, and Natural History of Lower Extremity Peripheral Arterial Disease: http://www.utdol.com

3. Bates ER, Babb JD, Casey DE, et al: ACCF/SCAI/SVMB/SIR/ASITN 2007 clinical expert consensus document on carotid stenting: a report of the American College of Cardiology Foundation Task Force on Clinical Expert Consensus Documents, *J Am Coll Cardiol* 49:126-70, 2007.

4. Hiatt WR: Medical treatment of peripheral arterial disease and claudication. *N Engl J Med* 344(21):1608-1621.

5. Hirsch AT, Haskal ZJ, Hertzer NR, et al: ACC/AHA guidelines for the management of patients with peripheral arterial disease, *J Am Coll Cardiol* 47(6):1239-312, 2006.

6. Norgren L, Hiatt WR, Dormandy JA, et al: Inter-Society Consensus for the Management of Peripheral Arterial Disease (TASC II), *Eur J Vasc Endovasc Surg* 33(Suppl 1):S1-75, 2007.

7. Sacco RL, Adams R, Albers G, et al: AHA/ASA guidelines for prevention of stroke in patients with ischemic stroke or transient ischemic attack, *Stroke* 37:577-617, 2006.

8. White CJ, Jaff MR, Haskal ZJ, et al: Indications for renal arteriography at the time of coronary arteriography: a science advisory from the American Heart Association Committee on Diagnostic and Interventional Cardiac Catheterization, Council on Clinical Cardiology, and the Councils on Cardiovascular Radiology and Intervention and on Kidney in Cardiovascular Disease, *Circulation* 114(17):1892-1895, 2006.

CHAPTER 60

DEEP VEIN THROMBOSIS

Geno J. Merli, MD, FACP

1. **What three primary factors promote thromboembolic disease?**
   Development of venous thrombosis is promoted by the following:
   - Venous blood stasis
   - Injury to the intimal layer of the venous vasculature
   - Abnormalities in coagulation or fibrinolysis

2. **List the risk factors for thromboembolic disease.**
   The numerous risk factors for thromboemoblic disease include surgery, trauma, immobility, cancer, pregnancy, prolonged immobilizaiton, estrogen-containing oral contraceptives or hormone replacement therapy, and acute medical illnesses. A more complete listing of these risk factors is given in Box 60-1.

BOX 60-1. RISK FACTORS FOR DEEP VENOUS THROMBOEMBOLISM

- Surgery
- Trauma (major or lower extremity)
- Immobility, lower extremity paresis
- Cancer (active or occult)
- Cancer therapy (hormonal, chemotherapy, angiogenesis inhibitors, or radiotherapy)
- Venous compression (tumor, hemotoma, arterial abnormality)
- Previous history of thromboembolic disease
- Obesity
- Pregnancy and postpartum period
- Prolonged immobilization
- Lower-extremity or pelvic trauma or surgery
- Surgery with greater than 30 minutes of general anesthesia
- Congestive heart failure
- Nephrotic syndrome
- Estrogen-containing oral contraceptives or horomone replacement therapy
- Selective estrogen receptor modulators
- Inflammatory bowel disease
- Acute medial illness
- Myeloproliferative disorders
- Paroxysmal nocturnal hemoglobinuria
- Central venous catheter
- Inherited or acquired thrombophilia
- Increasing age

---

3. **What is the natural history of venous thrombosis?**

Resolution of fresh thrombi occurs by endogenous fibrinolysis and organization. *Fibrinolysis* results in actual clot dissolution. *Organization* reestablishes venous blood flow by reendothelializing and incorporating into the venous wall residual clot not dissolved by fibrinolysis. In the absence of new clot formation, the two processes generally are complete in 7 to 10 days.

4. **Can patients with deep venous thrombosis be accurately diagnosed clinically?**

No. The clinical diagnosis of deep venous thrombosis is neither sensitive nor specific. Less than 50% of patients with confirmed deep venous thrombosis present with the classic symptoms and signs of deep vein thrombosis (DVT), which include pain, tenderness, redness, swelling, and Homan's sign (calf pain with dorsiflexion of the foot). This sole use of clinical findings is artificial because clinicians couple the medical and surgical history, concomitant medical problems, medications, and risk factors to decide on further testing to confirm DVT.

5. **Where is the most common origin for thrombi that result in pulmonary emboli?**

Thromboses in the deep veins of the lower extremities account for 90% to 95% of pulmonary emboli. Less common sites of origin include thromboses in the right ventricle; in upper extremity, prostatic, uterine, and renal veins; and, rarely, in superficial veins.

6. **How is the diagnosis of lower extremity deep vein thrombosis confirmed?**

Diagnostic evaluation of suspected DVT includes a clear correlation among clinical probability, test selection, and test interpretation.

Contrast venography is no longer appropriate as the initial diagnostic test in patients exhibiting DVT symptoms, although it remains the gold standard for confirmatory diagnosis of DVT. It is nearly 100% sensitive and specific and provides the ability to investigate the distal and proximal venous system for thrombosis. Venography is still warranted when noninvasive testing is inconclusive or impossible to perform but its use is no longer widespread because of the need for administration of a contrast medium and the increased availability of noninvasive diagnostic strategies.

Ultrasound is safe and noninvasive and has a higher specificity than impedance plethysmography for the evaluation of suspected DVT. With color flow doppler and compression ultrasound, DVT is diagnosed based on the inability to compress the common femoral and popliteal veins. In patients with lower extremity symptoms, the sensitivity is 95% and specificity 96%. The diagnostic accuracy of ultrasound in asymptomatic patients, those with recurrent DVT, or those with isolated calf DVT is less reliable. The sensitivity of ultrasound improves with serial testing in untreated patients. Repeat testing at 5 to 7 days will identify another 2% of patients with clots not apparent on the first ultrasound. Serial testing can be particularly valuable in ruling out proximal extension of a possible calf DVT. Because the accuracy of ultrasound in diagnosing calf DVT is acknowledged to be lower (81% for DVT below the knee versus 99% for proximal DVT), follow-up ultrasounds at 5 to 7 days are reasonable because most calf DVTs that extend proximally will do so within days of the initial presentation.

7. **When should prophylaxis of deep venous thromboses be considered?**

Two factors must be weighed in deciding to initiate prophylaxis of deep venous thrombosis: the degree of risk for thrombosis (see Questions 1 and 2) and the risk of prophylaxis. The risk factors for deep venous thrombosis are cumulative. The primary risk of pharmacologic prophylaxis is hemorrhage, which is generally uncommon if no coagulation defects or lesions with bleeding potential exist.

8. **What prophylactic measures are available?**

Approaches to prophylaxis of deep venous thrombosis (DVT) include antithrombotic drugs and pneumatic-compressive devices. Heparin, low-molecular-weight heparin (LMWH), and warfarin are effective in preventing DVT. Subcutaneous heparin has been the mainstay of DVT prophylaxis with efficacy in multiple surgical and medical scenerios. The LMWHs have been shown to be as effective or superior to unfractionated heparin in different clinical circumstances. Warfarin dosing to maintain an international normalized ratio [INR] between 2 to 3 also has a low risk of bleeding and is effective in patients with total hip arthroplasty, total knee arthroplasty, and hip fracture surgery. However, it takes several days to develop a full antithrombotic effect. Antiplatelet drugs such as aspirin are not effective in DVT prophylaxis.

Intermittent pneumatic-compressive devices effect prophylaxis by maintaining venous flow in the lower extremities and are especially efficacious in patients who cannot receive anticoagulant medications. Modalities available include compressive devices applied to the feet alone, covering the calves, or extending to the thighs. No version has been shown to provide superior prophylaxis.

9. **What is the approach to DVT prophylaxis in the hospitalized, medically ill patient?**
The acutely ill medical patient admitted to the hospital with congestive heart failure or severe respiratory disease, or who is confined to bed and has one or more additional risk factors, including active cancer, previous venous thromboembolism, sepsis, acute neurologic disease, or inflammatory bowel disease, should receive DVT prophylaxis with the following agents:
  - Unfractionated heparin: 5000 units subcutaneously (SC) every 8 hours
  - LMWH:
    ○ Dalteparin: 5000 IU SC every 24 hours
    ○ Enoxaparin: 40 mg SC every 24 hours
    ○ Fondaparinux: 2.5 mg SC every 24 hours

10. **Should patients undergoing surgery receive DVT prophylaxis based on specific recommendations for each respective procedure?**
Yes. The following surgical procedures have defined recommendations for preventing DVT in the postoperative period:

General Surgery

The following regimens are for gynecologic patients undergoing major surgical procedures for benign or malignant disease and associated DVT risk factors:
  - Unfractionated heparin: 5000 units SC every 8 hours
  - LMWH: enoxaparin 40 mg SC every 24 hours, dalteparin 5000 IU SC every 24 hours or external pneumatic compression sleeves plus one of the above regimens

Urologic Surgery

The following regimens are for urology patients undergoing major open procedures for benign or malignant disease and with associated DVT risk factors:
  - Unfractionated heparin: 5000 units SC every 8 hours
  - LMWH: enoxaparin 40 mg SC every 24 hours, dalteparin 5000 IU SC every 24 hours or external pneumatic compression sleeves plus one of the above regimens
  - For patients who are actively bleeding, the use of mechanical devices is recommended until one of the above pharmacologic regimens can be initiated.

Orthopedic Surgery

The following regimens are for patients undergoing orthopedic surgery:
  - Total hip replacement:
    ○ LMWH: enoxaparin 30 mg SC every 12 hours, dalteparin 5000 IU SC every 24 hours, fondaparinux 2.5 mg SC every 24 hours
    ○ Warfarin 5 mg the evening of surgery; then adjust dose to achieve an INR of 2 to 3
  - Total knee replacement:
    ○ LMWH: enoxaparin 30 mg SC every 12 hours, dalteparin 5000 IU SC every 24 hours, fondaparinux 2.5 mg SC every 24 hours.
    ○ Warfarin: 5 mg the evening of surgery; then adjust dose to achieve an INR of 2 to 3

Hip Fracture

The following regimens are for patients undergoing surgery for hip fracture:
- LMWH: enoxaparin 30 mg SC every 12 hours, dalteparin 5000 IU SC every 24 hours, fondaparinux 2.5 mg SC every 24 hours
- Unfractionated heparin: 5000 units SC every 8 hours
- Warfarin: 5 mg the evening of surgery; then adjust dose to achieve an INR of 2 to 3

Neurosurgery

The following regimens are for patients undergoing neurosurgery:
- External pneumatic compression sleeves are the prophylaxis of choice.
- Combination therapy with either unfractionated heparin (5000 units SC every 8 or 12 hours) or LMWH (enoxaparin 40 mg SC every 24 hours) can be used.

Coronary Artery Bypass Surgery

The following regimens are for patients undergoing coronary artery bypass surgery:
- LMWH (preferred over unfractionated heparin): enoxaparin 40 mg SC every 24 hours or dalteparin 5000 IU SC every 24 hours
- Unfractionated heparin: 5000 units, SC every 8 hours

11. **Are there specific surgical groups that require extended DVT prophylaxis following hositpal discharge?**
    - For a patient undergoing total hip replacement, total knee replacement, and hip fractures, extended DVT prophylaxis is recommended for up to 35 days after surgery. LMWH: enoxaparin 40 mg SC every 24 hours, dalteparin 5000 IU SC every 24 hours, fondaparinux 2.5 mg SC every 24 hours; or warfarin with dose adjusted to achieve a target INR of 2 to 3.
    - For selected high-risk gynecology patients undergoing cancer surgery or who have previously had DVT, it is recommended that DVT prophylaxis be continued with LMWH: enoxaparin 40 mg SC every 24 hours or dalteparin 5000 IU SC every 24 hours for 28 days.
    - For selected high-risk general surgery patients undergoing major cancer surgery or who have previously had venous thromboembolism, it is recommended that DVT prophylaxis be continued with LMWH: enoxaparin 40 mg SC every 24 hours or dalteparin 5000 IU SC every 24 hours for 28 days.

12. **What treatment regimens are available for the treatment of DVT?**

Unfractionated Heparin

- Administer intravenous bolus (80 units/kg or 5000 units) followed by continuous infusion of 18 unit/kg/hr or 1300 units/hr.
- The activated partial thromboplastin time (aPTT) is checked every 6 hours to adjust the infusion to achieve the therapeutic aPTT of the hospital laboratory.
- Subcutaneous unfractionated heparin at 333 units/kg is the initial dose, followed in 12 hours by 250 units/kg SC every 12 hours. Monitoring of the APTT is not necessary.

LMWH

- Enoxaparin 1 mg/kg, subcutaneous, every 12 hours or 1.5 mg/kg, subcutaneous every 24 hours
- Dalteparin 200 IU/kg SC every 24 hours
- Tinzaparin 175 IU/kg SC every 24 hours
- Fondaparinux dosed by weight range: less than 50 kg, 5 mg SC; 50 to 100 kg, 7.5 mg SC every 24 hours; more than 100 kg, 10 mg SC every 24 hours

13. **Which LMWHs are renally excreted?**
All the LMWHs are renally excreted. Enoxaparin is the only LMWH that has a recommended dose for creatinine clearance less than 30 ml/min (1 mg/kg SC every 24 hours). All other LMWHs listed here should not be used with creatinine clearance less than 30 ml/min.

14. **When should warfarin be started with the regimens of treatment of DVT listed earlier?**
In patients with acute DVT, warfarin should be administered on the first day of unfractionated heparin or LMWH at a dose of 5 or 10 mg.

15. **When should these therapeutic regimens for treating DVT be discontinued and warfarin remain as the sole therapy?**
These therapies must be used for at least 5 days and until the INR is more than 2 for 24 hours.

16. **What is the target INR for treating patients with DVT?**
The target INR for the treatment of DVT to prevent recurrent disease is 2 to 3.

17. **How long should patients with acute DVT be treated with warfarin?**
For patients with DVT secondary to a transient risk factor, 3 months of warfarin is appropriate. Idiopathic proximal DVT in patients without risk factors for bleeding should receive long-term warfarin therapy with a target INR of 2 to 3. Patients with DVT and cancer should receive LMWH for 3 to 6 months as the initial approach to management and long-term treatment with either warfarin or LMWH until the cancer is resolved.

18. **When can patients with acute DVT ambulate?**
Patients can ambulate with acute DVT and should not be placed on bed rest unless the lower extremity is painful and cannot bear weight.

19. **Can patients with acute DVT be treated as outpatients?**
Yes. The LMWH regimens listed here can be used to treat patients in the outpatient setting. The same principles of management should be followed using these agents as with inpatient treatment.

20. **When should catheter-directed thrombolysis be used to treat acute DVT?**
In selected patients with extensive acute proximal ilofemoral DVT in which symptoms have been present for less than 14 days, who are functionally active, and who have a low bleeding risk, the use of pharmacomechanical thrombolysis is recommended if the appropriate expertise and resources are available.

21. **Are inferior vena caval filters indicated for the initial treatment of acute DVT?**
No. Vena caval filters are indicated when the patient cannot receive anticoagulation for the treatment of acute DVT. In certain cases (temporary contraindication to anticoagulant therapy) the use of retrievable vena caval filters have been placed, with the plan to remove them in a defined time (2 to 4 weeks), after which anticoagulation therapy can be reinstituted.

22. **When are gradient elastic stockings recommended as part of the treatment of acute DVT?**
For patients with symptomatic DVT the use of gradient elastic stockings with an ankle pressure of 30 to 40 mm Hg is recommended. The pressure may not be tolerated because of the degree of lower extremity edema. Elastic bandages may be used because they can be adjusted to control swelling and the pain that is associated with increased external pressure. The elastic bandages can be used initially, but as the swelling recedes, gradient elastic stockings at 20 to 30 mm Hg or 30 to 40 mm Hg may be applied.

CONTROVERSIES

23. **When is a low-intensity INR indicated for the treatment of DVT?**
For patients with idiopathic (unprovoked) DVT who have a strong preference for less frequent INR testing to monitor their therapy, it is recommended that after the first 3 months of therapy low-intensity therapy at an INR of 1.5 to 1.9 with less frequent INR monitoring be employed instead of stopping warfarin anticoagulation.

24. **Are there other INR ranges for DVT prophylaxis in orthopedic surgery?**
The American Academy of Orthopedic Surgery recommends an INR of between 1.5 and 2.0. This is not supported in randomized prospective trials in this surgical population. The INR range of 2 to 3 is recommend range.

25. **Should compression ultrasound be used as routine screening in the total joint replacement surgery patient at the time of discharge?**
Asymptomatic joint replacement surgery patients should not have compression ultrasound on discharge as screening test for DVT because the ultrasound is not as sensitive and specific in asymptomatic patients. Appropriate DVT prophylaxis should be the approach to management.

BIBLIOGRAPHY, SUGGESTED READINGS, AND WEBSITES

1. Grant BJB: Diagnosis of Suspected Deep Vein Thrombosis of the Lower Extremity: http://www.utdol.com

2. Landaw SA, Bauer KA: Approach to the Diagnosis and Therapy of Deep Vein Thrombosis: http://www.utdol.com

3. Turpie AGG: Deep Venous Thrombosis: http://www.merck.com/mmpe

4. British Thoracic Society Standards of Care Committee: Pulmonary Embolism Guideline Development Group: British Thoracic Society guidelines for the management of suspected acute pulmonary embolism, *Thorax* 58(6):470-483, 2003.

5. Decousus H, Leizorovicz A, Parent F, et al: A clinical trial of vena caval filters in the prevention of pulmonary embolism in patients with proximal deep-vein thrombosis, *N Engl J Med* 338:409-415, 1998.

6. Geerts WH, Bergqvist D, Pineo G, et al: Prevention of venous thromboembolism, *Chest* 133:381S-453S, 2008.

7. Kearon C, Ginsberg JS, Julian JA, et al: Comparison of fixed-dose weight adjusted unfractionated heparin and low-molecular weight heparin for acute treatment of venous thromboembolism, *JAMA* 296: 935-942, 2006.

8. Kearon C, Kahn SR, Agnelli G, et al: Antithrombotic therapy for venous thromboembolic disease: the Eighth ACCP Conference on Antithrombotic and Thrombolytic Therapy, *Chest* 133:54-545, 2008.

9. Koopman MM, Prandoni P, Piovella F, et al: Treatment of venous thrombosis with intravenous unfractionated heparin administered in the hospital as compared with subcutaneous low-molecular-weight heparin administered at home, *N Engl J Med* 334:682-687, 1996.

10. Levine M, Gent M, Hirsh J, et al: A comparison of low-molecular-weight heparin administered primarily at home with unfractionated heparin administered in the hospital for proximal deep vein thrombosis, *N Engl J Med* 334:677-681, 1996.

11. Merli GJ: Pathophysiology of venous thrombosis and the diagnosis of deep vein thrombosis-pulmonary embolism in the elderly, *Cardiol Clin* 26:203-219, 2008.

12. Merli G, Spiro T, Olsson CG, et al: Subcutaneous enoxaprain once or twice daily compared with intravenous unfractionated heparin for treatment of venous thromboembolic disease, *Ann Intern Med* 134: 191-202, 2001.

13. Prevention and treatment of venous thromboembolism. International consensus statement (guidelines according to scientific evidence), *Int Angiol* 25(2):101-161, 2006.

14. Snow V, Qaseem A, Barry P, et al: Management of venous thromboembolism: a clinical practice guideline from the American College of Physicians and the American Academy of Family Physicians, *Ann Intern Med* 146(3):204-210, 2007.

15. The Matisse Investigators. Subcutaneous fondaparinux versus intravenous unfractionated heparin in the initial treatment of pulmonary embolism, *N Engl J Med* 349:1695-1702, 2003.

16. Wells PS, Anderson DR, Rodger MA, et al: A randomized trial comparing 2 low-molecular-weight heparins for the outpatient treatment of deep vein thrombosis and pulmonary embolism, *Arch Intern Med* 165:733-738, 2005.

CHAPTER 61

PULMONARY EMBOLISM

Gregg J. Stashenko, MD and Victor F. Tapson, MD

1. **Who first described pulmonary embolism?**
   Pulmonary embolism (PE) was probably first reported in the early 1800s clinically, but Rudolf Virchow elucidated the mechanism by describing the connection between venous thrombosis and PE in the late 1800s. He also coined the term *embolism*.

2. **What is Virchow's triad?**
   These are the three broad categories of risk factors which contribute to thrombosis:
   - Endothelial injury
   - Stasis or turbulence of blood flow
   - Blood hypercoagulability

3. **What percentage of patients with acute PE have clinical evidence of deep vein thrombosis in the legs?**
   In the Prospective Investigation of Pulmonary Embolism Diagnosis (PIOPED) study of 251 patients with angiographically documented PE, only 11% had evidence of deep vein thrombosis (DVT) by physical examination. However, the majority of patients with proven PE do have residual DVT present. More than 90% of PEs originate in the deep veins of the legs.

4. **What percentage of patients with DVT will develop PE?**
   Approximately 50%.

5. **What is the usual cause of death in PE?**
   It is well established that right ventricular (RV) failure is the cause of cardiovascular collapse in acute massive PE. Registry data have also suggested that patients with RV dysfunction on echocardiogram are at increased risk of all-cause mortality at 3 months.

6. **What are the major risk factors for venous thromboembolism?**
   Risk factors are crucial in raising suspicion for acute venous thromboembolism (VTE), although the disease may be idiopathic. Previous thromboembolism, immobility, cancer, advanced age, major surgery, trauma, and acute medical illness impart significant risk. A list of risk factors is shown in Box 61-1.

7. **How should a patient with suspected DVT be initially evaluated?**
   The symptoms and signs of DVT are nonspecific, and although clinical prediction rules can be useful, there should be a low threshold to proceed to compression ultrasonography. D-dimer testing may be useful; the diagnosis of DVT can be excluded without the need for ultrasound by using a combination of low or moderate clinical probability estimate and a negative D-dimer result. If the patients falls into the high clinical pretest probability or has a positive D-dimer test, further evaluation with ultrasound is advised. The enzyme-linked immunosorbent assay (ELISA)–based D-dimer tests have superior sensitivity (96% to 98%). DVT is also discussed in Chapter 60 on DVT.

BOX 61-1. RISK FACTORS FOR VENOUS THROMBOEMBOLISM*

Hereditary
Antithrombin deficiency
Protein C deficiency
Protein S deficiency
Factor V Leiden
Activated protein C resistance without factor V Leiden
Prothrombin gene mutation
Dysfibrinogenemia
Plasminogen deficiency

Acquired
Reduced mobility
Advanced age
Cancer/myeloproliferative disorders
Acute medical illness
Nephrotic syndrome
Major surgery
Trauma
Spinal cord injury
Pregnancy/postpartum period
Polycythemia vera
Antiphospholipid antibody syndrome
Oral contraceptives
Hormonal replacement therapy
Heparins
Chemotherapy
Obesity
Central venous catheters
Immobilizer/cast

Probable/Not Certain
Low tissue factor pathway inhibitor levels
Elevated levels of the following:
   1. Homocysteine
   2. Factors VIII, IX, XI
   3. Fibrinogen
   4. Thrombin-activatable fibrinolysis inhibitor
   5. Lipoprotein (a)

*The hereditary versus acquired nature of some disorders listed remains unclear and may involve both.

8. **What are the symptoms and signs of acute PE?**
   The symptoms and signs of PE are generally nonspecific but may include the following:
   - Dyspnea (either sudden in onset or evolving over days)
   - Chest pain (often pleuritic)
   - Hemoptysis (the two latter findings generally occur with pulmonary infarction)
   - Palpitations
   - Light-headedness
   - Syncope
   - Tachypnea
   - Tachycardia
   - Pleural rub
   - Fever
   - Wheezing
   - Rales

   If PE is associated with pulmonary hypertension, then elevated neck veins, a loud P2, RV heave, or a right-sided gallop may be noted.

9. **What are three clinical syndromes seen with acute PE?**
   - **Massive pulmonary embolism/acute cor pulmonale:** Not all patients with acute cor pulmonale will go on to develop hypotension (which defines massive PE), but such a presentation should raise concern.
   - **Pulmonary infarction/pulmonary hemorrhage:** Because of dual blood supply and free anastomosis between the pulmonary capillaries, emboli usually don't cause infarction in a healthy lung. Pulmonary infarction is uncommon when emboli obstruct central arteries but much more common when distal arteries are occluded. Obstruction of distal arteries can result in pulmonary hemorrhage as a result of an influx of bronchial arterial blood at systemic pressure. Hemorrhage causes symptoms and radiographic changes usually attributed to pulmonary infarction. However, hemorrhage appears to usually resolve without infarction in patients without heart disease; that is, of the patients who do develop hemorrhage, cardiac patients appear more likely to progress to pulmonary infarction.
   - **Acute unexplained dyspnea:** A diagnosis of PE should be considered in patients with dyspnea of unclear cause and may merit consideration even when there is another potential explanation.

10. **What is the Wells score for suspected acute PE?**
    First described in 1998, the Wells score is a clinical prediction score based on simple, noninvasive clinical parameters. It has evolved over the years and been validated and is useful in determining pretest probability for suspected acute PE. The score is calculated based on specific variables (Table 61-1). If the patient has a score of 4 or less and the D-dimer test is negative, no further testing appears to be necessary. A score greater than 4 requires further evaluation, and computed tomographic angiography (CTA) is usually performed. High clinical suspicion, however, should always take precedence, even if the Wells score is low.

11. **What are the most common findings on electrocardiography (ECG) in acute PE?**
    Sinus tachycardia is commonly present in acute PE. The "classic" S1Q3T3 pattern (Fig. 61-1) is seen in a minority of patients. Other ECG findings include the following:
    - Arrhythmias (premature atrial and ventricular beats)
    - First-degree atrioventricular block
    - Supraventricular tachycardia
    - RV strain (right axis deviation)
    - RV hypertrophy
    - Right bundle branch block
    - Depression, elevation, or inversion of ST segments and T waves

    ST-T changes, when present, are often most marked in the right precordial leads. Although the ECG may be suggestive of PE, it is by no means diagnostic.

TABLE 61-1. THE WELLS SCORE IN SUSPECTED ACUTE PULMONARY EMBOLISM

	Number of Points:
DVT symptoms and signs	3.0
PE as likely as or more likely than alternative diagnosis	3.0
Heart rate > 100 beats/min	1.5
Immobilization or surgery in previous 4 weeks	1.5
Previous DVT or PE	1.5
Hemoptysis	1.0
Cancer	1.0

Total score: < 2.0—low pretest probability; 2.0–6.0—moderate pretest probability; and > 6.0—high pretest probability. (More recently, a dichotomized score has been validated, with ≤ 4 points suggesting a low likelihood for acute PE, and > 4 points, a high likelihood).

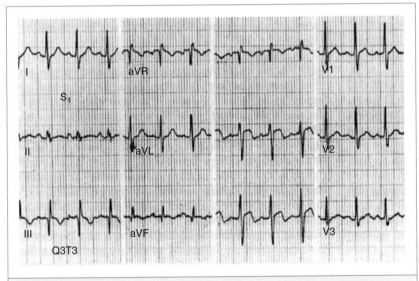

Figure 61-1. ECG in acute pulmonary embolism. The classic S1Q3T3 pattern seen here is not, however, diagnostic.

12. **What are the common chest radiographic findings in patients with acute PE?**
The chest radiograph is commonly abnormal in acute PE, although a significant minority of patients have a normal film. When it is abnormal, however, the findings are nonspecific and include an elevated hemidiaphragm, focal or multifocal infiltrates, pleural effusion, platelike atelectasis, enlarged pulmonary arteries, focal oligemia (Westermark's sign), and RV enlargement.

Hampton and Castleman described in detail the radiographic findings in PE and pulmonary infarction in 1940, having assembled 370 cases of PE and infarction. In pulmonary infarction, they suggested that the cardiac margin of the opacity of a pulmonary infarction on chest radiograph is rounded or *hump*-shaped (i.e., Hampton's hump).

13. **What are typical arterial blood gas (ABG) findings in patients with PE?**
Low Pa_{O2}, low P_{CO2}, high alveolar-arterial difference. Alhough nonspecific, one of these findings is likely to be present in up to 97% of cases. A normal ABG does not absolutely exclude PE.

14. **When should the ventilation-perfusion (V/Q) scan be performed?**
The V/Q scan is most useful when the chest radiograph is normal and there is no cardiopulmonary disease. In this setting, it has the highest likelihood of being either normal or high probability. Diagnostic tests (and especially those for PE) must be interpreted in light of the clinician's pretest probability. It is crucial to remember that commonly the V/Q scan is low or intermediate probability, even when PE is present.

15. **Does a negative CTA indicate that PE is not present with *certainty*?**
No, but a good quality CTA is quite sensitive. We learned from the Prospective Investigation of Pulmonary Embolism Diagnosis (PIOPED) II, published in 2006, that clinical probability is extremely important when considering CTA results. Approximately 60% (9/15) of patients who had high clinical pretest probability but a negative CTA were ultimately diagnosed with PE. Similarly, 16/38 (42%) of patients with a low clinical pretest probability and a positive CTA did not have PE. A recent study of more than 3000 patients with suspected acute PE by the Christopher Investigators suggested that if CTA is negative, outcome at 3 months is excellent without therapy. Nonetheless, it is prudent to consider additional imaging when a negative CTA is accompanied by high clinical suspicion; furthermore, imaging quality is not uniformly high in all clinical settings. A large PE, documented by CTA, is shown in Figure 61-2. A diagnostic algorithm, which can be used as a guide, is offered in Figure 61-3.

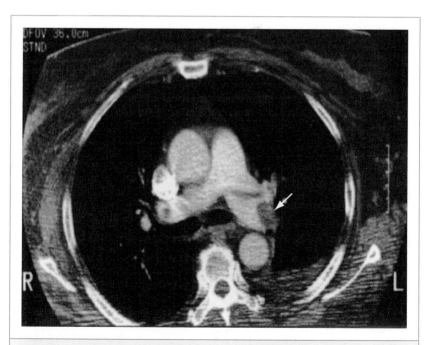

Figure 61-2. A large left pulmonary artery PE is shown by CTA *(white arrow)*.

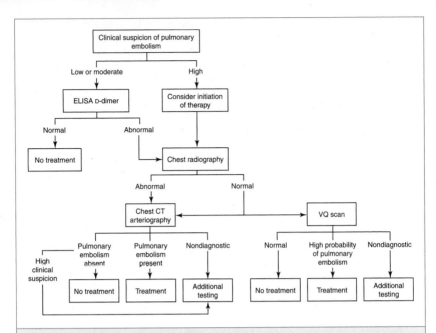

Figure 61-3. A diagnostic strategy for suspected acute pulmonary embolism. The use of a clinical prediction score and D-dimer may reduce the need for imaging. If suspicion for acute PE is high and the bleeding risk deemed low, initiation of anticoagulant therapy should be considered. The V/Q scan is most useful when the chest radiograph is normal or minimally abnormal. When significant renal insufficiency is present, CTA is contraindicated and the V/Q scan may be useful. (Modified from Tapson VF: *N Engl J Med* 358: 1037-1052, 2008.)

16. **What is the most appropriate initial therapy for patients with documented acute PE?**
    In patients with acute PE, a therapeutic level of anticoagulation should ideally be achieved within 24 hours because this appears to reduce the risk of recurrence. The 8th American College of Chest Physicians Evidence-Based Clinical Practice (ACCP) Guidelines from 2008 recommend initiation of treatment while awaiting diagnostic tests if clinical suspicion is deemed high. Initial treatment with low-molecular-weight heparin (LMWH), unfractionated heparin (UFH), or fondaparinux for at least 5 days and until the international normalized ratio (INR) is 2.0 or more for at least 24 hours is recommended. Initiation of a vitamin K antagonist (VKA), such as warfarin, should also be started on the first treatment day rather than delaying it. The ACCP also recommends that in patients with acute nonmassive PE, initial treatment with LMWH rather than intravenous UFH be used, if feasible, based on advantages of LMWH, including subcutaneous rather than intravenous delivery, much less need for monitoring, and a lower rate of heparin-induced thrombocytopenia. Anticoagulation clearly improves survival in patients with acute symptomatic PE. Finally, bed rest is not recommended for DVT unless there is substantial pain or swelling. The data for PE are not sufficient to support this recommendation.

17. **What is the primary indication for thrombolytic therapy?**
    Proven pulmonary embolism with cardiogenic shock. The 8th ACCP Guidelines also note that in selected high-risk patients without hypotension who are judged to have a low risk of bleeding, thrombolytic therapy can be considered. This received a grade 2B recommendation—that is,

> ## BOX 61-2. SYNOPSIS OF KEY THROMBOLYTIC THERAPY RECOMMENDATIONS FROM THE 8TH ACCP CONSENSUS
>
> Recommendations are graded based on the evidence. Grade 1 indicates that benefit appears to outweigh potential harm, whereas with Grade 2, this is less certain. The lettered recommendation indicates the quality of the methodology used to make the recommendation. *A* recommendations are the strongest and are based on data from very good quality prospective, randomized trials.
>
> 1. All PE patients should undergo rapid risk stratification (grade 1C).
> 2. When there is hemodynamic compromise, thrombolytic therapy is recommended, unless there are major contraindications owing to bleeding risk (grade 1B).
> 3. Thrombolysis in patients with hemodynamic compromise should not be delayed because irreversible cardiogenic shock may ensue.
> 4. In selected high-risk patients without hypotension deemed to have a low risk of bleeding, administration of thrombolytic therapy is suggested (grade 2B).
> 5. The decision to use thrombolytic therapy depends on the clinician's assessment of PE severity, prognosis, and risk of bleeding.
> 6. In patients with acute PE, when a thrombolytic agent is used, peripheral vein administration rather than direct pulmonary artery infusion is recommended (grade 1B).
> 7. In patients with acute PE, with administration of thrombolytic therapy, we recommend use of regimens with short infusion times (e.g., a 2-hour infusion) over those with prolonged infusion times (e.g., a 24-hour infusion) (grade 1B).
>
> Modified from Kearon C, Kahn SR, Agnelli G, et al: Antithrombotic therapy for venous thromboembolic disease, *Chest* 133:454S-545S, 2008.

there were no large prospective, randomized trials to support the suggestion. An example would be in submassive PE (RV dilation and hypokinesis without hypotension). The decision to use thrombolytic therapy depends on the clinician's assessment of PE severity, prognosis, and risk of bleeding. It is often also considered in patients with hypotension but without shock. Box 61-2 summarizes the recommendations with regard to thrombolytic therapy in PE.

18. **What are some complications and contraindications of thrombolytic therapy?**
    Intracranial hemorrhage is the most devastating complication of thrombolytic therapy and has been reported in less than 1% of patients in clinical trials but in about 3% of patients in data from the International Cooperative Pulmonary Embolism Registry (ICOPER). Other complications include retroperitoneal and gastrointestinal bleeding and bleeding from surgical wounds or from sites of recent invasive procedures.
    Contraindications to thrombolytic therapy include the following:
    - Intracranial, ocular, or spinal surgery
    - Injury
    - Disease
    - Recent major surgery or other invasive procedures
    - Active or recent major bleeding
    - Pregnancy
    - Clinically obvious risk of bleeding

    In a patient with life-threatening PE, thrombolytic therapy should not be withheld solely because of pregnancy.

19. **Has thrombolytic therapy been shown to improve mortality from PE?**
No. Thrombolytic therapy has never been shown to improve mortality from PE in a clinical trial. It has been shown to improve hemodynamics and lung scans with a suggestion that younger (less than 50 years old) patients, new emboli (less than 48 hours old), and larger emboli respond better (Urokinase Pulmonary Embolism Trial [UPET]). Thrombolytic therapy, when given to patients with evidence of RV strain on echocardiography but without hypotension, was shown to decrease the need for treatment escalation, but a mortality endpoint was not reached.

20. **What are the indications for inferior vena caval (IVC) filter placement?**
The primary indications for placement of an IVC filter include contraindications to anticoagulation, major bleeding complications during anticoagulation, and recurrent PE despite adequate anticoagulation. Alhough there are no firm trial data, some experts suggest filter placement in the case of massive PE when it is believed that additional emboli might be lethal, particularly if thrombolytic therapy is contraindicated.

21. **What are some complications of IVC filter placement?**
IVC filters increase the subsequent incidence of DVT (in about 20% of patients) and have not been shown to increase overall survival. The other complications of IVC filters include procedural-related complications of insertion site thrombosis (8%), pneumothorax, air embolism, or hematoma, and late complications of IVC thrombosis (2% to 10%), postthrombotic syndrome, IVC penetration, and filter migration. Certain models of IVC filters are retrievable, typically within several months of insertion, and may alleviate some of the late complications of IVC filter placement.

22. **Can PE be treated as an outpatient?**
Although the use of LMWH as outpatient therapy for DVT is well established, the data for outpatient treatment of acute PE are less robust. Recent data suggest that early discharge in acute PE can be done safely if patients are carefully screened. Initial admission, even if brief, is clearly the most common practice today.

23. **How well are recommended VTE prevention measures used?**
Recent data suggest that worldwide, prophylaxis is underused. A recent study including more than 67,000 patients, the Epidemiologic International Day for the Evaluation of Patients at Risk for Venous Thromboembolism in the Acute Hospital Care Setting (ENDORSE) registry, indicated that in many countries less than half of patients deemed appropriate candidates for prophylaxis measures actually received them.

BIBLIOGRAPHY, SUGGESTED READINGS, AND WEBSITES

1. Christopher Study Investigators: Effectiveness of managing suspected pulmonary embolism using an algorithm combining clinical probability, D-dimer testing, and computed tomography, *JAMA* 295:172-179, 2006.
2. Chunilal SD, Eikelboom JW, Attia J, et al: Does this patient have pulmonary embolism? *JAMA* 290(21): 2849-2858, 2003.
3. Cohen AT, Tapson VF, Bergmann JF, et al: Venous thromboembolism risk and prophylaxis in the acute hospital care setting (ENDORSE study): a multinational cross-sectional study, *Lancet* 371:387-394, 2008.
4. Dalen JE: Pulmonary embolism: what have we learned since Virchow? Natural history, pathophysiology, and diagnosis, *Chest* 122:1440-1456, 2002.
5. Dalen JE: Pulmonary embolism: what have we learned since Virchow? Treatment and prevention, *Chest* 122:1801-1817, 2002.
6. Dong B, Jirong Y, Liu G, et al: Thrombolytic therapy for pulmonary embolism, *Cochrane Database System Rev* 2:CD004437 DOI: 10.1002/14651858.CD004437.pub2, 2006.

7. Goldhaber SZ, Visani L, De Rosa M: Acute pulmonary embolism: clinical outcomes in the International Cooperative Pulmonary Embolism Registry (ICOPER), *Lancet* 353:1386-1389, 1999.

8. Hanna CL, Michael B, Streiff MB: The role of vena caval filters in the management of venous thromboembolism, *Blood Rev* 19:179-202, 2005.

9. Kearon C, Kahn SR, Agnelli G, et al: Antithrombotic therapy for venous thromboembolic disease, *Chest* 133:454S-545, 2008.

10. Konstantinides S, Geibel A, Heusel G, et al: Heparin plus alteplase compared with heparin alone in patients with submassive pulmonary embolism, *N Eng J Med* 347:1143-1150, 2002.

11. PIOPED Investigators: Value of the ventilation/perfusion scan in acute pulmonary embolism, *JAMA* 263(20):2753-2759, 1990.

12. Simonneau G, Sors H, Charbonnier B, et al: A comparison of low-molecular weight heparin with unfractionated heparin for acute pulmonary embolism, *N Engl J Med* 337:663-669, 1997.

13. Stein PD, Alnas M, Skaf E, et al: Outcomes and complications of retrievable inferior vena cava filters, *Am J Cardiol* 94:1090, 2004.

14. Stein PD, Fowler SE, Goodman LR, et al: Multidetector computed tomography for acute pulmonary embolism (PIOPED II), *N Engl J Med* 354(22):2317-2327, 2006.

15. Tapson VF: Acute pulmonary embolism, *N Engl J Med* 358:1037-1052, 2008.

16. Wells PS, Owen C, Doucette S, et al: Does this patient have deep vein thrombosis, *JAMA* 295:199-207, 2006.

CHAPTER 62

PULMONARY HYPERTENSION

Zeenat Safdar, MD, FCCP

1. **What is the hemodynamic criteria used in the National Institute of Health Registry to define pulmonary arterial hypertension?**
   The widely accepted hemodynamic definition of pulmonary arterial hypertension (PAH) is a mean pulmonary arterial pressure of more than 25 mm Hg at rest or more than 30 mm Hg during exercise with a pulmonary capillary or left atrial pressure of less than 15 mm Hg. A right-sided heart catheterization is the diagnostic gold standard for PAH because the echocardiogram may be inacccurate in determining pulmonary artery pressures and, in addition, does not measure the mean pulmonary artery pressure.

2. **What are the usual physical findings in patients with pulmonary hypertension?**
   The most common findings on physical examination might include the following:
   - Loud pulmonic valve closure sound (P_2)
   - Right ventricular heave
   - Murmur of tricuspid regurgitation (a systolic murmur over the left lower sternal border)
   - Murmur of pulmonic insufficiency (a diastolic murmur over the left sternal border)
   - Jugular venous distension (indicating elevated central venous pressures)
   - Peripheral edema
   - Hepatomegaly
   - Hepatojugular reflux
   - Ascites
   - Cyanosis
   - Clubbing

3. **How is PAH classified?**
   At the third World Conference on Pulmonary Hypertension held in Venice (2003), the term *primary pulmonary hypertension* was replaced by the current classification outlined in Box 62-1. Pulmonary hypertension is classified as pulmonary arterial hypertension, pulmonary venous hypertension, pulmonary hypertesnion associated with hypoxemia, pulmonary hypertension caused by chronic thrombotic or embolic disease, and miscellaneous causes.

4. **Is pulmonary hypertension a genetic disease?**
   About 6% of patients with PAH have familial PAH. The mutations in the gene encoding the bone morphogenetic receptor 2 (BMPR2) were found in approximately 50% of families with familial pulmonary hypertension and in 25% of patients thought to have sporadic PAH. Because penetrance of this gene is low, most patients with this mutation never acquire the disease. A subject with a mutation has a 10% to 20% lifetime risk of acquiring FPAH.

5. **What should the clinical evaluation for possible pulmonary hypertension include?**
   Evaluation should begin with a thorough history and physical examination. Possible causes of secondary pulmonary hypertension should be addressed in the history. In addition, travel to or residence in an area endemic for schistosomiasis should be considered. All patients should receive a basic initial screening evaluation, consisting of collagen vascular disease serologic testing, human immunodeficiency virus (HIV) testing, chest radiograph, pulmonary function testing, ventilation-perfusion (V/Q) scan, electrocardiogram, and echocardiogram.

BOX 62-1. THIRD WORLD CONFERENCE ON PULMONARY HYPERTENSION CLASSIFICATION OF PULMONARY HYPERTENSION

Group I: Pulmonary Arterial Hypertension
- Idiopathic
- Familial
- PAH associated with:
  - Collagen vascular disease
  - Congenital heart disease
  - HIV
  - Drugs or toxins
  - Portal hypertension
- Associated with significant venous or capillary involvement
  - Pulmonary venoocclusive disease
  - Pulmonary capillary hemangiomatosis

Group II: Pulmonary Venous Hypertension
- Left-sided atrial or ventricular disease
- Left-sided valvular disease

Group III: Pulmonary Hypertension Associated with Hypoxemia
- Chronic obstructive pulmonary disease
- Interstitial lung disease
- Sleep-disordered breathing
- Alveolar hypoventilation disorders
- Chronic exposure to high altitude

Group IV: PH Associated with Chronic Thrombotic or Embolic Disease
- Thromboembolic obstruction of proximal pulmonary artery
- Thromboembolic obstruction of distal pulmonary artery
- Pulmonary embolism (tumor, parasites, foreign material)

Group V: Miscellaneous
- Sarcoidosis
- Histocytois X
- Lymphangiomatosis
- Compression of pulmonary vessels (tumors, adenopathy, fibrosing mediastinitis)

Patients with no clues to the cause on history or physical examination are given a broad, *detailed* evaluation; patients with a suspected secondary cause receive a *focused* evaluation to verify that cause, followed by the broad evaluation if necessary. In addition to these tests, arterial blood gases and pulmonary angiography may be indicated. If undertaken, pulmonary angiography should be performed by someone experienced in working with pulmonary hypertension patients. An assessment of the patient's functional status should also be performed (Table 62-1).

6. **Which connective tissue diseases most commonly cause pulmonary hypertension?**
   - Scleroderma (especially CREST syndrome)
   - Mixed connective tissue disease
   - Systemic lupus erythematosus
   - Rheumatoid arthritis
   - Dermatomyositis

TABLE 62-1. WORLD HEALTH ORGANIZATION CLASSIFICATION OF FUNCTIONAL STATUS OF PATIENTS WITH PULMONARY HYPERTENSION

Class	Description
I	Patients with pulmonary hypertension but without resulting limitation of physical activity. Ordinary physical activity does not cause undue dyspnea or fatigue, chest pain, or near syncope.
II	Patients with pulmonary hypertension resulting in slight limitation of physical activity. They are comfortable at rest. Ordinary physical activity causes undue dyspnea or fatigue, chest pain, or near syncope.
III	Patients with pulmonary hypertension resulting in marked limitation of physical activity. They are comfortable at rest. Less than ordinary activity causes undue dyspnea or fatigue, chest pain, or near syncope.
IV	Patients with pulmonary hypertension with inability to carry out any physical activity without symptoms. These patients manifest signs of right-sided heart failure. Dyspnea or fatigue may even be present at rest. Discomfort is increased by any physical activity.

Modified from Rubin LJ: Diagnosis and management of pulmonary arterial hypertension: ACCP evidence-based clinical practice guidelines, *Chest* 126:7S-10S, 2004.

7. **What population group is most commonly affected by PAH?**
   Although PAH occurs in both sexes and virtually all age groups, it has a tendency to affect young females. The female-to-male predominance is 1.7:1.

8. **Is surgical therapy now an option for patients with pulmonary hypertension secondary to chronic recurrent thromboembolism?**
   A patient with PAH and a V/Q scan suggestive of chronic thromboembolic disease is required to have a pulmonary angiogram for accurate diagnosis and assessment of operability. It is now possible to surgically remove organized thrombus from the proximal pulmonary arteries of patients with pulmonary hypertension secondary to chronic recurrent thromboembolism. Operative mortality is low in most experienced centers, and lifelong anticoagulation and inferior vena cava (IVC) filter placement are essential for such patients.

9. **What is the average survival for a PAH patient?**
   According to the National Institutes of Health Registry on Primary Pulmonary Hypertension, in the past the median survival was approximately 2.8 years from the date of diagnosis. With the availability of new therapeutic modalites, survival has significantly increased. According to the French registry, the 1-year survival is now 88%.

10. **What is now considered *conventional therapy* for patients with PAH?**
    Conventional therapy includes the following:
    - *Supplemental oxygen* as needed to maintain an oxygen saturation of at least 91%
    - *Diuretics* if the patient has clinically significant edema or ascites
    - *Vasodilators* (oral or intravenous)
    - *Anticoagulation* in the absence of contraindications, and occasionally *digitalis*

11. **Are calcium channel blockers used in the treatment of PAH?**
Calcium channnel blockers (CCBs) are only used in patients with a documented vasodilator response to a short vasodilator at the time of a right-sided heart catheterization. This comprises 6% of all PAH patients; of these patients, 50% turn out to be sustained responders. CCBs should not be empirically used in patients without the demonstration of vasoreactivity. If patients have a favorable response to acutely administered vasodilators, this predicts a response to calcium channel blockers. The 1-, 3-, and 5-year survival in patients on a CCB was 94%, 94%, and 94%, respectively, as compared with 68%, 47%, and 38% in those classified as nonresponders. If patients do not have a favorable response to acutely administered vasodilators, consider treatment with a endothelin receptor antagonist, phostodiesterase-5 inhibitor, or prostacyclin therapy.

12. **What is considered a favorable response to acutely administered vasodilators?**
A decrease in mean pulmonary artery pressure of at least 10 mm Hg to less than 40 mm Hg with an increased or unchanged cardiac output is considered a favorable response. Such patients should be considered candidates for a trial of an oral calcium channel antagonist. The agents used to determine vasoreactivity include intravenous adenosie and epoprostenol and inhaled nitric oxide.

13. **What are the approved therapies to treat PAH?**
Currently six Food and Drug Administration (FDA)-approved therapies target the three identified pathways involved in the pathogenesis of PAH.
- Endothelin-1, a potent vasoconstrictor, acts as a mitogen, induces fibrosis, and leads to the proliferation of vascular smooth muscle cells. The effects of endothelin-1 are mediated through the activation of ET_A and ET_B receptors. Differential activation of ET_A and ET_B receptors leads to the vasoconstricting and vascular proliferative actions of endothelin-1. Tracleer is a dual endothelin receptor blocker, whereas ambrisentan is an ET_A blocker.
- Prostacyclin is the main product of arachidonic acid in the vascular endothelium. By the production of cyclic adenosine monophosphate, prostacyclin promotes pulmonary vascular relaxation and inhibits growth of smooth muscle cells. In addition, prostacyclin is a powerful inhibitor of platelet aggregation. There are three prostacylins approved for therapy; these include intravenous epoprostenol and treprostinil and inhaled ventavis.
- Phosphodiestersae-5 (PDE-5) inhibitor blocks the breakdown of cyclic guanosine monophosphate in the vascular endothelium, resulting in increased activity of endogenous nitric oxide that enhances pulmonary vasodilation. Sildenafil is the PDE-5 inhibitor approved to treat PAH.

14. **What are the complications associated with prostaniod therapy?**
Because these are nonselective vasodilators, a common complication is systemic hypotension. Other commonly reported side effects include flushing, headaches, nausea, diarrhea, leg pain, and jaw pain. Because intravenous administration of prostacyclin requires central venous access, line infections and catheter-associated thrombosis are common. Careful care of the catheter and anticoagulation help lessen these risks, but there is still the chance for significant and life-threatening complications.

15. **How do I treat the pulmonary hypertension associated with CREST syndrome?**
Pulmonary hypertension is a common, life-threatening complication of the CREST syndrome and accounts for the significant morbidity and mortality of this disease. Orally available vasodilators have been notoriously ineffective in the treatment of pulmonary hypertension associated with CREST. Recently, infused prostacyclin has been shown to improve the functional status of patients with CREST and pulmonary hypertension and is being used in this clinical setting more commonly.

16. **Is transplantation possible in patients with PAH?**

    Yes. Lung transplantation is an additional option, especially for patients who do not respond to aggressive treatment. A combined heart and lung transplant is no longer believed to be required because the right ventricle appears to recover function after lung transplantation. Occasionally, heart-lung transplantation is required in patients with uncorrectable congenital heart defects with Eisenmenger's syndrome.

BIBLIOGRAPHY, SUGGESTED READINGS, AND WEBSITES

1. Oudiz RJ: Pulmonary Hypertension, Primary: http://www.emedicine.com

2. Rubin LJ, Hopkins W: Overview of Pulmonary Hypertension: http://www.utdol.com

3. Sharma S: Pulmonary Hypertension, Secondary: http://www.emedicine.com

4. Merck: http://www.merck.com

5. Barst RJ, Rubin LJ, Long WA, et al: A comparison of continuous intravenous epoprostenol (prostacyclin) with conventional therapy for primary pulmonary hypertension. The Primary Pulmonary Hypertension Study Group, *N Engl J Med* 334:296-302, 1996.

6. Channick RN, Simonneau G, Sitbon O, et al: Effects of the dual endothelin-receptor antagonist bosentan in patients with pulmonary hypertension: a randomised placebo controlled study, *Lancet* 358:1119-1123, 2001.

7. Galie N, Ghofrani HA, Torbicki A, et al: Sildenafil citrate therapy for pulmonary arterial hypertension, *N Engl J Med* 353:2148-2157, 2005.

8. Humbert M, Sitbon O, Chaouat A, et al: Pulmonary Arterial Hypertension in France: results from a National Registry, *Am J Respir Crit Care Med* 173(9):1023-1030, 2006.

9. McGoon M, Gutterman D, Steen V, et al: Screening, early detection, and diagnosis of pulmonary arterial hypertension: ACCP evidence-based clinical practice guidelines, *Chest* 126:14S-34S, 2004.

10. McLaughlin VV, Shillington A, Rich S: Survival in primary pulmonary hypertension: the impact of epoprostenol therapy, *Circulation* 106:1477-1482, 2002.

11. Miyamoto S, Nagaya N, Satoh T, et al: Clinical correlates and prognostic significance of six-minute walk test in patients with primary pulmonary hypertension. Comparison with cardiopulmonary exercise testing, *Am J Respir Crit Care Med* 161:487-492, 2000.

12. Olschewski H, Simonneau G, Galie N, et al: Inhaled iloprost for severe pulmonary hypertension, *N Engl J Med* 347:322-329, 2002.

13. Galiè N, Olschewski H, Oudiz RJ, et al. Ambrisentan for the treatment of pulmonary arterial hypertension: results of the ambrisentan in pulmonary arterial hypertension, randomized, double-blind, placebo-controlled, multicenter, efficacy (ARIES) study 1 and 2. *Circulation* 117(23):2966-2968, 2008.

14. Simonneau G, Barst RJ, Galie N, et al: Continuous subcutaneous infusion of treprostinil, a prostacyclin analogue, in patients with pulmonary arterial hypertension: a double-blind, randomized, placebo-controlled trial, *Am J Respir Crit Care Med* 165:800-804, 2002.

15. Sitbon O, Humbert M, Jais X, et al: Long-term response to calcium channel blockers in idiopathic pulmonary arterial hypertension, *Circulation* 111:3105-3111, 2005.

16. Sitbon O, Humbert M, Nunes H, et al: Long-term intravenous epoprostenol infusion in primary pulmonary hypertension: prognostic factors and survival, *J Am Coll Cardiol* 40:780-788, 2002.

CHAPTER 63

PREOPERATIVE CARDIAC EVALUATION

Lee A. Fleisher, MD, FACC

1. **What is the natural history of perioperative cardiac morbidity?**

   Perioperative cardiac morbidity occurs most commonly during the first 3 postoperative days and includes perioperative myocardial infarction, unstable angina, cardiac death, and nonfatal cardiac arrests. Traditionally, the peak incidence of perioperative myocardial infarction was during postoperative day 3, although recent studies have suggested it occurs earlier and may arise most commonly in the first 24 hours. Additionally, the mortality from a perioperative cardiac myocardial infarction has decreased from previous rates of 30% to 50% to approximately 20%.

2. **What is the cause of perioperative cardiac morbidity?**

   The cause of perioperative myocardial infarction is multifactorial. The postoperative period is associated with a stress response, which includes the release of catecholamines and cortisol, resulting in tachycardia and hypertension. The tachycardia can lead to supply/demand mismatches distal to a critical stenoses, causing myocardial ischemia, and, if prolonged, can lead to perioperative myocardial infarction. Tissue injury, tachycardia, and the hypercoagulable state also leads to plaque rupture and acute thrombosis, potentially resulting in a perioperative myocardial infarction. Therefore, many perioperative events will not be predicted by identifying critical stenoses or preoperative imaging. Additionally, perioperative strategies to reduce cardiac morbidity require a multimodal approach of both reducing supply/demand mismatches and reducing the risk of acute thrombosis.

3. **What are the strongest predictors of perioperative cardiac events?**

   For some specific patients, surgery represents a very high risk of cardiac complications and either therapy should be initiated preoperatively or the benefits of surgery must significantly outweigh the risks if the decision is to proceed to surgery. According to the 2007 American College of Cardiology/American Heart Association (ACC/AHA) Guidelines on Perioperative Cardiovascular Evaluation, these are considered active cardiac conditions. These conditions fall into the general categories of unstable coronary symptoms syndromes, active heart failure, severe valvular disease, and severe arrhythmias. Specific conditions within these general categories are shown in Table 63-1.

4. **What is the revised cardiac risk index (RCRI) and how is it used clinically?**

   Cardiac risk indices for perioperative risk stratification have been used in clinical practice for more than 30 years. These indices do not inform clinicians on how to modify perioperative care specifically, but they do provide a baseline assessment of risk and the value of different intervention strategies. Calculation of an index is not a substitute for providing detailed information of the underlying heart disease, its stability, and ventricular function. The RCRI was developed by studying more than 5000 patients and identifying six risk factors, including the following:

TABLE 63-1. ACTIVE CARDIAC CONDITIONS FOR WHICH THE PATIENT SHOULD UNDERGO EVALUATION AND TREATMENT BEFORE NONCARDIAC SURGERY (CLASS I, LEVEL OF EVIDENCE: B)

Condition	Examples
Unstable coronary syndromes	Unstable or severe angina* (CCS class III or IV)[†]
	Recent MI[‡]
Decompensated HF (NYHA functional class IV; worsening or new-onset HF)	
Significant arrhythmias	High-grade atrioventricular block
	Mobitz II atrioventricular block
	Third-degree atrioventricular heart block
	Symptomatic ventricular arrhythmias
	Supraventricular arrhythmias (including atrial fibrillation) with uncontrolled ventricular rate (HR > 100 beats/min at rest)
	Symptomatic bradycardia
	Newly recognized ventricular tachycardia
Severe valvular disease	Severe aortic stenosis (mean pressure gradient > 40 mm Hg, aortic valve area < 1.0 cm^2, or symptomatic)
	Symptomatic mitral stenosis (progressive dyspnea on exertion, exertional presyncope, or HF)

CCS, Canadian Cardiovascular Society; *HF*, heart failure; *HR*, heart rate; *MI*, myocardial infarction; *NYHA*, New York Heart Association

*According to Campeau.

[†]May include *stable* angina in patients who are unusually sedentary.

[‡]The American College of Cardiology National Database Library defines recent MI as more than 7 days but less than or equal to 1 month (within 30 days).

Modified from Fleisher LA, Beckman JA, Brown KA, et al: ACC/AHA guidelines on perioperative cardiovascular evaluation and care for noncardiac surgery: executive summary, *J Am Coll Cardiol* 50:1716, 2007.

- High-risk surgery
- Ischemic heart disease
- History of congestive heart failure
- History of cerebrovascular disease
- Preoperative treatment with insulin
- Preoperative serum creatinine greater than 2 mg/dl

In determining the need and value of preoperative testing and interventions, the ACC/AHA guidelines incorporate the number of risk factors from the RCRI, other than high-risk surgery, which is incorporated elsewhere. Importantly, diabetes (without regard to type of treatment) is considered one of the risk factors, as opposed to insulin treatment.

5. **What is the importance of exercise capacity?**
Numerous studies have demonstrated the importance of exercise capacity on overall perioperative morbidity and mortality. Based on several of these studies, patients can be dichotomized into poor functional capacity (less than four METS) versus moderate or excellent exercise capacity. Patients with moderate to excellent exercise capacity rarely need further testing before noncardiac surgery.

6. **What is the influence of the surgical procedure on the decision to perform further diagnostic testing?**

In all patients, regardless of the type of surgery, determination of the presence of active cardiac conditions is first and foremost because proceeding to surgery should only be done after assessing and potentially treating these conditions. Low-risk surgeries, those associated with a perioperative cardiac morbidity and mortality less than 1%, rarely, if ever, require a change in management based on the results of a diagnostic test. The most common such procedures are those performed on an outpatient basis. Multiple studies have focused on patients undergoing vascular surgery, particularly open aortic and lower extremity revascularization. Therefore, these patients are treated uniquely in the assessment of the need to perform diagnostic testing based on the extensive evidence and the high perioperative cardiac morbidity and mortality, often in the range of 5% or greater. In the intermediate group of procedures, a gradation of risk is based on the specific surgical procedures and the institution-specific risk is critical to determine if further diagnostic testing would add value.

7. **How do the ACC/AHA guidelines suggest an approach to preoperative evaluation?**

The algorithm from the 2007 guidelines can be found in Fig. 63-1. Importantly, any decision to perform diagnostic testing based the algorithm must incorporate the value of the information

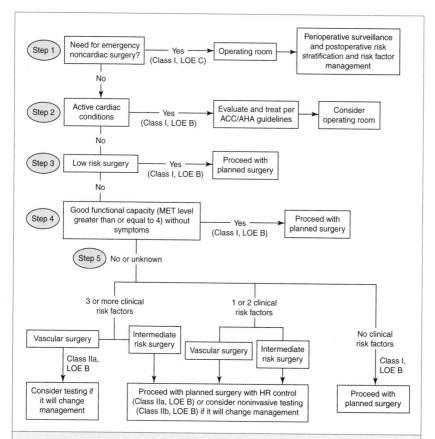

Figure 63-1. Algorithm from the ACC/AHA for the decision for preoperative cardiovascular testing in patients undergoing noncardiac surgery. *HR,* Heart rate; *LOE,* level of evidence; *MET,* metabolic equivalent. (Modified from Fleisher LA, Beckman JA, Brown KA, et al: ACC/AHA guidelines on perioperative cardiovascular evaluation and care for noncardiac surgery: executive summary, *J Am Coll Cardiol* 50:1718, 2007.)

to change perioperative management. Changes in management can include the decision to undergo coronary revascularization but may also include decisions by the patient to forego surgery and decisions by the surgeon to change the type of procedure. The algorithm incorporates the urgency of surgery, clinical risk factors, and functional status. For patients with risk factors undergoing vascular surgery, the studies demonstrate no difference between coronary revascularization before noncardiac surgery or proceeding directly to the noncardiac surgery, incorporating heart rate control perioperatively. The class of recommendation and strength of evidence, based on the ACC/AHA criteria, is shown on the algorithm.

8. **What is the value of coronary revascularization before noncardiac surgery?**
Traditionally it was thought that patients who'd had prior coronary artery bypass grafting (CABG) had a lower rate of perioperative cardiac morbidity compared with patients with a similar extent of coronary disease who had not undergone revascularization. Several randomized trials have questioned the value of acute revascularization before noncardiac surgery. In the Coronary Artery Revascularization Prophylaxis (CARP) trial, 500 patients were randomized to coronary revascularization versus medical therapy and followed for up to 6 years. Importantly, patients with left main disease, severe triple vessel disease with depressed ejection fraction, and severe comorbidities were excluded. Two thirds of the patients who underwent coronary revascularization had percutaneous coronary interventions (PCI). There was no difference in either perioperative or long-term morbidity and mortality. In the DECREASE-II trial, patients with one to two clinical risk factors were randomized to preoperative testing and revascularization or proceeded directly to vascular surgery with tight heart rate control; again no difference in outcome was detected. In the DECREASE–V pilot study of 101 patients with extensive coronary artery disease, no difference in perioperative cardiac morbidity and mortality was seen between the revascularization and medical therapy arms of the trial, although the study was underpowered. Therefore, currently high-quality evidence suggests that coronary revascularization before major noncardiac surgery is of limited or no benefit in stable patients; however, this cannot be generalized to patients with left main or severe triple vessel disease because of the absence of data in these groups.

9. **What is the concern regarding surgery in patients with a previous PCI?**
Patients who have previously undergone PCI have not been shown to have a significant difference in perioperative outcomes compared with case-matched controls. Importantly, the risk of thrombosis after PCI is high and the hypercoagulable perioperative state increases the probability of this occurring. Multiple cohort studies and case reports now show acute thrombosis and perioperative myocardial infarction at the site of coronary stents. In patients with bare metal stents, this most commonly occurs in patients who have undergone noncardiac surgery within 30 days. In patients with drug-eluting stents, the higher rate of acute thrombosis can be seen for at least 1 year, and there are case reports of it occurring after this period. Therefore, the current recommendation is to delay elective surgery for at least 14 days after percutaneous transluminal coronary angioplasty, 30 days after placement of bare metal stents, and 1 year after placement of drug-eluting stents.

10. **How should antiplatelet agents be managed in the perioperative period?**
The recent consensus statement from the ACC/AHA in 2007, as well as the perioperative guidelines, advocate continuing aspirin in all patients who have had a previous PCI. In patients currently taking a thienopyridine, particularly those within 30 days of placement of a bare metal stent or 1 year for drug-eluting stents, the agent should either be continued or discontinued for a short period, if possible, and restarted as quickly as possible in the postoperative period.

11. **How should beta-blockers be managed in the perioperative period?**
Based on cohort studies and consensus opinion, patients who are receiving chronic beta-blocker therapy at the time of surgery should be continued on these agents to avoid the risk of

beta-blocker withdrawal, which is associated with tachycardia and an increased incidence of perioperative myocardial infarction. Currently, controversy exists regarding the acute administration of beta-blocker therapy for those patients at high risk but not taking these agents. The DECREASE trial and subsequent cohort studies from the Erasmus group have demonstrated improved outcome in patients with known coronary heart disease by administration of bisoprolol at lower doses, started a minimum of 7 days prior to surgery and titrated to a heart rate less than 80 beats/min. In the Perioperative Ischemic Evaluation (POISE) study, 8351 patients were randomized to high-dose metoprolol succinate, a long-acting agent, compared with placebo. Although nonfatal perioperative myocardial infarctions were reduced, the incidence of death and stroke was significantly increased and was associated with higher rates of hypotension. Therefore, initiating high-dose beta-blocker therapy in the perioperative period without titration to heart rate and blood pressure could lead to greater harm than benefit and should not be considered. However, heart rate control remains a critical approach to reducing perioperative cardiac morbidity and initial treatment should focus on treating the cause of tachycardia, including pain management, after which careful titration of beta-blockers is appropriate. In patients who should be taking beta-blockers independent of noncardiac surgery for underlying coronary artery disease, initiation and titration a week or more in advance has been advocated by some authors, but the safest protocol is controversial.

12. **How should statins be managed in the perioperative period?**
    Traditionally there was concern that continuation of statins in the perioperative period could lead to an increased incidence of rhabdamyolysis, and most clinicians stopped these agents before surgery. Evidence has accumulated that statin therapy is protective and that withdrawal is harmful. In the 2007 perioperative guidelines, the committee advocated continuing statins in all patients currently taking these agents.

BIBLIOGRAPHY, SUGGESTED READINGS, AND WEBSITES

1. Devereaux PJ, Yang H, Yusuf S, et al: Effects of extended-release metoprolol succinate in patients undergoing non-cardiac surgery (POISE trial): a randomised controlled trial, *Lancet* 371:1839-1847, 2008.

2. Fleisher LA, Beckman JA, Brown KA, et al: ACC/AHA 2007 guidelines on perioperative cardiovascular evaluation and care for noncardiac surgery: a report of the American College of Cardiology/American Heart Association Task Force on Practice Guidelines (Writing Committee to Revise the 2002 Guidelines on Perioperative Cardiovascular Evaluation for Noncardiac Surgery), *J Am Coll Cardiol* 50:e159-e241, 2007.

3. McFalls EO, Ward HB, Moritz TE, et al: Coronary-artery revascularization before elective major vascular surgery, *N Engl J Med* 351:2795-2804, 2004.

4. Poldermans D, Boersma E, Bax JJ, et al: The effect of bisoprolol on perioperative mortality and myocardial infarction in high-risk patients undergoing vascular surgery. Dutch Echocardiographic Cardiac Risk Evaluation Applying Stress Echocardiography Study Group, *N Engl J Med* 341:1789-1794, 1999.

5. Poldermans D, Bax JJ, Schouten O, et al: Should major vascular surgery be delayed because of preoperative cardiac testing in intermediate-risk patients receiving beta-blocker therapy with tight heart rate control? *J Am Coll Cardiol* 48:964-969, 2006.

CHAPTER 64

COCAINE AND THE HEART

James McCord, MD

1. **How common is cocaine use in the United States?**

   Cocaine is the second most commonly used illicit drug in the United States, with marijuana being used more often. In 2005 there were approximately 450,000 cocaine-related emergency department visits in the United States. The most frequent age group for these visits was 35 to 44 years of age, accounting for 37% of all cocaine-related emergency department encounters.

2. **What are the typical symptoms after cocaine ingestion?**

   Cardiopulmonary complaints are the most commonly reported symptoms in patients after cocaine use, occurring in 56% of cases. Chest pain is the most common symptom and is typically described as a pressure sensation. Other common symptoms include dyspnea, anxiety, palpitations, dizziness, and nausea.

3. **How often does acute myocardial infarction (AMI) occur after cocaine ingestion?**

   The overall incidence of AMI in patients presenting to the emergency department after cocaine ingestion is 0.7% to 6%. The variance in the incidence of AMI in studies likely relates to difference in patient populations and AMI diagnostic criteria.

4. **What else should be considered in the differential diagnosis after cocaine use?**

   Because patients who present to the emergency department after cocaine use are commonly hypertensive and tachycardic, aortic dissection needs to be considered. Information concerning cocaine-induced aortic dissection is limited, but one study of 38 consecutive cases of aortic dissection demonstrated a surprisingly high number 17 (37%) were associated with cocaine use. However, among 921 patients in the International Registry of Aortic Dissection (IRAD), only 0.5% of aortic dissection cases were associated with cocaine use. In addition, an acute pulmonary syndrome, *crack lung* has been described after inhalation of freebase cocaine, which involves hypoxemia, hemoptysis, respiratory failure, and diffuse pulmonary infiltrates.

   Chronic cocaine use can lead to decreased left ventricular systolic function and congestive heart failure. This may relate to accelerated atherosclerosis or myocarditis, both of which are associated with cocaine use.

5. **How does cocaine ingestion lead to AMI?**

   Cocaine can lead to AMI in a multifactorial fashion, including the following: (1) increasing myocardial oxygen demand by increasing heart rate, blood pressure, and contractility; (2) decreasing oxygen supply as a result of vasoconstriction; (3) inducing a prothrombotic state by altering the balance between procoagulant and anticoagulant factors; and (4) accelerating the atherosclerotic process.

6. **Should younger patients with chest pain have a cocaine screening test?**

   The American Heart Association (AHA) recommends that establishing cocaine use should depend primarily on self-reporting. Because the use of cocaine influences treatment strategies, patients being evaluated for possible acute coronary syndrome (ACS) should be queried about cocaine use; this applies especially to younger patients. Enough information has not been published to definitively recommend screening of particular subgroups that are being evaluated for possible ACS.

7. **Are there any specific electrocardiogram findings in patients that use cocaine?**

Abnormal electrocardiograms (ECGs) have been reported in 56% to 84% of patients with cocaine-associated chest pain. Many of these patients are younger and have the normal variant findings of early repolarization. In a study of 101 patients who had used cocaine, 42% manifested ST-segment elevation on the ECG, but all of them ultimately had AMI excluded by serial cardiac marker testing. Left ventricular hypertrophy can also be noted on the ECG. In a series of 238 individuals who used cocaine, 33% had a normal ECG, 23% had nonspecific findings, 13% had left ventricular hypertrophy, 6% had left ventricular hypertrophy and early repolarization, and 13% had early repolarization alone.

8. **Should all patients with cocaine-associated chest pain be admitted to the hospital?**

No. Most patients with cocaine-associated chest pain do not have ACS and can safely and efficiently be evaluated in a chest pain observation unit. In a prospective study of 344 patients with cocaine-associated chest pain, 42 (12%) high-risk patients with ST-segment elevation or depression, elevated cardiac markers, or hemodynamic instability were directly admitted. The other 302 were evaluated in an observation unit over 9 to 12 hours with telemetry monitoring, serial troponin I measurement, and selective stress testing. Among the patients in the observation unit there were no cardiac deaths, 4 (2%) nonfatal AMIs, and 158 (52%) patients who underwent stress testing.

9. **Should all patients with cocaine-associated chest pain have a stress test?**

No. The AHA states that stress testing is optional in patients who have an uneventful 9 to 12 hours of observation. Patients should be counseled about cessation of cocaine use. Patients can be followed as an outpatient and stress testing considered later depending on cardiac risk factors and ongoing symptoms.

10. **How should patients with ST-elevation myocardial infarction (STEMI) be treated in the setting of cocaine use?**

Rapid reperfusion by percutaneous coronary intervention (PCI) in a high-volume center by experienced operators is preferred over fibrinolytic therapy in the setting of STEMI, and this is even more desirable in the setting after cocaine use. Many young patients will have early repolarization, and only a small percentage of these patients will actually be experiencing an AMI. Furthermore, hypertensive patients after cocaine use are at higher risk for significant bleeding complications. There have been case reports of intracranial hemorrhage after fibrinolytic therapy in the setting of STEMI. Fibrinolytic therapy should only be considered for patients who are clearly having a STEMI who cannot receive timely PCI. Patients with non–ST-elevation myocardial infarction (NSTEMI) should be treated in similar fashion as patients without cocaine with a notable exception regarding beta-blockers (see Question 12).

11. **How should patients with cocaine-associated chest pain be treated?**

Patients who ingest cocaine are commonly hypertensive, tachycardic, and anxious. In patients who use cocaine, the AHA recommends the early use of intravenous benzodiazepines (Fig. 64-1). The use of benzodiazepines has been shown to relieve chest pain and have beneficial hemodynamic effects. Many times the hypertension and tachycardia will not need to be directly treated after the use of benzodiazepines. In patients who remain hypertensive, nitroglycerin can be administered. Aspirin should also be given. Calcium channel blockers have not been well studied in this population but can be considered in patients who do not respond to benzodiazepines and nitroglycerin. However, short-acting nifedipine should never be used, and verapamil and diltiazem should be avoided in the setting of heart failure or decreased left ventricular systolic function.

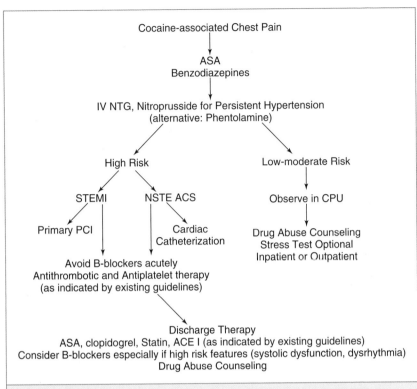

Figure 64-1. Therapeutic and diagnostic recommendations in cocaine-associated chest pain. *ASA,* aspirin; *NTG,* nitroglycerin; *STEMI,* ST-segment elevation MI; *NSTE ACS,* non–ST-segment-elevation ACS; *CPU,* chest pain unit; *PCI,* percutaneous coronary intervention; *B-blockers,* beta-blockers; *ACE,* angiotensin-converting enzyme.

12. **Should beta-blockers be given to patients with cocaine-associated chest pain?**
    No. The AHA recommends that beta-blockers not be administered acutely in patients with ACS or undifferentiated chest pain in the setting of cocaine use. After cocaine use the administration of propranolol leads to the worsening of coronary vasoconstriction. The unopposed α-adrenergic effect in this setting can lead not only to worsening of coronary vasoconstriction but increased systemic blood pressure. Multiple experimental animal models have shown in this setting that beta-blockers decrease coronary blood flow, increase seizure activity, and increase mortality. There have been case reports of sudden cardiac death in humans shortly after the administration of beta-blockers in the setting of cocaine use.
    Although theoretically more attractive, the administration of labetolol in the setting of cocaine use is not recommended by the AHA. Labetolol has substantially more beta-blocking than alpha-blocking effects. In animal models, labetolol leads to increased seizure activity and death after cocaine administration and does not reverse coronary vasoconstriction in humans. The β_1-selective agent metoprolol has not been evaluated in the setting of cocaine, but the β_1-selective agent esmolol has been associated with an increase in systemic blood pressure after cocaine use (Table 64-1).

13. **How should tachyarrhythmias be treated after cocaine use?**
    Sinus tachycardia and atrial tachyarrhythmias may respond to benzodiazepines. In cases of atrial tachyarrhythmias that do not respond to benzodiazepines, verapamil or diltiazem can be

Continued on p. 418

TABLE 64-1. SCIENTIFIC STRENGTH FOR TREATMENT RECOMMENDATIONS FOR INITIAL MANAGEMENT OF COCAINE-ASSOCIATED MYOCARDIAL ISCHEMIA OR INFARCTION

Therapy	Classification of Recommendation/ Level of Evidence	Controlled Clinical Trials	Cardiac Catheterization Laboratory Studies	Case Series or Observational Studies	Case Reports	Controlled In Vivo Animal Experiments
Benzodiazepines	I/B	X			X	X
Aspirin	I/C			X		
Nitroglycerin	I/B	X	X	X		
Calcium channel blocker	IIb/C		X			X
Phentolamine	IIb/C		X		X	X
β-Blockers	II/C		X		X	X
Labetalol	II/C		X		X	X

No. of patients in studies/reports: benzodiazepines, 67; nitroglycerin, 67; phentolamine, 45; calcium channel blocker, 15; β-blockers without α-blocking properties, 30; labetalol, 15; and fibrinolytics, 66.

From McCord J, Jneid H, Hollander JE, et al: Management of cocaine-associated chest pain and myocardial infarction, *Circulation* 117(14):1897-1907, 2008.

considered. Ventricular arrhythmias that occur immediately after cocaine use are thought to result from effects on the sodium channel and may respond to the administration of sodium bicarbonate, similar to arrhythmias associated with type IA and IC agents.

Ventricular arrhythmias that occur several hours after cocaine use usually are due to ischemia, which should be treated as directed earlier. In case of persistent ventricular arrhythmias, lidocaine can be used.

14. How should patients be managed after discharge?

The cessation of cocaine use should be the primary goal. The combination of intensive group and individual drug counseling has been shown to be effective. The recurrence of chest pain is unlikely, and the prognosis is good in patients who discontinue cocaine use. Aggressive modification of risk factors is indicated for patients with AMI or coronary artery disease similar to patients who do not use cocaine.

Although beta-blockers should be avoided acutely, special consideration needs to be given in selected patients for chronic use. In patients with left ventricular systolic dysfunction, AMI, or ventricular arrhythmias, the long-term use of beta-blockers should be strongly considered. The AHA recommends that this decision be individualized on the basis of risk-benefit assessment and recommends counseling the patient about the potential negative effects of the use of beta-blockers and cocaine ingestion.

BIBLIOGRAPHY, SUGGESTED READINGS, AND WEBSITES

1. Baumann BM, Perrone J, Hornig SE, et al: Randomized, double-blind, placebo-controlled trial of diazepam, nitroglycerin, or both for treatment of patients with potential cocaine-associated acute coronary syndromes, *Acad Emerg Med* 7:878-885, 2000.

2. Boehrer JD, Moliterno DJ, Willard JE, et al: Hemodynamic effects of intranasal cocaine in humans, *J Am Coll Cardiol* 20:90-93, 1992.

3. Brogan WC, Lange RA, Kim AS, et al: Alleviation of cocaine-induced coronary vasoconstriction by nitroglycerin, *J Am Coll Cardiol* 18:581-586, 1991.

4. Feldman JA, Fish SS, Beshansky JR, et al: Acute cardiac ischemia in patients with cocaine-associated complaints: results of a multicenter trial, *Ann Emerg Med* 36:469-476, 2000.

5. Hollander JE: The management of cocaine-associated myocardial ischemia, *N Engl J Med* 333:1267-1272, 1995.

6. Hollander JE, Hoffman RS: Cocaine-induced myocardial infarction: an analysis and review of the literature, *J Emerg Med* 10:169-177, 1992.

7. Hollander JE, Hoffman RS, Burstein JL, et al: Cocaine-associated myocardial infarction. Mortality and complications. Cocaine-Associated Myocardial Infarction Study Group, *Arch Intern Med* 155:1081-1086, 1995.

8. Hollander JE, Hoffman RS, Gennis P, et al: Prospective multicenter evaluation of cocaine-associated chest pain. Cocaine Associated Chest Pain (COCHPA) Study Group, *Acad Emerg Med* 1:330-339, 1994.

9. Hollander JE, Lozano M, Fairweather P, et al: "Abnormal" electrocardiograms in patients with cocaine-associated chest pain are due to "normal" variants, *J Emerg Med* 12:199-205, 1994.

10. Hsue PY, Salinas CL, Bolger AF, et al: Acute aortic dissection related to crack cocaine, *Circulation* 105:1592-1595, 2002.

11. Isner JM, Estes NA 3rd, Thompson PD, et al: Acute cardiac events temporally related to cocaine abuse, *N Engl J Med* 315:1438-1443, 1986.

12. Lange RA, Cigarroa RG, Yancy CW Jr, et al: Cocaine-induced coronary-artery vasoconstriction, *N Engl J Med* 321:1557-1562, 1989.

13. Lange RA, Hillis LD: Cardiovascular complications of cocaine use, *N Engl J Med* 345:351-358, 2001.

14. McCord J, Jneid H, Hollander JE, et al: Management of cocaine-associated chest pain and myocardial infarction, *Circulation* 117(14):1897-1907, 2008.

15. Weber JE, Shofer FS, Larkin GL, et al: Validation of a brief observation period for patients with cocaine-associated chest pain, *N Engl J Med* 348:510-517, 2003.

CHAPTER 65

HEART DISEASE IN WOMEN

Brandi J. Witt, MD and C. Noel Bairey Merz, MD, FACC, FAHA

Despite the fact that cardiovascular disease is the leading cause of death in the developed world, less than 50% of women are aware that heart disease is the biggest threat to their health. Additionally, not all physicians think of the cardiovascular system when presented with a female patient. Understanding the unique aspects of cardiovascular disease in women will help one better diagnose and treat this common problem, as well as educate one's patients.

1. **Is cardiovascular disease as big a concern for women as it is for men?**
   Yes. Incidence rates (new cases) for coronary disease in given aged men are similar to incidence rates among women who are on average 10 years older. However, prevalence (existing cases) is higher in older women and younger men.

2. **Is treadmill exercise testing in women as useful as it is in men?**
   Generally, no. As criteria used to evaluate the response to exercise stress testing, the occurrence of chest pain and ST-segment changes have lower sensitivity for obstructive coronary disease among women. The finding of poor exercise capacity has similar predictive value in men and women.

3. **Are all women good candidates for treadmill exercise testing?**
   No. Because of older age, decreased functional capacity at presentation with coronary heart disease, and male-pattern exercise protocols, women more often require pharmacologic stress testing compared with men.

4. **Are stress echocardiography and stress radionuclide scanning useful in women?**
   Yes. Diagnostic and prognostic accuracy of both exercise and pharmacologic stress echocardiography and exercise and pharmacologic stress radionuclide scanning are similar in men and women. Both stress echocardiography and stress radionuclide scanning provide incremental value over treadmill exercise testing or risk factor assessment alone in both men and women.

5. **Is cardiac computed tomography (CT) useful in women?**
   Yes. Detection of coronary calcium is an excellent tool in asymptomatic women because of a negative predictive value of 100%. Furthermore, the overall calcium burden as measured by the Agatston score has more prognostic value in women compared with men. However, the risk of cumulative radiation dose to breast tissue and lungs must be weighed against the benefit of testing.

6. **Does ischemic heart disease have similar presentation in women as in men?**
   No. Women delay seeking medical attention for symptoms longer than men, perhaps because of a lack of recognition that the symptoms are heart related. Additionally, women more often present with back, neck, or jaw pain; dyspnea; nausea or vomiting; indigestion; anorexia; weakness or fatigue; dizziness; or palpitations compared with men, who are more likely to present with typical chest pain. When chest pain is present in women, it is more likely to be nonexertional.

7. **Are women at risk for sudden cardiac death from ischemic heart disease?**
Yes. Although sudden cardiac death is more common in men, women who do experience cardiac arrest are more likely to die compared with men.

8. **What are the risk factors for cardiovascular disease in women?**
Although the risk factors for cardiovascular disease are similar for men and women, including smoking, central obesity, diabetes, hyperlipidemia, hypertension, and family history, the distribution of these factors are not equal among men and women.

9. **Which risk factors are more common in women?**
Total cholesterol greater than 200 mg/dl and obesity (BMI greater than 30) are more prevalent among women, whereas diabetes and low high-density lipoprotein (HDL) are more prevalent among men. Hypertension (systolic blood pressure [BP] greater than 140, diastolic BP greater than 90) is more prevalent among men in persons younger than 45 years of age, whereas hypertension becomes more prevalent among women in persons older than 55 years of age. Metabolic syndrome and smoking prevalence are similar between men and women.

10. **Are any risk factors associated with greater risk in women than men?**
Yes. High triglycerides are more predictive of coronary disease in women compared with men. Additionally, diabetic women are at increased risk of cardiovascular disease compared with diabetic men and must be aggressively treated to modify risk factors.

11. **Is age a risk factor for cardiovascular disease in women?**
Yes, although the age at which risk increases differs between men and women. The risk of coronary disease increases after age 45 for men but not until after 55 for women. An increased risk of cardiovascular disease exists if cardiovascular disease is present in a first-degree male relative older than age 55 or female relative older than age 65.

12. **Are nontraditional risk factors predictive of cardiovascular disease in women?**
Elevated high-sensitivity C-reactive protein (hsCRP) and B-type natriuretic peptide (BNP) provide incremental prognostic value in women beyond measuring "traditional" risk factors such as blood pressure, cholesterol, and weight. However, measurement of homocysteine and lipoprotein A do not.

13. **Are women treated the same as men for cardiovascular disease?**
No. Women are less likely to undergo or be treated with coronary angiography, fibrinolytics, and coronary artery bypass grafting (CABG) compared with men. Among coronary angiograms performed, nondiagnostic coronary angiography is more common among women. This may be due to a higher prevalence of microvascular coronary disease and endothelial dysfunction in women, compared with higher prevalence of macrovascular obstructive coronary disease in men.

14. **Should women receive the same medications as men after a myocardial infarction?**
Yes. Beta-blockers, angiotensin receptor blockers, statins, and aspirin are equally beneficial in women and men.

15. **Are the recommendations for primary prevention of cardiovascular disease similar between men and women?**
Although many of the recommendations are similar, there are some differences. The recommendations in women are summarized in Box 66-1.

BOX 65-1. RECOMMENDATIONS FOR THE PREVENTION OF CARDIOVASCULAR DISEASE IN WOMEN*

Class I

- Complete avoidance of tobacco products
- 30 minutes of moderate activity all most or all days of the week
- Diet high in fruits, vegetables, whole grains
- Diet with < 10% calories from saturated fat, < 300 mg/day cholesterol, salt < 2.3 g/day
- Less than one alcoholic drink daily
- Cardiac rehabilitation with angina, ACS, PCI, stroke, heart failure, or peripheral vascular disease
- Maintain body mass index (BMI) 18.5–24.9
- Blood pressure < 120/80
- Antihypertensives for BP > greater than 140/90 (beta-blocker, ACE inhibitor if CHD present, thiazide diuretic if no CHD)
- LDL < 100 (statins if LDL > 100 and CHD present, LDL > 130 and ≥ 2 RFs present, LDL > 160 and 1 RF present, LDL > 190 and no RF)
- HDL > 50, triglycerides < 150
- Beta-blockers for all women with CHD
- ACE inhibitors for all women with diabetes or CHD with EF < 40%
- Aspirin (75–325 mg/day) in women at high risk for the development of cardiovascular disease or with established atherosclerotic disease.

Class II

- 1 g/day omega-3 fatty acids in all women with CHD
- 2–4 g/day omega-3 fatty acids in women with triglycerides > 150
- Aspirin (81 mg daily or 100 mg every other day) for (1) women > 65 if the blood pressure is controlled and the benefit for ischemic stroke and MI prevention is likely to outweigh risks of gastrointestinal bleeding and hemorrhagic stroke or (2) women < 65 years of age when the benefit for ischemic stroke prevention is likely to outweigh adverse effects of therapy
- Screen for depression in all women with CHD

Class III

- Hormone replacement therapy or SERMs
- Antioxidants (vitamins E or C, betacarotene)
- Folate
- Aspirin for women < 65 and no RF for stroke

ACE, Angiotensin-converting enzyme; ACS, acute coronary syndrome; CHD, coronary heart disease; EF, ejection fraction; LDL, low-density lipoprotein; RF, risk factor; SERMS, selective estrogen receptor modulators.
*Class I recommendations are those interventions that are *useful and effective*; class II recommendations encompass those where the weight of evidence/opinion is in favor of usefulness/ efficacy (class IIa) or the intervention is considered less well established by evidence/opinion (class IIb); class III is where the intervention is felt to not be useful/effective and may be harmful.

Based on recommendations in Mosca L, Banka CL, Benjamin EJ, et al: Evidence-based guidelines for cardiovascular disease prevention in women: 2007 update, *J Am Coll Cardiol* 49(11):1230-1250, 2007.

16. **Should women without cardiovascular disease take aspirin to prevent it (primary prevention)?**

    Aspirin (75–325 mg/day) is recommended in women at high risk for the development of cardiovascular disease or with established atherosclerotic disease (class I recommendation). Aspirin (81 mg daily or 100 mg every other day) should be considered for women older than 65 if BP is controlled and the benefit for ischemic stroke and myocardial infarction (MI) prevention is likely to outweigh risks of gastrointestinal bleeding and hemorrhagic stroke (class IIa recommendation) and in women younger than 65 years of age when the benefit for ischemic stroke prevention is likely to outweigh adverse effects of therapy (class IIb recommendation).

17. **Should women take estrogen (hormone replacement therapy) after menopause to prevent cardiovascular disease?**

    No. Hormone replacement therapy with estrogen or selective estrogen receptor modulators (SERMs) are *not* recommended for prevention of coronary disease (class III).

18. **Are antioxidants helpful in preventing coronary disease in women?**

    No. There is no proven benefit from antioxidant vitamins (E, C, and B) or folate in men or women.

19. **Is the prognosis after MI similar for men and women?**

    No. Mortality after MI is greater in women. Additionally, women are more likely to have recurrent MI and heart failure, as well as clinically significant depression, compared with men after MI.

20. **Is the prognosis after percutaneous coronary intervention (PCI) or CABG similar for men and women?**

    No. Short-term survival after PCI and CABG is worse in women, perhaps because of their older age, smaller vessel size, lack of weight-based thrombolytic regimens, and increased risk of comorbid conditions. Women also have more in-hospital complications after PCI and CABG compared with men. However, long-term survival is similar in men and women.

21. **What is microvascular coronary artery disease?**

    Traditional coronary artery disease is obstructive plaque in one of the major three epicardial coronary arteries or one of their major branches. Microvascular coronary artery disease is diffuse dysfunction in the small branch vessels that cannot be visualized by coronary angiogram. Women, especially younger women, are more likely to have microvascular, *nonobstructive* coronary disease.

22. **Is microvascular coronary artery disease a problem in women?**

    Yes. Microvascular coronary disease in women can result in demonstrable ischemia. However, because of the diffuse atherosclerotic burden with microvascular disease as compared with focal macrovascular obstructive coronary plaques often observed in men, angiography in this subset of women with microvascular disease is less accurate, leading to a group of women with ischemic coronary disease and *normal coronaries*. These women often go untreated for cardiovascular disease because the symptoms are labeled as *noncardiac*.

23. **What is endothelial vasomotor dysfunction, and is it a concern in women?**

    Endothelial vasomotor dysfunction is inappropriate contraction of vascular endothelium leading to vasoconstriction. Similar to microvascular coronary disease, endothelial vasomotor dysfunction can also lead to demonstrable ischemia. There is a high positive predictive value of endothelial vasomotor dysfunction testing in women for adverse outcomes.

24. **Are diastolic heart failure and heart failure with preserved systolic function concerns in women?**

    Yes. Heart failure with preserved left ventricular systolic function is more common among older women than men, perhaps because of a higher prevalence of hypertension in women at older ages. Mortality from heart failure after MI is higher among women, perhaps related to "diastolic" heart failure. Furthermore, although the treatments for systolic heart failure are well established, these same treatments are not as well proven or effective for diastolic heart failure. Thus, although the mortality for heart failure has leveled off, it continues to increase in women, possibly related to the presence of diastolic heart failure.

BIBLIOGRAPHY, SUGGESTED READINGS, AND WEBSITES

1. American Heart Association: Heart Disease and Stroke Statistics: 2008 Update: http://www.americanheart.org/statistics

2. Bairey Merz CN: Insights from the NHLBI-Sponsored Women's Ischemia Syndrome Evaluation (WISE) Study, *J Am Coll Cardiol* 47:S21-S29, 2006.

3. Canto JG: Symptom presentation of women with acute coronary syndromes, *Arch Intern Med* 167:2405-2413, 2007.

4. Collins P: HDL-C in post-menopausal women, *Int J Cardiol* 124:275-282, 2008.

5. Grady D: Cardiovascular disease outcomes during 6.8 years of hormone therapy (HERS II), *JAMA* 288(1):49-57, 2002.

6. Kim C: A systematic review of gender differences in mortality after coronary artery bypass graft surgery and percutaneous coronary intervention, *Clin Cardiol* 30:491-495, 2007.

7. Makaryus AN: Diagnostic strategies for heart disease in women, *Cardiol Rev* 15:279-287, 2007.

8. Meijboom WB: Comparison of diagnostic accuracy of 64-slice computed tomography coronary angiography in women versus men with angina pectoris, *Am J Cardiol* 100:1532-1537, 2007.

9. Mieres JH, Shaw LJ, Arai A, et al: Role of noninvasive testing in the clinical evaluation of women with suspected coronary artery disease: Consensus statement from the Cardiac Imaging Committee, Council on Clinical Cardiology, and the Cardiovascular Imaging and Intervention Committee, Council on Cardiovascular Radiology and Intervention, American Heart Association. *Circulation* 111(5):682-696, 2005.

10. Mosca L: Evidence-based guidelines for cardiovascular disease prevention in women, *Circulation* 115:1-21, 2007.

11. Mosca L, Banka CL, Benjamin EJ, et al: Evidence-based guidelines for cardiovascular disease prevention in women: 2007 update, *J Am Coll Cardiol* 20:49(11):1230-1250, 2007.

12. Owan TE: Trends in prevalence and outcome of heart failure with preserved ejection fraction, *N Engl J Med* 355:251-259, 2006.

13. Shaw LJ: Insights from the NHLBI-sponsored Women's Ischemia Syndrome Evaluation (WISE) study, *J Am Coll Cardiol* 47:S4-S20, 2006.

14. Wenger NK: Coronary heart disease in women, *Nature Clin Practice* 3:194-202, 2006.

CHAPTER 66

HEART DISEASE IN THE ELDERLY

Matthew A. Cavender, MD and E. Magnus Ohman, MD

1. **Who are the elderly and how do the guidelines suggest this population be treated?**

   Although the elderly population is typically considered to be those more than 75 years old, this population represents a heterogenous population of people with a wide variety of life expectancies, comorbidities, and goals. Optimal treatment in this group is difficult because chronologic age is influenced by many other factors, such as frailty, physical reserve, and cognitive status. For this reason, current guidelines regarding the care of the elderly emphasize the individualization of health care based on the patient's overall life goals, expectations, and needs.

2. **Are common risk factors (diabetes, tobacco use, hypertension, hyperlipidemia) important in the elderly?**

   Risk factors such as diabetes, tobacco abuse, and hyperlipidemia are common in the general population of patients with coronary artery disease. In older patients, the overall prevalence of these risk factors decreases, but the relative risk of these risk factors resulting in coronary events actually increases. In patients with no known coronary disease, the use of statin medications has not been shown to provide benefit. However, in patients with known coronary artery disease, aggressive risk factor modification has been shown to be highly beneficial. A meta-analysis of the effectiveness of statin therapy in elderly patients with coronary disease has shown a 22% reduction in all cause mortality, 30% reduction in coronary disease mortality, and 25% reduction in nonfatal myocardial infarction (MI). Interestingly, older patients with coronary disease have been shown to obtain a greater relative risk reduction from the use of statin medications than do younger patients.

3. **Should we treat elderly patients with isolated hypertension?**

   In the elderly, the long-term effects of hypertension on the heart (left ventricular hypertrophy, diastolic function) are commonly seen. However, aggressive treatment of hypertension in the elderly is often avoided because of the potential risk of falls or hypotension. Recent evidence suggests that the treatment of hypertension in the elderly is beneficial and can improve mortality. In the HYpertension in the Very Elderly Trial (HYVET), 3845 patients more than 80 years old were randomized to indapamide and prendolapril versus placebo. Patients actively treated for hypertension had an average blood pressure that was 15.0/6.1 mm Hg lower than the group treated with placebo. Most importantly, this group had a 21% decrease in all-cause mortality, 30% reduction in fatal and nonfatal strokes, and 64% reduction in the rate of heart failure. Based on these results, blood pressure should continue to be treated even in the elderly.

4. **What is the most common arrhythmia in the elderly, and how should it be treated?**

   Atrial fibrillation occurs in up to 9% of patients older than 80 and is the most common arrhythmia in the elderly population. If patients are able to tolerate atrial fibrillation, rate control with atrioventricular (AV) nodal blocking drugs (beta-blockers, non–dihydropyridine calcium channel blockers) is preferred to rhythm control with the antiarrhythmic agents currently available. Elderly patients are at an increased risk of stroke (8% annual risk in patients older than 75). Comorbidities that are common in the elderly, such as diabetes, hypertension, and congestive heart failure (CHF), can increase this risk further.

5. **What is the preferred method of stroke prevention in the elderly with atrial fibrillation?**
Reduction in the risk of stroke can be achieved through the use of either aspirin or coumadin (target international normalized ratio [INR] 2.0–3.0). Although coumadin has been shown to be more effective in reducing the risk of stroke when compared with aspirin, it is also associated with a higher rate of bleeding. Unfortunately, coumadin is often underutilized in the elderly because of the higher rates of bleeding. Current American College of Cardiology/American Heart Association (ACC/AHA) guidelines support the use of coumadin in patients between 65 and 75 years old with at least one risk factor (diabetes, coronary artery disease) and in all women greater than 75 even if no other risk factors are present. In men older than 75 with no other risk factors, either aspirin or coumadin is acceptable. In patients with absolute or relative contraindication to coumadin (previous life threatening bleeding, frequent falls, etc.), aspirin is the preferred alternative.

6. **Do elderly patients with acute coronary syndrome present differently than younger patients?**
Younger patients are much more likely than the elderly to present with typical chest pain symptoms (substernal chest pain radiating to the left jaw/arm). In contrast, elderly patients will often present with dyspnea, diaphoresis, nausea/emesis, or syncope. A proportion of the elderly will have silent MI and never seek medical care. This makes the management of acute coronary syndrome (ACS) in the elderly particularly challenging. Patients with atypical symptoms are diagnosed with ACS later in the course of care, resulting in longer time before evidence-based therapies are initiated. The elderly are also more likely to develop an acute MI during the course of another illness (e.g., gastrointestinal [GI] bleeding, pneumonia, sepsis). The pathophysiology of MI in this setting is fundamentally different than typical ACS, given that these events are due to subendocardial ischemia as a result of increased myocardial oxygen demand.

7. **Have guidelines been published to help clinicians manage elderly patients with non–ST-elevation acute coronary syndrome?**
ACC/AHA guidelines for the treatment of ACS in the elderly recommend treating all patients with antiplatelet agents (ASA, clopidogrel) and with antithrombotic agents (enoxaparin, heparin). In addition, glycoprotein IIb/IIIa inhibitors are also recommended for patients in whom left-sided heart catheterization and percutaneous coronary intervention (PCI) is planned. Elderly patients with non–ST-elevation myocardial infarction (NSTEMI) treated with early revascularization (less than 48 hours) have been shown to have improved outcomes as compared with patients in whom revascularization is delayed or used only if recurrent ischemia occurs. Unfortunately, elderly patients are less likely to receive guideline-based care and be treated with an early invasive strategy despite the fact that they receive a larger absolute benefit. Although all patients should be treated based on their individual risks and benefits, improved accessibility to revascularization and earlier treatment with guideline-based therapies should be the focus in the care of elderly patients with ACS.

8. **How can adverse events be minimized in the elderly with ACS?**
Although the treatment of patients with evidence-based antiplatelet and antithrombotic medications combined with an early invasive revascularization strategy improves clinical endpoints and is associated with a greater absolute benefit than the same therapy in younger, lower risk patients, these treatments are associated with a higher risk of complications. Although the risk/benefit ratio should be an individualized decision, minimizing complications

TABLE 66-1. PHARMACOLOGIC AGENTS AND DOSING RECOMMENDATIONS FOR ACUTE CORONARY SYNDROMES

Agent	Indication	Standard	Renal Adjustment*
Aspirin	NSTEMI STEMI	325 mg on presentation, followed by 81 mg daily	None
Clopidogrel	NSTEMI STEMI	300–600 mg on presentation, followed by 75 mg daily	None
Heparin	NSTEMI STEMI	IV bolus of 60 U/kg followed by an infusion of 12 U/kg per hour for goal aPTT of 50–70. Maximum suggested dose of 4000 U bolus and 900 U/hr infusion or 5000 U bolus and 1000 U/hr infusion if patient is >100 mg	None
Enoxaparin	NSTEMI STEMI	1 mg/kg subcutaneously every 12 hours	If CrCl $\leq$ 30 ml/min, 1 mg/kg every 24 hours
Fondaparinux	NSTEMI	2.5 mg subcutaneously daily (if no PCI planned)	Contraindicated if CrCl $\leq$ 30 ml/min
Bivalirudin	NSTEMI STEMI	Initial management: 0.1 mg/kg bolus, 0.25 mg/kg/h infusion	
		During PCI: 0.5 mg/kg bolus, increase infusion to 1.75 mg/kg/hr for patients who received initial medical management or 0.75 mg/kg bolus, then 1.75 mg/kg/hr infusion for those who did not receive initial medical management	
Eptifibatide	NSTEMI	180 µg/kg initial dose followed by maintenance infusion of 2.0 µg/kg/min	Reduce infusion rate by 50% (1 µg per kg/min) in patients with creatinine clearance* $\leq$ 50 ml/min
Tirofiban	NSTEMI	12 µg/kg bolus, then 0.1 µg/kg/min	Decrease dose by 50% if CrCl < 30 ml/min (6 µg/kg bolus the 0.05 µg/kg per min)
Abciximab	STEMI	0.25 mg/kg IV bolus (max. 10 µg/min), then 0.125 µg/kg/min infusion	None

aPTT, activated partial thromboplastin time; *CrCl*, creatinine clearance; *IV*, intravenous; *STEMI*, ST-segment-elevation myocardial infarction.
*Creatinine clearance is based on the Cockcroft-Gault formula: Glomerular filtration rate = [(140 − age) × (Wt in kg) × (0.85 if female)]/ (72 × Cr)

such as bleeding are likely to improve clinical outcomes. Bleeding can be minimized through proper dosing of antithrombotic medications based on weight and creatinine clearance. Elderly patients have a high incidence of renal insufficiency; therefore, all patients should have a current weight and creatinine clearance calculated using the Cockcroft-Gault formula before the initiation of antithrombotic medications (Table 66-1). Pharmacotherapy dosing and dosing adjustments in chronic kidney disease are summarized in Table 66-1.

9. **What is the preferred treatment for ST-segment-elevation myocardial infarction in the elderly?**
   Treating the elderly with ST-segment-elevation myocardial infarction (STEMI) is difficult given the large proportion of patients with atypical or no symptoms, late time from the onset of symptoms, or a nondiagnostic electrocardiogram (ECG). Given these factors, as well as the high rate of absolute or relative contraindications to fibrinolytic therapy, elderly patients are less likely to be treated with either fibrinolytics or PCI. In patients without contraindications, revascularization should be attempted because patients treated for STEMI have improved outcomes when compared with patients who do not receive therapy. Ideally, patients should be treated with primary PCI when possible given the large absolute mortality benefit seen with PCI as compared with fibrinolytic therapy (85 years or older, −6.9%; 75–84 years old, −5.1%). For this reason, current ACC/AHA guidelines for the treatment of STEMI in the elderly give preference to PCI over fibrinolytics. Fibrinolytic therapy is most effective in the first 3 hours from symptom onset and should be used when transfer to a center with primary PCI capabilities is not feasible in less than 90 minutes.

BIBLIOGRAPHY, SUGGESTED READINGS, AND WEBSITES

1. Afilalo J, Duque G, Steele R, et al: Statins for secondary prevention in elderly patients: a hierarchical bayesian meta-analysis, *J Am Coll Cardiol* 51(1):37-45, 2008.

2. Alexander KP, Newby LK, Cannon CP, et al: Acute coronary care in the elderly, part I: non–ST-segment-elevation acute coronary syndromes: a scientific statement for healthcare professionals from the American Heart Association Council on Clinical Cardiology: in collaboration with the Society of Geriatric Cardiology, *Circulation* 115(19):2549-2569, 2007.

3. Alexander KP, Newby LK, Armstrong PW, et al: Acute coronary care in the elderly, part II: ST-segment-elevation myocardial infarction: a scientific statement for healthcare professionals from the American Heart Association Council on Clinical Cardiology: in collaboration with the Society of Geriatric Cardiology, *Circulation* 115(19):2570-2589, 2007.

4. Alexander KP, O'Connor CM: The elderly and aging. In Topol EJ, Califf RM, Isner J, editors: *Textbook of cardiovascular medicine*, ed 3, Philadelphia, 2007, Lippincott Williams & Wilkins.

5. Beckett NS, Peters R, Fletcher AE, et al: Treatment of hypertension in patients 80 years of age or older, *N Engl J Med* 358(18):1887-1898, 2008.

HEART DISEASE IN PREGNANCY

Sheilah A. Bernard, MD

CHAPTER 67

1. **What cardiac physiologic changes occur during pregnancy?**

   Both the mother's plasma volume (from water and sodium retention) and red blood cell volume (from erthyrocytosis) increase because of hormonal changes during normal pregnancy. Disproportionate increases explain the *physiologic anemia of pregnancy*. Maternal heart rate (HR) also increases throughout the 40 weeks, in part mediated by increased sympathetic tone and normal heat production. Stroke volume subsequently continues to increase until the third trimester, when venal caval return may be compromised by the gravid uterus. Maternal cardiac output (CO) increases by 30% to 50% during a normal pregnancy.

2. **Are there independent vascular changes that occur during a normal pregnancy?**

   The vascular wall weakens during pregnancy as a result of estrogen and prostaglandin. As the placenta develops, it creates a low-resistance circulation. These factors, in addition to heat production, contribute to the reduced systemic vascular resistance (SVR) that is a normal part of pregnancy.

3. **What are normal cardiac signs and symptoms of pregnancy?**
   - *Hyperventilation* (as a result of increased minute ventilation)
   - *Edema* (from volume retention and compressed inferior vena cava [IVC] by the uterus)
   - *Dizziness/lightheadedness* (from reduced SVR and venal caval compression)
   - *Palpitations* (normal HR increases by 10–15 beats/min)

4. **What are pathologic cardiac signs and symptoms of pregnancy?**
   - *Anasarca*, or generalized edema, and *paroxysmal nocturnal dyspnea* (PND) are not components of normal pregnancy and warrant workup.
   - *Syncope* should be evaluated for hypotension, obstructive valvular pathology (aortic, mitral or pulmonic stenosis), pulmonary hypertension, pulmonary embolism, or tachybradyarrhythmias.
   - *Chest pain* may be due to aortic dissection, pulmonary embolism, angina, or even myocardial infarction. Women are delaying their child-bearing years, with a higher incidence of preexisting cardiac risk factors in the older pregnant woman.
   - *Hemoptysis* may be a harbinger of occult mitral stenosis, although rheumatic heart disease is becoming less common in developed countries.

5. **How does the cardiac examination change during a normal pregnancy?**

   Blood pressure (BP) will decline and HR will increase. The point of maximum impulse (PMI) will be displaced laterally as the uterus enlarges. S3 is common because of increased rapid filling of the left ventricle (LV) in early diastole. S4 is unusual and may reflect underlying hypertension. A physiologic pulmonic flow murmur is common because of elevated stroke volume passing through a normal valve. Systolic murmurs of 1/6–2/6 can be explained by these physiologic changes. A mammary soufflé and venous hum are two continuous, superficial murmurs that can be obliterated by compressing the site with the diaphragm of the stethoscope. If the murmur does not change, consider patent ductus arteriosus or coronary atrioventricular (AV) fistula.

6. **What are abnormal cardiac findings during pregnancy?**
   - *Clubbing* and *cyanosis* are not a part of normal pregnancy; desatuaration for any reason is abnormal and warrants investigation.
   - *Elevated jugular venous pressure* is abnormal, reflecting elevated right atrial pressure; it is important to evaluate neck veins in any pregnant woman who has peripheral edema.
   - *Pulmonary hypertension* (right ventricular heave, loud P2, JVP elevation) evidence should be investigated early. Women with pulmonary hypertension (pulmonary pressure greater than 75% of systemic pressure) should be counseled in general as to the risks of pregnancy.
   - *Systolic murmur 3/6 or louder* and any *diastolic murmur* audible in pregnancy are considered abnormal and warrant evaluation.

7. **What are the cardiac changes that occur during labor and delivery?**
   With each contraction, 300 to 500 ml of blood are autotransfused from the uterus into the maternal system. CO drops less with vaginal delivery than cesarean, so this form of delivery is recommended most commonly in patients with cardiac disease. Vacuum-assisted delivery is used to shorten stage II of labor for women who may not tolerate pushing. After delivery, intravascular volume increases from release of the vena caval compression and HR slows. BP, CO, and HR normalize over the next 5 to 6 weeks as hormonal changes return to the pregravid state.

8. **Which women should undergo infective endocarditis (IE) prophylaxis at the time of delivery?**
   IE prophylaxis is optional in vaginal delivery for patients with prior IE, prosthetic valves, congenital heart disease (CHD) within the first 6 months of repair or after 6 months if there is residual shunting, surgically constructed systemic-pulmonary shunts or conduits, and posttransplantation valvulopathy. It is not indicated in cesarean section per 2007 American Heart Association (AHA) guidelines, although it is often given.

9. **What maternal cardiac tests can be performed safely?**
   - Electrocardiograms and echocardiograms are safe.
   - Chest radiographs can be performed with proper pelvic shielding.
   - Low-level exercise tolerance testing to 70% of maternal maximal heart rate is safe with low risk of fetal distress/bradycardia.
   - Transesophageal echocardiography (TEE) can be performed with appropriate sedation and monitoring if risks/benefits are justified.
   - Cardiac catheterization, balloon valvuloplasty, angioplasty, and percutaneous intervention are invasive diagnostic and therapeutic tests that may be life saving to the mother with appropriate pelvic shielding for the fetus.
   - Computerized tomography and magnetic resonance imaging (MRI) are contraindicated.

10. **What are the highest risk maternal valvular lesions during pregnancy?**
    Moderate to severe mitral, aortic, and pulmonic stenosis are tolerated poorly during pregnancy. Patients should be counseled, with consideration of valvuloplasty or valve replacement before conception. These procedures can be performed during pregnancy at higher risk if the patient decompensates. Pulmonary hypertension is also a high-risk condition.

11. **Are regurgitant lesions equally risky?**
    Both mild to moderate aortic insufficiency and mitral regurgitation are tolerated well during pregnancy. The reduction in SVR can lessen the degree of regurgitation. Only patients with severe symptomatic regurgitation (New York Heart Association [NYHA] class III–IV or greater) should be considered for valve replacement before pregnancy, and the only indication for valve replacement for regurgitation in the gravid patient is infective endocarditis.

12. **What are predictors of maternal or fetal complications for pregnant women with cardiac disease?**
Maternal pulmonary edema, stroke, arrhythmia, or cardiac death were complications noted in a study of 599 such pregnancies. Fetal complications were seen with maternal symptoms more than NYHA class II or cyanosis, left heart obstruction, anticoagulation, smoking, and multiple gestations.

13. **How are pregnant women anticoagulated during pregnancy?**
Because warfarin is contraindicated during the first trimester and at term, 2004 American College for Chest Physicians (ACCP) guidelines recommend one of the following grade 1C strategies:
- Aggressive adjusted dose unfractionated heparin (UFH) every 12 hours to activated partial thromboplastin time (aPTT) two to three times normal *or*
- Aggressive adjusted dose low-molecular-weight heparin (LMWH) twice daily to anti-factor Xa level 0.7 to 1.2 U/ml *or*
- UFH or LMWH (as earlier) until the thirteenth week, change to warfarin until the middle of the third trimester, and then restart UFH or LMWH. Long-term anticoagulants should be resumed postpartum with all regimens, as early as the same evening. Low-dose aspirin can be optionally added for high-risk patients with mechanical heart valves. Mothers taking warfarin may nurse after delivery.

14. **How are the common congenital lesions tolerated during pregnancy?**
Congenital heart disease (CHD) has superseded rheumatic heart disease as the most common preexisting heart disease in pregnancy. Repaired atrial septal defects (ASD) and ventricular septal defects (VSD) confer no increased cardiac risk. Unrepaired left-to-right intracardiac shunts (ASD and VSD) are well tolerated because of the reduction in SVR, which decreases left-to-right shunting during pregnancy. Patients are at an increased risk for paradoxical embolization if they develop deep venous thrombosis.

Right-to-left (cyanotic) shunting is poorly tolerated in pregnancy. Women with tetralogy of Fallot should undergo repair before contemplating pregnancy. Right-to-left shunting worsens during pregnancy because of reduction of SVR. Women with Eisenmenger's syndrome risk a 30% to 50% maternal mortality with pregnancy. Such high-risk women are counseled to avoid pregnancy or undergo therapeutic termination. There is a growing literature on women with extensive corrected CHD who are surviving into adulthood and completing successful pregnancies; they are advised to undergo fetal ultrasound. Because of prenatal identification of abnormal fetal cardiac examinations and elective terminations, the incidence of CHD is decreasing.

15. **Which cardiac arrhythmias can complicate pregnancy?**
Patients may develop atrial and ventricular ectopy because of myocardial stretch. Reentrant pathways can emerge and be treated acutely with vagal maneuvers or adenosine if the mother is unstable. Recurrent supraventricular arrhythmias can be prevented with digitalis or beta-blockers. Symptomatic ventricular arrhythmias are treated medically or with implantable cardioverter defibrillators. If a pregnant woman suffers a cardiac arrest, the viable baby should be delivered after 15 minutes if there is no return of spontaneous maternal circulation.

16. **How do you treat a pregnant woman with an acute myocardial infarction?**
Pregnant women with ST-segment-elevation myocardial infarction (STEMI) should be taken to the catheterization laboratory for primary balloon angioplasty. Heparin can be used safely; however, there is little data on the use of stents because clopidrogel has not been studied in pregnancy. Beta-blockers and aspirin can be used in pregnancy, but angiotensin-converting enzyme (ACE) inhibitors, angiotensin-receptor blockers (ARBs), and statins should be avoided. Risk factors should be treated.

17. **How do women with hypertrophic cardiomyopathy (HCM) tolerate pregnancy?**
    Women with HCM will experience left ventricular end-diastolic pressure (LVEDP) elevations
    because of increased volume of pregnancy. Outflow obstruction may improve if the LV can dilate.
    Management is similar to the nongravid state. At the time of delivery, anesthesia is critical to
    reduce sympathetic stimulation from pain; most anesthetic agents reduce myocardial contractility.
    Preload and afterload changes during delivery must be minimized to avoid increased outflow
    obstruction. Short-acting vasoconstrictors, diuretics, or volume adjustments may be necessary.

18. **What are the recommendations for patients with Marfan syndrome?**
    Women with Marfan syndrome are at risk for aortic dissection because of the vascular
    changes of pregnancy. Genetic counseling should be performed before pregnancy because of
    autosomal dominant transmission. Those with an aortic root diameter of more than 40 mm are
    at highest risk and are advised to avoid pregnancy. Management includes beta-blockers,
    serial echocardiograms, and bedrest to avoid further root dilation. If dissection is suspected,
    TEE is recommended over MRI for diagnosis. Type A dissection (involving the ascending aorta)
    should be managed surgically, with delivery of the viable fetus before repair. Type B dissection
    (descending aortic involvement) can be managed medically with labetalol or nitroprusside.

19. **Which commonly used cardiac medications should be avoided during pregnancy?**
    - Women should be counseled that warfarin and statins are currently Food and Drug
      Administration (FDA) class X. Investigations on the use of statins in pregnancy are
      underway.
    - ACE inhibitors, ARBs, atenolol, and amiodarone are class D.
    - LMWH or UFHs should replace warfarin at certain periods of pregnancy, at discussed
      earlier.
    - Hydralazine with nitrates should replace ACE inhibitors/ARBs in patients with heart failure.
    - ACE inhbitors can be used in nursing mothers.
    - Metoprolol, propranolol, or labetalol should be used instead of atenolol.

20. **What is peripartum cardiomyopathy (PCMP)?**
    This is a syndrome of congestive heart failure diagnosed in the last month of pregnancy up to 5
    months postpartum, with demonstration of reduced systolic function by echocardiogram,
    without identifiable or reversible cause. Preexisting cardiac disease usually presents before the
    final month due to physiologic changes of pregnancy. Women are treated with standard
    heart failure medications (hydralazine/nitrates while pregnant; ACE inhibitors are safe after
    delivery in nursing mothers). Prognosis is determined by degree of systolic function recovery.
    Maternal risk is higher during subsequent pregnancies if LVEF persists at less than 40%. B-type
    natriuretic peptide (BNP) levels do not rise with normal pregnancy; levels increase in women
    with myopathy, preeclampsia, eclampsia, and diabetes.

BIBLIOGRAPHY, SUGGESTED READINGS, AND WEBSITES

1. Drenthen W, Pieper P, Roos-Hesselink J, et al: Outcome of pregnancy in women with congenital heart disease:
   a literature review, *J Am Coll Card* 49:2303-2311, 2007.
2. Elkayam U, Bitar F: Valvular heart disease in pregnancy, parts I (native) and II (prosthetic), *J Am Coll Cardiol*
   46:223-230, 46:403-410, 2005.
3. Reimold SC, Rutherford JD: Clinical practice: valvular heart disease in pregnancy, *N Eng J Med* 349:52-59,
   2003.
4. Bonow RO, Carabello BA, et al: ACC/AHA Guidelines for management of patients with valvular heart disease,
   Circulation 114:493-496, 2006.
5. Wilson W, Taubert K, Gewitz M, et al: Prevention of infective endocarditis: Guidelines from the AHA, *Circulation*
   116:1736-1754, 2007.

CHAPTER 68

CARDIOVASCULAR MANIFESTATIONS OF CONNECTIVE TISSUE DISORDERS AND THE VASCULITIDES

Nishant R. Shah, MD

1. **What is the leading cause of death in patients with rheumatoid arthritis, and what are its most common cardiac manifestations?**
   The leading cause of death in patients with rheumatoid arthritis (RA) is ischemic heart disease. Risk factors attributable to RA include chronic proinflammatory and prothrombotic states, endothelial dysfunction, dyslipidemia, insulin resistance, increased oxidative stress, and nonsteroidal antiinflammatory drug (NSAID)/corticosteroid use. Other cardiac manifestations of RA include increased risk of congestive heart failure (CHF), pericarditis, and conduction block as a result of myocardial rheumatoid nodules.

2. **What are the cardiovascular manifestations of systemic lupus erythematosus?**
   The most common cardiac complication of systemic lupus erythematosus (SLE) is pericarditis. Clinically evident myocarditis also occurs in 8% to 25% of patients. Libman-Sacks endocarditis is discussed in Question 5. Finally, premature atherosclerosis, as a result of many of the same independent risk factors noted for RA, is now recognized as a major cause of morbidity/mortality.

3. **What are the cardiovascular consequences of NSAIDs with predominantly cyclooxygenase-2 inhibition?**
   Cyclooxygenase-2 (COX-2) inhibitors cause a shift toward thrombosis through reduced endothelial production of prostacyclin (a COX-2–mediated antithrombotic process) and relative sparing of platelet production of thromboxane A_2 (a COX-1–mediated prothrombotic process). For this reason, concurrent low-dose aspirin is recommended for patients taking COX-2 inhibitors. Secondly, COX-2 inhibitors increase sodium/water retention, predisposing patients to edema, CHF exacerbations, and hypertension. Finally, COX-2 inhibitors prevent protective COX-2 upregulation in the setting of myocardial ischemia/infarction, leading to larger infarct size and increased risk of myocardial rupture. Of note, NSAIDs with predominantly COX-1 inhibition are associated with increased risk of gastrointestinal (GI) bleeding. For this reason, concurrent proton pump inhibitor therapy is recommended for patients on COX-1 inhibitors.

4. **What is the major cardiovascular concern associated with tumor necrosis factor (TNF)-α antagonists?**
   Results from the Anti-TNF Therapy Against Congestive Heart Failure (ATTACH) trial suggest that high-dose TNF-α antagonist therapy actually *increases* death from any cause and heart failure hospitalization in patients with New York Heart Association (NYHA) class III-IV CHF.

5. **What are the clinical manifestations of antiphospholipid antibody syndrome?**
   Antiphospholipid antibodies (APAs) promote intravascular clotting and can be found in primary APA syndrome or secondary to other conditions, most commonly SLE. Clinical manifestations of APA syndrome include spontaneous venous/arterial thromboses, strokes/neurologic syndromes, digital/extremity ischemia, livedo reticularis, thrombocytopenia, and recurrent

spontaneous abortions. From a cardiac standpoint, acute coronary thromboses and diffuse small vessel clotting resulting in global myocardial dysfunction have been described. In addition, Libman-Sacks endocarditis, defined by sterile vegetations on the mitral > aortic/tricuspid > pulmonary valves, is thought to arise from organization of thrombi and can cause valvular regurgitation or stenosis requiring surgical correction. Treatment for APA syndrome is warfarin (goal international normalized ratio [INR] 2.0–3.0) with or without daily low-dose aspirin and hydroxychloroquine.

6. **What is neonatal lupus erythematosus syndrome?**
   Neonatal lupus erythematosus (NLE) syndrome is most commonly manifested as a transient lupus rash in a newborn infant. The major cause of morbidity and mortality is development of complete congenital heart block in the fetus between 18 and 30 weeks, causing intrauterine death or need for postpartum pacemaker placement. Transplacental transfer of maternal anti-Ro (SS-A) and anti-La (SS-B) IgG autoantibodies to the fetus has been implicated in the pathophysiology of NLE.

7. **How is drug-induced lupus different from SLE, and what drugs can cause it?**
   With exceptions for select medications, antihistone antibodies *without* the presence of anti-dsDNA/anti-Sm antibodies is the predominant autoantibody pattern in drug-induced lupus. Although rash, central nervous system (CNS) disease, and renal disease are much less common in drug-induced lupus than in SLE, pulmonary infiltrates are more common. Additionally, drug-induced lupus is reversible on discontinuation of the offending medication. Drugs associated with drug-induced lupus are listed in Table 68-1.

TABLE 68-1. DRUGS ASSOCIATED WITH DRUG-INDUCED LUPUS

Drugs *definitively* known to cause drug-induced lupus:	Cardiovascular medications that *probably* cause drug-induced lupus:
■ Procainamide	■ Beta-blockers
■ Hydralazine	■ Captopril
■ Diltiazem	■ Hydrochlorothiazide
■ TNF-α antagonists	■ Amiodarone
■ Minocycline	
■ Chlorpromazine	
■ Quinidine	
■ D-penicillamine	
■ Isoniazid	
■ Methyldopa	
■ Interferon-α	

TNF, Tumor necrosis factor.

---

8. **Describe the characteristic myocardial lesions of scleroderma/systemic sclerosis and their clinical manifestations.**
   Scleroderma of the myocardium manifests as biventricular random patchy fibrosis. Evidence thus far suggests that fibrosis results from recurrent ischemia and reperfusion injury caused by transient recurrent vasospasm of intramural small arteries/arterioles (myocardial Raynaud's

phenomenon). For this reason, calcium channel blocker therapy is appropriate for these patients. Clinically, patients with scleroderma are at increased risk for exercise-induced arrhythmias and biventricular heart failure. Of note, although a septal pseudoinfarct pattern and other conduction abnormalities can be seen on electrocardiogram (ECG), a normal ECG is the most common finding.

9. **What is the most common cardiac complication of scleroderma/systemic sclerosis?**
Cor pulmonale. Intimal proliferation of the small pulmonary arteries causes pulmonary hypertension and subsequent right-sided heart failure. For this reason, pulmonary function test (PFT) screening for measurement of carbon monoxide diffusion in the lung (DLCO) has become standard in the treatment of scleroderma. Prostacyclin analogs and bosentan have been shown to reduce pulmonary vascular resistance and improve outcomes. Lung transplantation is another treatment option when medical management fails.

10. **What is a scleroderma renal crisis, and how should it be treated?**
Severe systemic hypertension and microangiopathic hemolytic anemia are the first signs of a scleroderma renal crisis. Increased plasma renin and rapid deterioration of renal function then develop over days to weeks. Left ventricular heart failure can also develop. Aggressive and prompt lowering of blood pressure with angiotensin-converting enzyme (ACE) inhibitors can reverse/stabilize the renal failure. Hemodialysis and renal transplantation are reserved for severe and irreversible cases.

11. **What are the most common cardiac findings associated with the seronegative spondyloarthropathies?**
Aortic regurgitation (AR) occurs as a result of aortic root thickening/dilation, thickening/shortening of the aortic valve cusps, and development of a fibrous "bump". Mitral regurgitation (MR) is less common but is due to a similar thickening at the basal portion of the anterior mitral leaflet (or secondary to AR). Complete atrioventricular (AV) nodal or bundle branch block can develop when the fibrosing process extends into the muscular septum. Interestingly, the combination of lone AR and severe conduction system disease in patients not known to have seronegative spondylarthritis is highly correlated with the presence of human leukocyte antigen B27 (HLA-B27).

12. **Name the clinical manifestations of polyarteritis nodosa, including the most common cardiovascular complications.**
Polyarteritis nodosa (PAN) is a nongranulomatous, patchy, necrotizing vasculitis of medium-sized muscular arteries. Constitutional symptoms (fever, malaise, myalgias, arthralgias, weight loss) are common. Focal tissue ischemia and infarction can cause one of four cutaneous findings (painful subcutaneous nodules, nonblanching livedo reticularis, skin ulceration, and digital ischemia), asymmetric mononeuritis multiplex, hyperreninemic hypertension/renal insufficiency, or mesenteric infarction/aneurysmal rupture. Vasculitis in the distal coronary arteries cause recurrent small myocardial infarctions that variably manifest as angina, acute myocardial infarction, congestive heart failure, or arrhythmias. Treatment for PAN is high-dose corticosteroids and cytotoxic therapy (cyclophosphamide, azathioprine, or methotrexate).

13. **What are the most common findings in Takayasu's arteritis, and how should these patients be managed?**
Takayasu's arteritis is a granulomatous vasculitis of the aorta and its branches most common in young Asian women. Resultant arterial stenosis is much more common than aneurysm formation. Claudication, especially in the upper extremities, is the most common symptom. The most common findings include bruits, hypertension, and upper extremity blood pressure/ pulse asymmetry. Aneurysms, when they occur, are most common in the aortic root and can cause significant AR. Angiographic evaluation of the entire aorta and its primary branches to

determine the distribution and severity of vascular lesions is recommended. When contraindications to angiography exist, magnetic resonance or computed tomography (CT) angiography are acceptable alternatives. High-dose corticosteroids and anatomic correction of clinically significant lesions are the treatments of choice. Cyclophosphamide, methotrexate, and anti–tumor necrosis factor (TNF) agents are reserved for severe disease.

14. **What are the most common cardiac manifestations of Kawasaki disease?**
    Kawasaki disease is an acute systemic febrile illness most common in infants and young children. Defining symptoms include high-spiking fever, cervical lymphadenopathy (nontender, greater than 1.5 cm in diameter, usually unilateral), erythematous/desquamative skin rash, and mucous membrane lesions (oropharyngeal injection, strawberry tongue, bilateral nonexudative conjunctivitis). Typical laboratory abnormalities include leukocytosis, elevated erythrocyte sedimentation rate (ESR) and C-reactive protein (CRP), and late thrombocytosis. Thrombosis of coronary artery aneurysms (Fig. 68-1) (especially larger than 8 mm) is the most common cause of death. For this reason, serial echocardiography to evaluate coronary artery anatomy and other parameters is crucial. Treatment consists of high-dose aspirin and intravenous immune globulin.

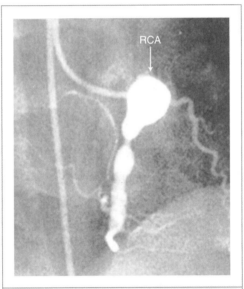

Figure 68-1. Coronary angiogram demonstrating giant aneurysm of the right coronary artery in 6-year-old boy. (From Newburger JW, Takahashi M, Gerber MA, et al: Diagnosis, treatment, and long-term management of Kawasaki disease, *Pediatrics* 114:1708-1733, 2004.)

15. **What is the most common cardiovascular complication of Marfan syndrome?**
    Marfan syndrome (MFS) is caused by an autosomal-dominant fibrillin gene defect. The most common cardiovascular complication is asymptomatic progressive aortic root enlargement beginning at the sinuses of Valsalva. The development of an ascending aortic aneurysm subsequently places patients at high risk for type A aortic dissection, aortic rupture, or aortic regurgitation (AR). Of note, mitral valve prolapse is present in 70% to 90% of MFS patients and progresses to mitral regurgitation in up to 50%.

16. **How should Marfan syndrome be managed from a cardiovascular standpoint?**
    Annual imaging with transthoracic/transesophageal echocardiography or CT/magnetic resonance angiography is required to detect and assess aortic dilation. When the aortic diameter reaches 5 cm, prophylactic aortic root replacement should be considered. Criteria for earlier consideration of surgery include aortic diameter growth greater than 1 cm/year, family history of dissection less than 5 cm, or moderate to severe AR. Finally, MFS patients should receive beta-blocker therapy, which has been shown to improve survival.

17. **How is Ehlers-Danlos Syndrome type IV different from the other types?**
    Ehlers-Danlos Syndrome (EDS) type IV patients have type III collagen defects, resulting in thin, translucent skin absent the hyperextensibility characterizing other EDS patients. Additionally, EDS type IV patients are at high risk for life-threatening spontaneous arterial rupture, most commonly in the abdominal cavity and the gravid uterus. Bleeding should be managed as conservatively as possible because these patients's tissues don't hold sutures well and angiography should be avoided because of a high rate of complications.

BIBLIOGRAPHY, SUGGESTED READINGS, AND WEBSITES

1. Schur PH, Rose BD: Drug-Induced Lupus: http://www.utdol.com
2. Andrews J, Mason JC: Takayasu's arteritis—recent advances in imaging offer promise, *Rheumatology (Oxford)* 46(1):6-15, 2007.
3. Antman EM, Bennett JS, Daugherty A, et al: Use of nonsteroidal antiinflammatory drugs: an update for clinicians: a scientific statement from the American Heart Association, *Circulation* 115(12):1634-1642, 2007.
4. Arnett FC, Willerson JT: Connective tissue diseases and the heart. In Willerson JT, Cohn JN, Wellens HJJ, et al, editors: *Cardiovascular medicine*, ed 3, London, 2007, Springer-Verlag.
5. Chung ES, Packer M, Lo KH, et al: Randomized, double-blind, placebo-controlled, pilot trial of infliximab, a chimeric monoclonal antibody to tumor necrosis factor-alpha, in patients with moderate-to-severe heart failure: results of the anti-TNF Therapy Against Congestive Heart Failure (ATTACH) trial, *Circulation* 107(25): 3133-3140, 2003.
6. Levine JS, Branch DW, Rauch J: The antiphospholipid syndrome, *N Engl J Med* 346(10):752-763, 2002.
7. Mandell BF, Hoffman GS: Rheumatic diseases and the cardiovascular system. In Libby P, Bonow R, Mann D, et al, editors: *Braunwald's heart disease: a textbook of cardiovascular medicine*, ed 8, Philadelphia, 2008, Saunders.
8. Milewicz DM: Inherited disorders of connective tissue. In Willerson JT, Cohn JN, Wellens HJJ, et al, editors: *Cardiovascular medicine*, ed 3, London, 2007, Springer-Verlag.
9. Milewicz DM: Treatment of aortic disease in patients with Marfan syndrome, *Circulation* 111(11):e150-e157, 2005.
10. Newburger JW, Takahashi M, Gerber MA, et al: Diagnosis, treatment, and long-term management of Kawasaki disease, *Circulation* 110(17):2747-2771, 2004.
11. Roman MJ, Salmon JE: Cardiovascular manifestations of rheumatologic diseases, *Circulation* 116(20): 2346-2355, 2007.
12. Sattar N, McCarey DW, Capell H, McInnes IB: Explaining how "high-grade" systemic inflammation accelerates vascular risk in rheumatoid arthritis, *Circulation* 108(24):2957-2963, 2003.
13. Stone JH: Polyarteritis nodosa, *JAMA* 288(13):1632-1639, 2002.

CHAPTER 69

CARDIAC MANIFESTATIONS OF HIV/AIDS

Sheilah A. Bernard, MD

1. **How have the cardiac manifestations of human immunodeficiency virus/ acquired immunodeficiency syndrome (HIV/AIDS) changed over the years?**
   Until the early 1990s, cardiologists saw AIDS-related pericardial disease, myocarditis, dilated and infiltrative cardiomyopathy, pulmonary disease with pulmonary hypertension, arrhythmias, and marantic or infectious endocarditis. Because patients tended to be younger, very little atherosclerosis was noted. As effective HIV treatment has become available this century, late-stage cardiac complications are seen only in untreated patients with advanced AIDS. HIV patients have a higher incidence of traditional cardiovascular risk factors, such as male gender, smoking, advanced age, glucose intolerance, insulin resistance, and dyslipidemia. They additionally have a higher incidence of nontraditional cardiac risk factors, including polysubstance abuse, lifestyle choices, immune dysregulation, and effects of antiretroviral therapy (ART). Atherosclerotic disease is becoming more common in the HIV population as patients are surviving longer with treated disease. Over the next decades, children born with vertically transmitted HIV will survive to adulthood, with attendant cardiac complications from chronic inflammation, drug therapy, and immunosuppression.

2. **What are the clinical manifestations of AIDS in the heart?**
   In untreated patients (historically in the 1980s to 1990s in the United States, or currently in underdeveloped countries), advanced AIDS can cause the following:
   - Pericardial effusion/tamponade
   - Myocarditis/cardiomyopathy (systolic and diastolic dysfunction)
   - Marantic (thrombotic) or infectious endocarditis
   - Cardiac tumors (Kaposi's sarcoma, lymphoma)
   - Right ventricular (RV) dysfunction from pulmonary hypertension or opportunistic infections

   In HIV patients undergoing treatment with ART, there are emerging metabolic disorders (including dyslipidemias, insulin resistance, lipodystrophy) with an attendant increase in atherosclerosis. Also, arrhythmias are seen with some HIV antibiotics.

3. **How common is pericardial effusion?**
   Pericardial effusion is an incidental finding in about 11% of HIV-infected patients and up to 30% of AIDS patients with CD4 counts less than 400 who have cardiac echocardiograms. It only rarely progresses to tamponade, which is more common in end-stage, cachexic patients who develop elevated intrapericardial pressures caused by low right-sided filling pressures *(low-pressure tamponade)*. The effusion is mostly transudative, but *T. mycobacterium* and *T. aviarum* are the principal causes of infectious pericarditis. Rarely, Kaposi's sarcoma can bleed into the pericardium, causing tamponade physiology. It is unusual to isolate an infectious agent from pericardial fluid that is not elsewhere in the body.

4. **Is HIV myocarditis common?**
   In one series, more than 50% of patients undergoing endomyocardial biopsy had myocarditis before ART. Additionally, up to 10% of endomyocardial specimens in HIV patients have evidence of other infections (Coxsackie B, Epstein-Barr virus, adenovirus, cytomegalovirus). HIV is thought to cause myocarditis from direct action of HIV on myocytes or indirectly through toxins.

5. **What is the incidence of HIV cardiomyopathy?**
   It appears to be rare in ART-treated HIV patients referred for echocardiography (less than 1%), all of whom had other causes for left ventricular (LV) dysfunction (coronary artery disease [CAD], alcohol history, sepsis, polysubstance abuse, adriamycin exposure). Patients with cardiomyopathy can present with New York Heart Association (NYHA) class I to IV symptoms, which are often obscured by the underlying untreated disease or active infection, malignancy, or cachexia. Echocardiogram is most sensitive for detecting myopathy because screening electrocardiograms and chest radiographs are nondiagnostic. About 8% of patients with CD4 greater than 400 developed a left ventricular ejection fraction (LVEF) less than 45% over 60 months with NYHA class I symptoms; almost all had CD4 less than 400 at time of diagnosis. This projects to an incidence of 16 cases/1000 patients. Vertical transmission of HIV in children has been associated with LV dilation or LV hypertrophy.

6. **Can nutritional deficiencies be responsible for HIV myopathy?**
   Nutritional deficiencies are seen in late-stage, untreated AIDS. Malabsorption can cause diarrhea and attendant electrolyte losses. Selenium deficiency increases the virulence of Coxsackie virus to cardiac tissue and is reversed by repleting selenium. Low levels of B_{12}, carnitine, growth hormone, and T4 can cause a reversible myopathy.

7. **How is AIDS cardiomyopathy treated?**
   Standard heart failure regimen should be used as tolerated, including angiotensin-converting enzyme (ACE) inhibitors or angiotensin-receptor blockers (ARBs), beta-blockers, aldosterone antagonists, diuretics for volume overload, and digoxin for advanced disease. Additionally, nutritional and electrolyte deficiencies should be repleted.

8. **Why is infective valvular endocarditis a rarity in AIDS?**
   Valvular devastation usually seen with bacterial infections does not occur in HIV patients because of impairment of autoimmune response. Patients who have hemodynamically significant valvular disease warrant valve replacement if their HIV is well controlled. Fulminant infective endocarditis can occur in late AIDS with high mortality. Patients with AIDS rarely develop marantic, or noninfectious, endocarditis, with large, friable, sterile thrombotic vegetations. These can be associated with disseminated intravascular coagulation (DIC) and systemic embolization.

9. **Can cardiothoracic surgery be performed safely in HIV patients?**
   HIV patients can undergo cardiothoracic surgery (valve replacement, coronary artery bypass) with similar mortality to non-HIV patients but slightly higher morbidity (as a result of sepsis, sternal infection, bleeding, prolonged intubation, and readmission). CD4 counts do not drop postoperatively. Needle sticks remain a health care issue in all patients.

10. **What malignancies can affect the heart in AIDS/HIV?**
    Kaposi's sarcoma is associated with herpesvirus-8 in homosexual AIDS patients. This tumor is often found in the subepicardial fat around surface coronary arteries. About 25% of AIDS patients with systemic Kaposi's had incidental cardiac involvement, with death as a result of underlying opportunistic infections. Non-Hodgkin's lymphoma is more common in HIV-positive patients, with a poor prognosis. Leiomyosarcoma is rarely associated with Epstein-Barr virus in AIDS patients.

11. **What causes RV dysfunction in AIDS?**
    RV failure is most commonly caused by pathology that increases pulmonary vascular resistance, including LV failure, opportunistic pulmonary infections, contaminants from intravenous drug use, microvascular emboli, and pulmonary arteritis from immunologic effects. Primary pulmonary hypertension can be seen in less than 1% of patients with AIDS, with

lung biopsy showing plexigenic pulmonary arteriopathy. This is felt to be due to cytokine release because no viruses can be identified. Therapy includes that used for primary pulmonary hypertension, including intravenous epoprostenol and endothelin antagonists. Anticoagulation and pulmonary vasodilators can also be considered.

12. **What is the mechanism of accelerated atherosclerosis more recently noted in treated HIV patients?**

    Postmortem studies in young AIDS patients identified a high incidence of advanced atherosclerosis in patients who had no traditional cardiovascular risk factors or cocaine exposure. It was not clear whether this was due to direct HIV toxicity, cytokine release with inflammatory response, or alteration in lipid metabolism from protease inhibitor therapy. Protease inhibitors (PIs) act on the mitochondria in liver, muscle, and adipose cells to cause dyslipidemia, lipodystrophy, and insulin resistance.

13. **What dyslipidemias occur with HIV disease?**

    Triglycerides increase and high-density lipoprotein (HDL) and low-density lipoprotein (LDL) levels decline in PI-treated HIV patients. The triglycerides cannot be stored in subcutaneous fat depots and so accumulate in liver and skeletal muscle, which contributes to insulin resistance. Initially a hyperinsulinemic response compensates for insulin resistance, followed by atrophy leading to type II diabetes. Low HDL is also associated with premature atherosclerosis. As patients improve on therapy, LDL levels may rise slightly as a result of improved diet and genetic influences.

14. **What is acquired lipodystrophy?**

    This is a disorder characterized by selective loss of adipose tissue from subcutaneous areas of the face, arms, and legs, with redistribution to the posterior neck *(buffalo hump)* and visceral abdomen. Visceral adipose is associated with increased inflammatory markers. This may also relate to insulin resistance, with attendant development of diabetes mellitus (DM), dyslipidemia, hepatic steatosis, and acanthosis nigricans. It can occur in 20% to 40% of HIV patients taking PIs for more than 1 to 2 years.

15. **How are these dyslipidemias treated?**

    PIs can be replaced with other ART (nucleoside or nonnucleoside reverse transcriptase inhibitors). Changing PI agents may alter fat and triglyceride deposition because each PI has a different metabolic profile. Many statins (simvastatin, lovastatin, atorvastatin) are degraded by cytochrome P450 isoform 3A4, which is inhibited by protease inhibitors. Pravastatin, ezetimibe, or plant stanos or sterols, which are not metabolized by the cytochrome P450 pathway, may be more effective in reducing LDL levels. The goal of therapy is to control diabetes and its complications (recurrent pancreatitis, cirrhosis, atherosclerotic vascular disease) by doing the following:
    - Eating a diet with less than 15% (extremely low) fat to reduce chylomicronemia
    - Exercising to improve insulin sensitivity and lipids
    - Maintaining euglycemia with oral agents or insulin
    - Using fibrates or high-dose fish oils containing n-3 polyunsaturated fats
    - Avoiding estrogen and alcohol, which raise triglyceride levels

16. **What oral hypoglycemics are recommended?**

    Metformin is an attractive agent to use for glucose control because it reduces appetite, induces weight loss, and treats steatosis. The nucleoside analog abacavir and metformin can both cause lactic acidosis, so this combination of agents should be used cautiously. Insulin is used for more difficult DM management.

17. **What other drugs used in AIDS/HIV treatment can have cardiac complications?**

    All protease inhibitors can cause dyslipidemia, lipodystrophy, insulin resistance, and accelerated atherosclerosis as described. The PI ritonavir increases triglyceride level the most; stavudine and efavirenz may also have this effect. These same PIs can cause insulin resistance. The nucleoside analogues abacavir can cause hypotension and lactic acidosis, and zidovudine can cause skeletal myopathy. The antiparasitic pentamadine, antiviral gancyclovir, and antibiotic erythromycin have been associated with QT prolongation and torsades (polymorphic ventricular tachycardia). Chemotherapeutic agents such as vincristine, interferon, interleukin, and doxorubicin can cause cardiomyopathy.

18. **How should HIV patients be screened for coronary artery disease?**
The Framingham Risk Score (age, gender, blood pressure, total cholesterol, HDL, diabetes, and smoking) has been applied to HIV patients on therapy and reasonably predicts CAD events. The Data Collection on Adverse Events of Anti-HIV Drugs (DAD) group is validating other risk scores that incorporate ART and other HIV-specific factors. Diagnostic stress testing can be performed in patients with an intermediate (10%–20%) risk of CAD. Carotid intimal medial thickening and coronary artery calcium scores are also being investigated in the HIV population to predict early CAD. Other risk factors, such as highly sensitive C-reactive protein (CRP) and adiponectin, may emerge to further risk stratify the HIV patient.

BIBLIOGRAPHY, SUGGESTED READINGS, AND WEBSITES

1. Cheitlin, MD: Cardiac Involvement in HIV-Infected Patients: http://www.utdol.com
2. Barbazo G, Lipshultz SE: Pathogenesis of HIV-associated cardiomyopathy, *Ann N Y Acad Sci* 946:57-81, 2001.
3. Cotter BR: Epidemiology of HIV cardiac disease, *Progress Cardiovasc Dis* 45:319-326, 2003.
4. Friis-Moller N, Reiss P, Sabin CA, et al: Class of antiretroviral drugs and the risk of myocardial infarction, *N Engl J Med* 356:1723-1735, 2007.
5. Green MI: Evaluation and management of dyslipidemia in patients with HIV infection, *J Gen Int Med* 17: 797-810, 2002.
6. Grinspoon SK, Grunfeld C, Kotler DP, et al: State of the Science Conference: initiative to decrease cardiovascular risk and increase quality of care for patients living with HIV/AIDS, Executive summary, *Circulation* 118:198-210, 2008.
7. Katz AS, Sadaniantz A: Echocardiography in HIV cardiac disease, *Progress Cardiovasc Dis* 45:285-292, 2003.

INDEX

Page numbers in **boldface type** indicate complete chapters. Page numbers followed by *t* indicate tables; *f,* figures.